DOUBLE
CONTRAST
GASTROINTESTINAL
RADIOLOGY

DOUBLE CONTRAST GASTROINTESTINAL RADIOLOGY

Igor Laufer, M.D.

Professor of Radiology
University of Pennsylvania School of Medicine
Chief, Gastrointestinal Radiology Section
Hospital of the University of Pennsylvania
Philadelphia, Pennsylvania

Marc S. Levine, M.D.

Professor of Radiology
University of Pennsylvania School of Medicine
Gastrointestinal Radiology Section
Hospital of the University of Pennsylvania
Philadelphia, Pennsylvania

2nd Edition

W. B. SAUNDERS COMPANY
Harcourt Brace Jovanovich, Inc.

Philadelphia London Toronto
Montreal Sydney Tokyo

W. B. SAUNDERS COMPANY
Harcourt Brace Jovanovich, Inc.

The Curtis Center
Independence Square West
Philadelphia, Pennsylvania 19106

Library of Congress Cataloging-in-Publication Data

Laufer, Igor.

Double contrast gastrointestinal radiology/Igor Laufer,
Marc S. Levine.—2nd ed.

p.   cm.

Rev. ed. of: Double contrast gastrointestinal radiology with
endoscopic correlation/Igor Laufer. 1979.

Includes index.

1. Digestive organs—Diseases—Diagnosis.   2. Radiography.
   Double-contrast.   I. Levine, Marc S.   II. Laufer, Igor.
   Double contrast gastrointestinal radiology with endoscopic
   correlation.   III. Title. [DNLM: 1. Contrast Media.
   2. Gastrointestinal System—radiography.

   WI 141 L373d]   RC804.R6L38 1992   616.3'30757—dc20

ISBN 0–7216–5649–8

DNLM/DLC   91–14971

Editor: Lisette Bralow
Designer: Dorothy Chattin
Production Manager: Ken Neimeister
Manuscript Editors: Jody Murphy and Alison Kelley
Illustration Coordinator: Cecelia Roberts
Cover Designer: Joan Wendt
Indexer: Linda Van Pelt

Double Contrast Gastrointestinal Radiology, 2nd Edition   ISBN   0–7216–5649–8

Printed in the United States of America

Last digit is the print number: 9   8   7   6   5   4   3   2   1

To Miriam and Jacob

"Every person born into the world represents
something new, something that never existed before,
something original and unique."

Martin Buber

IGOR LAUFER

To my parents, Helen and Wilfred Levine,
for a lifetime of love and guidance

MARC S. LEVINE

CONTRIBUTORS

Clive I. Bartram, F.R.C.P., F.R.C.R.

Consultant Radiologist, St. Mark's and St. Bartholomew's Hospitals, London, England.

Hans Herlinger, M.D., F.R.C.R.

Professor of Radiology (Emeritus), University of Pennsylvania School of Medicine; Gastrointestinal Radiology Section, Hospital of the University of Pennsylvania, Philadelphia, Pennsylvania.

Herbert Y. Kressel, M.D.

Professor of Radiology, University of Pennsylvania School of Medicine; Director, David W. Devon Medical Imaging Center, Hospital of the University of Pennsylvania, Philadelphia, Pennsylvania.

Masakazu Maruyama, M.D.

Visiting Professor, Korea University School of Medicine, Seoul, Korea; and Honorary Professor, University of Montevideo, Faculty of Medicine, Montevideo, Uruguay; Chief of Mass Survey Division and Vice-Chief of Departments of Internal Medicine and Radiology, Cancer Institute Hospital, Tokyo, Japan.

J. Odo Op den Orth, M.D.

Consultant Radiologist, St. Elisabeth's of Groote Gasthuis, Haarlem, The Netherlands.

Stephen E. Rubesin, M.D.

Associate Professor of Radiology, University of Pennsylvania School of Medicine; Gastrointestinal Radiology Section, Hospital of the University of Pennsylvania, Philadelphia, Pennsylvania.

Giles W. Stevenson, M.D., F.R.C.R., F.R.C.P.(c)

Professor and Chairman of Radiology, McMaster University; Head of Radiology Section, McMaster University Medical Center, Hamilton, Ontario.

Akiyoshi Yamada, M.D.

Professor of Surgery and Radiology, Institute of Gastroenterology, Tokyo Women's Medical College, Tokyo, Japan.

PREFACE

Twelve years have passed since the publication of the first edition of *Double Contrast Gastrointestinal Radiology*. Although there have been increasingly urgent requests for a new edition for more than 5 years, the demands of everyday life and living have always seemed to postpone the pursuit of this project. Besides, the pace of change seemed to be slow, and surely not that much had changed.

As I look back now on the contents of this new edition compared with its predecessor, it is clear that there has been a great deal of change. Techniques have been refined and streamlined; the world has been rocked by the emergence of new diseases, most notably HIV infection; our understanding of various pathologic processes has been sharpened; and it is now possible to make many new diagnoses radiologically, including those of conditions such as drug-induced esophagitis, nonsteroidal anti-inflammatory drug (NSAID) gastritis, and carpet lesions of the colon and rectum. As interest in swallowing disorders has increased, so has our understanding of the function and morphology of the pharynx. This is beautifully illustrated in the new chapter by my colleague Stephen E. Rubesin, who has made an exquisite study of the anatomy and morphology of the pharynx as seen on double contrast radiographs.

In 1979, Marc Levine was still a resident in the Department of Radiology at the Hospital of the University of Pennsylvania. Since that time, he has joined our faculty and has quickly risen to the rank of Professor of Radiology. His observations, writings, and teachings have led to many of the new developments that are found in this second edition. Therefore, it is particularly appropriate and a particular pleasure to welcome Marc as co-author of this text.

I want to thank again those mentors responsible for kindling and nourishing my interest in gastrointestinal radiology. Dr. Norman Joffe at the Beth Israel Hospital in Boston impressed on me the contribution an individual can make to patient care by virtue of attention and expertise. Dr. W. Peter Cockshott, my chairman at McMaster University in Hamilton, Ontario, had the foresight and provided the encouragement to explore different approaches to the radiologic examination of the gastrointestinal tract. My chairman at the University of Pennsylvania for the past 16 years, Dr. Stanley Baum, has provided the support and freedom to develop our Gastrointestinal Radiology section and to pursue our areas of interest. I also want to pay tribute to two of the deceased giants of our field who provided inspiration in their own ways: Dr. Richard Marshak of New York, whose writings and teachings brought gastrointestinal radiology to life; and Dr. Roscoe E. Miller of Indianapolis, whose enthusiasm for double contrast studies affected me deeply.

I hope that readers of this book will find in it a coherent approach to barium studies of the gastrointestinal tract and that they will appreciate not only the book's logic and content but its aesthetic qualities as well.

IGOR LAUFER

I was deeply honored when Igor Laufer invited me to be the co-author for the second edition of *Double Contrast Gastrointestinal Radiology*. The first edition, published in 1979, was a classic. Nevertheless, the field of double contrast gastrointestinal radiology has evolved dramatically during the past decade. As our technical and interpretive skills have improved, it has become possible to diagnose a host of conditions that were beyond the realm of gastrointestinal radiology 12 years ago. The time has arrived for a second edition.

I feel fortunate to have been part of the tradition of gastrointestinal radiology at the Hospital of the University of Pennsylvania. Under the leadership of Stanley Baum and Igor Laufer, this section has set a standard of excellence and innovation. It has also been a privilege to work with my other colleagues in the gastrointestinal section, Hans Herlinger and Stephen E. Rubesin, who themselves have made important contributions to the field. Without a doubt, it has been for me an exciting and fulfilling time to be involved in gastrointestinal radiology.

I would like to thank the radiology residents who over the years performed many of the studies included in the book. I am also indebted to Steven Strommer and Juanita James for their excellent reproductions of the radiographs and to Elizabeth Gordon for her meticulous preparation of the manuscript. Finally, I would like to thank my wife, Deborah, for her complete and unwavering support and for her understanding and patience during the long hours I worked on the book. With the impending birth of our fourth child, this was no small sacrifice on her part. Thank you, Deb.

MARC S. LEVINE

CONTENTS

INTRODUCTION

1

Igor Laufer, M.D.
Marc S. Levine, M.D.

GENERAL COMMENTS

The status of barium studies of the gastrointestinal tract is no longer as secure as it was in previous generations. Some of the diagnostic burden has been allocated to newer diagnostic modalities such as ultrasound and computed tomography (CT). In addition, diagnostic endoscopy has gained a major role in the diagnosis of gastrointestinal diseases. Thus, barium studies no longer clearly represent the first choice for gastrointestinal diagnosis.[1] In view of the increasing competition for the diagnostic dollar, it is vital that radiologists emphasize the value of double contrast studies for the diagnosis of early or minimal disease.

The detection of early or minimal disease requires the ultimate in radiologic technique and a thorough familiarity with normal appearances and their variations. For this reason, the emphasis in this book will be on technical details, on normal appearances and their variations, and on the early manifestations of the multitude of neoplastic and inflammatory lesions that affect the gastrointestinal tract.

There are three basic components of barium contrast studies in the gastrointestinal tract. These are (1) barium-filled views with compression, (2) mucosal relief, and (3) double contrast. Figure 1–1 illustrates these three components in the examination of the colon. The ideal examination technique would utilize each of these components to best advantage. However, in practice this is not feasible because optimal results in the various phases of the examination require different types of barium suspensions and radiographic technique. Therefore, the examiner must choose a basic approach to gastrointestinal contrast studies, giving emphasis to one or two of the basic components. The examiner will then choose materials that are appropriate to this type of study, realizing that the other phases of the examination may be compromised but are not eliminated.

Many authors have shown that a combination of techniques produces the best achievable results.[2–4] Nevertheless, the double contrast radiographs allow detection of the smallest and most subtle lesions.

CONVENTIONAL BARIUM STUDIES

Principles

The most prevalent approach to barium contrast studies of the gastrointestinal tract in the Western world still emphasizes barium-filled views with compression and mucosal relief views. We shall refer to these as "conventional barium studies." Because of the need to penetrate the opacity of the barium column, these films are exposed at a relatively high kVp. Mucosal relief films are obtained with the organ collapsed either after the administration of a small volume of barium, as in the stomach, or after evacuation of the barium, as in the colon. Even here, there must be a compromise in the choice of barium suspension, since a low-density barium chosen for its suitability for barium-filled compression studies will not give the optimal coating for mucosal relief views. "Air contrast" views are frequently obtained to supplement the information obtained during the earlier phases of the examination. In the upper gastrointestinal study the volume of gas that happens to be in the stomach is utilized, and on occasion adequate distention of the antrum and duodenum can be obtained. However, the quality of mucosal coating is seldom high, and there is rarely sufficient distention for an adequate study of the body and fundus of the stomach. In the colon, double contrast views are frequently obtained by insufflation of air after the patient has evacuated the barium. This type of "secondary air contrast study" has many deficiencies. The type of barium used for the single contrast enema does not produce good mucosal coating. The degree of evacuation is variable, and therefore the volume of residual barium is variable. The time interval during which the patient is evacuating the barium may result in flocculation or flaking of the barium coating. In addition there is frequently flooding of the small bowel, which obscures the sigmoid colon.

Drawbacks

It is clear that the accuracy of the type of examination just described depends primarily on the quality of the barium-filled and mucosal relief films. Several major problems are encountered in using the conventional barium technique.

1. In order to obtain greater distention of the organ, it is necessary to increase the volume of barium. Therefore, increasing distention results in increasing opacity, which can obscure lesions that are not caught in profile. This problem also applies to the examination of segments of the gastrointestinal tract with a wide caliber, such as the gastric fundus or the right colon.

2. Areas of the gastrointestinal tract that are not accessible for palpation cannot be examined optimally. This generally includes areas such as the gastric fundus, the colonic flexures, and the rectum. This problem also exists in any patient in whom

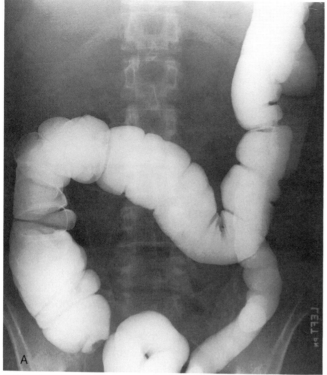

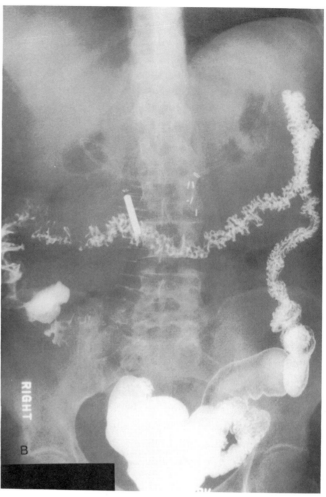

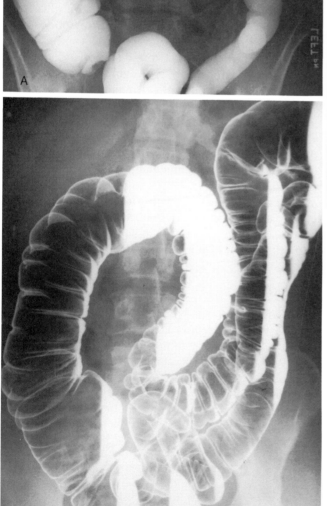

FIGURE 1–1

The three basic elements in barium examinations illustrated in the examination of the colon are barium filling (A), mucosal relief (B), and double contrast (C).

effective compression cannot be applied, either because of obesity, anatomic abnormalities, or local tenderness.

3. In the colon, high quality mucosal relief films are not obtained reproducibly. The degree of evacuation is variable. In some patients the entire barium enema is evacuated, leaving no mucosal relief, whereas in others very little is evacuated, and again no mucosal relief is seen. Even when the mucosal relief is well seen in one part of the colon, it is usually not possible to map the state of the mucosa thoroughly throughout the entire colon. This may be of particular importance in the assessment of patients with inflammatory bowel disease and in the differentiation between ulcerative and granulomatous colitis.

4. Single contrast technique depends heavily on diagnostic fluoroscopy. It relies on the keenness of the fluoroscopist's powers of observation to detect a lesion, and in many cases a diagnostic conclusion is based on fluoroscopic impression. This may pose no problem if the fluoroscopist is extremely skilled and experienced. However, there is no possibility in many cases for an intelligent second opinion, since the critical information may have been fluoroscopic. This poses a particular problem in departments in which many studies are performed by residents and trainees whose fluoroscopic skills are not fully developed.

Diagnostic Accuracy

Despite these theoretical deficiencies, conventional barium studies were thought to be generally quite accurate. This is understandable, since evidence of radiologic error was usually found only at surgery or autopsy when advanced lesions missed by radiologic study would have been discovered. It would be reasonable to assume that smaller lesions were missed in many patients who did not come to surgery or autopsy. The development of fiberoptic endoscopy has provided a valuable tool with which to evaluate the accuracy of our contrast studies in the gastrointestinal tract. Endoscopic experience has shown that the majority of small lesions and even a disturbing number of large lesions are missed by conventional barium studies.

Upper Gastrointestinal Tract

Several endoscopic studies have assessed the accuracy of the conventional barium examination of the stomach and duodenum.[5–9] The results are summarized in Table 1–1. Radiologic errors were made in an average of 29% of patients coming to endoscopy. In 22%, the radiologic error was a false negative, in which a significant lesion was not detected. For the

TABLE 1–1. Radiologic Error Rates With Conventional Barium Study

Series	Number of Patients	False Negative (%)	False Positive (%)	Total (%)
Laufer et al.[5]	175	11	11	22
Cotton[6]	518	27	6	35
Papp[7]	85	18	6	24
Dellipiani[8]	137	19	5	24
Barnes et al.[9]	50	14	4	18
Total	965	22	7	29

From Laufer, I.: Assessment of the accuracy of double contrast gastroduodenal radiology. Gastroenterology 71:874, 1976, with permission.

purpose of these statistics, mucosal inflammation and erosions were not included as significant lesions. In an additional 7% of patients, a lesion diagnosed radiologically could not be confirmed by endoscopy. It is likely that in some of these cases the radiologic diagnosis was correct, and the lesion may have been overlooked at endoscopy. However, it is probable that in most cases the endoscopic diagnosis was accurate. The major causes of false-negative errors are failure to recognize an abnormality on the film and the small size of some of the lesions.[10] Most false-positive diagnoses are due to deformity or to prominent mucosal folds, which are mistaken for or which simulate pathologic lesions.[5] It seems to us that many of these errors can be avoided by using a technique that makes gross pathology more obvious, allows for detection of smaller lesions, and results in better gastric distention and effacement of normal mucosal folds.

Colon

Colonoscopy has had a dramatic effect on our approach to colonic polyps. A major fringe benefit of the development of colonoscopy has been the opportunity to assess the accuracy of radiologic examination of the colon, particularly with respect to polyp detection, but also with respect to inflammatory bowel disease. Several studies have indicated that 40% to 50% of all colonic polyps are missed on the conventional barium enema.[11, 12] These results are particularly important because of the increasing evidence that many colonic carcinomas arise in benign polypoid tumors.[13]

Of course it is difficult to distinguish between errors due to imperfect performance or interpretation and errors due to inherent limitations of technique.[14] Nevertheless, it seems safe to suggest that the conventional barium enema has definite limitations in the examination of segments not accessible to palpation, such as the rectum and the colonic flexures; in the differentiation of extraneous material from true pathologic findings; and in the detection of the early changes in inflammatory bowel disease, such as mucosal granularity in ulcerative colitis and aphthoid ulcers in Crohn's disease.[15, 16]

DOUBLE CONTRAST STUDIES

The accumulation of evidence regarding the deficiencies of these conventional studies led many radiologists to reconsider their gastrointestinal radiologic techniques. This search renewed interest in the development of double contrast techniques, either for routine use or for supplementation of the standard examination. In response to this renewed interest, new barium suspensions and other accessories were developed to make possible an efficient, high quality double contrast examination on a routine basis.[17–21] With increasing use of these techniques, many new and confusing radiologic appearances have been seen. In this respect, fiberoptic endoscopy has been an invaluable tool for clarifying the nature and significance of these findings and for sharpening interpretative skills.

Advantages

Double contrast diagnosis depends primarily on gaseous distention and mucosal coating with a thin layer of high-density barium. In theory, many of the deficiencies associated with the conventional barium study can be overcome. (a) Increasing distention is obtained without increasing opacity and therefore without loss of surface detail. Thus the wide caliber portions of the gastrointestinal tract are easily examined. (b) The segments of the gastrointestinal tract that are inaccessible to palpation are easily examined. (c) Excellent mucosal detail is achieved routinely. (d) Diagnostic fluoroscopy is minimized. The emphasis is placed on a series of routine radiographs obtained in standard projections. Fluoroscopy is used primarily for determining the correct volume of contrast media for positioning and timing spot films. Of course, if an abnormality is detected at fluoroscopy, additional views are taken. Further opinions can usually be obtained in the absence of fluoroscopic information.

Double contrast techniques have another advantage that has not been widely appreciated. They make it much easier to distinguish between true pathology and extraneous material. This distinction is made by the use of gravity and horizontal beam films. The extraneous material almost always flows to the dependent segment with barium, leaving the air-filled segments clean. Even on recumbent view double contrast radiographs, it is possible to differentiate filling defects on the elevated wall from those on the dependent wall (see Chapter 2). Thus any filling defect on the elevated wall is almost certainly a true polyp, because extraneous material would be expected only on the dependent wall. Because of these factors it has frequently been possible to find small polypoid lesions in the colon even in the presence of extensive fecal residue.

Because of the interest in surface detail, the radiographic exposures in a double contrast study are considerably lighter and can be exposed at a lower kV than the single contrast study. Therefore, it is usually possible to obtain high quality spot films even when using equipment capable of very low mA and kV output. The exposures are shorter and there is less scatter because there is no need to penetrate the opaque barium column.

Historical Development
Double Contrast Enema

The history of gastrointestinal radiology has been reviewed recently by Margulis and Eisenberg.[22, 23] The principles of double contrast technique were first applied to the colon in 1923 by Fischer in Germany and subsequently by Weber at the Mayo Clinic. Major advances in the understanding, performance, and interpretation of these studies were contributed by Welin in Malmö, Sweden, where over 70,000 such examinations have been performed.[24] Despite its high polyp detection rate and exquisite demonstration of minute mucosal abnormalities in neoplastic and inflammatory disease, the technique did not become popular in North America. It is likely that many radiologists tried the double contrast technique but could not reproduce the results obtained by Welin. This is probably the result of failure to obtain the same degree of colonic cleansing and failure to appreciate the need for specific types of barium suspensions, different diagnostic maneuvers, and variations in the appearance of various pathologic lesions on the double contrast films.

In the 1960's the message of the double contrast enema was taken up by the late Roscoe Miller, who was largely responsible for the development of new apparatus, barium suspensions, and accessories.[25, 26] These developments made it possible to perform efficient double contrast studies of high quality. There has therefore been a renewed interest in this technique. Recent surveys confirm the continuing increase in double contrast examinations of the colon at the expense of the single contrast study.[27, 28]

Upper Gastrointestinal Tract

The potential value of the double contrast technique as an alternative to the palpation method was recognized by Hampton in 1937.[29] Utilizing swallowed air and a barium suspension of creamy consistency, he showed examples of duodenal ulcers and a prepyloric carcinoma. Schatzki described the importance of en face views with air contrast for diagnosis of gastric ulcers.[30] In 1952 Ruzicka and Rigler described a method for double contrast examination of the stomach.[31] Their examination required nasogastric intubation. The quality of the coating was not excellent because of the barium suspensions available at that time.

In about 1950 a group of gastroenterologists in Japan, under the leadership of Professor Hikoo Shirakabe, were studying the pathologic morphology of intestinal tuberculosis, using double contrast examination of the colon. This study led them to develop a double contrast technique for the examination of the stomach.[32] Their initial interest was in the demonstration of gastric ulcers, particularly linear ulcers that had not been demonstrated on conventional studies. This experience led them to further refinements of the technique for the radiologic diagnosis of early gastric cancer.[33] Double contrast examination became standard in Japan during the 1960's, and spectacular results have been achieved in both mass screening programs and the evaluation of symptomatic patients. As a result, patients with early gastric ulcer have had a 5-year survival of 90% or more.[34]

The Japanese work seemed to attract little interest in the West because of its emphasis on early gastric cancer, a disease with a much lower incidence in the West. In the late 1960's and early 1970's several short papers appeared describing modifications of the Japanese technique.[35, 36] The quality of mucosal coating in these early radiographs was suboptimal because of the poor effervescent agents available and the relatively poor coating produced by the barium suspensions at that time. In the early 1970's more attention was directed to technical details of the examination and in particular to the quality of the barium preparations. This led to the development of new barium suspensions specifically designed to produce high quality double contrast examinations of the stomach.[21] Several papers then reported that subtle pathologic lesions that had not been seen before were now being diagnosed. These included superficial gastric erosions,[37, 38] linear ulcers,[39, 40] and ulcer scars.[40, 41] A report by Quizlbash and co-workers[42] suggested that an increased incidence of early gastric cancer in their hospital could be attributed at least in part to the institution of double contrast examination of the stomach.

Diagnostic Accuracy

Colon

Several studies have shown that the double contrast enema can be highly accurate for the detection of polypoid lesions greater than 5 mm in diameter. Ninety per cent or more of such polyps are detected on high quality double contrast enema examinations.[43] This type of study has also been shown to be accurate in reflecting the visual mucosal abnormalities in patients with inflammatory bowel disease.[15, 44]

Upper Gastrointestinal Tract

Several studies have compared the radiologic diagnoses using double contrast technique with endoscopic findings. In these series the double contrast method has been found to be more than 90% accurate.[40, 45, 46] In hospitalized patients the studies tend to be less accurate because these patients are less able to cooperate for the examination.[47] Furthermore, we found that radiologic errors were generally predictable, in that they were usually confined to those studies that were considered to be unreliable by the examiner. With increasing confidence in the radiologic diagnosis, the endoscopic examination can be reserved for those patients in whom the results of radiologic study either are equivocal or demonstrate a lesion requiring confirmation or histologic diagnosis.

Drawbacks

Despite the advantages of increased resolution with double contrast studies, there are a number of significant drawbacks. For the practicing radiologist the method represents a commitment of time and energy to learn new techniques. It requires a revised concept of the relative roles of fluoroscopy and radiography in gastrointestinal diagnosis. It also requires a reorientation to interpretation of the films, since there is much more emphasis on the en face appearance of lesions than on their appearance in profile. The examiner may find that the old familiar pathology may have different appearances, and that self-retraining is necessary to find the more subtle lesions that are diagnosable by these techniques.

It is likely that the double contrast examinations are slightly more time-consuming than the conventional barium studies. This is particularly true during the early stages when the examiner is becoming familiar with these techniques. However, if one considers the increased yield and the fewer number of repeat examinations, we believe that the extra time is more than justified.

The technical quality of a double contrast study is highly dependent on the materials used and in particular on the quality of the barium suspension. Thus the radiologist must constantly monitor the quality of barium preparations and must be willing to try new products that might improve the quality of the study.

A high quality double contrast study can provide aesthetic pleasure approaching that of a work of art. However, a poor study, whether the fault of the examiner or the patient or both, may not only be useless but misleading.[48] It is probably true that a poor quality double contrast examination is more dangerous than a poor quality single contrast examination. Therefore, the utilization of double contrast techniques requires a commitment to the development of technical excellence.

STATE OF THE ART: SINGLE VERSUS DOUBLE CONTRAST

Although the volume of barium studies has decreased by 25% to 30% over the past decade,[49] double contrast examinations now represent greater than 40% of all barium studies.[50] This proportion has doubled over the past decade. Indeed, the absolute number of double contrast examinations has actually increased over this period.

It must be re-emphasized that the term *double contrast examination* refers to an examination relying primarily on double contrast films but also incorporating the elements of single contrast and, where possible, mucosal relief. In the majority of studies, this type of double contrast examination has been shown to be clearly superior to the type of examination relying primarily on single contrast. The difficulty of comparing statistics regarding the diagnostic accuracy of these two types of studies has been described by Gelfand and Ott.[51] Nevertheless, in his own work, Gelfand also has found that the double contrast views are the single most informative part of the examination.[3] We believe that there is strong feeling in the general medical community that single contrast studies, as they have been performed, cannot compete effectively with the results achieved by endoscopy.[51–53] At the same time, there is increasing evidence that the double contrast examination can be competitive, particularly in this era of cost containment.[54, 55]

CONCLUSION

We feel certain that the radiologist who spends the time and effort to master these techniques will be rewarded by gastrointestinal studies of increased diagnostic value and in many cases of great aesthetic quality. Our experience suggests that this combination stimulates interest in gastrointestinal radiology not only for the radiologist but also for students, technologists, and referring physicians. This can only result in greater diagnostic accuracy and an enhanced appreciation of the role of radiology in the diagnosis of gastrointestinal disorders.

REFERENCES

1. Op den Orth, J. O: Use of barium in evaluation of disorders of the upper gastrointestinal tract: Current status. Radiology 173:601, 1989.
2. Montagne, J. P., Moss, A. A., and Margulis, A. R.: Double-blind study of single and double contrast upper gastrointestinal examinations using endoscopy as a control. AJR 130:1041, 1978.
3. Gelfand, D. W., Chen, Y. M., and Ott, D. J.: Multiphasic examinations of the stomach: Efficacy of individual techniques and combinations of techniques in detecting 153 lesions. Radiology 162:829, 1987.
4. Dekker, W., and Op den Orth, J. O.: Biphasic radiologic examination and endoscopy of the upper gastrointestinal tract. J. Clin. Gastroenterol. 10(4):461, 1988.
5. Laufer, I., Mullens, J. E., and Hamilton, J.: The diagnostic accuracy of barium studies of the stomach and duodenum—correlation with endoscopy. Radiology 115:569, 1975.
6. Cotton, P. B.: Fiberoptic endoscopy and the barium meal—results and implications. Br. Med. J. 2:161, 1973.
7. Papp, J. P.: Endoscopic experience in 100 consecutive cases with the Olympus GIF endoscope. Am. J. Gastroenterol. 60:466, 1973.
8. Dellipiani, A. W.: Experience with duodenofiberscopes. Scott. Med. J. 19:7, 1974.
9. Barnes, R. J., Gear, M. W. L., and Nicol, A.: Study of dyspepsia in a general practice as assessed by endoscopy and radiology. Br. Med. J. 4:214, 1974.
10. Gelfand, D. W., Ott, D. J., and Tritico, R.: Causes of error in gastrointestinal radiology. Gastrointest. Radiol. 5:91, 1980.
11. Wolff, W. I., Shinya, H., Geffen, A., et al.: Comparison of colonoscopy and the contrast enema in five hundred patients with colo-rectal disease. Am. J. Surg. 129:181, 1975.
12. Thoeni, J. F., and Menuck, L.: Comparison of barium enema and colonoscopy in the detection of small colonic polyps. Radiology 124:631, 1977.
13. Lane, N., Fenoglio, C. M.: The adenoma-carcinoma sequence in the stomach and colon. 1. Observations on the adenoma as precursor to ordinary large bowel carcinoma. Gastrointest. Radiol. 1:111, 1976.
14. Kelvin, F. M., Gardiner, R., Vos, W., et al.: Colorectal carcinoma missed on double contrast barium enema study: A problem in perception. AJR 137:307, 1981.
15. Laufer, I.: Air contrast studies of the colon in inflammatory bowel disease. CRC Crit. Rev. Diagn. Imaging 9:421, 1977.
16. Laufer, I., and Costopoulos, L.: Early lesions of Crohn's disease. AJR 130:307, 1978.
17. Miller, R. E.: Barium enema examination with large bore tubing and drainage. Radiology 82:905, 1964.
18. Gelfand, D. W., and Hachiya, J.: The double contrast examination of the stomach using gas-producing granules and tablets. Radiology 93:1381, 1969.
19. Miller, R. E., Chernish, S. M., Skucas, J., et al.: Hypotonic roentgenography with glucagon. AJR 121:264, 1974.
20. Laufer, I.: A simple method for routine double-contrast study of the upper gastrointestinal tract. Radiology 117:513, 1975.
21. Gelfand, D. W.: High density, low viscosity barium for fine

mucosal detail on double-contrast upper gastrointestinal examinations. AJR 130:831, 1978.

22. Margulis, A. R., and Eisenberg, R. L.: Gastrointestinal radiology from the time of Walter B. Cannon to the 21st century. Radiology 178:297, 1991.

23. Eisenberg, R. L., and Margulis, A. R.: Brief history of gastrointestinal radiology. Radiographics 11:121, 1991.

24. Welin, S.: Results of the Malmö technique of colon examination. JAMA 199:369, 1967.

25. Miller, R. E.: Examination of the colon. Curr. Probl. Radiol. 5(2):3, 1975.

26. Miller, R. E.: Recipes for gastrointestinal examinations. AJR 137:1285, 1981.

27. Semelka, R. C., and MacEwan, D. W.: Changes in diagnostic investigation and improved detection of colon cancer, Manitoba 1964–1984. J. Can. Assoc. Radiol. 38:251, 1987.

28. Thoeni, R. F., and Margulis, A. R.: The state of radiographic technique in the examination of the colon: A survey in 1987. Radiology 167:7, 1988.

29. Hampton, A. O.: A safe method for the roentgen demonstration of bleeding duodenal ulcers. AJR 38:565, 1937.

30. Schatzki, R., and Gary, J. E.: Face-on demonstration of ulcers in the upper stomach in a dependent position. AJR 79:722, 1958.

31. Ruzicka, F. F., and Rigler, L. G.: Inflation of the stomach with double contrast: Roentgen study. JAMA 145:696, 1951.

32. Shirakabe, H.: Double Contrast Studies of the Stomach. Stuttgart, Georg-Thieme Verlag, 1972.

33. Shirakabe, H., Ichikawa, H., Kumakura, K., et al.: Atlas of X-Ray Diagnosis of Early Gastric Cancer. Philadelphia, J. B. Lippincott, 1966.

34. Yamada, E., Nagazato, H., Koite, A., et al.: Surgical results of early gastric cancer. Int. Surg. 59:7, 1974.

35. Obata, W. G.: A double-contrast technique for examination of the stomach using barium sulfate with simethicone. AJR 115:275, 1972.

36. Scott-Harden, W. G.: Radiological investigation of peptic ulcer. Br. J. Hosp. Med. 10:149, 1973.

37. Laufer, I., Hamilton, J., and Mullens, J. E.: Demonstration of superficial gastric erosions by double contrast radiology. Gastroenterology 68:387, 1975.

38. Poplack, W., Paul, R. E., Goldsmith, M., et al.: Demonstration of erosive gastritis by the double contrast technique. Radiology 117:519, 1975.

39. Poplack, W., Paul, R. E., Goldsmith, M., et al.: Linear and rod-shaped peptic ulcers. Radiology 122:317, 1977.

40. Laufer, I.: Assessment of the accuracy of double contrast gastroduodenal radiology. Gastroenterology 71:874, 1976.

41. Gelfand, D. W.: The Japanese-style double contrast examination of the stomach. Gastrointest. Radiol. 1:7, 1976.

42. Quizlbash, A., Harnorine, C., and Castelli, M.: Early gastric carcinoma: Value of combined use of endoscopy, air contrast x-ray films, cytology and multiple biopsy specimens. Arch. Pathol. 101:610, 1977.

43. Laufer, I., Smith, N. C. W., and Mullens, J. E.: The radiological demonstration of colorectal polyps undetected by endoscopy. Gastroenterology 70:167, 1976.

44. Simpkins, K. C., and Stevenson, G. W.: The modified Malmö double-contrast enema in colitis: An assessment of its accuracy in reflecting sigmoidoscopic findings. Br. J. Radiol. 45:486, 1972.

45. Moule, E. B., Cochrane, K. M., Sokhi, G. S., et al.: A comparative study of the diagnostic value of upper gastrointestinal endoscopy and radiology. Gut 16:411, 1975.

46. Herlinger, H., Glanville, J. N., and Kreel, L.: An evaluation of the double contrast barium meal (DCBM) against endoscopy. Clin. Radiol. 28:307, 1977.

47. Dooley, C. P., Larson, A. W., and Stace, N. H., et al.: Double-contrast barium meal and upper gastrointestinal endoscopy. Ann. Intern. Med. 101:438, 1984.

48. Hartzell, H. V.: To err with air. JAMA 187:455, 1964.

49. Gelfand, D. W., Ott, D. J., and Chen, Y. M.: Decreasing numbers of gastrointestinal studies: Report of data from 69 radiologic practices. AJR 148:1133, 1987.

50. Ominsky, S. H., and Margulis, A. R.: Radiographic examination of the upper gastrointestinal tract. Radiology 139:11, 1981.

51. Gelfand, D. W., and Ott, D. J.: Single- vs. double-contrast gastrointestinal studies: Critical analysis of reported statistics. AJR 137:523, 1981.

52. Tedesco, F. J., Griffin, J. W. Jr., Crisp, W. L., and Anthony, H. F. Jr.: "Skinny" upper gastrointestinal endoscopy—the initial diagnostic tool: A prospective comparison of upper gastrointestinal endoscopy and radiology. J. Clin. Gastroenterol. 2:27, 1980.

53. Martin, T. R., Vennes, J. A., Silvis, S. E., and Ansel, H. J.: A comparison of upper gastrointestinal endoscopy and radiography. J. Clin. Gastroenterol. 2:21, 1980.

54. Young, J. W., Ginthner, T. P., and Keramati, B.: The competitive barium meal. Clin Radiol. 36:43, 1985.

55. Chandie Shaw, M. P.: Biphasic radiological examination of the stomach and duodenum compared with fiberoptic endoscopy. Doctoral thesis. University of Leiden, 1987.

PRINCIPLES OF DOUBLE CONTRAST DIAGNOSIS

Igor Laufer, M.D.
Herbert Y. Kressel, M.D.

2

INTRODUCTION
Why Double Contrast?

Despite the data outlined in Chapter 1 regarding the consistent superiority of double contrast techniques throughout the gastrointestinal tract, many radiologists have chosen not to change their gastrointestinal techniques. Perhaps the most convincing argument for switching to double contrast is illustrated in Figure 2–1. The example is that of a conventional Styrofoam cup examined by single contrast in which no "lesions" are seen. Using double contrast technique, a complete ring of artificial erosions is seen both en face and in profile. Even in retrospect, none of these lesions can be recognized in the barium-filled cup. This example illustrates the number of lesions that may be present and obscured by barium and yet are clearly demonstrated by double contrast.

Orientation

Successful application of double contrast techniques in gastrointestinal radiology requires the development of skill both in the performance and in the interpretation of these studies. The transition from single contrast to double contrast radiology requires more than a minor adjustment in technique. Indeed, the double contrast approach requires a major reorientation to the performance and interpretation of gastrointestinal studies.

The purpose of this chapter is to outline general principles in the performance and interpretation of double contrast examinations. When properly performed, they make it possible to provide a precise translation from the radiographic abnormalities to the gross pathology and, in many cases, to the microscopic pathology. Some of these principles are illustrated in vitro using Styrofoam cups and simulated pathologic lesions. This work was performed by Dr. Miriam C. Green during a student elective in our department. In addition, examples and illustrations are drawn from the entire gastrointestinal tract to stress the general applicability of these principles. Their specific applications are discussed in detail in the appropriate chapters. We would also like to stress the causes of potential error in the use of double contrast techniques and to suggest some approaches whereby some of these errors can be avoided.

DIFFERENCES BETWEEN SINGLE AND DOUBLE CONTRAST STUDIES

In order to understand the double contrast approach to gastrointestinal radiology, it is important to clarify the basic differences between single and double contrast studies. The single contrast study concentrates on examination of the contour and lumen of the gastrointestinal tract.[1] Its most important component is the fluoroscopic study whereby the volume of barium is monitored, graded compression is applied,

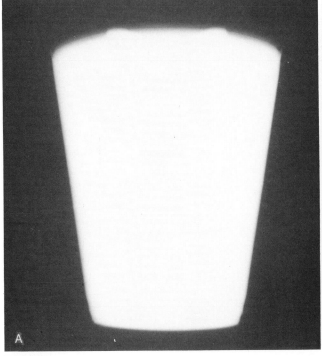
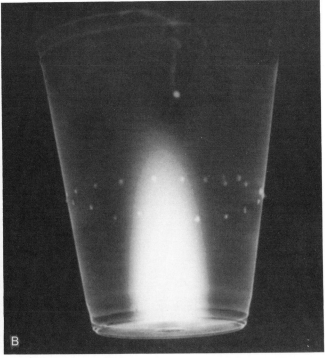

FIGURE 2–1

THE ADVANTAGE OF DOUBLE CONTRAST. A, The Styrofoam cup is examined by single contrast. No lesion is seen.
    B, With double contrast, a ring of "erosions" is clearly seen both en face and in profile.

and in most cases a diagnostic impression is reached. The purpose of multiple radiographs is to provide complementary views of the same lesion or the same surface. In general we expect to see a lesion on all or most radiographs that incorporate the area in question. We are generally content to identify an abnormality and suggest its pathologic nature. We are usually not interested in precise three-dimensional reconstruction or localization, and in particular we are rarely concerned with differentiation between the dependent and the nondependent surfaces.

By comparison, the double contrast examination is concerned primarily with delineation of mucosal detail, and secondarily with abnormalities of the contour and lumen. Fluoroscopy is used primarily for monitoring of the volume of contrast materials and for accurate localization and timing of spot films. Diagnostic fluoroscopy is minimized. The mainstay of diagnosis is careful examination of multiple radiographs. The multiple radiographs taken in different projections are additive rather than complementary, since each film presents a certain proportion of the mucosal surface for diagnostic evaluation while the remainder of the mucosal surface is obscured by the high-density barium. Thus the total examination requires the interpolation and integration of the information obtained from the multiple radiographs.[2] It is not surprising that some lesions may be visible on only one or two of a dozen or more films.

The adequacy of the double contrast study is judged by the en face appearance of the mucosal surface and not by the visibility of the contour of the bowel. Similarly, diagnostic interpretation is based largely on an analysis of the en face appearance of the mucosal surface. Accurate interpretation of these radiographic findings depends on a clear understanding of the differing appearances of structures and lesions on the dependent and nondependent surfaces. This understanding allows for an accurate translation from radiographic abnormalities to pathologic condition. It also allows for an appreciation of the limitations of each radiograph and suggests maneuvers for demonstrating suspected lesions in greater detail.

Finally, these new techniques present a variety of artifactual appearances.[3] These are discussed in general terms and are also illustrated in specific chapters in conjunction with the types of pathology they may simulate.

COMPONENTS OF THE DOUBLE CONTRAST EXAMINATION

Patient Preparation

Adequate cleansing of the mucosal surface throughout the gastrointestinal tract is of obvious importance in preparing the patient for double contrast examination, so that the barium coating will provide an accurate reflection of the mucosal surface. Residual debris obscures the mucosal surface, and residual fluid results in dilution of the barium suspension, producing poor mucosal coating as well as artifacts because of patchy coating (Fig. 2–2).

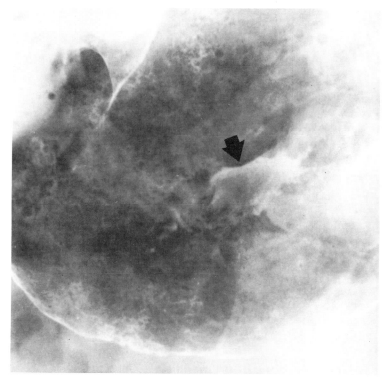

FIGURE 2–2

PATCHY COATING SIMULATING AN ULCER. There is poor coating owing to fluid and debris within the stomach. This has resulted in an irregular collection on the posterior wall resembling an ulcer (arrow). A repeat study with good mucosal coating showed no abnormality.

Mucosal Coating

High-Density Barium

Relatively little is known about the ingredients and additives in the various commercial barium suspensions.[4, 5] In particular, the physical and chemical properties that produce good mucosal coating are unknown. One would expect the ideal barium suspension for double contrast studies to have low viscosity and high density. However, there are other important factors, such as the resistance of a suspension to acid, mucin, or alkali. Because of these many factors, there is no single barium suspension that produces good results throughout the gastrointestinal tract. As a result, in our barium kitchen we have a "menu" from which we choose a barium suspension best suited for the examination being performed. In general terms, the upper gastrointestinal study requires a high-density (200% to 250% w/v), low-viscosity barium suspension, whereas the colon examination gives best results with an intermediate-density (85% to 100% w/v), higher-viscosity suspension. The requirements for the small bowel examination are still different (see Chapter 11).

The important point is that barium cannot be considered a homogeneous product with differences only in concentration, flavoring, and coloring. There are variations in viscosity, as well as other differences related to the addition of unspecified ingredients, that may affect the quality of mucosal coating. Therefore, the radiologist interested in performing double contrast examinations must be familiar with the properties of these suspensions and must be able to choose a product appropriate to the specific study being performed.

Criteria for Good Mucosal Coating

When there is good mucosal coating, the mucosal surface has a uniform grayness that fades at the edge to blend with the continuous smooth white line at the periphery, representing the profile view of the mucosa. The coating must be continuous, with no artifacts resulting from patchy coating. In the stomach, demonstration of the areae gastricae pattern serves as an additional criterion for good coating.[6] A similar surface pattern, the innominate grooves, may be seen in the colon, but with much less frequency (Fig. 2–3).[7]

Poor mucosal coating can be recognized by a lack of grayness in the en face appearance of the mucosa, with contrast provided only by the gas. The profile view of the mucosa may show thin, irregular, or interrupted coating (see Fig. 2–2). This type of coating

may be the result of incorrect choice of barium or of improper preparation of the barium suspension or of fluid, acid, or mucus within the bowel. In the colon such poor coating, with flaking of the barium suspension, may be seen on postevacuation films.

In the presence of poor or patchy coating, lesions are easily missed[8] (Fig. 2–4A). Therefore, in such cases the barium bolus must be washed across the area of poor coating until adequate coating is achieved (Fig. 2–4B).

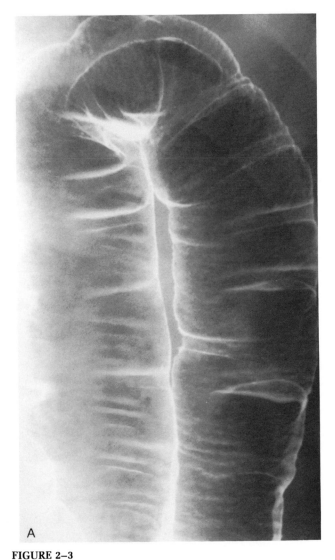

A

FIGURE 2–3

NORMAL SURFACE PATTERNS. A, The innominate lines and pits representing the surface pattern of the colon.

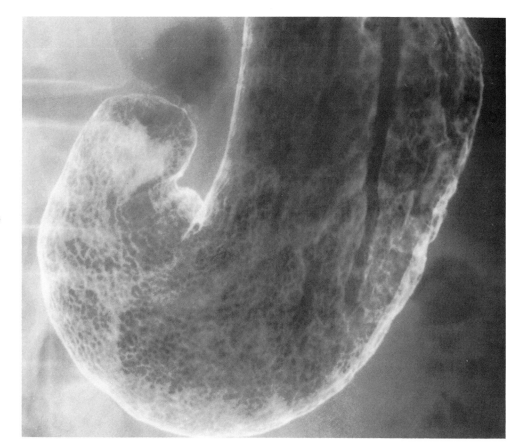

FIGURE 2–3 *Continued*

B, The areae gastricae. The fine reticular appearance of the normal surface pattern of the stomach is seen particularly in the gastric antrum.

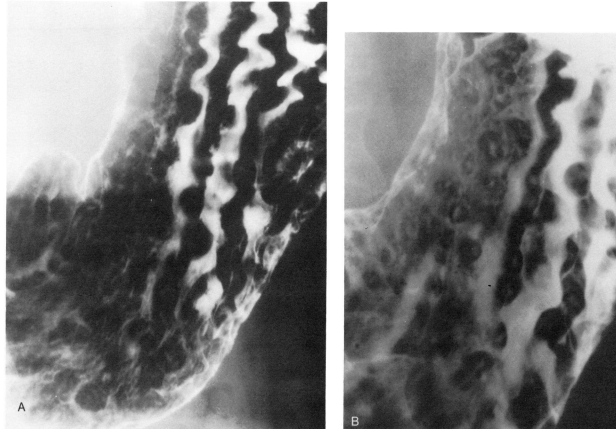

FIGURE 2–4

THE HAZARDS OF SUBOPTIMAL MUCOSAL COATING. *A*, A supine film of the stomach with suboptimal coating shows only thickening of the gastric rugal folds.

B, With improvement in mucosal coating, a diffuse erosive gastritis becomes obvious.

Distention

Gaseous distention is produced by different means throughout the gastrointestinal tract. The common goal is to separate the surfaces of the viscus and to efface the mucosal folds. In some areas, such as the gastric fundus, this is difficult to achieve, but at least the mucosal folds should be straightened.

It is easy to appreciate that inadequate gaseous distention may hide lesions (Fig. 2–5). However, it may not be so obvious that overdistention may also obscure lesions (Fig. 2–6). Figure 2–7 shows that varying degrees of distention give different information about the lesion. With overdistention, an area of rigidity is accentuated, whereas with partial collapse, the appearance of the mucosal surface may be appreciated more readily. This is particularly true in lesions with a submucosal component. Therefore, when evaluating a complex or subtle lesion, it is important to use the concept of varying degrees of distention and to examine the lesion with overdistention, adequate distention, and partial collapse. One can then synthesize the information obtained from each of these views to come to a final conclusion regarding

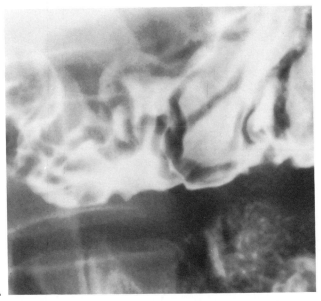
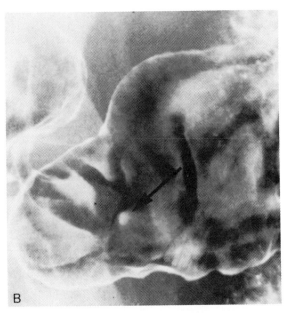

A

B

FIGURE 2–5

THE HAZARDS OF UNDERDISTENTION. *A,* Film of the gastric antrum collapsed shows only prominent folds and no definite ulcer can be identified.

   B, With adequate distention, a small ulcer *(arrow)* becomes obvious with its radiating folds. (*B,* From Laufer, I., et al.: The diagnostic accuracy of barium studies of the stomach and duodenum—correlation with endoscopy. Radiology 115:569–573, 1975, with permission.)

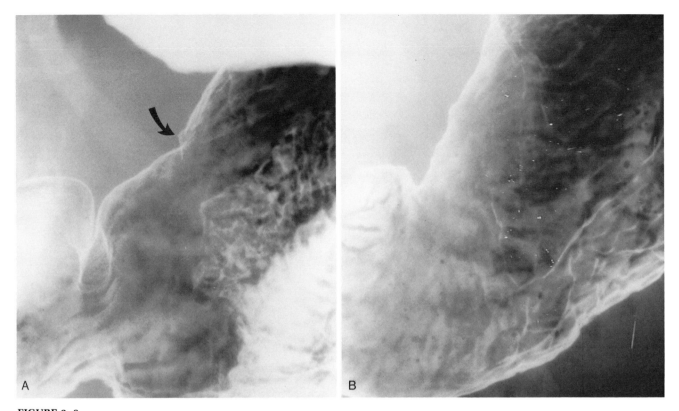

FIGURE 2–6

RISKS OF OVERDISTENTION. *A,* With moderate distention, a small ulcer crater is seen along the lesser curve of the stomach *(arrow).*
  B, With overdistention, the ulcer becomes unrecognizable.

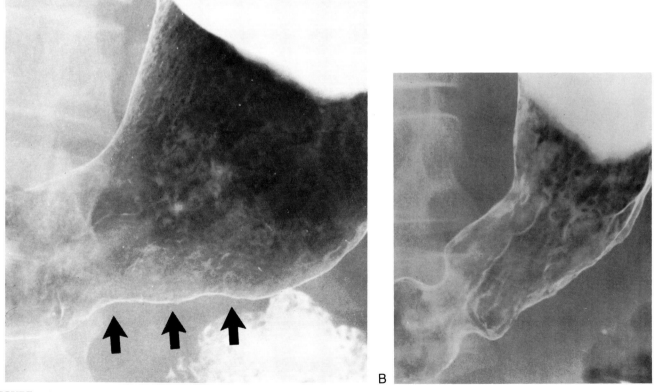

FIGURE 2–7

VALUE OF VARYING DEGREES OF DISTENTION. *A,* With the stomach overdistended, the rigidity along the greater curvature is clearly seen *(arrows).*
  B, With the stomach partially collapsed, the nodularity of the mucosal surface is more easily appreciated but the area of rigidity is not as evident. These findings were due to a scirrhous carcinoma of the stomach.

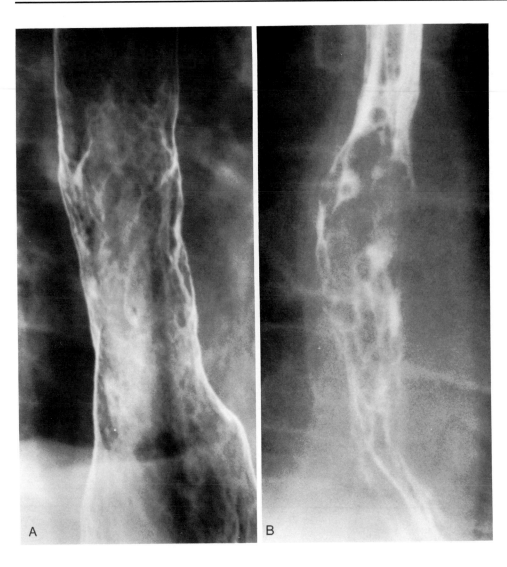

A   B

FIGURE 2–8

ADENOCARCINOMA OF BARRETT'S ESOPHAGUS. *A,* The double contrast view shows ulceration and slight rigidity of the contour.

B, The mucosal relief film shows the polypoid nature of the lesion.

the nature and extent of the lesion. This concept is illustrated in Figure 2–8 in a patient with adenocarcinoma of the distal esophagus in Barrett's epithelium. The double contrast film, with the esophagus well distended, shows slight rigidity, abnormality of the contour, and areas of ulceration (Fig. 2–8A). With the esophagus collapsed the polypoid nature of the lesion is more clearly shown (Fig. 2–8B). Thus, we cannot say that either one of the films is better than the other, but we can say that the combination of the two gives us the most information about the nature and extent of the lesion.

Projection

For each examination, attempts should be made to keep the number of films to a minimum. The minimum number of films is that required to show each area free of overlapping loops of bowel. A series of maneuvers must therefore be designed to optimize mucosal coating and to yield the required spot films. The purpose of these maneuvers is to optimize mu-

cosal coating by removing mucus and debris from the mucosal surface. The more frequent the washing, the better the mucosal coating. The maneuvers should also be designed to avoid loss of contrast material and to avoid overlapping loops of bowel until spot films of any given segment have been obtained. If there are overlapping loops, additional spot films in different obliquities are required (Fig. 2–9). The procedure must be executed quickly to prevent both overlap and deterioration in the quality of coating.

Compression

The compression study is not as critical in the double contrast study as it is in the single contrast study. Nevertheless, in some cases a lesion may be seen only on the compression spot films, whereas in others it may be appreciated and defined more easily on the compression radiograph (Fig. 2–10). Therefore, it must be emphasized that compression spot films are a routine and indispensable component of the complete double contrast examination.

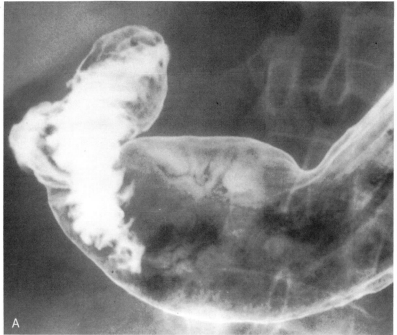

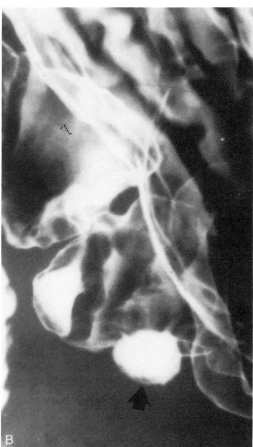

FIGURE 2–9

THE IMPORTANCE OF PROJECTION. *A,* In the supine projection the duodenum overlaps the distal antrum and pylorus.

B, In the left posterior oblique projection this area is clearly seen, and the large greater curvature ulcer is identified *(arrow).*

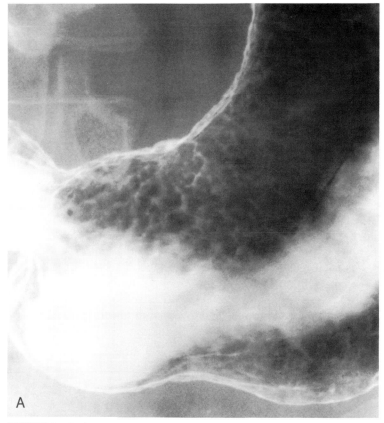

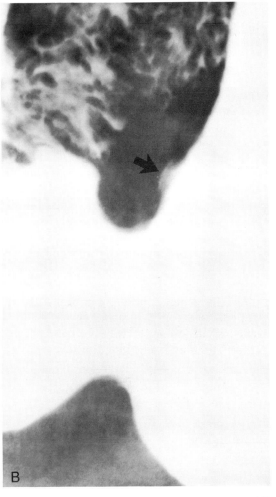

FIGURE 2–10

THE IMPORTANCE OF COMPRESSION. *A,* The double contrast film shows a coarse areae gastricae pattern along the lesser curvature. An ulcer crater is difficult to recognize.

B, Barium filling with compression shows a small ulcer crater *(arrow)* in this area.

Relaxant Drugs

There is no doubt that the use of relaxant drugs results in a higher-quality double contrast examination. In the examination of the colon it has the additional advantage of decreasing patient discomfort.[9, 10] However, the use of an injectable drug presents a slight nuisance and delay in the examination as well as an increase in cost. With the use of glucagon there are virtually no side effects except for the remote possibility of a hypersensitivity reaction.[11] However, glucagon in the upper gastrointestinal tract may delay filling of the duodenum, which may prolong the examination. It must be appreciated that the various organs differ in their sensitivity to glucagon. The upper gastrointestinal tract is very sensitive to glucagon in doses as low as 0.05 mg, whereas in the colon we believe that a dose of at least 1 mg is required to be effective.[12]

At the present time we tend to use intravenous glucagon 0.10 mg routinely for our upper gastrointestinal studies. We do not use a relaxant drug for the double contrast enema unless we encounter severe patient discomfort, spasm, or persistent stricture. Occasionally we require a relaxant drug for the examination of the esophagus. For this purpose we use propantheline bromide (Pro-Banthine), 15 to 30 mg intravenously, since glucagon is ineffective in abolishing esophageal peristalsis.[13]

Radiographic Technique

Attention to radiographic technical details is of utmost importance, since surface detail can easily be obscured by faulty technique. Theoretically, the smaller the focal spot size, the better the resolution on the films. However, in practice we have been able to obtain more than satisfactory studies with focal spot sizes as large as 1.2 and 2.0 mm, provided that the exposure time is short enough. The mA should be set as high as possible to obtain the shortest exposure time. We have been able to obtain satisfactory studies of most patients with equipment capable of providing only 200 mA. Short exposure time is particularly important in the examination of the esophagus, where motion is more prominent.

For the demonstration of surface detail a low kV would be desirable. However, this lengthens the exposure and may result in a film that shows too much contrast, such that a small area of the film is well exposed while the rest is poorly exposed. The exposure is particularly sensitive to the position of the phototimer cell. We have used approximately 105 kV for our films to shorten the exposure and to provide greater latitude. The modern rare earth screens with 400-speed film screen combinations seem to provide the optimal combination of radiographic detail and short exposure.

Endoscopic and Pathologic Correlation

With the use of double contrast techniques many unfamiliar appearances will be encountered. We have relied heavily on endoscopic and pathologic correlation for clarification of the nature and significance of new radiologic findings.[14, 15] It is important for the radiologist to actually see the specimen or to look through the endoscope to appreciate the mucosal surface, rather than to rely on a written report. By recognizing the normal appearances and their variations throughout the gastrointestinal tract as well as the gross pathologic appearances of various types of surface abnormalities the radiologist will come to appreciate the limitations and confidence limits of endoscopic and pathologic diagnosis. With the development of technical and interpretative skills, the radiologist can help the endoscopist and the pathologist to appreciate more subtle anatomic and pathologic details. We consider constant endoscopic and pathologic correlation an indispensable tool in the development of technical and interpretative skills in gastrointestinal radiology.

ESSENTIALS OF INTERPRETATION

Elements of the Double Contrast Image

In general terms, there are three elements contributing to each double contrast image. These are the dependent surface, the nondependent surface, and the barium pool (Fig. 2–11). The specific surface that is in the dependent or nondependent position is determined by the position of the patient. The barium pool will be found in the most dependent segments.

Dependent Surface

The dependent surface is covered by a barium pool of varying depth. The radiographic sequence is designed to remove most of the barium from the surface before the radiograph is exposed. Under ideal conditions, just enough barium will be left to outline protrusions without covering over and obscuring shallow lesions. If the dependent surface has any undulations, barium will collect in puddles or pools within the valleys between the hills. The barium pool is discussed in detail later in this chapter.

Nondependent Surface

The nondependent surface has a thinner coating of barium because all the free barium falls off onto the dependent surface. Thus, there is no barium pool or puddle on the nondependent surface.

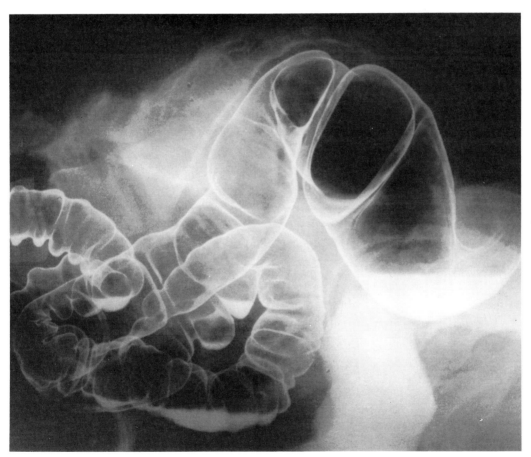

FIGURE 2–11

COMPONENTS OF THE DOUBLE CONTRAST IMAGE. Cross-table lateral view of the rectum and sigmoid with the patient prone. Dependent and nondependent surfaces can be identified. There are barium pools on the anterior wall of the distal rectum and sigmoid in addition to smaller barium puddles throughout the sigmoid colon.

Anterior Versus Posterior Wall Structures

Because of the differences in barium coating of the dependent and nondependent surfaces, anatomic structures on the anterior and posterior walls have different appearances. These differences are illustrated diagrammatically in Figure 2–12. For purposes of this discussion we will assume that the patient is in the supine position, and therefore the posterior surface is dependent and the anterior surface is nondependent. A rugal fold on the posterior wall of the stomach appears as a radiolucent defect in the barium pool on the posterior wall. However, a rugal fold on the anterior wall appears as two thin white lines, as the x-ray beam is attenuated by barium coating on the side of the fold. There is obviously no barium pool or puddle on the anterior surface. Thus the anterior wall fold is "etched in white." On the supine radiograph in Figure 2–13 it is possible to distinguish between posterior wall and anterior wall folds. Similar reasoning applies to any protrusion, whether it is a normal fold or a polypoid lesion. On the dependent surface it appears as a radiolucent filling defect, whereas on the nondependent surface the margin of the lesion is etched in white (Fig. 2–14).

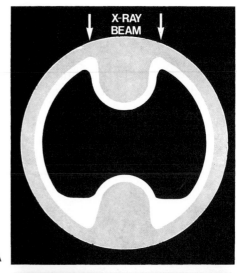

A

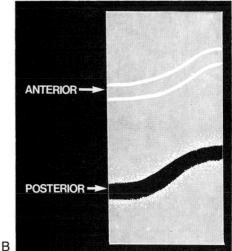

B

FIGURE 2–12

A and B, Diagrammatic representation of the appearances of a rugal fold on the anterior and posterior walls of the stomach.

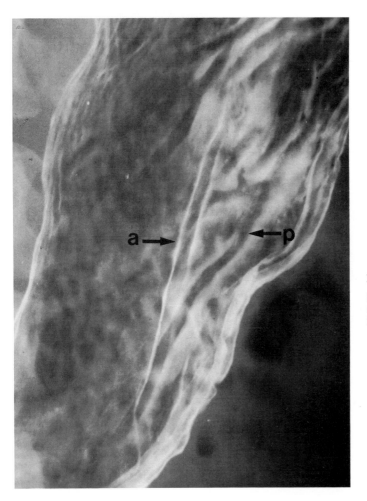

FIGURE 2–13

Supine view double contrast radiograph, showing the distinction between anterior (a) and posterior (p) wall rugal folds.

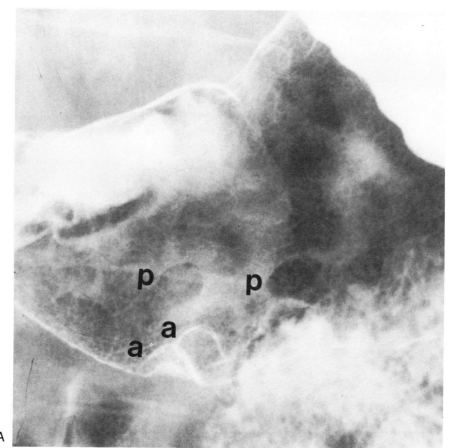

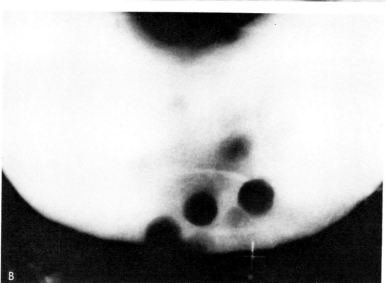

FIGURE 2–14

ANTERIOR AND POSTERIOR WALL POLYPS. *A*, On the supine view double contrast radiograph, the anterior wall polyps (*a*) are etched in white, whereas the posterior wall polyps (*p*) are seen as radiolucent filling defects.

B, The compression study shows the polyps to good advantage, but it is not possible to distinguish between the anterior and posterior wall lesions.

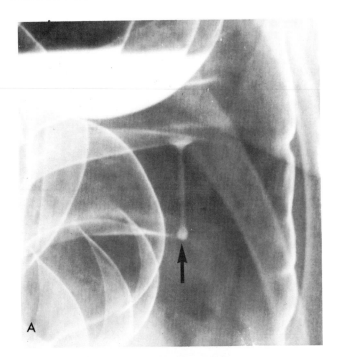

A

Stalactite Phenomenon

With these high-density barium suspensions, drops of barium are frequently seen hanging from protrusions on the nondependent surface (Fig. 2–15A). This has been termed the "stalactite phenomenon" by Op den Orth and Ploem.[16] An appreciation of the differences between dependent and nondependent wall structures makes it easy to recognize these stalactites and to differentiate them from ulcers. They are always seen in relation to a protrusion on the nondependent surface, and therefore they could not possibly represent ulcers. Furthermore, the presence of the stalactite indicates that there is a protrusion on the nondependent surface. This may be either a normal fold (Fig. 2–15B) or a polypoid lesion (Fig. 2–15C). In some cases, the stalactite may be the first and only clue to the presence of a protruded lesion on the nondependent surface. Additional films can then be obtained that will confirm the presence of the lesion.[17]

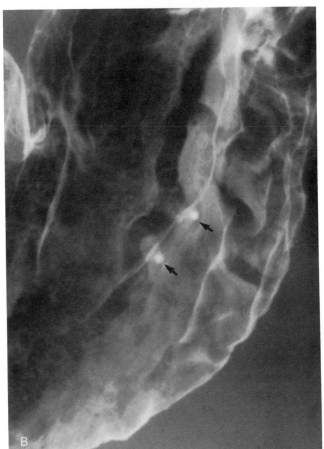

B

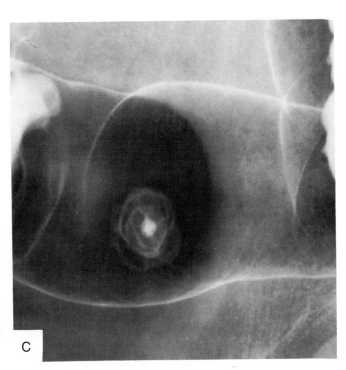

C

FIGURE 2–15

THE STALACTITE PHENOMENON. *A,* A film of the colon in the upright position shows a long droplet of barium hanging from a haustral fold.

B, Two stalactites (*arrows*) hanging from a rugal fold on the anterior wall.

C, Sigmoid polyp with a stalactite. There is a polypoid lesion in the sigmoid colon. The lesion is etched in white and is therefore on the nondependent surface. The central density represents a hanging droplet or stalactite.

Basic Roentgen Pathology

Two basic types of pathologic processes are encountered in the gastrointestinal tract. These are protruded lesions, such as polyps, inflammatory swellings, or malignant tumors, and depressed lesions, such as ulcers and diverticula. The basic roentgen manifestations of these types of lesions are similar throughout the gastrointestinal tract.

Protruded Lesions

The basic appearance of a polypoid lesion on the anterior or posterior wall has been described earlier. A polyp on the dependent surface appears as a radiolucent filling defect, whereas a polyp on the nondependent surface is "etched in white" (Fig. 2–14). This distinction is clearly seen in a Styrofoam cup with "polyps" on both the anterior and posterior walls (Fig. 2–16). Several additional features of polypoid lesions are frequently seen. The "bowler hat sign" indicates that the filling defect forms an acute angle with the bowel wall.[18] This sign is illustrated and explained diagrammatically in Figure 2–17. It consists basically of a ring, representing the barium in the angle between the polyp and the bowel wall, and a curvilinear density, representing the dome of the polyp. When the two densities are caught at a particular oblique angle, the bowler hat sign is produced. At other angles differing appearances are produced, and when the lesion is seen en face, only a single ring shadow is visible (see Fig. 2–17).

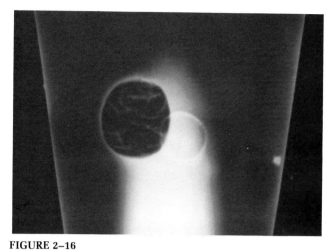

FIGURE 2–16

STYROFOAM CUP WITH "POLYPS" ON THE DEPENDENT AND NONDEPENDENT SURFACES. The large filling defect represents a polyp on the dependent surface whereas the polyp on the nondependent surface is etched in white.

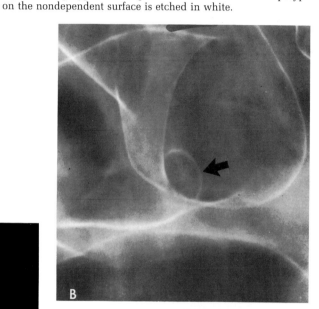

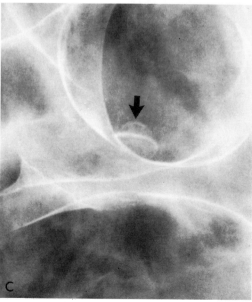

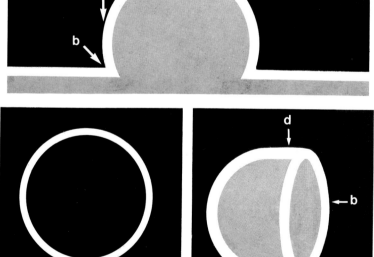

FIGURE 2–17

THE BOWLER HAT SIGN. A, Diagrammatic representation of the bowler hat sign showing the base (b) and the dome (d).
B, With the dome of the polyp and its base overlapping, a ring shadow is produced.
C, A typical bowler hat sign is produced when a sigmoid polyp is viewed obliquely.

Although the bowler hat sign was originally described as a sign of a polypoid lesion, Tobin and Young pointed out that in most cases, the bowler hat sign is due to a diverticulum.[19] Miller and co-workers showed clearly in a model as well as in clinical studies that the distinction between a polyp and a diverticulum could be made using the axis of the bowler hat.[20] When the bowler hat faces toward the axis of the bowel, it is a polyp. When the bowler hat faces away from the axis of the bowel, it represents a diverticulum (Fig. 2–18).

Ament and Alfidi have explored some aspects of the radiologic appearance of sessile polyps using a phantom.[21] They showed that basal indentation is simply a reflection of the proportion of the circumference of the bowel that is covered by the polyp. The larger the lesion, the more likely the base is to be seen in profile as a basal indentation. Therefore, the relationship of basal indentation to carcinoma is related only to the size of the lesion. Ament and Alfidi also described the "figure 8" sign as a variation of the basal indentation.

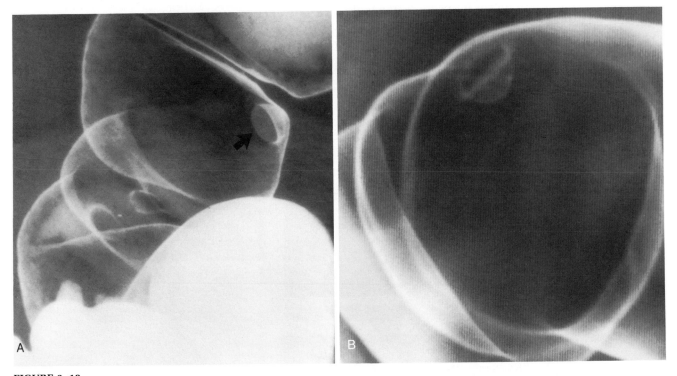

FIGURE 2–18

BOWLER HAT: DIVERTICULUM OR POLYP? A, When the dome of the hat points away from the axis of the bowel, it is a diverticulum. B, When the dome of the hat points toward the lumen of the bowel, it is a polyp.

The demonstration that a filling defect has a stalk is also conclusive proof that it is a true polypoid lesion. The stalk may be seen in profile, but it may also be seen end-on through the head of the polyp, producing the "Mexican hat sign"[18] (Fig. 2–19). The bowler hat and the Mexican hat signs are helpful in the distinction between true polyps and extraneous material. In addition, if a protruding lesion can be demonstrated to be on the nondependent surface either because it is etched in white or because it is associated with a stalactite, it almost certainly represents a true polypoid lesion, since extraneous material would usually be expected only on the dependent surface. However, in some cases fecal residue may be adherent to the nondependent surface and cannot be differentiated from a true polyp.

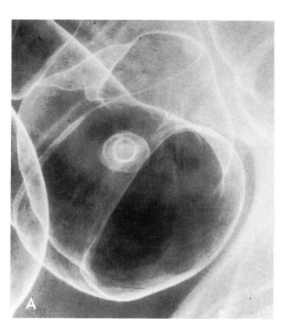
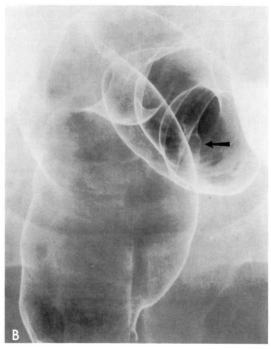

FIGURE 2–19

THE MEXICAN HAT SIGN. *A*, With the patient supine, the pedunculated polyp is seen hanging from the anterior wall. The central ring represents the stalk seen end-on, whereas the outer ring represents the head of the polyp.
  B, With the patient in the upright position, the polyp and its stalk are clearly seen *(arrow)*.

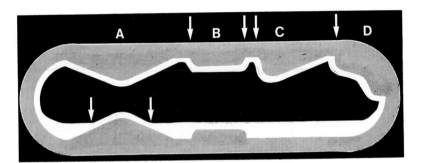

FIGURE 2–20

DIAGRAMMATIC REPRESENTATION OF THE EFFECT OF THE SHAPE OF THE POLYP ON ITS ROENTGEN APPEARANCE. A polypoid lesion with sloping edges on the nondependent surface (A) will probably not be seen on the radiograph in the supine position because no edge will be visible tangentially. A similar lesion on the dependent surface may be detected, although it may appear to be smaller than its true size because the peripheral portion of the lesion may be obscured by barium. A flat plaque-like lesion on the nondependent surface (B) will produce a very fine white etching which may be difficult to detect. A similar lesion on the dependent surface may be obscured by the barium pool, but will be seen if the barium pool is thinned out. A polypoid lesion with a sloping margin (C) may be seen as only a single line representing the nonsloping edge. See Figure 2–21. A plaque-like lesion on a curved surface (D). Only the edge of the lesion tangential to the x-ray beam will be seen. See Figure 2–22.

The appearance of protrusion is determined not only by the lesion's location but also by its shape, and in particular by the configuration of its margins. Figure 2–20 illustrates diagrammatically various types of polypoid lesions. Lesion A is a protruded lesion with gradually tapered margins. When it is located on the dependent surface, it is seen as a radiolucent filling defect. However, it appears to be smaller than it really is because the peripheral parts of the lesion are obscured by the barium pool. If this lesion with gradually tapered margins is located on the nondependent surface, it may be invisible because there is no edge for the x-ray beam to catch tangentially. A stalactite may be hanging down from the tip of this lesion, which may be the only clue to its presence on the nondependent surface.[17] Lesions such as this are best demonstrated by turning the patient over so that the lesion is situated on the dependent surface. In addition, a protruded lesion may be demonstrated by compression; that is, a lesion may be compressed into the barium pool and then seen as a filling defect.

Lesion B is a flat, plaque-like lesion. When situated on the dependent surface, it may be covered over and rendered invisible by the barium pool. As the barium pool is thinned out, the lesion may appear. When the barium pool disappears completely, the lesion may again be invisible. Lesions such as this are, in fact, best demonstrated with a very shallow barium pool using "flow technique."[22] With this technique, the barium pool flows around or across lesions on the dependent surface, and spot films should be exposed when the lesion is seen to best advantage. When such a lesion is on the nondependent surface, it is faintly etched in white. The density of the etching depends on the thickness of the lesion. If the lesion is flat enough, the etching may be so faint as to be invisible. In addition, if there is a significant barium pool on the opposite wall, it may obscure the etching of this lesion.

Lesion C has one abrupt margin and one tapered margin. In cases in which the lesion is on the nondependent surface, only the portion of the lesion with an abrupt margin can be seen. Therefore the lesion may be manifested only as a line or semicircle (Fig. 2–21).

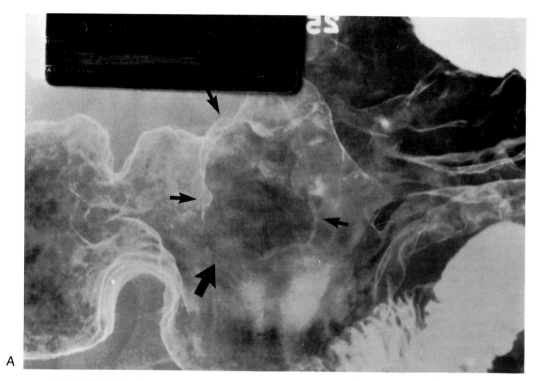

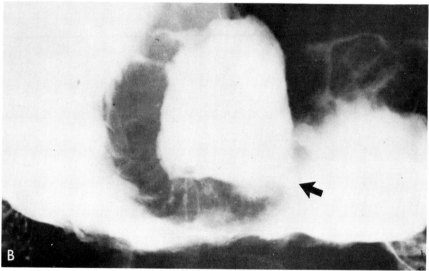

FIGURE 2–21

ULCERATED, PLAQUE-LIKE CARCINOMA ON THE ANTERIOR WALL. *A,* The supine view double contrast radiograph shows an irregular ring density representing the ulcerated mass on the anterior wall *(small arrows).* The distal margin of the lesion is ill defined *(large arrow)* because of its sloping margin.

B, A film taken with patient in prone position shows the large ulcer, filled with barium, and the core of tumor tissue surrounding it except at its distal edge *(arrow),* where the tumor mass becomes less prominent.

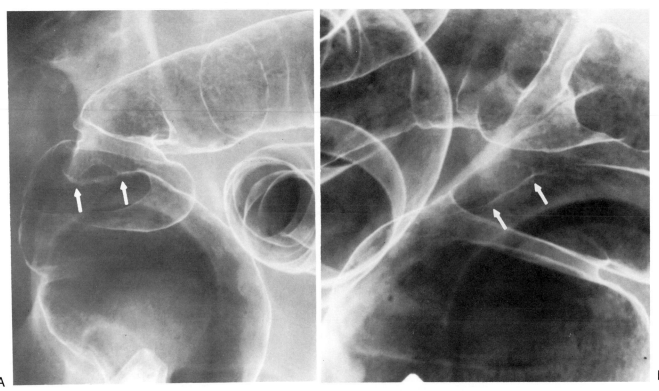

FIGURE 2–22

PLAQUE-LIKE LESION ON A CURVED SURFACE. *A,* An oblique film of the rectum shows a linear density *(arrows)* adjacent to the normal bowel wall. This is the subtle manifestation of a plaque-like carcinoma on a curved surface.

B, The presence of the plaque-like carcinoma is confirmed in the lateral projection.

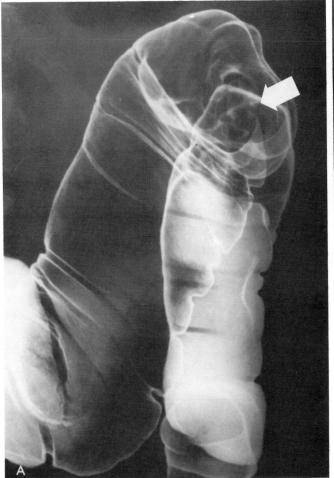

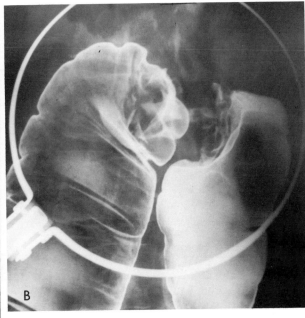

FIGURE 2–23

ANNULAR CARCINOMA SEEN EN FACE AND IN PROFILE. *A,* The irregularity of the lumen seen end-on *(arrow)* is the result of an annular carcinoma.

B, Carcinoma is confirmed on the appropriate oblique projection.

Lesion D is a plaque-like lesion located on a curved surface. Medially, the margin of the lesion can be seen, but laterally, only the normal bowel wall can be seen. On single contrast studies, such colonic tumors are recognized either as filling defects in the barium pool or as contour defects. Therefore, those unaccustomed to interpreting double contrast radiographs may have difficulty recognizing such a lesion. It is important to realize that polypoid lesions may appear on double contrast studies as abnormal lines seen only en face as well as the traditional filling defect or contour defect.

Annular lesions can be recognized as contour defects on double contrast studies, just as on the single contrast examination. In addition, they can be recognized end-on when seen through overlapping loops of bowel (Fig. 2–23). The irregularity and nodularity of the lumen are clearly apparent and can be confirmed by the appropriate oblique projection.

Submucosal lesions (Fig. 2–24) form a right angle with the bowel wall and stretch the overlying mucosa. Therefore, they have a very smooth surface in profile and very sharp margins en face. In addition, mucosal folds may appear to fade out as they approach the lesion (Fig. 2–24C).

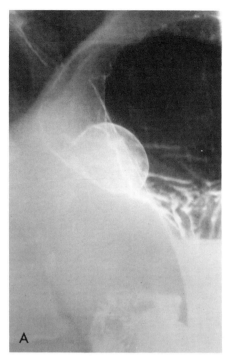

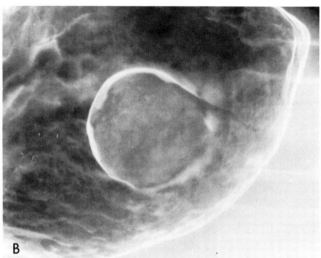

FIGURE 2–24

TYPICAL SUBMUCOSAL LESION. A, The profile view shows the right angle formed by the mass and the gastric wall and the smooth mucosal surface.

B, En face view shows the very abrupt, well-defined edge of the tumor.

C, Another projection shows mucosal folds fading out at the edge of the lesion.

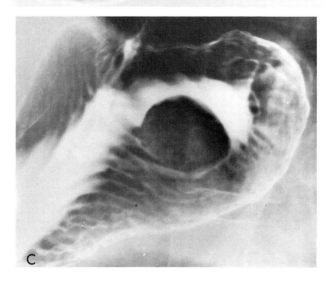

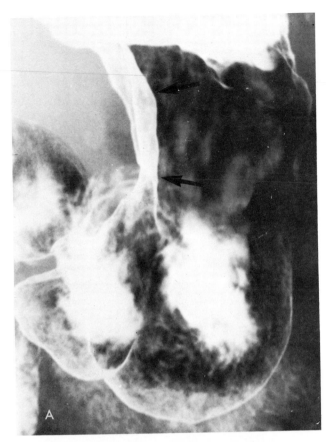

Extrinsic masses (Fig. 2–25) may be seen in profile or en face as an ill-defined radiolucency. When such a mass is viewed in an oblique projection, only a white line representing one edge of the extrinsic mass may be seen (Fig. 2–25C). Because of the marked gastric distention, the stomach may appear to surround an extrinsic mass, which may simulate an intramural lesion[23] (Fig. 2–25D).

FIGURE 2–25

EXTRINSIC MASS DUE TO CARCINOMA OF THE PANCREAS. A, Lateral view, showing extrinsic compression on the posterior wall of the stomach (arrows).

B, Frontal view, showing an ill-defined radiolucency caused by the retro-gastric mass.

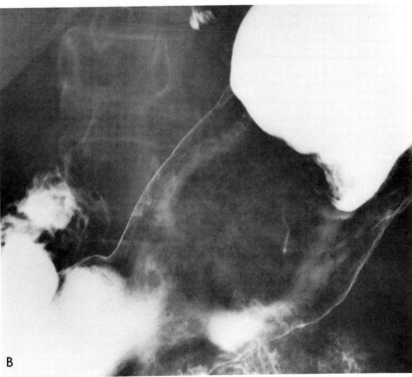

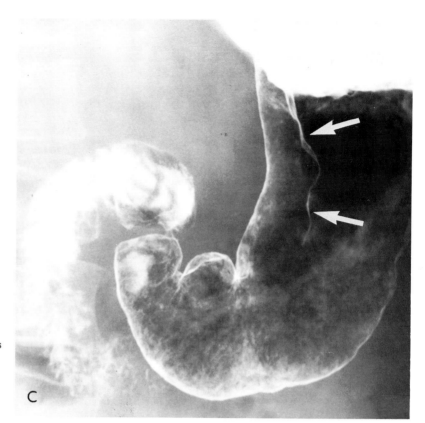

FIGURE 2–25 *Continued*

C, Oblique projection, showing a curving line representing the edge of the retrogastric mass *(arrows).*

D, In another patient, there is a prominent impression owing to an enlarged caudate lobe of the liver *(arrow).* The appearance simulates an intramural gastric lesion.

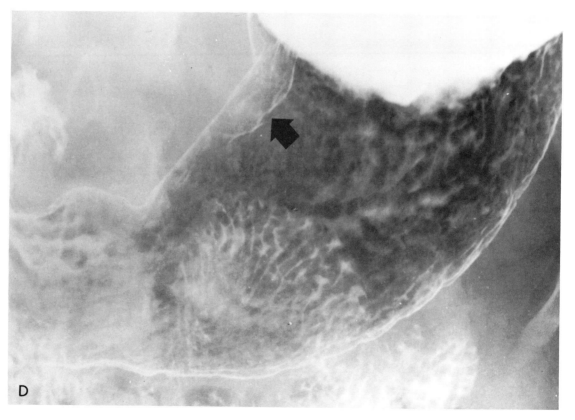

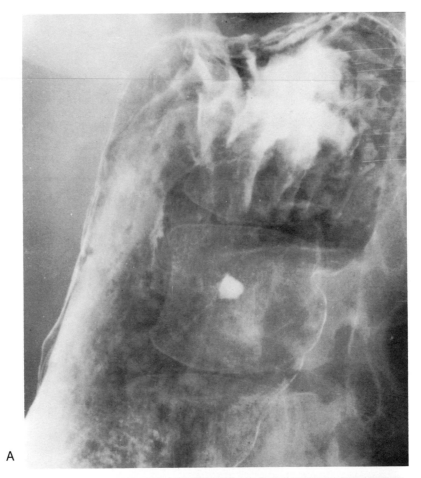

A

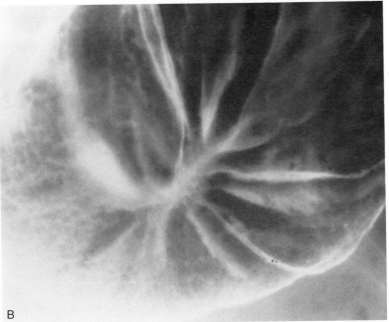

B

FIGURE 2–26

DEPRESSED LESIONS ON THE DEPENDENT SURFACE. *A,* Film of the
stomach in the right posterior oblique (RPO) projection shows a typical high
lesser curve ulcer en face.

B, In another patient, prominent radiating folds are seen on the posterior wall
in relationship to a healing posterior wall ulcer.

Depressed Lesions

Depressed lesions are lesions that extend beyond the mucosal surface, most typically ulcers or diverticula. A depressed lesion on a dependent surface is easily recognized by the familiar barium collection or niche (Fig. 2–26A). If there are associated radiating folds, these also will have the characteristics of dependent wall structures; that is, they will be seen as radiolucent filling defects (Fig. 2–26B). When an ulcer is situated on a nondependent surface, the barium empties out, leaving the sides and base of the ulcer coated with barium. The resulting radiographic appearance is a ring shadow that can be considered to be an empty crater (Fig. 2–27). Radiating folds associated with such a lesion are etched in white.

Therefore, the appearance of a ring shadow may cause diagnostic confusion. It may represent either a depressed or protruded lesion on the nondependent surface. In addition, either type of lesion may produce a ring shadow when it is situated on the dependent surface and when there is absolutely no barium pool. A careful analysis of the radiographs can usually reveal whether the ring shadow is due to a protrusion

or a depression. A depressed lesion has a sharp outer border and fades to the inside (Fig. 2–28), whereas a protruded lesion has a sharp inner border and fades to the outside[18] (Fig. 2–29).

A ring shadow may also be caused by several types of depressed lesions, such as an empty diverticulum (Fig. 2–30A) or an empty ulcer crater on either the dependent (Fig. 2–28A) or nondependent surface (Fig. 2–30B). It may also be the result of a filling defect, such as a blood clot within an ulcer crater (Fig. 2–31). For further evaluation of a ring shadow the patient can be turned to demonstrate the lesion in profile. Attempts should also be made to wash the lesion with barium to demonstrate its appearance in the barium pool.

Occasionally a double ring shadow may be seen and usually indicates a lesion on the nondependent surface. It may indicate an ulcer or diverticulum, with the inner ring representing the neck and the outer ring the base (Fig. 2–32), or it may indicate an ulcerated protruded lesion, with the inner ring representing the ulcer and the outer ring representing the edge of the protrusion (see Fig. 2–36).

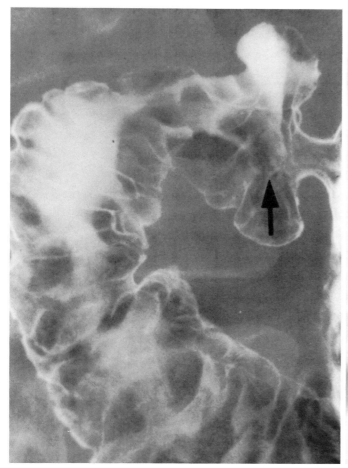
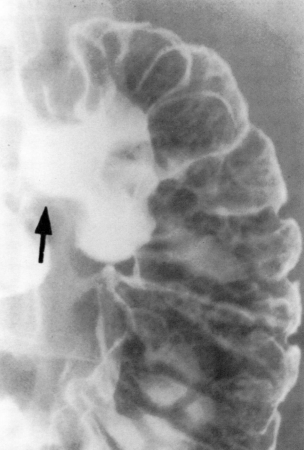

A
B

FIGURE 2–27

ANTERIOR WALL ULCER. *A*, A film in the left posterior oblique (LPO) projection shows a ring shadow in a deformed duodenal cap. *B*, With patient in prone position, the ring shadow fills with barium *(arrow)* indicating an anterior wall duodenal ulcer.

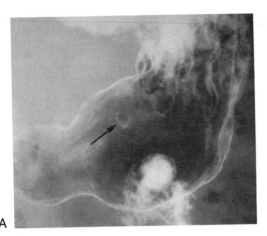
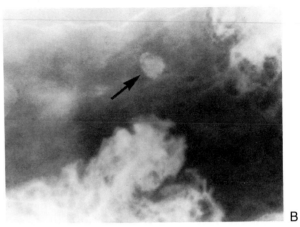

A   B

FIGURE 2–28

RING SHADOW DUE TO AN ULCER. *A*, A shallow posterior wall ulcer with an empty crater. The ring shadow is the result of coating of the sides of the ulcer crater. Note that the ring shadow has a sharp outer border and fades to the inside. (From Laufer, I.: Simple method for routine double contrast study of the upper gastrointestinal tract. Radiology *117*:513–518, 1975, with permission.)

B, With further manipulation of the barium pool, the ulcer crater can be filled with barium *(arrow)*.

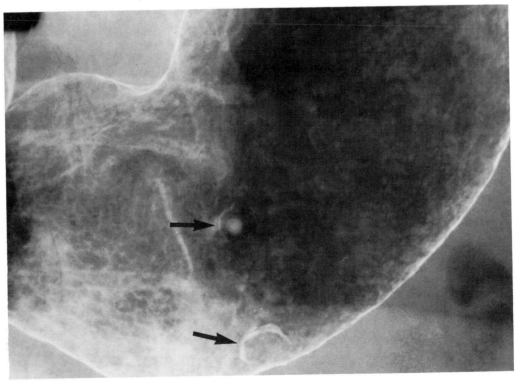

FIGURE 2–29

RING SHADOWS DUE TO ANTERIOR WALL POLYPS *(arrows)*. The central polyp also exhibits the stalactite phenomenon.

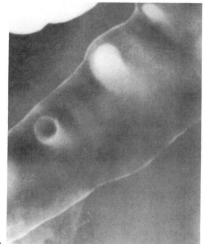

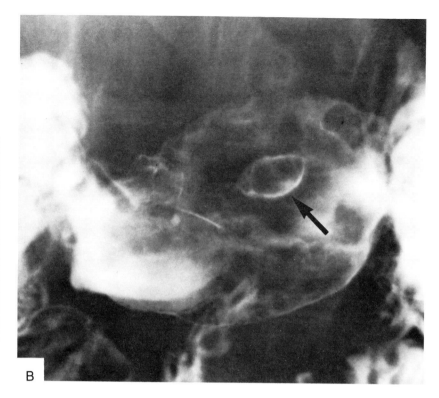

FIGURE 2–30

OTHER CAUSES OF RING SHADOWS. *A*, An empty diverticulum.

    B, Anterior wall duodenal ulcer. With patient in supine position, a ring shadow is seen in the center of the duodenal cap. This could be filled only in the prone position, indicating that it is an ulcer on the anterior wall.

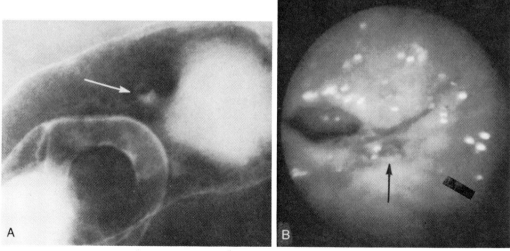

FIGURE 2–31

RING SHADOW DUE TO BLOOD CLOT IN A SMALL ULCER. *A*, Close-up view of the antrum shows partial filling of a shallow ulcer in the distal antrum with a radiolucency representing the blood clot (*arrow*).

    B, The endoscopic photograph shows the blood clot (*arrow*) adherent to the base of the ulcer. (From Laufer, I., Hamilton, J., and Mullens, J. E.: Demonstration of superficial gastric erosions by double contrast radiography. Gastroenterology 68:387, 1975, with permission.)

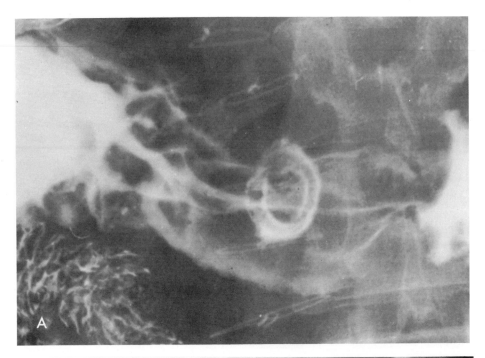

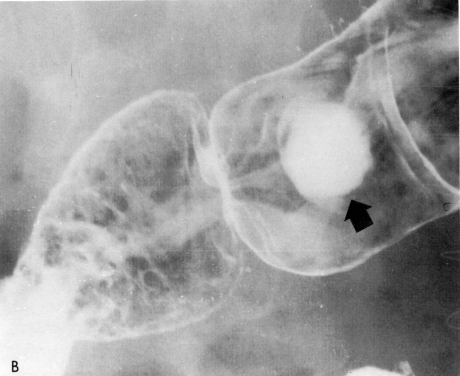

FIGURE 2–32

DOUBLE RING SHADOW DUE TO AN ULCER. A, In the prone position, a double ring is seen. The inner ring represents the neck of the ulcer, whereas the outer ring represents the outer margins of the ulcer crater, where it is wider in diameter.

B, The corresponding film in the supine position confirms that the ulcer crater is on the posterior wall.

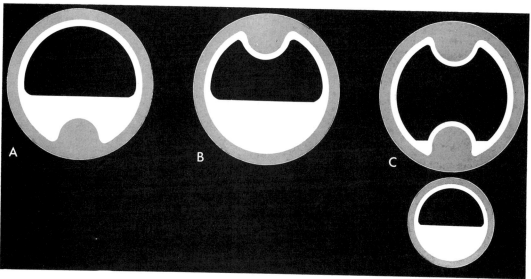

FIGURE 2–33

DIAGRAMMATIC REPRESENTATION OF THE HAZARDS OF THE BARIUM POOL. *A*, Barium pool obscures the lesion on the dependent surface. See Figure 2–35.

B, The barium pool obscures the fine white etching of the lesion on the nondependent surface. See Figure 2–36.

C, The barium pool in the overlapping loop of bowel may obscure a lesion on either the dependent or the nondependent surface. See Figure 2–9.

The Barium Pool

The barium pool is the bolus of free barium that is not adherent to the mucosal surface. The major portion of the bolus, which we shall call the barium pool, is found in the most dependent segments of the bowel. In addition, small "puddles" may be found in any segment where there are minor depressions. The barium pool is of critical importance, since it is used to wash and coat the mucosal surface and to fill any depressed lesions. It can also be used to demonstrate posterior wall protrusions more clearly. Indeed, the entire double contrast examination rests on skillful manipulation of the barium pool. Nevertheless, the barium pool or puddle can lead to serious error in several different ways (Fig. 2–33). A dependent wall protrusion may not be seen because it is covered over by the barium pool (Fig. 2–34). However, even a

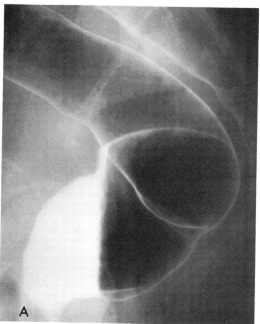
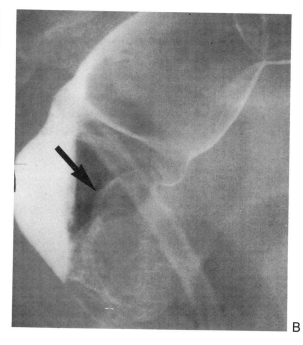

FIGURE 2–34

DEPENDENT WALL LESION OBSCURED BY BARIUM. *A*, The patient is prone. The barium pool on the anterior wall of the rectum obscures a large polypoid tumor.

B, With the patient supine, the barium pool has shifted to the posterior wall and the polypoid tumor is clearly seen (*arrow*).

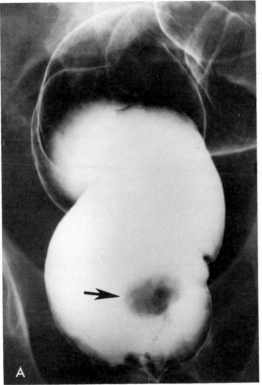

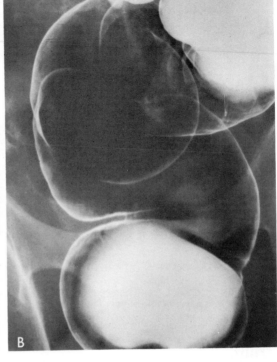

FIGURE 2–35

A, A film taken in the supine position shows a large filling defect in the rectum. This must be on the posterior wall.

B, In the prone position no abnormality can be detected because the barium pool on the anterior wall obscures the fine white etching of the polypoid tumor on the posterior surface.

C, A cross-table lateral film confirms the posterior wall location of the early polypoid carcinoma and shows the barium pool on the anterior wall.

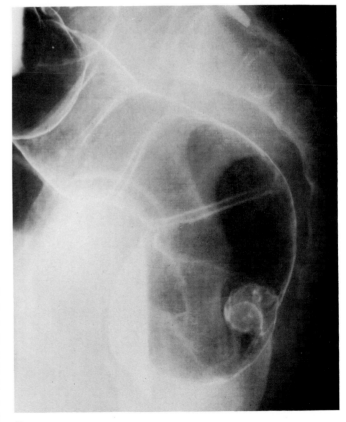

C

small barium puddle may obscure or veil the fine white etching of a relatively large polypoid lesion on the nondependent surface. This principle is illustrated in Figure 2–35. In the supine position a large polypoid tumor on the posterior wall of the rectum is clearly seen as a filling defect in the barium pool on the posterior wall (Fig. 2–35A). With the patient in the prone position the lesion is now on the nondependent surface and should be etched in white (Fig. 2–35B). However, the delicate etching of this polypoid lesion is entirely obscured by the barium pool on the anterior wall. A lateral view confirms the posterior wall location of this lesion and shows the barium pool (Fig. 2–35C).

In addition, a barium pool may collect in an overlapping structure and obscure a pathologic lesion (see Fig. 2–9). Some of the problems associated with the barium pool can be avoided by compression, as illustrated in Figures 2–36 and 2–37. A lesion on the nondependent surface may be seen only faintly (Fig. 2–36). However, with compression it is immersed in the barium pool and is clearly seen as a radiolucent filling defect (Fig. 2–37).

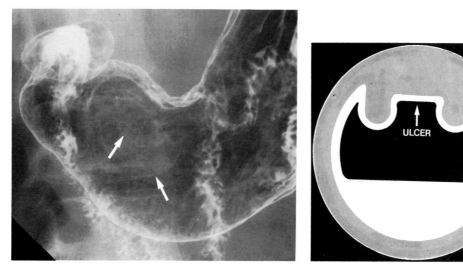

FIGURE 2–36

VALUE OF COMPRESSION IN ANTERIOR WALL LESIONS. The plaque-like lesion on the anterior wall and the central ulcer are faintly seen.

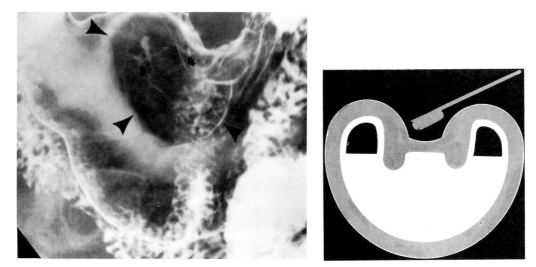

FIGURE 2–37

With compression the tumor is pushed into the barium pool, causing a radiolucent filling defect and making the tumor (arrowheads) and the ulcer (small arrow) more apparent.

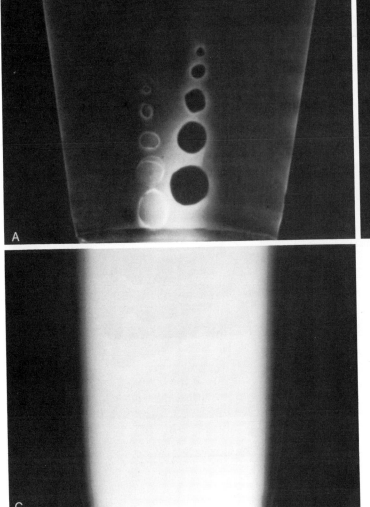

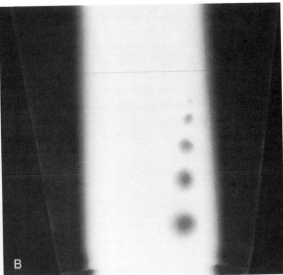

FIGURE 2-38

HAZARDS OF THE BARIUM POOL. *A,* Styrofoam cup has a row of "polyps" on both the anterior wall and the posterior wall.

B, With 10 ml barium added, the polyps on the anterior wall are totally obscure.

C, With 40 ml barium, the polyps on both the anterior and the posterior walls are hidden.

Thus a barium pool or puddle may be either a blessing or a curse. It improves mucosal coating; it may fill an ulcer crater on the dependent surface; and it helps to demonstrate dependent wall protrusions. On the other hand, it can obscure lesions on both the dependent and nondependent surfaces. This concept is illustrated in Figure 2-38. With the Styrofoam cup coated and all the free barium poured off, two rows of "polyps" can be identified, one on the dependent surface and one on the nondependent surface (Fig. 2-38A). With the addition of 10 ml of high-density barium, the polyps on the nondependent surface are entirely obscured (Fig. 2-38B) and with 40 ml of barium, both the dependent and nondependent wall polyps become invisible (Fig. 2-38C). This shows clearly the hazards of the barium pool and the importance of thinning out this barium pool. An understanding of the potential value as well as the hazards of the barium pool is an important step in mastering double contrast techniques.

ARTIFACTS

In addition to becoming familiar with a new array of normal and pathologic appearances, the radiologist starting to use double contrast techniques must also learn to recognize a variety of artifacts that may be peculiar to double contrast techniques.[3] The causes of these artifacts are listed in Table 2-1. Many artifacts can be attributed to the high viscosity of the barium suspension and to the variations in mucosal coating. Some of these artifacts, such as patchy coating (see Fig. 2-2) and the stalactite phenomenon (see Fig. 2-15), have already been mentioned. Some barium suspensions may cause precipitation or flaking, which may simulate diffuse mucosal ulceration (Fig. 2-39). In many cases these artifacts can be avoided by the choice of an appropriate barium suspension. However, in some patients with excessive fluid and debris they may be unavoidable. Cho and colleagues[25] described a peculiar artifactual appearance in the

TABLE 2–1. Causes of Double Contrast Artifacts		
Barium-Related	**See-Through Effect**	**Extraneous or Foreign Material**
High viscosity—stalactite phenomenon[16]	Normal anatomic structures	Gas bubbles
Patchy coating	Calcified structures	Effervescent agent
Precipitation and flaking	Contrast-filled structures	Adherent fecal material
"Kissing" artifact		Others—mineral oil, Telepaque
Pseudo-intraluminal diverticulum[25]		

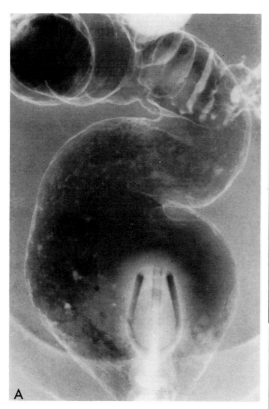

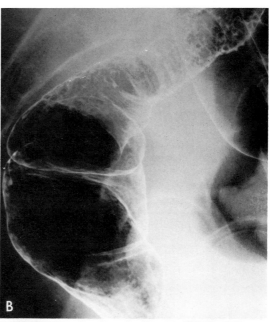

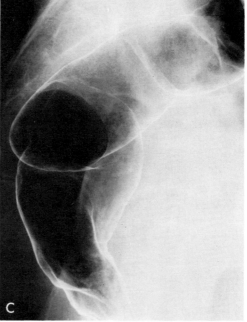

FIGURE 2–39

ARTIFACTS DUE TO POOR BARIUM SUSPENSIONS. *A,* Barium precipitation, simulating inflammatory bowel disease.

B, Flaking of the barium suspension, simulating inflammatory bowel disease.

C, In the same patient, a film taken 10 minutes before shows a perfectly normal mucosal surface. (Reprinted with permission from Laufer, I.: Air contrast studies of the colon in inflammatory bowel disease. CRC Crit. Rev. Diagn. Imaging 9:421, 1977. Copyright CRC Press, Inc., Boca Raton, FL.)

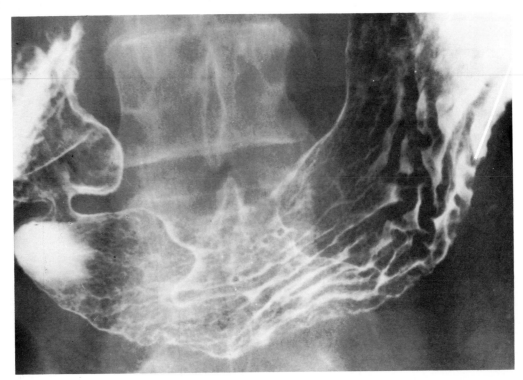

FIGURE 2–40

Kissing artifact in the antrum due to adherence of the anterior and posterior walls of the stomach as it crosses in front of the aorta.

esophagus simulating an intraluminal diverticulum. This artifact is caused by the interaction of barium with debris and mucus in the esophagus.

In some patients there is insufficient gas to separate the anterior and posterior walls. The area of contact between the anterior and posterior walls may produce an irregular outline that may simulate an ulcer or polypoid lesion[8] (Fig. 2–40). With further distention of the area, the artifact disappears. We have termed this a "kissing" artifact.

The segment of the gastrointestinal tract outlined by double contrast becomes transparent. Therefore, opacities overlying any segment can be clearly seen and may simulate an intrinsic lesion. These opacities may be normal skeletal structures (Fig. 2–41); calcified structures, such as lymph nodes, uterine fibroids, or phleboliths; or contrast-filled structures, such as diverticula or lymph nodes.

Extraneous material in the lumen must be differentiated from polypoid lesions in both single and double contrast techniques. However, with double contrast techniques there are additional artifacts, such as gas bubbles and undissolved effervescent pills or granules (Fig. 2–42), that must be recognized.

Table 2–2 lists the various types of pathologic conditions that may be simulated by artifacts. Some of these artifacts are discussed in further detail in the specific chapters under the lesions they simulate.

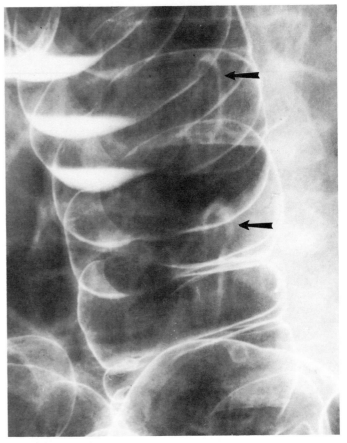

FIGURE 2–41

SEE-THROUGH ARTIFACTS. Spinous processes seen through the gas-filled colon may simulate polypoid lesions.

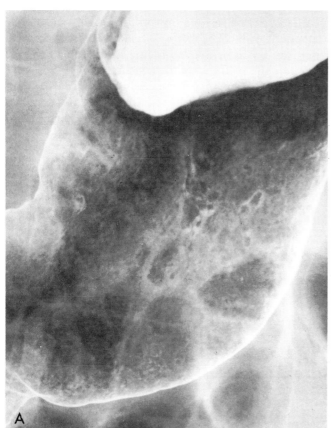
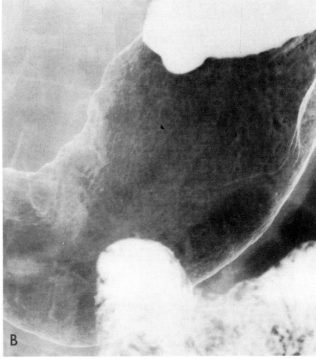

FIGURE 2–42

ARTIFACT DUE TO EXTRANEOUS MATERIAL. *A,* The early film from a double contrast study shows small filling defects in the stomach due to undissolved effervescent agent.

B, A later film shows that the filling defects are no longer present.

TABLE 2–2. Pathologic Conditions That May Be Simulated by Artifacts		
Diffuse Superficial Ulceration	**Discrete Ulceration**	**Polypoid Lesion**
Barium precipitation	Colonic or duodenal	See-through effect
Flaking	diverticulum	Extraneous material
Debris	Patchy coating	"Kissing" artifact
	Stalactite phenomenon	
	"Kissing" artifact	
	Pseudo-intraluminal	
	diverticulum	

SUMMARY

The use of double contrast techniques requires an understanding of the basic differences in approach between single and double contrast studies of the gastrointestinal tract. The transition from one approach to the other demands a major reorientation to the performance and interpretation of gastrointestinal radiologic studies. It also requires an understanding of the elements that combine to form the double contrast image—the dependent wall, the nondependent wall, and the barium pool. Great attention must be paid to the quality of mucosal coating as a criterion of the adequacy of the study. Materials such as barium suspensions, which are designed for double contrast studies, must be used. Although gaseous distention is generally desirable, it is important to understand the value of varying the degree of distention to best demonstrate certain types of lesions. Management of the barium pool is a critical aspect of double contrast technique. The examiner must be aware of the importance of the barium pool and of its potential hazards.

Interpretation of these studies requires a clear understanding of the difference in appearances between structures and lesions on the dependent and nondependent walls. The examiner should aim at a precise translation from the radiologic findings to the gross pathologic features of the lesion. He or she must concentrate on a basic analysis of the lines, points, and shadows on the film. Endoscopic and pathologic correlation should be viewed as an extension of the radiologic examination whereby the radiologist can improve the quality of his or her studies and the precision of interpretation.

Figures 2–43 to 2–52 illustrate additional examples of the application of these principles to the performance and interpretation of double contrast studies.

Text continued on page 54

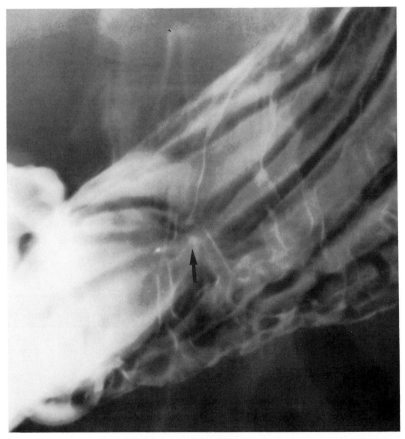

FIGURE 2–43

SEPARATION OF ANTERIOR AND POSTERIOR WALL FOLDS. On the supine film of the stomach, the normal anterior wall folds are seen etched in white and running transversely. The posterior wall folds are seen as radiolucent filling defects with an area of convergence toward a very small ulcer (*arrow*). Thus, the separate analysis of anterior and posterior walls allows for correct diagnosis of small posterior wall ulcer with converging folds.

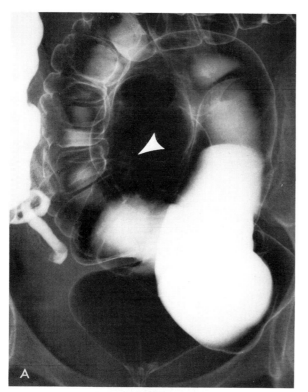

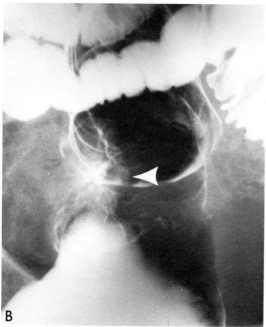

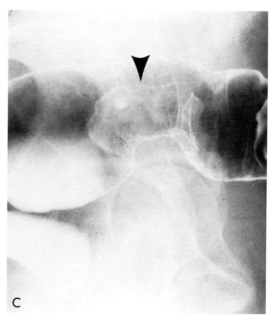

FIGURE 2–44

DANGERS OF INCORRECT EXPOSURE.
A, Frontal view with overexposure. An
abnormality on the right lateral aspect of the
sigmoid can only be suspected.

B, With a lighter exposure the irregular,
plaque-like lesion on the right lateral wall of
the sigmoid is clearly seen.

C, Left lateral projection in which the
plaque-like lesion on the nondependent
surface is etched in white.

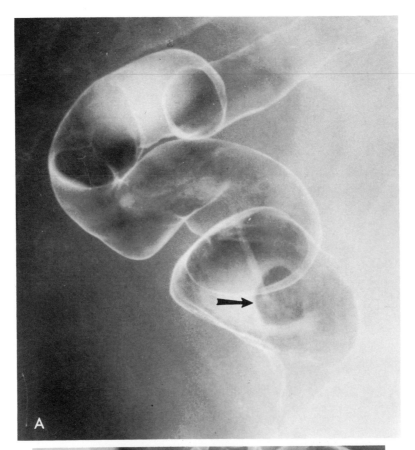

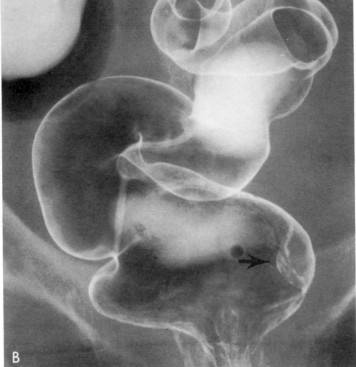

FIGURE 2–45

A, Left lateral view of the rectum shows a rounded filling defect in the barium pool. Therefore, the polypoid lesion must be on the dependent surface, i.e., the left lateral wall of the rectum.

B, This is confirmed in the frontal projection.

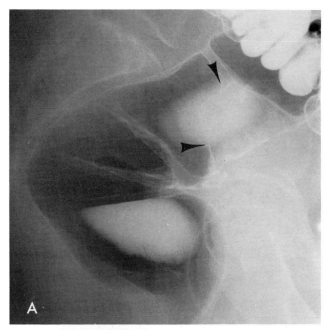

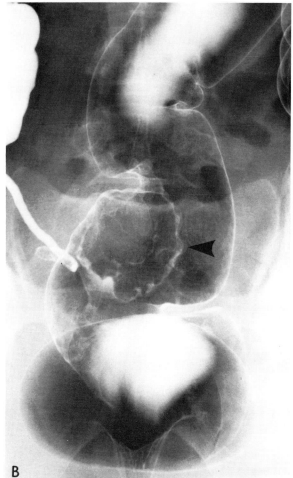

FIGURE 2–46

A, In the left lateral projection the fine white etching (*arrowheads*) is almost obscured by a small barium puddle. Because of the etched outline of the lesion, it must be on the nondependent (right lateral) wall.

B, The location of the lesion is confirmed on the frontal projection, which shows an ulcerated mass on the right lateral wall of the rectosigmoid (*arrowhead*).

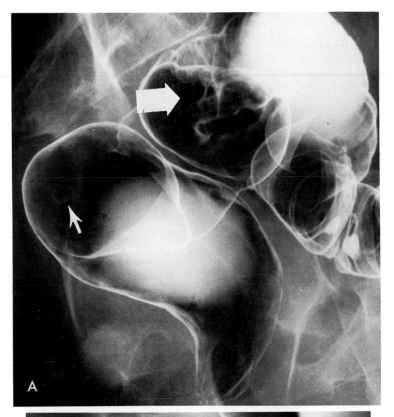

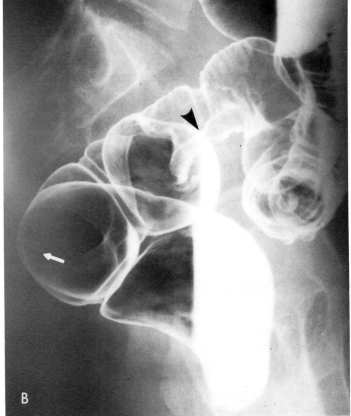

FIGURE 2–47

A, Oblique view of the rectosigmoid is suggestive of an abnormality at the rectosigmoid junction. The abnormality is seen through overlapping loops of bowel (*large arrow*). There is also a small polypoid lesion in the rectum (*small arrow*).

   B, Lateral view shows more clearly a plaque-like lesion at the rectosigmoid junction (*black arrowhead*) due to carcinoma. The small polyp on the posterior wall of the rectum (*white arrow*) is faintly seen.

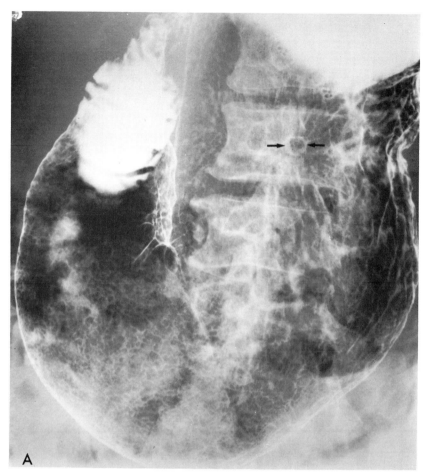

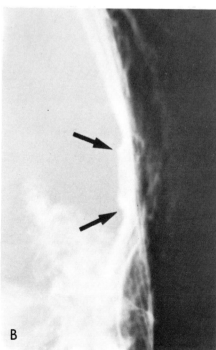

FIGURE 2–48

A, Double contrast view of the stomach in RPO projection. A ring shadow *(arrows)* is seen on the dependent surface, i.e., the lesser curvature. Because this represents an empty crater, the ulcer is probably very shallow.

B, Tangential view confirms presence of broad, shallow crater *(arrows)*. (Courtesy of Hans Herlinger, M.D., Philadelphia, Pennsylvania.)

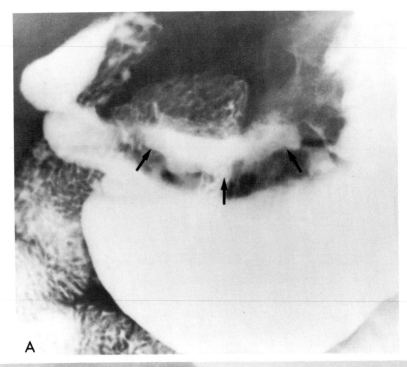

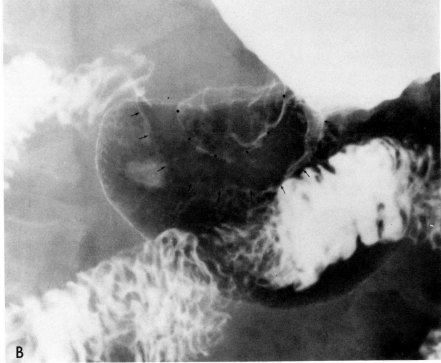

FIGURE 2–49

CARMAN'S MENISCUS SIGN SEEN ON CONVENTIONAL STUDY AND WITH DOUBLE CONTRAST. *A*, Conventional view of the lesser curvature ulcer *(arrows)* and the surrounding rim of tumor tissue.

B, The double contrast view shows the rim of tumor tissue *(arrows)* and the outline of the ulcer *(dots)*. Note the absence of the areae gastricae over the tumor tissue. (Courtesy of Hans Herlinger, M.D., Philadelphia, Pennsylvania.)

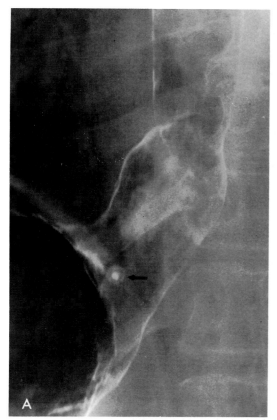

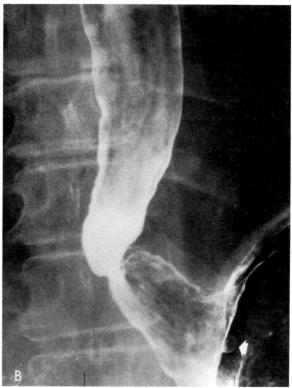

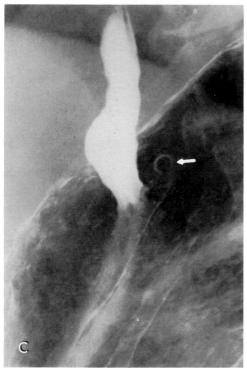

FIGURE 2–50

BARIUM STALACTITE POINTING TO A POLYPOID LESION. *A,* Prone position. There is a ring shadow *(arrow)* with a central radiodensity, representing the stalactite. This indicates that the ring shadow must be due to a protruded lesion on the nondependent (posterior) surface of the hiatal hernia.

B, Another view confirms the presence of a small polypoid lesion *(arrow).*

C, Steep RPO projection, with the hiatal hernia reduced back into the stomach. The polypoid lesion is seen to lie posteriorly *(arrow).*

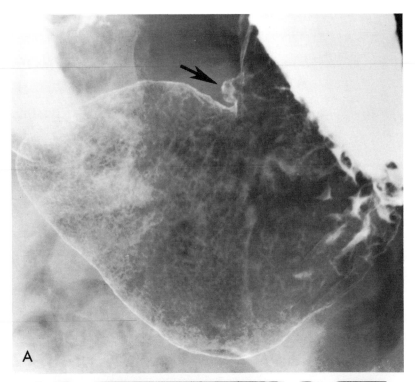

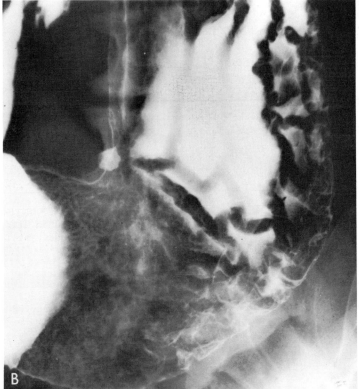

FIGURE 2–51

THE VALUE OF FLOW TECHNIQUE FOR DEMONSTRATION OF POSTERIOR WALL STRUCTURES. *A,* Supine view double contrast radiograph shows a lesser curvature ulcer *(arrow).* The surrounding folds are not well seen.

B, In a slight RPO projection the ulcer crater is filled with barium, and the surrounding mucosal folds are seen much more clearly.

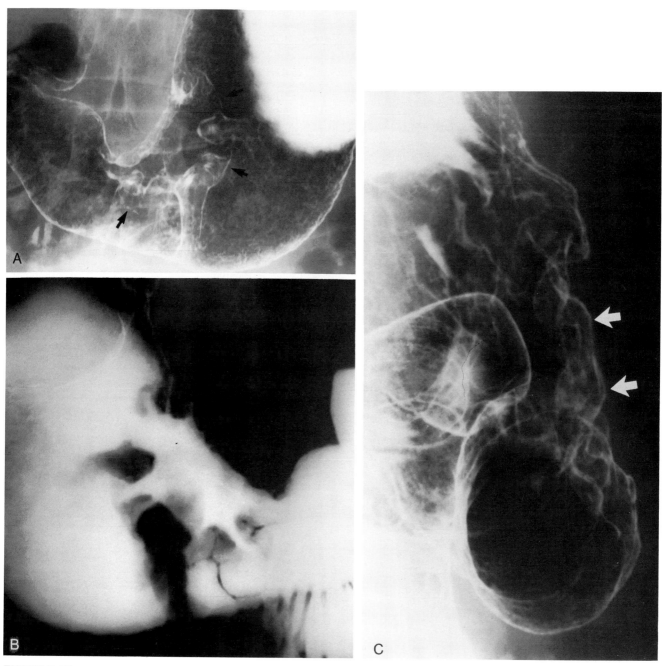

FIGURE 2–52

ANALYSIS OF A COMPLEX CASE. *A,* The supine film shows the edge of a lesion etched in white *(arrows).* There are also radiating folds etched in white. The tips of the folds are clubbed and stalactites are hanging down from the folds. This film suggests that there is an anterior wall lesion associated with ulceration and clubbing of the radiating folds.

B, The prone film confirms the presence of a large ulcer with a rim of tumor tissue. The radiating folds are now seen as filling defects.

C, The left lateral film confirms the presence of a large mass on the anterior wall with a large central ulcer *(arrows).* These findings were due to an excavated adenocarcinoma of the anterior wall of the stomach.

REFERENCES

1. James, W. B.: Double contrast radiology in the gastrointestinal tract. Clin. Gastroenterol. 7:397, 1978.
2. Ichikawa, H.: What is double contrast radiography? *In* Shirakabe, H. (ed.): Double Contrast Studies of the Stomach. Stuttgart, Georg Thieme Verlag, 1972, pp 4–6.
3. Gohel, V. K., Kressel, H. Y., and Laufer, I.: Double contrast artifacts. Gastrointest. Radiol. 3:139, 1978.
4. Skucas, J.: Gastrointestinal agents. *In* Skucas, J. (ed.): Radiographic Contrast Agents, ed. 2. Rockville, MD, Aspen Publishers, 1989, pp. 10–82.
5. Rubesin, S. E., and Herlinger, H.: The effect of barium suspension viscosity on the delineation of areae gastricae. AJR 146:35, 1986.
6. Mackintosh, C. E., and Kreel, L.: Anatomy and radiology of the areae gastricae. Gut 18:855, 1977.
7. Matsuura, K., Nakata, H., Takeda, N., et al.: Innominate lines of the colon. Radiology 123:581, 1977.
8. Laufer, I.: A simple method for routine double contrast study of the upper gastrointestinal tract. Radiology 117:513, 1975.
9. Miller, R. E., Chernish, S. M., Skukas, J., et al.: Hypotonic roentgenography with glucagon. AJR 121:264, 1974.
10. Meeroff, J. C., Jorgens, J., and Isenberg, J. I.: The effect of glucagon on barium enema examination. Radiology 115:5, 1975.
11. Gelfand, D. W., Sowers, J. C., DePonte, K. A., et al.: Anaphylactic and allergic reactions during double-contrast studies: Is glucagon or barium suspension the allergen? AJR 144:405, 1985.
12. Feczko, P. J., Simms, S. M., Lorio, J., and Halpert, R.: Gastroduodenal response to low-dose glucagon. AJR 140:935, 1983.
13. Hogan, W. J., Dodds, W. J., Hoke, S. E., et al.: The effect of glucagon on esophageal motor function. Gastroenterology 69:160, 1975.
14. Laufer, I., Mullens, J. E., and Hamilton, J.: The diagnostic accuracy of barium studies of the stomach and duodenum—correlation with endoscopy. Radiology 115:569, 1975.
15. Laufer, I., Mullens, J. E., and Hamilton, J.: Correlation of endoscopy and double contrast radiography in the early stages of ulcerative and granulomatous colitis. Radiology 118:1, 1976.
16. Op den Orth, J. O., and Ploem, S.: The stalactite phenomenon in double contrast studies of the stomach. Radiology 117:523, 1975.
17. Aronchick, J., Laufer, I., and Glick, S.: Barium stalactites: Observations on their nature and significance. Radiology 149:588, 1983.
18. Youker, J. E., and Welin, S.: Differentiation of true polypoid tumors of the colon from extraneous material: A new roentgen sign. Radiology 84:610, 1965.
19. Tobin, K. D., and Young, J. W. R.: The bowler hat: a valid sign of colonic polyps? Gastrointest. Radiol. 12:250, 1987.
20. Miller, W. T., Jr., Levine, M. S., Rubesin, S. E., and Laufer, I.: Bowler-hat sign: A simple principle for differentiating polyps from diverticula. Radiology 173:615, 1989.
21. Ament, A. E., and Alfidi, R. J.: Sessile polyps: Analysis of radiographic projections with the aid of a double-contrast phantom. AJR 139:111, 1982.
22. Kikuchi, Y., Levine, M. S., Laufer, I., et al: Value of flow technique for double-contrast examination of the stomach. AJR 147:1183, 1986.
23. Battle, W. M., Laufer, I., Moldofsky, P. J., et al.: Anomalous liver lobulation as a cause of perigastric masses. Am. J. Dig. Dis. 24:65, 1979.
24. Laufer, I., Hamilton, J., and Mullens, J. E.: Demonstration of superficial gastric erosions by double contrast radiography. Gastroenterology 68:387, 1975.
25. Cho, S. R., Henry, D. A., Shaw, C. I., et al.: Vanishing intraluminal diverticulum of the esophagus. Gastrointest. Radiol. 7:315, 1982.
26. Laufer, I.: Air contrast studies of the colon in inflammatory bowel disease. CRC Crit. Rev. Diagn. Imaging 9:421, 1977.

UPPER GASTROINTESTINAL TRACT: TECHNICAL ASPECTS

Marc S. Levine, M.D.
Igor Laufer, M.D.

3

BASIC REQUIREMENTS

The routine double contrast upper gastrointestinal examination should be performed as a biphasic study with double contrast and single contrast views of the esophagus, stomach, and duodenum to optimize the diagnostic yield of the procedure. In the double contrast portion of the study, a series of maneuvers is required to achieve adequate gaseous distention while a thin layer of high-density barium is spread on the mucosa. The effects of gravity are utilized to manipulate the barium pool so that each portion of the upper gastrointestinal tract is visualized en face and in profile. The double contrast study is facilitated by the routine use of hypotonic agents. The examination is then completed by obtaining prone and/or upright single contrast views of the esophagus, stomach, and duodenum with low-density barium and varying degrees of compression.

It should be emphasized that double contrast views permit a more detailed assessment of the appearance of the mucosa en face than conventional single contrast techniques. The basic elements of the double contrast examination are (1) gaseous distention, (2) mucosal coating, (3) hypotonia, (4) attention to technical details, and (5) a routine set of maneuvers for performing the study. These are discussed separately in the sections below.

Gaseous Distention

Gaseous distention is required to efface normal folds so that the overlying mucosa can be adequately visualized. If distention is inadequate, prominent folds may obscure small lesions, and barium trapped between folds may simulate ulcers. At the same time, overdistention may impair mucosal coating or obliterate abnormal folds, such as those radiating toward an ulcer or ulcer scar. Similarly, varices may be effaced or even obliterated by overdistention. Thus, it is critical to obtain the proper degree of gaseous distention (i.e., just enough to efface normal folds without interfering with mucosal coating).

A variety of methods can be used to introduce gas into the stomach and duodenum. The ideal method for distending these structures is nasogastric intubation. However, intubation techniques would meet with considerable patient resistance if applied on a routine basis. Instead, the simplest method for introducing gas is to have the patient swallow effervescent granules, powder, or tablets that rapidly release 300 to 400 ml of carbon dioxide on contact with fluid in the stomach.[1-3] Unfortunately, bubble formation may occur as an undesirable artifact as gas is liberated in the esophagus or stomach. Because of this problem, most effervescent agents contain simethicone, an an-

tifoaming agent that disperses bubbles.[3] We prefer to chase the granules with 10 ml of water before giving barium. This appears to promote more rapid release of carbon dioxide without trapping bubbles in the barium.[4]

While the stomach and duodenum are readily distended by effervescent agents, the patient must gulp the high-density barium suspension as quickly as possible to achieve adequate gaseous distention of the esophagus. With rapid swallowing, the peristaltic sequence is interrupted, and the esophagus becomes hypotonic. As the patient gulps the high-density barium, swallowed air also distends the esophagus, contributing further to the double contrast effect. Nevertheless, some elderly or debilitated patients may be able to take only small sips of barium, so that adequate distention of the esophagus cannot always be achieved.

Mucosal Coating

Adequate mucosal coating is obtained by washing a high-density barium suspension over the mucosa. The quality of mucosal coating depends on a variety of factors, including the properties of the barium suspension, the volume of barium and gas, the frequency of washing, and the amount of fluid or secretions in the stomach. In general, a larger volume of barium results in better mucosal coating. If there is too much barium, however, only a small portion of the mucosa can be seen in double contrast. Optimal coating is achieved by turning the patient through 360 degrees to wash the barium suspension across all surfaces of the stomach. However, the quality of mucosal coating tends to deteriorate rapidly during the fluoroscopic examination, so that repeated turning of the patient is required to manipulate the barium pool and obtain a fresh coating before each exposure. In the absence of good mucosal coating, small or even large lesions may be missed. Uneven coating may also simulate lesions (see Chapter 2).

Because mucosal coating depends on the physical and chemical properties of the barium suspension, the choice of barium directly affects the quality of the double contrast examination.[4-7] In general, the best results are obtained with a high-density barium (250% w/v) of intermediate viscosity.[8] Adequate mucosal coating is usually present when a thin, uniform white line is observed along the contour of the stomach. The quality of coating can also be judged on the basis of whether or not an areae gastricae pattern is visible in the stomach. With standard barium suspensions, the areae gastricae can be detected in about 70% of patients.[9] However, visualization of these structures depends on many factors, including the amount and viscosity of mucus in the stomach, so that failure to demonstrate an areae gastricae pattern does not necessarily indicate that coating is inadequate.

Excess fluid or secretions in the stomach also impair mucosal coating. Patients with gastric outlet obstruction, gastroparesis, or hypersecretory states are more likely to have excess fluid. In such cases, the properties of the barium suspension become even more important, as some suspensions precipitate rapidly on contact with acid in the stomach and others are more resistant to acid.[6] When excessive fluid is present, the patient may be given additional high-density barium and rotated several times to wash the barium across the stomach and improve the coating. If adequate coating is still not achieved, the stomach can be filled with a low-density barium suspension for a conventional single contrast study, or the examination can be repeated at a later date after fluid is aspirated from the stomach with a nasogastric tube.

Hypotonia

A variety of hypotonic agents can be used to facilitate the double contrast examination. In the past, Pro-Banthine (propantheline bromide) was used to induce gastric hypotonia,[10] but because of its anticholinergic side effects, this drug has been largely supplanted by glucagon. A standard dose of 0.1 mg of glucagon administered intravenously produces adequate gastric hypotonia within 45 seconds of the injection in most patients.[11, 12] As a result, it is possible to obtain better double contrast views of the antrum and body of the stomach in a relaxed, hypotonic state. Glucagon also tends to contract the pylorus and delay gastric emptying, so that the stomach can be visualized in double contrast before it is obscured by overlapping loops of barium-filled duodenum or small bowel. Because glucagon delays filling of the duodenum, however, the examination may be prolonged in some patients.

Glucagon is an extremely safe drug that has virtually no side effects, except for the remote possibility of a hypersensitivity reaction.[11, 12] However, some patients may have nausea or vomiting if the drug is injected too rapidly.[13] There is also the occasional patient who has a vasovagal reaction to the sight of the needle. The only contraindications to the use of glucagon are pheochromocytoma, insulinoma, brittle, insulin-dependent diabetes, and a history of allergy to glucagon.

In the evaluation of known gastric lesions (e.g., healing of gastric ulcers), larger doses of glucagon (usually 1.0 mg) should be given intravenously to achieve greater levels of gastric hypotonia for a more detailed examination. In patients who have undergone partial gastrectomy, a large dose of intravenous

glucagon should also be given to prevent rapid spillage of barium through the gastroenterostomy into the proximal small bowel (see Chapter 9). To obtain a more detailed examination of the duodenum, 0.5 to 1.0 mg of glucagon should be given intravenously only after barium has entered the duodenum. This "tubeless" hypotonic duodenogram is a valuable technique for evaluating known or suspected lesions in or around the duodenum (see Chapter 10).

Although glucagon is a useful hypotonic agent for the stomach and duodenum, it has no effect on esophageal peristalsis and does not produce better double contrast views of the esophagus. However, it has been shown that glucagon relaxes the lower esophageal sphincter[14] and therefore increases the frequency of spontaneous gastroesophageal reflux.[15] Alternatively, Pro-Banthine may be given intravenously in doses of 20 to 30 mg to paralyze the esophagus. This drug is particularly helpful for visualizing esophageal varices.[16] However, as indicated earlier, Pro-Banthine is rarely used because of its many side effects.

Buscopan (hyoscine N-butyl bromide) is another anticholinergic agent that is frequently used in double contrast examinations.[2] This drug produces effective but transient hypotonia of the esophagus, stomach, and duodenum. It has the additional advantage of relaxing the pylorus, so that excellent double contrast views of the duodenum can be obtained. Buscopan appears to be free of the major side effects of Pro-Banthine, although blurred vision is still a common complaint. It should also be recognized that Buscopan markedly prolongs small bowel transit time, so that a small bowel study becomes impractical in these patients. Buscopan is a popular hypotonic agent in Europe but is not available in the United States.

Attention to Technical Details

Meticulous attention to technical details is required to achieve consistently high-quality double contrast studies.[4] The preparation of the barium is critical. The suspension is prepared by adding a precise amount of water (usually 65 to 70 ml) measured in a syringe or graduated cylinder to a cup of powdered, high-density barium.[9] This results in a 250% w/v barium suspension that is ideal for double contrast studies of the upper gastrointestinal tract. Most high-density barium settles quickly from the suspension, so that the cup of barium must be vigorously stirred or shaken immediately before starting the examination. We prefer to expose our spot films at about 110 kVp, although lower kVp can be used with the rare earth intensifying screens. The density settings on the phototimer should generally be lower than those used on conventional barium studies to avoid washing out the surface detail of the mucosa.

Maneuvers

A standard set of maneuvers is required to achieve adequate mucosal coating of all surfaces of the esophagus, stomach, and duodenum and to produce unobscured double contrast views of each area.[17] The examination must be performed quickly, since overlapping loops of barium-filled small bowel may impair visualization of the stomach and duodenum. The major purpose of fluoroscopy is to determine the volume of barium and gas, to assess mucosal coating, and to insure accurate positioning and timing of spot films. Because careful fluoroscopic positioning of the patient is required, the routine double contrast study consists only of fluoroscopic spot films. In general, overhead radiographs have not been found to contribute additional information to the study.[18] However, we do obtain overhead films when a surgical lesion is encountered or when a large extrinsic mass is seen displacing the esophagus, stomach, or duodenum.

Flow technique refers to the fluoroscopic observation of the flow of barium across the dependent wall of the stomach in order to provide a barium pool of varying thickness.[19] By turning the patient one way or the other, barium can be made to flow "uphill" from the antrum into the fundus or "downhill" from the fundus into the antrum. It is an ideal technique for detecting relatively subtle lesions in the stomach as barium flows around small protrusions or fills small ulcers on the dependent surface (see Chapter 7).[19]

Although it is important to develop a standard routine for performing the fluoroscopic examination, additional maneuvers or spot films may be required if an abnormality is suspected at fluoroscopy. When the double contrast portion of the study has been completed, prone or upright compression views of the esophagus, stomach, and duodenum should be obtained with a low-density barium suspension to supplement the double contrast examination. These views are particularly important for showing small polypoid lesions or ulcers on the anterior wall of the stomach and duodenum (see Chapters 7, 8, and 10).

THE ROUTINE EXAMINATION

Our routine procedure for examining the upper gastrointestinal tract is described in the following section. Of course, this routine can be altered as dictated by the indications for the examination or by findings during the examination.

Patient Preparation

Retained fluid in the stomach may significantly interfere with the quality of mucosal coating. Patients are therefore instructed to fast overnight before undergoing the examination in order to minimize the amount of fluid or secretions in the stomach. They should also be discouraged from smoking on the day of the examination, because cigarette smoke increases gastric secretions and therefore compromises mucosal coating in the stomach and duodenum.[20, 21] Finally, antacids or other medications that coat the mucosal surface of the stomach should not be taken until the examination has been completed. For obvious reasons, insulin-dependent diabetics should have their study done early in the day and should not receive their insulin injections until they are free to eat after the examination.

Materials

1. Barium: E-Z-HD or HD 85 (E-Z-EM Co., Westbury, NY).
2. Effervescent agent: E-Z Gas or Baros (E-Z-EM Co.).
3. Glucagon: 0.1 mg of glucagon diluted to 0.25 cc with sterile water in a tuberculin syringe with a 25-gauge needle.

Procedure

Our routine technique is designed to evaluate the upper gastrointestinal tract with the greatest economy in patient movement and film utilization while still obtaining a thorough examination.[17] It is important to be aware that each spot film is taken after patient turning has provided a fresh coating of barium on the mucosal surface being studied.

1. A standard dose of 0.1 mg of glucagon is given intravenously.
2. The patient swallows one packet of effervescent granules or "fizzies" followed by 10 ml of water. The patient is instructed to swallow repeatedly in order to avoid belching.
3. The patient rapidly gulps a cup of high-density barium (120 ml) as one 3-on-1 or two 2-on-1 left posterior oblique (LPO) spot films are obtained in rapid sequence to visualize the entire esophagus (Fig. 3–1A). (All radiographic projections are indicated with respect to the tabletop.)
4. The table is brought to the horizontal position with the patient's back to the tabletop.
5. The patient is turned to the right through a 360-degree circle back to the supine position. If mucosal coating is adequate, a frontal spot film of the

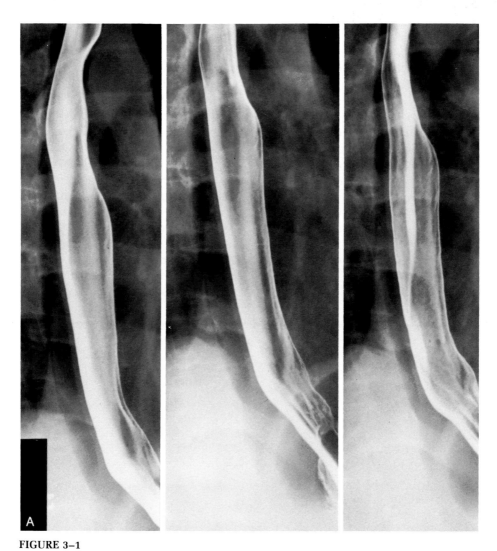

FIGURE 3–1

ROUTINE SERIES OF FILMS FOR DOUBLE CONTRAST UPPER GASTROINTESTINAL EXAMINATION. A, Three-on-one upright LPO views of esophagus. (From Levine, M.S.: Radiology of the Esophagus. Philadelphia, W.B. Saunders, 1989, p. 5, with permission.)

Illustration continued on following page

stomach is obtained for a double contrast view of the antrum and body (Fig. 3–1B), since barium pools in the fundus in the supine position.

6. The patient is turned through another 360-degree rotation, and a spot film of the antrum and body of the stomach is obtained in the LPO projection (Fig. 3–1C).

7. The patient is turned to the right lateral position for a double contrast view of the gastric cardia and fundus (Fig. 3–1D). This view also permits visualization of the retrogastric area.

8. "Uphill" flow technique is performed by turning the patient onto the back and then slowly to the LPO position. Four-on-one spot films are deliberately taken while the posterior wall of the body and antrum are covered by a thin layer of barium (Fig. 3–1E). Downhill flow technique is performed by slowly turning the patient to the right posterior oblique (RPO) position and obtaining 4-on-1 spot films of the high lesser curvature and gastric cardia in a steep RPO and right lateral position.

9. With the table semi-upright, the patient is turned to the RPO position for a double contrast view of the upper body and lesser curvature of the stomach (Fig. 3–1F). The gastric cardia can also be studied in more detail in this position.

10. By this time, barium usually has emptied into the duodenum. With the table semi-upright or horizontal, the patient is turned to the LPO position for 4-on-1 or 2-on-1 spot films of the duodenal bulb and descending duodenum in double contrast (Fig. 3–1G).

11. The table is lowered to the horizontal position, and the patient drinks a low-density barium suspension in the prone right anterior oblique (RAO) position. The patient is initially instructed to take single swallows of barium, so that esophageal peristalsis can be evaluated. A single 3-on-1 or two 2-on-1 spot films of the esophagus are then obtained during continuous drinking to permit optimal distention of the distal esophagus and gastroesophageal junction (Fig. 3–1H).

12. With the patient in the prone or prone RAO position, 4-on-1 spot films of the gastric antrum and body and duodenal bulb are obtained with varying degrees of compression using an inflatable balloon or other prone compression device positioned beneath the patient's abdomen (Fig. 3–1I).

13. The patient is turned to the left side and then onto the back, so that barium pools in the gastric fundus. The gastroesophageal junction is then monitored fluoroscopically as the patient is turned slowly to the right to elicit spontaneous gastroesophageal reflux. A straight-leg-raising maneuver or Valsalva maneuver can also be performed to provoke reflux.

14. The table is fully elevated with the patient in

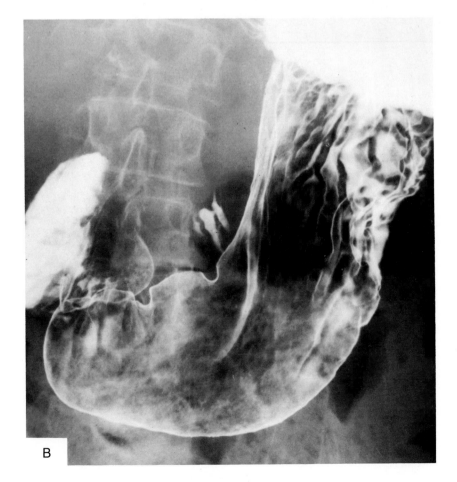

FIGURE 3–1 Continued

B, Supine view of gastric antrum and body.

B

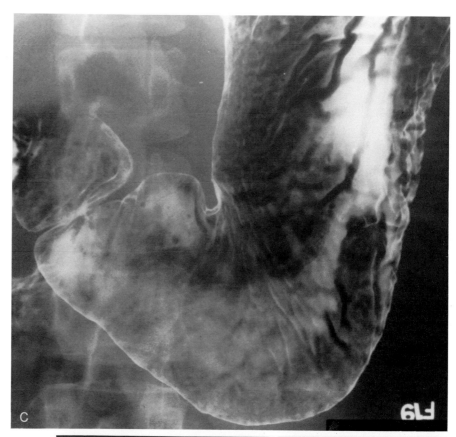

FIGURE 3–1 *Continued*

C, LPO view of gastric antrum and body.

D, Right lateral view of gastric cardia and fundus.

Illustration continued on following page

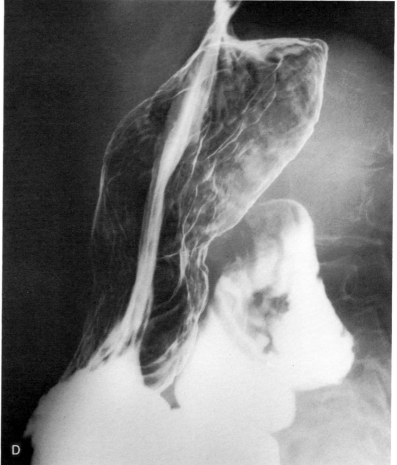

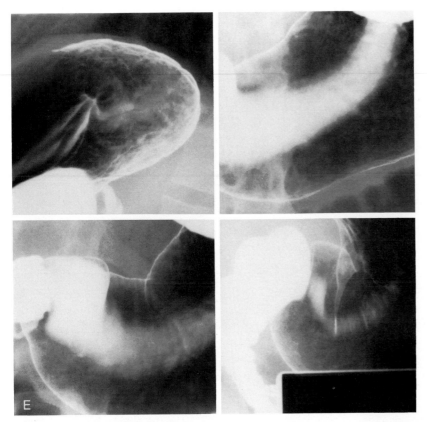

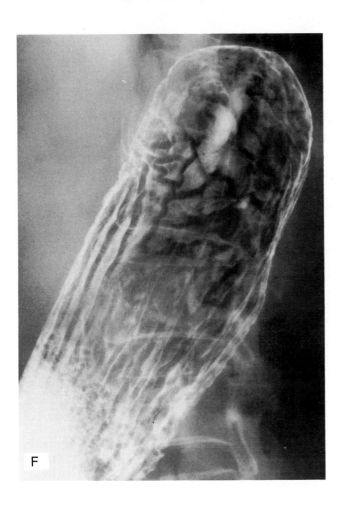

FIGURE 3–1 *Continued*

E, Flow technique with 4-on-1 spot films showing thin barium pool on posterior wall of stomach.

F, Semi-upright RPO view of high lesser curvature, upper body, and fundus.

G, LPO view of duodenum.

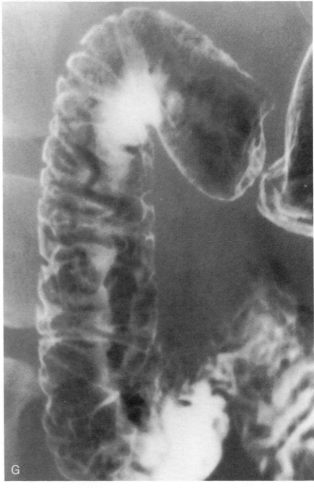

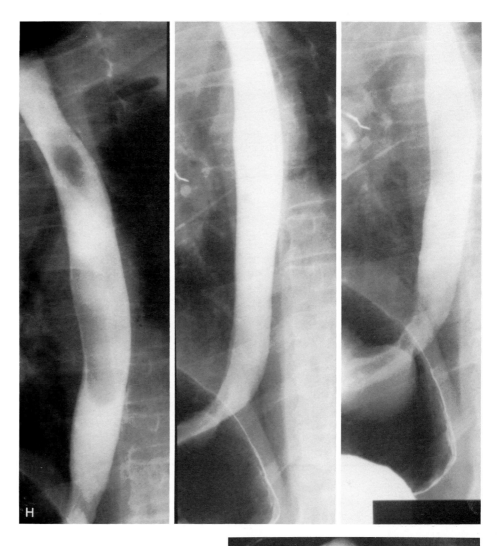

FIGURE 3–1 *Continued*

H, Three-on-one prone RAO views of barium-filled esophagus.

I, Prone RAO view of barium-filled duodenum.

Illustration continued on following page

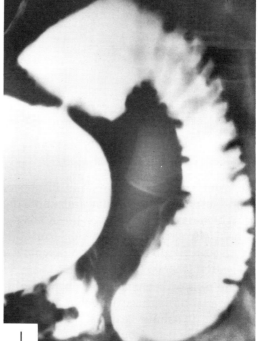

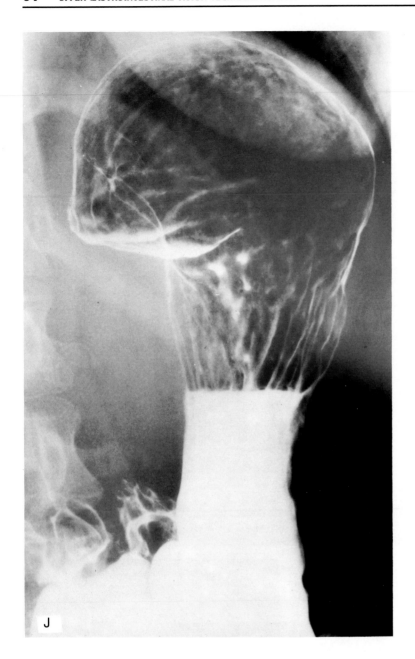

FIGURE 3–1 *Continued*

J, Upright, slightly LPO view of gastric fundus. (From Laufer, I.: A simple method for routine double contrast study of the upper gastrointestinal tract. Radiology 117:513, 1975, with permission.)

the right lateral position. This maneuver tends to keep barium in the antrum and duodenum, so that upright 4-on-1 spot films of these areas can be obtained with graded compression. An upright film of the gastric fundus can also be obtained in the LPO projection (Fig. 3–1*J*).

The filming sequence and purpose of each radiograph are summarized in Table 3–1. With some experience, it should be possible to complete the examination in 3 to 4 minutes of fluoroscopy time and about 10 minutes of room time. When a lesion is suspected at fluoroscopy, the barium study should be tailored to demonstrate the lesion en face and in profile with both single and double contrast techniques. Ultimately, each radiologist should develop a set routine for performing the examination. Although individual maneuvers or filming sequences may vary, the end result should be a thorough and efficient evaluation of all surfaces of the upper gastrointestinal tract.

TABLE 3–1. Summary of Filming Sequence for Biphasic Examination of Upper Gastrointestinal Tract		
View	**No. of Films**	**Purpose**
Upright LPO	1 (3-on-1)	Double contrast, esophagus
Supine	1	Double contrast, antrum and body
LPO	1	Double contrast, antrum and body
Right lateral	1	Double contrast, cardia and fundus; retrogastric area
Flow technique	1 (4-on-1)	Posterior wall of antrum and body
Semi-upright RPO	1	Double contrast, upper body, fundus, and cardia
Semi-upright or recumbent LPO	1 (4-on-1)	Double contrast, duodenum
Prone RAO	1 (3-on-1)	Single contrast, esophagus and gastroesophageal junction
Prone compression	1 (4-on-1)	Single contrast, stomach and duodenum
Upright compression	1 (4-on-1)	Single contrast, stomach and duodenum
Upright LPO	1	Double contrast, fundus

LPO, Left posterior oblique; RPO, right posterior oblique; RAO, right anterior oblique.

Variations

If the initial 360-degree rotation of the patient fails to produce adequate mucosal coating in the stomach, the patient may be rotated one or more additional turns before obtaining a film. Although some barium may spill into the duodenum during this maneuver, 360-degree rotation of the patient permits optimal coating of all mucosal surfaces of the stomach by high-density barium. If the patient cannot be rotated 360 degrees because of age, debilitation, or other reasons, a gentle rocking maneuver can be performed to achieve adequate mucosal coating in most cases.

Many lesions on the anterior wall of the stomach can be shown by the combination of supine double contrast and prone compression radiographs. Although routine double contrast views of the anterior wall do not appear to be warranted, a more detailed double contrast study of the anterior wall may be performed on patients who have equivocal findings on the initial examination or a high index of suspicion of a gastric lesion.[22] These views are obtained by placing the patient in the prone position, so that barium pools on the anterior wall of the stomach, outlining the rugal folds (Fig. 3–2A). The table is then tilted head down while the patient is turned to the prone left anterior oblique (LAO) position, allowing barium to drain into the fundus. This maneuver

FIGURE 3–2

DOUBLE CONTRAST EXAMINATION OF THE ANTERIOR WALL. *A,* Prone view shows barium outlining rugal folds on anterior gastric wall.

Illustration continued on following page

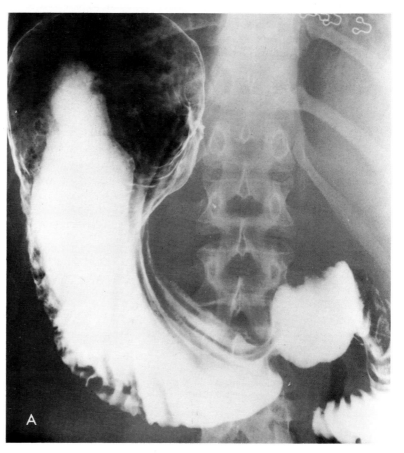

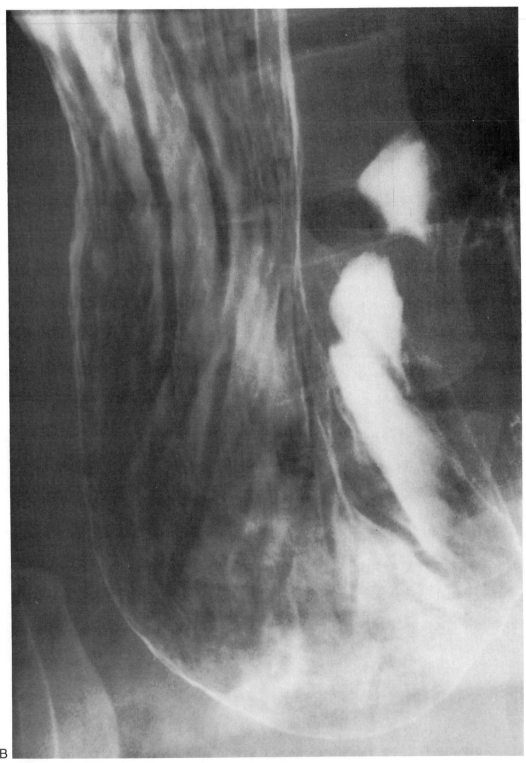

B

FIGURE 3–2 *Continued*

B, Double contrast view of anterior wall of antrum and body in prone LAO projection with table tilted 20 to 30 degrees head down.

leaves only a thin residual layer of high-density barium on the anterior wall of the antrum and body, so that excellent double contrast views of this region can be obtained (Fig. 3–2B). The head of the table is then elevated for double contrast views of the anterior wall of the upper body and fundus (Fig. 3–2C). A profile view of the anterior wall can also be obtained by turning the patient to the left lateral position (Fig. 3–2D). This particular view often permits visualization of the duodenum through the gas-filled stomach. Finally, the anterior wall may be demonstrated by a supine cross-table horizontal beam view of the stomach.

Anterior wall views of the duodenum may also be helpful in some patients. Starting in the LPO position for double contrast views of the duodenum, the patient is turned to the left side and then to the prone position. This causes barium to coat the anterior wall of the duodenum while gas is trapped in the descending duodenum. An inflatable balloon or pad may be used to displace the barium-filled antrum if it overlaps the duodenum. This maneuver permits recognition of the minor duodenal papilla (an anterior wall structure) as well as anterior wall lesions that may not be demonstrated on the routine study.

Additional variations in technique are described elsewhere for the evaluation of the postoperative stomach[23, 24] (see Chapter 9).

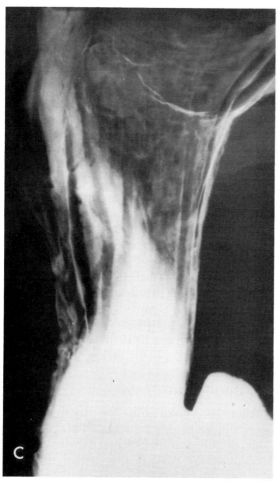

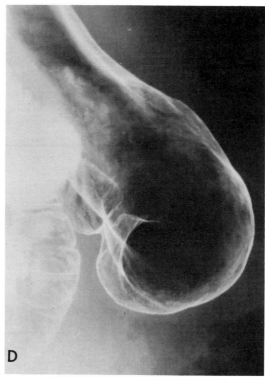

FIGURE 3–2 *Continued*

C, Double contrast view of anterior wall of upper body with head of table elevated.

D, Profile view of anterior wall of antrum in left lateral projection.

PROBLEMS AND PITFALLS

Esophagus

Technical factors related to the amount of barium and gas in the esophagus may greatly affect the quality of the double contrast study. Because double contrast radiographs of the esophagus are obtained with the patient in an upright position, pooling of barium in the distal esophagus may obscure mucosal detail. As barium enters the stomach, a residual layer of high-density barium in the esophagus may also obscure the mucosa. When this "flow artifact" is observed at fluoroscopy, additional views obtained moments later should better delineate mucosal lesions as the layer of residual high-density barium on the mucosa thins out[25] (see Fig. 5–16). At the same time, esophageal peristalsis causes the esophagus to collapse almost immediately after passage of the barium bolus into the stomach. The fluoroscopist therefore must time the exposures to capture the esophagus during the relatively brief period of optimal distention and coating. With some experience, it is possible to obtain satisfactory double contrast views of the esophagus in 75% to 85% of patients.[26, 27]

When esophageal disease is believed to be present, the cup of high-density barium may be split into two portions for a more detailed double contrast study. By having the patient drink half of the barium in the typical LPO projection and half in the RPO projection, protruded or depressed lesions in the esophagus may be evaluated both en face and in profile. Alternatively, a tube esophagram may be performed when the routine double contrast study is inconclusive[28] (see Chapter 5).

Whereas mucosal disease is best evaluated with double contrast technique, abnormalities of the longitudinal folds are better seen on mucosal relief views of the collapsed or partially collapsed esophagus. Esophageal varices may be effaced or even obliterated by esophageal distention, so that mucosal relief views are particularly important when varices are suspected.[29] Various types of esophagitis may also be recognized by the presence of thickened, irregular longitudinal folds in the collapsed esophagus.

When a ring or stricture is suspected in the distal esophagus, particular emphasis should be placed on prone single contrast views of the esophagus during continuous drinking of a low-density barium suspension to produce better distention of the distal esophagus and gastroesophageal junction. Schatzki rings or peptic strictures that are not visible on double contrast radiographs may be detected when the esophagus is optimally distended by this technique[30, 31] (Fig. 3–3).

Stomach

The proper volume of barium and gas are required for optimal double contrast views of the stomach. Although a single 120-ml cup of high-density barium is usually adequate for this purpose, barium occasionally may empty rapidly from the stomach despite intravenous administration of glucagon. In such cases, additional barium may be given to the patient in a recumbent LPO position to obtain better mucosal coating. Similarly, if the patient belches during the examination, an additional half packet of effervescent agent may be required to produce adequate gaseous distention. Conversely, the patient may be asked to belch if the stomach is overdistended with gas, since overdistention may efface abnormal folds associated with ulcers or ulcer scars.

In patients who are relatively unresponsive to glucagon, rapid emptying of barium into the duodenum may cause portions of the stomach to be obscured by overlapping loops of barium-filled duodenum or small bowel. This overlap may particularly impair visualization of the distal antrum. If it is a frequent problem, the first part of the double contrast study may be modified so that the table is returned to the horizontal position with the patient facing the table immediately after swallowing the high-density barium suspension. The patient then may be turned from the prone position onto the left side and back to obtain unobscured double contrast views of the distal antrum before barium spills into the duodenum. The usual routine then may be followed for the rest of the examination.

In patients who are unusually sensitive to glucagon, gastric hypotonia may significantly delay spillage of barium into the duodenum, prolonging the examination. When this problem is encountered, the patient may be asked to wait outside the examining room for 10 or 15 minutes until the glucagon effect has subsided. Because another study can be performed while the patient is waiting, the fluoroscopy schedule need not be delayed by a glucagon-sensitive person.

Duodenum

After the duodenum has filled with high-density barium, adequate double contrast views of the duodenal bulb and descending duodenum usually can be obtained by placing the patient in a recumbent or semi-upright LPO position to distend the bulb with gas. If, however, the bulb is inadequately distended with gas or obscured by barium, the table may be elevated further (even to a fully upright position). This maneuver causes barium to pool in the antrum or descending duodenum and air to rise into the duodenal bulb, which tends to assume a vertical

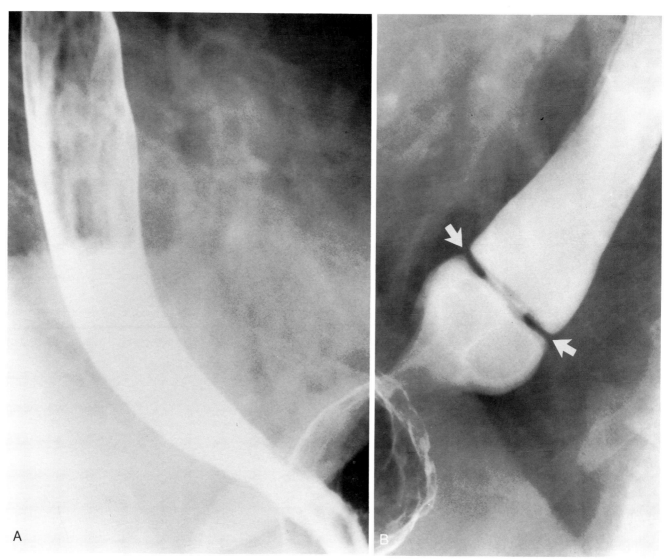

FIGURE 3–3

IMPORTANCE OF PRONE SINGLE CONTRAST VIEWS FOR DEMONSTRATING LOWER ESOPHAGEAL RINGS. *A,* Upright double contrast view of esophagus shows no evidence of lower esophageal ring. However, note pooling of barium in distal esophagus with suboptimal distention of this region.

B, Prone single contrast view from same examination shows hiatal hernia with unequivocal Schatzki ring *(arrows)* above hernia.

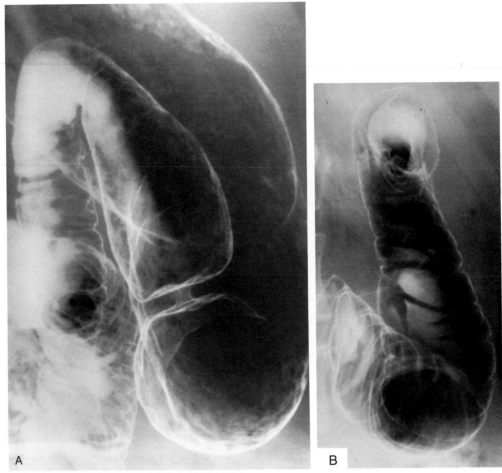

FIGURE 3–4

Double contrast views of duodenum in left lateral (A) and prone LAO (B) positions.

configuration, so that adequate double contrast views of the bulb can be obtained. If the duodenal bulb is located in a posterior position, the patient may also be turned to the left lateral or even the prone LAO position to achieve adequate gaseous distention of the bulb and descending duodenum (Fig. 3–4). If, despite these maneuvers, satisfactory double contrast views of the duodenum cannot be obtained, the fluoroscopist should proceed to the single contrast portion of the study rather than prolong the double contrast examination, because it usually is possible to obtain adequate prone or upright compression views of the duodenum. After these compression films have been taken, the table may be lowered with the patient in the LPO position. Gas is often seen to percolate from the antrum into the duodenum during this maneuver, providing a final opportunity for double contrast views of the bulb.

REFERENCES

1. Laufer, I.: A simple method for routine double contrast study of the upper gastrointestinal tract. Radiology 117:513, 1975.
2. Hunt, J.H., and Anderson, I.F.: Double contrast upper gastrointestinal studies. Clin. Radiol. 27:87, 1976.
3. Koehler, R.E., Weyman, P.J., Stanley, R.J., et al.: Evaluation of three effervescent agents for double-contrast upper gastrointestinal radiography. Gastrointest. Radiol. 6:111, 1981.
4. Miller, R.E.: Recipes for gastrointestinal examinations. AJR 137:1285, 1981.
5. Cumberland, D.C.: Optimum viscosity of barium suspension for use in the double contrast barium meal. Gastrointest. Radiol. 2:169, 1977.
6. Roberts, G.M., Roberts, E.E., Davies, R.L., et al.: Observations on the behaviour of barium sulfate suspensions in gastric secretion. Br. J. Radiol. 50:468, 1977.
7. Kormano, M., Makela, P., and Rossi, I.: Visualization of the areae gastricae in a double contrast examination—dependence on the contrast medium. Fortschr. Rontgenstr. 128:52, 1978.
8. Gelfand, D.W.: High density, low viscosity barium for fine mucosal detail on double-contrast upper gastrointestinal examinations. AJR 130:831, 1978.

9. Rubesin, S.E., and Herlinger, H.: The effect of barium suspension viscosity on the delineation of areae gastricae. AJR 146:35, 1986.
10. Merlo, R.B., Stone, M., Baugus, P., et al.: The use of Pro-Banthine to induce gastrointestinal hypotonia. Radiology 127:61, 1978.
11. Miller, R.E., Chernish, S.M., Greenman, G.F., et al.: Gastrointestinal response to minute doses of glucagon. Radiology 143:317, 1982.
12. Maglinte, D.D.T., Caudill, L.D., Krol, K.L., et al.: The minimum effective dose of glucagon in upper gastrointestinal radiography. Gastrointest. Radiol. 7:119, 1982.
13. Chernish, S.M., Maglinte, D.D.T.: Glucagon: Common untoward reactions—review and recommendations. Radiology 177:145, 1990.
14. Hogan, W.J., Dodds, W.J., Hoke, S.E., et al.: Effect of glucagon on esophageal motor function. Gastroenterology 69:160, 1975.
15. Haggar, A.M., Feczko, P.J., Halpert, R.D., et al.: Spontaneous gastroesophageal reflux during double-contrast upper gastrointestinal radiography with glucagon. Gastrointest. Radiol. 7:319, 1982.
16. Dalinka, M.K., Smith, E.H., Wolfe, R.D., et al.: Pharmacologically enhanced visualization of esophageal varices by Pro-Banthine. Radiology 102:281, 1972.
17. Levine, M.S., Rubesin, S.E., Herlinger, H., et al.: Double-contrast upper gastrointestinal examination: Technique and interpretation. Radiology 168:593, 1988.
18. Bova, J.G., Friedman, A.C., Hudson, T., et al.: Radiographs obtained during upper gastrointestinal fluoroscopy: Adequacy and comparison to postfluoroscopy images. Radiology 147:875, 1983.
19. Kikuchi, Y., Levine, M.S., Laufer, I., et al.: Value of flow technique for double-contrast examination of the stomach. AJR 147:1183, 1986.
20. Thoeni, R.F., and Goldberg, H.I.: The influence of smoking on coating of the gastric mucosa during double contrast examination of the stomach (abstract). Invest. Radiol. 15:388, 1980.
21. Rose, C., Somers, S., Mather, D.G., et al.: Cigarette smoking and duodenal coating with barium. J. Can. Assoc. Radiol. 33:77, 1982.
22. Goldsmith, M.R., Paul, R.E., Poplack, W.E., et al.: Evaluation of routine double-contrast views of the anterior wall of the stomach. AJR 126:1159, 1976.
23. Gold, R.P., and Seaman, W.B.: The primary double-contrast examination of the postoperative stomach. Radiology 124:297, 1977.
24. Gohel, V.K., and Laufer, I.: Double-contrast examination of the postoperative stomach. Radiology 129:601, 1978.
25. Maglinte, D.D.T., Lappas, J.C., Chernish, S.M., et al.: Flow artifacts in double-contrast esophagography. Radiology 157:535, 1985.
26. Balfe, D.M., Koehler, R.E., Weyman, P.J., et al.: Routine air-contrast esophagography during upper gastrointestinal examinations. Radiology 139:739, 1981.
27. Maglinte, D.D.T., Schultheis, T.E., Krol, K.L., et al.: Survey of the esophagus during the upper gastrointestinal examination in 500 patients. Radiology 147:65, 1983.
28. Levine, M.S., Kressel, H.Y., Laufer, I., et al.: The tube esophagram: A technique for obtaining a detailed double-contrast examination of the esophagus. AJR 142:293, 1984.
29. Nelson, S.W.: The roentgenologic diagnosis of esophageal varices. AJR 77:599, 1957.
30. Chen, Y.M., Ott, D.J., Gelfand, D.W., et al.: Multiphasic examination of the esophagogastric region for strictures, rings, and hiatal hernia: Evaluation of the individual techniques. Gastrointest. Radiol. 10:311, 1985.
31. Ott, D.J., Chen, Y.M., Wu, W.C., et al.: Radiographic and endoscopic sensitivity in detecting lower esophageal mucosal ring. AJR 147:261, 1986.

PHARYNX

4

Stephen E. Rubesin, M.D.

INTRODUCTION

The pharynx serves as the gateway to the gastrointestinal tract and as the crossroads of speech, respiration, and swallowing. During swallowing, the pharynx channels the bolus to enter the gastrointestinal tract and not the airway. During respiration, the pharynx actively maintains an open passage from the nasopharynx to the laryngeal aditus. During speech, the pharynx acts as a resonator, changing size and shape to alter sounds. The pharynx also participates in other activities, such as yawning, gagging, choking, and vomiting.

Pharyngeal disorders are common. Aspiration pneumonia, often due to pharyngeal dysmotility, is a frequent cause of increased morbidity and mortality. Approximately 8000 to 10,000 people die of choking yearly,[1] and 4% of malignant neoplasms in men are head and neck tumors.[1]

This chapter serves as an introduction to the complicated world of the pharynx. Because this textbook focuses on double contrast radiology, this chapter emphasizes the normal double contrast anatomy and the structural abnormalities of the pharynx. However, the radiologist should remember that most disorders of the pharynx are motility disorders. While double contrast studies can demonstrate structural correlates of functional disorders, high-resolution videofluoroscopy or cineradiography must be performed to evaluate pharyngeal function.

NORMAL APPEARANCES

A detailed knowledge of the complex anatomy of the pharynx is necessary for interpretation of the double contrast pharyngogram.[2–5] The major landmarks that can be identified radiographically include the soft

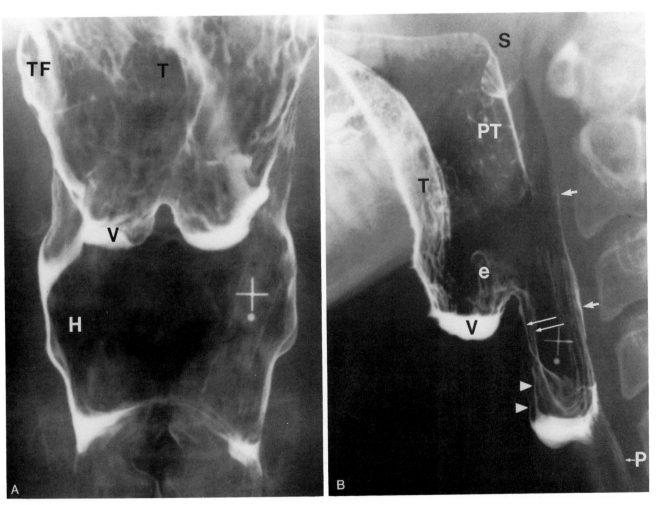

FIGURE 4–1

NORMAL PHARYNX. The frontal (A) and lateral (B) views of the pharynx are shown. On the frontal view, the contours of the tonsillar fossa (TF), valleculae (V), and hypopharynx (H) are demonstrated. The en face view of the surface of the base of the tongue (T) is seen. On the lateral view, the soft palate (S), palatine tonsil (PT), base of the tongue (T), valleculae (V), epiglottic tip (e), aryepiglottic folds (*long arrows*), and posterior pharyngeal wall (*short arrows*) are well imaged. The anterior walls of the piriform sinus are identified (*arrowheads*). The pharyngoesophageal segment (P) is collapsed. (Reprinted with permission from Rubesin, S.E., and Glick, S.N.: The tailored double-contrast pharyngogram. Crit. Rev. Diagn. Imaging 28:133, 1988. Copyright CRC Press, Inc., Boca Raton, FL.)

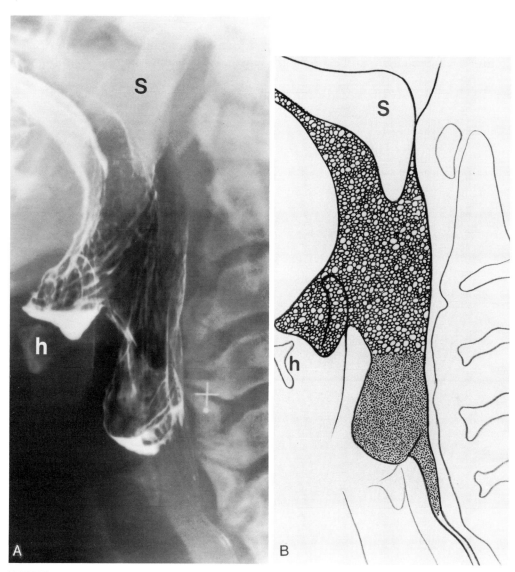

FIGURE 4–2

DIVISIONS OF THE PHARYNX. *A* and *B,* The pharynx is arbitrarily divided into three parts: the nasopharynx, the oropharynx *(bubble pattern),* and the hypopharynx *(granular pattern).* The division between the nasopharynx and the oropharynx is the soft palate (S); the division between the oropharynx and the hypopharynx is either the level of the hyoid bone (h) or the pharyngoepiglottic fold. (From Rubesin, S.E., et al.: Lines of the pharynx. Radiographics 7:217, 1987, with permission.)

palate, the base of the tongue, the valleculae, the epiglottis, and the piriform sinuses (Fig. 4–1).

The pharynx is arbitrarily divided into three parts: the nasopharynx, the oropharynx, and the hypopharynx (Fig. 4–2). The nasopharynx is purely a respiratory tract structure and is excluded from the digestive

tract by the soft palate. The oropharynx relates to the oral cavity and base of the tongue and extends from the soft palate to its arbitrary division from the hypopharynx at the level of the hyoid bone. Some anatomists regard the oropharynx as being divided from the hypopharynx by the pharyngoepiglottic fold

(Fig. 4–3), a mucosal fold overlying the stylopharyngeus.[2] The hypopharynx extends from the level of the hyoid bone to the lower portion of the cricopharyngeus at the inferior margin of the cricoid cartilage. These divisions are arbitrary because the soft palate and hyoid bone change position with phonation, swallowing, and respiration.

The pharynx is primarily a skeletal muscular tube extending 12 to 14 cm from the skull base to the lower border of the cricoid cartilage. The pharynx is confined posteriorly by the cervical spine and laterally by the muscles of the neck. The shape of the pharynx is determined by underlying musculature, impinging cartilages, the supporting skeleton, and the hyoid sling—the suspensory apparatus of the pharynx. The pharyngeal portion of the digestive tract (oropharynx and hypopharynx) has four openings: superiorly, the velopharyngeal portal between the

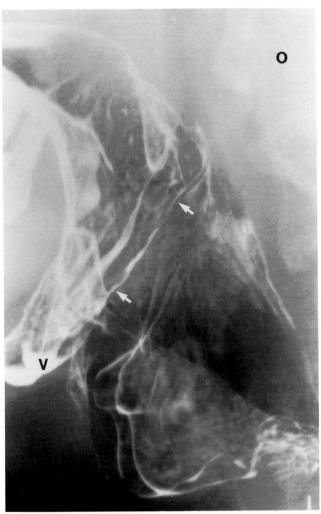

FIGURE 4–3

The pharyngoepiglottic fold (*arrows*) overlies the stylopharyngeus, which runs from the styloid process into the lateral wall of the pharynx. The pharyngoepiglottic fold is seen coursing obliquely across the pharynx from approximately the level of the odontoid (O) process to the junction of the base of the vallecula (V) and epiglottis. (Reprinted with permission from Rubesin, S.E., and Glick, S.N.: The tailored double-contrast pharyngogram. Crit. Rev. Diagn. Imaging *28*:133, 1988. Copyright CRC Press, Inc., Boca Raton, FL.)

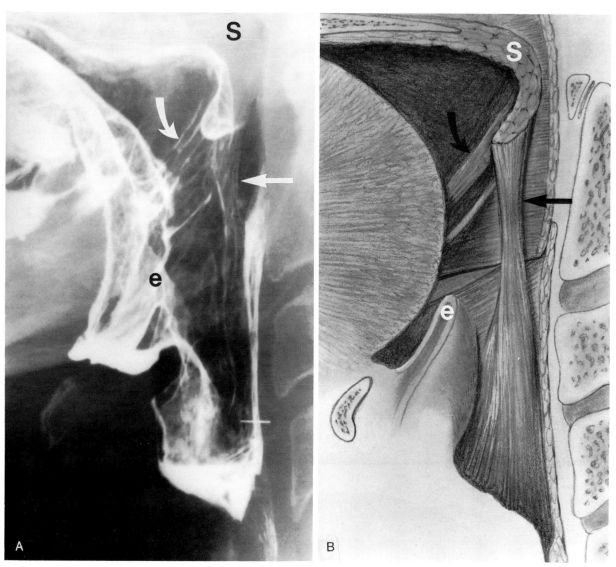

FIGURE 4–4

THE PALATOGLOSSAL AND PALATOPHARYNGEAL FOLDS. *A* and *B*, The palatoglossal fold (anterior tonsillar pillar) *(curved white arrow)* is formed by the palatoglossus *(curved black arrow)* and extends from the mid–soft palate (S) to the junction of the middle and posterior third of the tongue. The palatopharyngeal fold (posterior tonsillar pillar) *(straight white arrow)* overlies the palatopharyngeus *(straight black arrow)*. This muscle extends from the middle portion of the soft palate (S) to the lateral and posterior pharyngeal walls and is the major elevator of the pharynx. (e, Epiglottic tip.) (From Rubesin, S.E., et al.: Lines of the pharynx. Radiographics 7:217, 1987, with permission.)

nasopharynx and the oropharynx; anteriorly, the opening to the oral cavity; anteriorly, the laryngeal aditus; and inferiorly, the opening into the esophagus.

The muscular tube of the pharynx is divided into two layers: the outer circular (constrictor) layer and the inner longitudinal layer. The constrictor layer forms a ring that is incomplete anteriorly. It functions to push the bolus out of the pharynx. The major folds of mucosa (the palatoglossal, palatopharyngeal, and salpingopharyngeal folds) are determined by the inner longitudinal muscle layer (Fig. 4–4; see Fig. 4–3).[5] The double contrast appearance and landmarks of the pharynx, to a large extent, depend on the mucosa resting on the inner longitudinal muscle

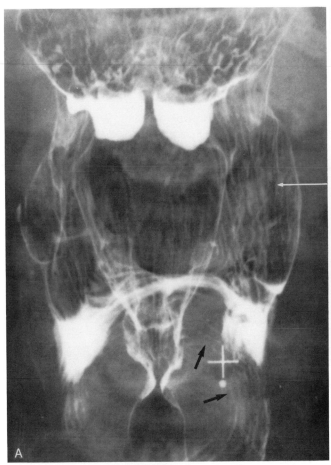

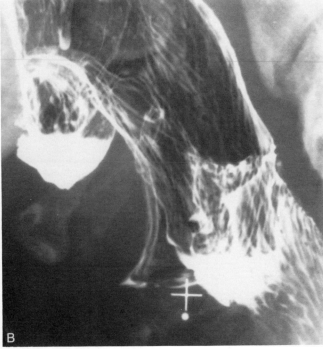

FIGURE 4–5

A and *B*, The squamous mucosa of the pharynx is closely apposed to the innermost layer of muscle. Laterally and posteriorly, the squamous mucosa is separated from the inner longitudinal layer of skeletal muscle by only a thin tunica propria. As a result, longitudinal striations (*white arrow*) appear on images obtained from double contrast pharyngography. Transverse folds (*black arrows*) along the anterior wall of the hypopharynx reflect redundant mucosa overlying the muscular processes of the mobile arytenoid cartilages and the cricoid cartilage. (Reprinted with permission from Rubesin, S.E., and Glick, S.N.: The tailored double-contrast pharyngogram. Crit. Rev. Diagn. Imaging 28:133, 1988. Copyright CRC Press, Inc., Boca Raton, FL.)

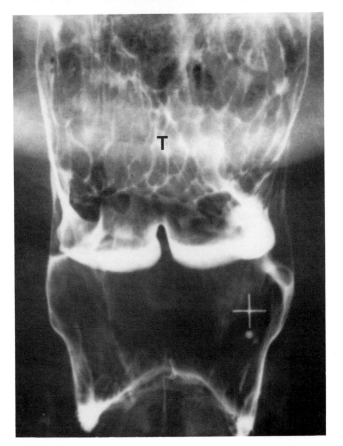

layer. Numerous transverse and longitudinal lines give the pharynx a striated appearance on double contrast radiographs (Fig. 4–5). Longitudinal lines reflect mucosa closely apposed to the longitudinally striated inner muscle layer (Fig. 4–5). Transverse folds overlying the muscular processes of the arytenoid cartilages and cricoid cartilage reflect the redundant mucosa overlying these structures.[5] Numerous round nodules on the vertical surface of the base of the tongue reflect the variable lymphoid tissue in the lingual tonsil (Fig. 4–6).[6]

FIGURE 4–6

LYMPHOID TISSUE AT THE BASE OF THE TONGUE. Normal lymphoid tissue lies at the base of the tongue (T) and appears on the frontal view as numerous round and ovoid lines that are approximately 2 to 4 mm in size. There is no definite criterion identifying normal variant lymphoid tissue versus lingual tonsil lymphoid hyperplasia. (Reprinted with permission from Rubesin, S.E., and Glick, S.N.: The tailored double-contrast pharyngogram. Crit. Rev. Diagn. Imaging 28:133, 1988. Copyright CRC Press, Inc., Boca Raton, FL.)

TECHNIQUE

The classic upper gastrointestinal examination begins at the level of the aortic arch. The act of swallowing, however, begins at the lips with the volitional carrying of a bolus to the mouth. Furthermore, peristalsis begins in the pharynx in the region of the superior constrictor. Thus, the radiologist is faced with the question, "Where do I start?" Patients with dysphagia, odynophagia, and chest pain should have an examination of both pharynx and esophagus. Patients who have a feeling of "a lump in the throat" need careful examination of the pharynx. Disorders of the pharynx may be manifested by respiratory and speech problems as well as by swallowing dysfunction. Recurrent pneumonia, asthma, chronic bronchitis, coughing, or choking may indicate a pharyngeal disorder. Nasal regurgitation or nasal quality of voice may indicate soft palate insufficiency. Because symptoms poorly reflect the level of a lesion in the pharynx and esophagus, the pharynx should be evaluated even if an esophageal pathologic process is suspected or discovered.[7] Barium studies are also useful in assessing pharyngeal function and morphologic features in patients with a known history of neuromuscular disease, stroke, pharyngeal tumor, or prior head and neck surgery or radiation.

Patient Preparation

Good barium coating requires dry pharyngeal mucosa. The patient is therefore instructed not to eat or drink after midnight. Activities that stimulate salivary secretion, such as smoking or chewing tobacco, gum, or throat lozenges, should be avoided. Diabetics should not take insulin the morning of the examination.

Plain Films

Contrast examination of the pharynx may be dangerous in patients with suspected airway obstruction, such as those with acute epiglottitis. A plain film of the neck should therefore constitute the initial examination if airway obstruction is suspected. Soft tissue scout-view films are also obtained when a foreign body, a fistula, an abscess, a perforation, or a palpable neck mass is suspected. The double contrast examination, however, obviates the need for plain films in most cases. Radiographic contrast between soft tissue and air is improved when barium coats the pharyngeal mucosa.

Routine Examination

Examination of the pharynx is tailored to the clinical problem and fluoroscopic results.[8, 9] The patient should be studied initially in the lateral position because this position is the best for visualizing the entrance of barium into the laryngeal vestibule, either during swallowing (penetration) or during normal breathing (aspiration). A videotape and double contrast spot-film examination are integrated to assess both motility and morphologic characteristics. The general principles of double contrast interpretation are the same in the pharynx as elsewhere in the gastrointestinal tract (see Chapter 2). The examination requires good mucosal coating, an adequate number of projections, and varying degrees of luminal distention.

Mucosal Coating

Adequate mucosal coating relies primarily on (1) dry pharyngeal mucosa and (2) properly prepared barium. A high-density barium (250% w/v) is used. If the barium is too "thin," the barium layer is of insufficient thickness and radiodensity to outline the pharyngeal mucosa. If the barium is too viscous, barium cannot wash mucus off the pharyngeal wall, resulting in artifactual strands of mucus.

Projection

In general, frontal and lateral films suffice for most diagnostic problems. Oblique films, however, help demonstrate the obliquely oriented aryepiglottic folds and the region of the cricopharyngeus.[10, 11] The frontal film shows the en face surface features of the base of the tongue, the median and lateral glossoepiglottic folds, and the contours of the palatine fossae, valleculae, and hypopharynx (see Fig. 4–1).

The lateral film (see Fig. 4–1) better examines the palatine fossae en face and the contour of the soft palate, base of the tongue, posterior pharyngeal wall, epiglottis, aryepiglottic folds, and anterior hypopharyngeal wall.[12] The lateral view is crucial for evaluating laryngeal vestibule penetration (Fig. 4–7) and the region of the cricopharyngeus.

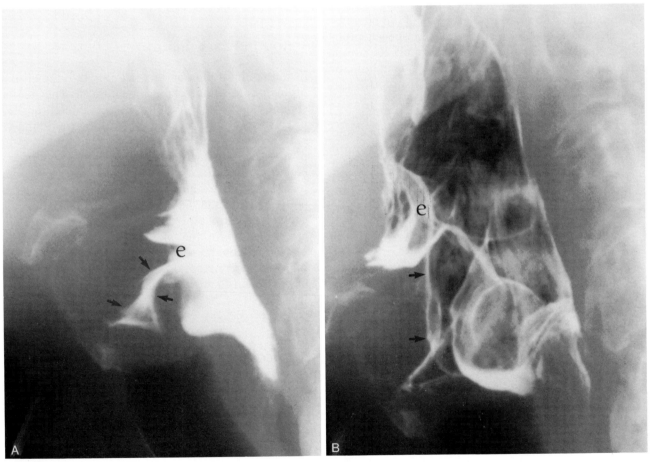

FIGURE 4–7

Laryngeal penetration is defined as barium entering the laryngeal vestibule while the patient is swallowing. Aspiration is defined as barium entering the laryngeal vestibule while the patient is breathing. *A,* Laryngeal penetration is best recorded in the lateral view during videofluoroscopy or cineradiography as barium enters the laryngeal vestibule (*arrows*). (e, Epiglottis.)

B, During suspended respiration, barium coats the open laryngeal vestibule (*arrows*). (e, Epiglottis.)

Distention

Adequate distention is crucial for demonstration of mucosal surfaces and contours. Air cannot be generated by effervescent agents, however, or instilled through tube insufflation, as in other regions of the gastrointestinal tract. Instead, pharyngeal distention is achieved either with phonation (long vowel sounds Eee . . . or Ooo . . .)[12] or with some form of modified Valsalva maneuver (Fig. 4–8). Pharyngeal distention results in better visualization of many structures, including the soft palate and asymmetry of the piriform sinus.[12]

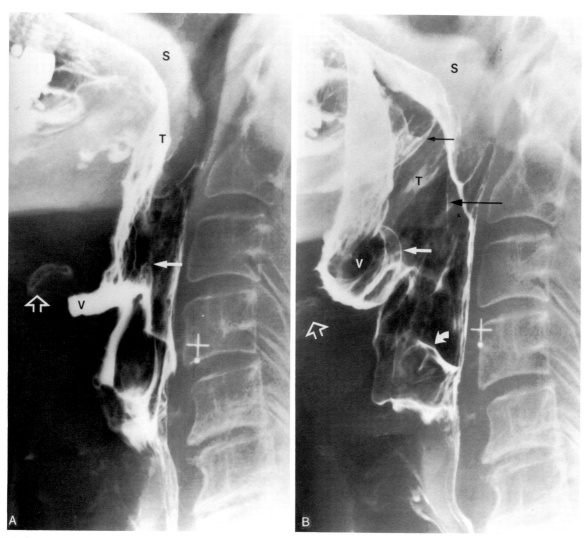

FIGURE 4–8

THE EFFECT OF PHONATION. *A,* During suspended respiration, the pharynx is partially collapsed. The soft palate (S) opposes the tongue, allowing communication of the nasopharynx and oropharynx. The pharyngoesophageal segment is closed to prevent swallowing of air or reflux of esophageal contents into the hypopharynx. (T, Tonsillar fossa; V, valleculae; *open arrow,* hyoid; *solid white arrow,* epiglottic tip.)

B, With phonation (*Eeee* . . .), the hyoid bone *(open arrow)* moves anteriorly and inferiorly, and the tongue moves anteriorly. The soft palate (S) elevates, closing the velopharyngeal portal, which prevents the voice from having a nasal quality. These movements result in expansion of the valleculae (V), oropharynx, tonsillar fossa (T), and upper hypopharynx. The pharyngoesophageal segment remains closed. Phonation by *Eeee* results in better visualization of the epiglottic tip *(white arrow),* aryepiglottic folds *(curved white arrow),* tonsillar fossa (T), and base of the tongue. The palatoglossal *(short black arrow)* and palatopharyngeal *(long black arrow)* folds are shown. (From Rubesin, S.E., et al.: Contrast pharyngography: The importance of phonation. AJR 148:269, 1987, with permission.)

POUCHES AND DIVERTICULA

Lateral Pharyngeal Pouches

Lateral pharyngeal pouches are *transient* protrusions of the lateral pharyngeal wall at sites of anatomic weakness, such as the posterior thyrohyoid membrane and the tonsillar fossa following tonsillectomy.[13] These pouches are common findings and usually occur as normal variants in asymptomatic patients. Rarely, some patients may complain of dysphagia, which is caused by the late spilling of pouch contents into the pharynx. The upper lateral pharyngeal wall is supported only by the superior constrictor muscle and tonsil. Following palatine tonsillectomy or atrophy of the tonsil with age, a transient protrusion may occur at this site. Pouches usually protrude in the upper hypopharyngeal wall near the site of penetration of the thyrohyoid membrane by the superior laryngeal nerve (Fig. 4–9).

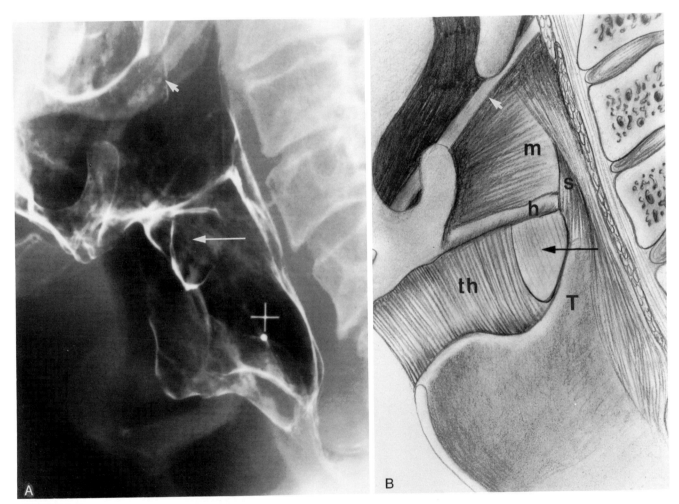

FIGURE 4–9

A and *B*, The lateral pharyngeal pouch *(long arrow)* is bounded superiorly by the hyoid bone (h) and the middle constrictor (m), posteriorly by the stylopharyngeus muscle (s) and the superior cornu of the thyroid cartilage (T), and anteriorly by the thyrohyoid muscle with its overlying thyrohyoid membrane (th). Calcified stylohyoid ligaments are also demonstrated *(short arrow)*. (From Rubesin, S.E., et al.: Lines of the pharynx. Radiographics 7:217, 1987, with permission.)

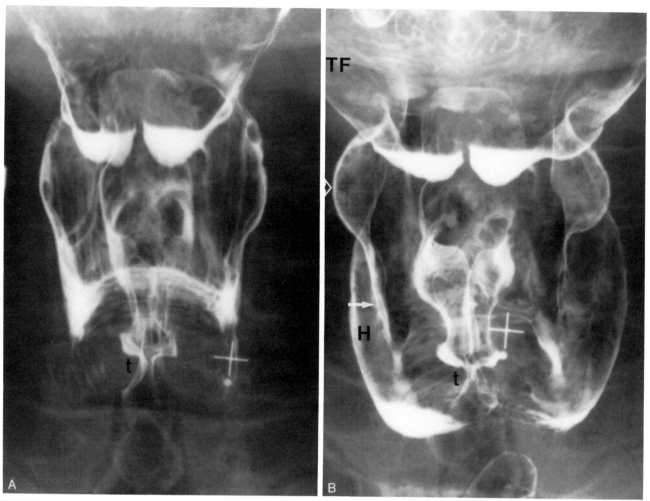

FIGURE 4–10

LATERAL PHARYNGEAL POUCHES. *A,* At the end of quiet inspiration, the pharynx is relatively collapsed. The true vocal cords (t) are slightly open.

B, During a modified Valsalva maneuver, the pharynx and oral cavity expand. The tonsillar fossae (TF) bulge laterally. Right and left lateral pouches are seen as smooth, hemispherical protrusions of the pharynx at the level of the thyrohyoid membrane *(open arrow).* The lateral hypopharyngeal wall (H) protrudes posteriorly around the lateral boundary of the thyroid cartilage *(white arrow).* The epiglottis is well coated. (t, True vocal cords.)

Lateral pharyngeal pouches (Fig. 4–10) appear on frontal views as transient, hemispherical protrusions in the upper hypopharynx above the calcified edge of the thyroid cartilage.[14] On lateral views, these pouches are recognized as ovoid barium collections or barium-coated rings in the anterior wall of the upper hypopharynx just below the hyoid bone, at the level of the valleculae (see Fig. 4–9).[14] They are seen only during swallowing or during periods of increased intrapharyngeal pressure. Lateral pharyngeal pouches disappear at rest.

Lateral pharyngeal diverticula are *persistent* pro-

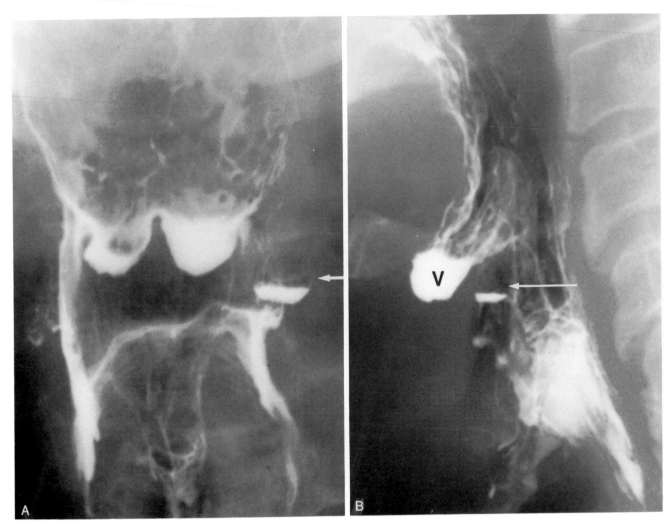

FIGURE 4–11

LATERAL PHARYNGEAL DIVERTICULUM. A round, barium- and air-filled structure (*arrow*) is lateral to the upper hypopharyngeal wall on the frontal view (*A*), and posterior to and at the level of the valleculae (V) on the lateral view (*B*). (Reprinted with permission from Rubesin, S.E., and Glick, S.N.: The tailored double-contrast pharyngogram. Crit. Rev. Diagn. Imaging 28:133, 1988. Copyright CRC Press, Inc., Boca Raton, FL.)

trusions from the tonsillar fossa or region of the thyrohyoid membrane (Fig. 4–11). These diverticula are much less common than lateral pharyngeal pouches; they frequently occur in individuals who have markedly elevated pharyngeal pressure (glass-blowers and wind instrument players).[13] When stasis occurs in pharyngeal pouches or diverticula, spillage of pouch contents into the hypopharynx may result in dysphagia or aspiration. Lateral pharyngeal diverticula may also appear as neck masses, or they may be sites of ulceration or neoplasia.

Radiographically, lateral pharyngeal diverticula appear as persistent pouches or saccular collections in the region of the posterior thyrohyoid membrane.

Zenker's Diverticulum

Zenker's diverticulum (posterior hypopharyngeal diverticulum) is an acquired mucosal herniation through an area of anatomic weakness in the region of the cricopharyngeus (Killian's dehiscence).[15] This area of anatomic weakness has been variably described as being located between the thyropharyngeus and cricopharyngeus[16] or between the oblique and horizontal fibers of the cricopharyngeal muscle.[17] Patients with Zenker's diverticulum complain of dysphagia referred to the suprasternal notch, coughing following swallowing, food regurgitation, and halitosis. Many patients with Zenker's diverticulum have an associated hiatal hernia, gastroesophageal reflux, or both. Rarely, these diverticula are complicated by ulceration or malignancy.

During swallowing, a Zenker's diverticulum appears as a posterior bulge of the distal pharyngeal wall above an anteriorly protruding cricopharyngeus (Fig. 4–12). At rest, the barium-filled diverticulum extends below the level of the cricopharyngeus, posterior to the proximal cervical esophagus. A large diverticulum may protrude to the left, compress the cervical esophagus, or do both.

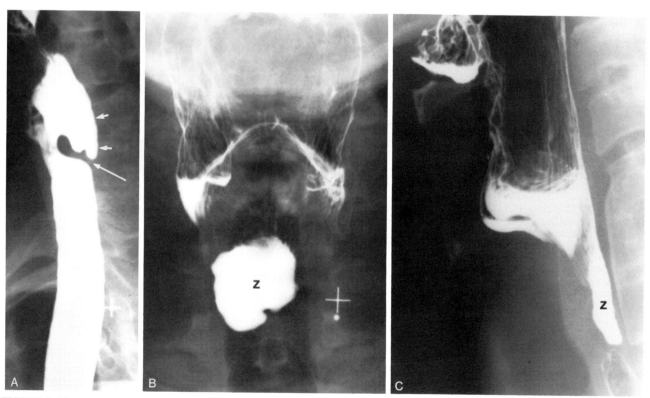

FIGURE 4–12

ZENKER'S DIVERTICULUM. A, During swallowing in the prone position, a Zenker's diverticulum appears as a contrast-filled bulge of the posterior pharyngeal wall *(short arrows)* above a protruding cricopharyngeal bar *(long arrow)*.

B, The frontal view of the pharynx shows a barium-filled saccular structure (z) in the midline, below the level of the hypopharynx.

C, In the lateral view, the Zenker's diverticulum (z) appears as a subtle, flat barium-filled collection behind the collapsed pharyngoesophageal segment and proximal cervical esophagus.

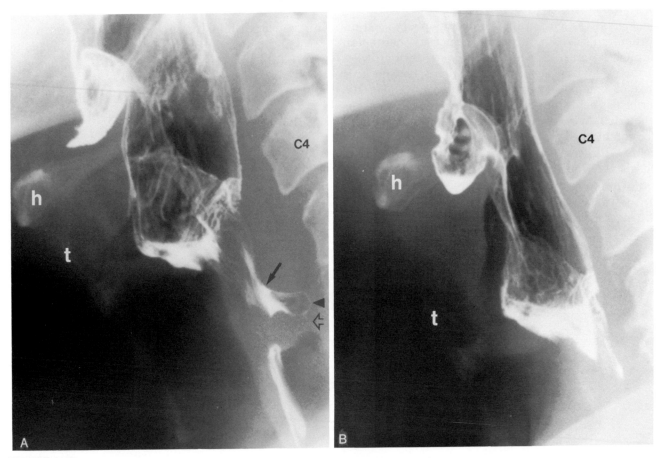

FIGURE 4–13

PSEUDO-ZENKER'S DIVERTICULUM. *A,* There is a small sac-like collection of barium *(arrowhead)* above a prominent cricopharyngeus *(open arrow).* Note that this collection is not a true diverticulum, but rather air and barium trapped between the pharyngeal peristaltic wave in the inferior constrictor *(arrow)* and the prominent cricopharyngeus. The pseudo-Zenker's diverticulum does not protrude posteriorly in relation to the expected pharyngeal contour. Note that this film has been taken near the end of a swallow: The epiglottis has returned to the upright position, but laryngeal elevation and thyrohyoid apposition are still occurring. The laryngeal vestibule is just beginning to open. Peristalsis is just about to pass the cricopharyngeus. (C4, fourth cervical vertebra; h, hyoid bone; t, thyroid cartilage.)

B, After the swallow, the pseudo-Zenker's diverticulum has disappeared. The larynx and pharynx are no longer elevated. The thyroid cartilage (t) and hyoid bone (h) have returned to their resting locations.

Barium trapped between a prominent cricopharyngeus and the pharyngeal peristaltic wave (contraction) may mimic Zenker's diverticulum. This small, trapped barium collection is termed a pseudo-Zenker's diverticulum (Fig. 4–13). The radiographic clues to differentiating true Zenker's diverticulum from pseudo-Zenker's diverticulum are (1) that the pseudo-Zenker's diverticulum is small and does not protrude from the expected contour of the posterior pharyngeal wall and (2) that the pseudo-Zenker's diverticulum disappears after the pharyngeal peristaltic wave passes the pharyngoesophageal segment.

Killian-Jamieson Diverticula

Another area of anatomic weakness lies just below the cricopharyngeus and is lateral to the insertion of the longitudinal tendon (muscle) of the esophagus on the cricoid cartilage. This area is known as the Killian-Jamieson space. Proximal cervical esophageal protrusions in this region are known as Killian-Jamie-son pouches or diverticula. Radiographically, these pouches or diverticula are seen on the anterolateral wall of the proximal cervical esophagus, just below the level of the cricopharyngeus (Fig. 4–14).[18] During fluoroscopy, these diverticula may easily be confused with Zenker's diverticula.

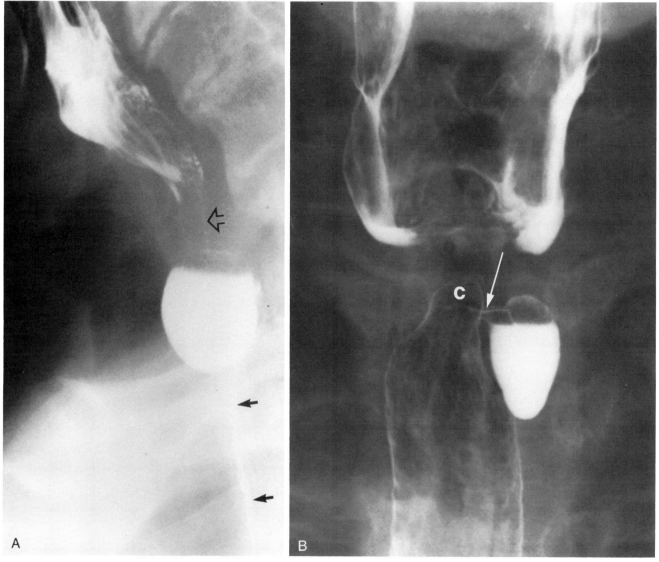

FIGURE 4–14

KILLIAN-JAMIESON DIVERTICULUM. *A,* On the lateral view, a round, barium-filled sac with an air–fluid level is seen just below the level of the pharyngoesophageal segment *(open arrow).* A radiographic clue that this diverticulum is not a Zenker's diverticulum is that the pouch protrudes anteriorly in relation to the cervical esophagus *(black arrows).*

B, The frontal view shows that the origin *(arrow)* of the Killian-Jamieson diverticulum is in the proximal cervical esophagus (c) along the lateral wall.

WEBS

Hypopharyngeal and cervical esophageal webs are thin folds composed of mucosa and submucosa.[19] Radiographically, webs appear as shelf-like filling defects that are 1 to 2 mm in width and that are seen along the anterior wall of the lower hypopharynx, pharyngoesophageal segment, or proximal cervical esophagus (Fig. 4–15).[19–22] Occasionally, webs are circumferential. Partial obstruction is suggested by a jet phenomenon or by dilatation of the esophagus or pharynx proximal to the web. Webs may be confused with redundant mucosa in the anterior wall of the hypopharynx at the level of the cricoid cartilage. This postcricoid impression has been attributed to a ve-nous plexus in the region,[23] but it more likely represents redundant mucosa.[5]

Most cervical esophageal webs are asymptomatic isolated findings. Some webs are associated with diseases of the esophagus that cause scarring, such as epidermolysis bullosa or benign mucous membrane pemphigoid. Some cervical esophageal webs may be due to gastroesophageal reflux. The association between cervical esophageal webs and iron deficiency anemia, termed the Plummer-Vinson or Paterson-Kelly syndrome, is controversial.[21–24] In some countries, this syndrome may be a premalignant condition associated with pharyngeal or esophageal carcinoma. In the United States, however, there is no association between webs and carcinoma.

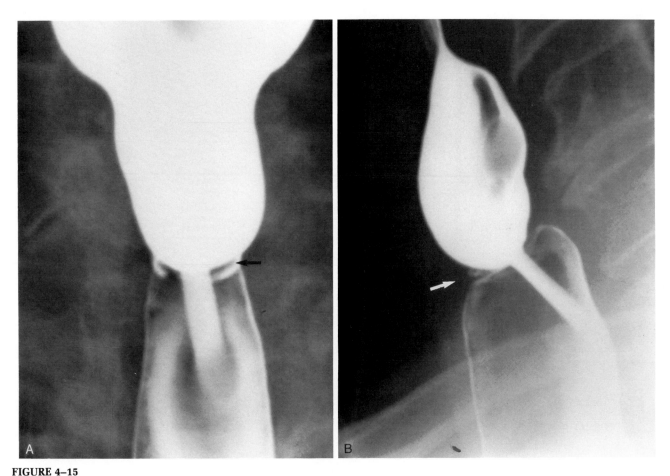

FIGURE 4–15

CERVICAL ESOPHAGEAL WEB. Frontal (A) and lateral (B) views during swallowing show a thin, 1-mm, radiolucent bar (arrow) encircling the cervical esophagus approximately 3 cm below the pharyngoesophageal junction. A jet of barium spurts through the center of the bar.

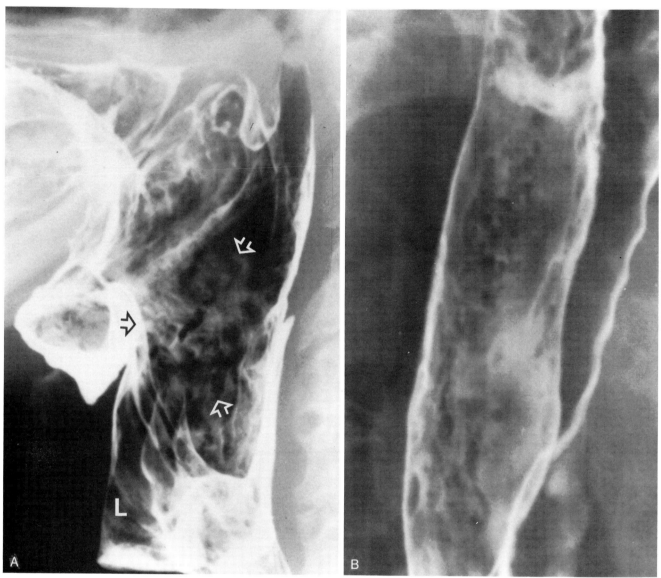

FIGURE 4–16

CANDIDA **PHARYNGITIS AND ESOPHAGITIS.** A, A lateral view of the pharynx during phonation shows multiple, irregular, 2- to 4-mm nodules *(arrows)* in the oropharynx and in the tonsillar fossa. Barium coating the laryngeal vestibule (L) and trachea reflects the motility disorder associated with severe pharyngeal inflammation.

B, A coned-down view of the midesophagus shows multiple small, well-circumscribed plaques aligned longitudinally along the mucosal folds.

INFLAMMATORY DISORDERS

Barium studies of the pharynx are usually of limited value in patients with acute sore throat due to viral, bacterial, or fungal infection.[25] Such patients have normal pharyngograms or nonspecific lymphoid hyperplasia of the palatine or lingual tonsils. A double contrast examination of the pharynx, however, may demonstrate the plaques of *Candida* pharyngitis (Fig. 4–16) or the ulcers of herpes pharyngitis, particularly in immunosuppressed patients or in patients with AIDS.[8] Barium studies may also be helpful in detecting underlying gastroesophageal reflux or reflux esophagitis in patients who have chronic sore throat.

Lymphoid Hyperplasia

Lymphoid hyperplasia of the palatine tonsil or base of the tongue is associated with aging, chronic infections, or allergic states.[6] In addition, lymphoid hyperplasia may be a compensatory response following tonsillectomy.

In lymphoid hyperplasia of the lingual tonsil, multiple smooth, round or ovoid nodules are seen along the vertical surface of the tongue (Fig. 4–17).[6] With severe lymphoid hyperplasia, nodules may extend into the valleculae or piriform sinuses. The nodules of lymphoid hyperplasia are usually small, uniform, and symmetrically distributed. In contrast, the nodules of a pharyngeal carcinoma are large, irregular, and associated with a focal mass and obliteration of the normal mucosal contour. Lymphoid hyperplasia can occasionally appear as a polypoid mass of the base of the tongue and may be confused with a carcinoma of the base of the tongue.[6]

Pharyngeal dysmotility is common in patients with marked gastroesophageal reflux or severe acute pharyngitis. Severe or longstanding inflammatory disorders of the pharynx can alter pharyngeal elevation, epiglottic tilt, or closure of the vocal cords and laryngeal vestibule. Thus, pharyngeal dysmotility due to a local inflammatory process may result in laryngeal penetration.

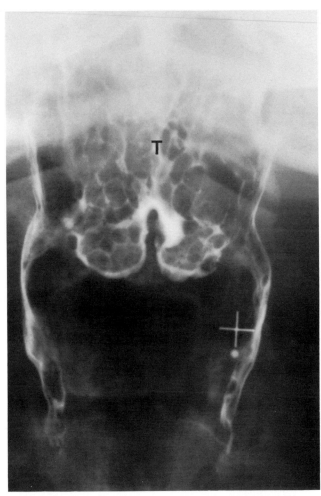

FIGURE 4–17

LYMPHOID HYPERPLASIA OF THE BASE OF THE TONGUE. A frontal view of the pharynx shows coarse nodularity of the tongue base (T).

DOUBLE CONTRAST MANIFESTATIONS OF PHARYNGEAL DYSMOTILITY

Review of double contrast spot films before review of the dynamic study aids in the interpretation of the videofluoroscopic images. Static radiographic signs of dysmotility are many. A coating of high-density barium on the laryngeal vestibule or vocal cords indicates penetration or aspiration. Barium coating of the posterior nasopharyngeal wall above the level of the soft palate indicates nasal regurgitation.[26] Excessive pooling of contrast agent in the valleculae or piriform sinuses may reflect unilateral or bilateral weakness. Smooth-surfaced, changeable asymmetry of the valleculae or lateral pharyngeal walls on the frontal view may indicate unilateral pharyngeal weakness. Excessive ballooning of the pharynx during the Valsalva maneuver may also indicate pharyngeal muscular weakness (Fig. 4–18). Distention of the normally tonically contracted pharyngoesophageal segment during the Valsalva maneuver also indicates muscular weakness (see Fig. 4–18). Rotation of the epiglottis may give it an asymmetric or a bulbous appearance on the lateral view.[27] A "ptotic" or posteriorly protruding epiglottis at rest may reflect epiglottic dysmotility.

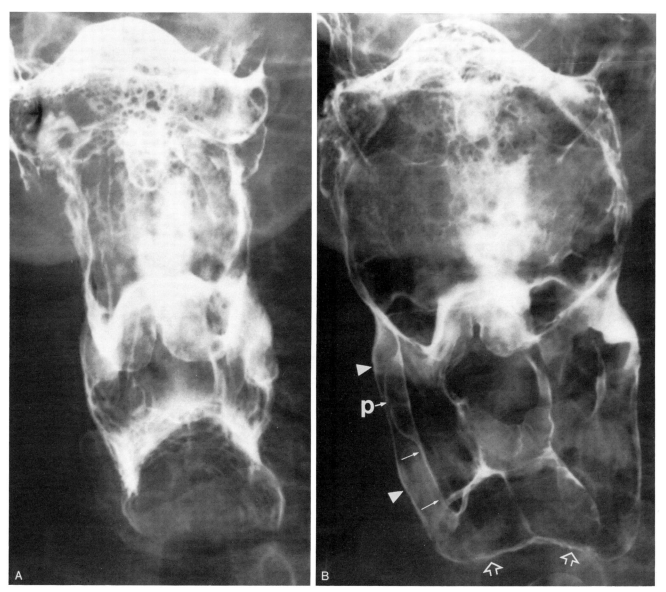

FIGURE 4–18

BALLOONING OF THE PHARYNX DUE TO MUSCLE WEAKNESS. *A,* During suspended respiration in the supine position, the pharynx shows barium pooling along the posterior pharyngeal wall.

B, During phonation, excessive distention of the pharynx occurs. The lateral pharyngeal walls *(arrowheads)* protrude laterally beyond the confines of the thyroid cartilage *(solid arrows)* and even beyond the anterolaterally located lateral pharyngeal pouch (P). The lower hypopharynx is usually collapsed, even during a Valsalva maneuver. In this patient, however, the lower hypopharynx is distended *(open arrows).* This distention is a sign of pharyngeal muscle weakness or hypotonicity.

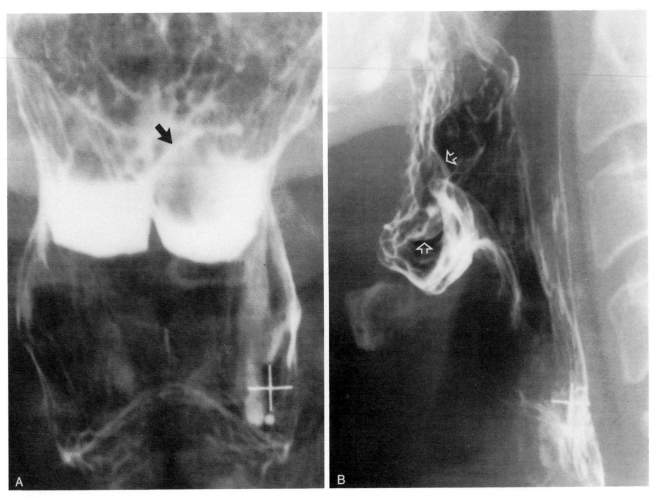

FIGURE 4–19

RETENTION CYST OF THE LEFT VALLECULA. The frontal view *(A)* shows a subtle filling defect *(arrow)* in the barium pool in the left vallecula. The lateral view *(B)* shows a smooth hemispheric line *(arrows)* protruding posteriorly in relation to the base of the tongue and partially obscured by the tip of the epiglottis.

BENIGN LESIONS

Whatever the underlying histologic characteristics, a benign pharyngeal tumor usually appears en face as a smooth, round, sharply circumscribed mass and in profile as a hemispheric line with acute angulation.[8] The most common benign lesions are retention cysts of the valleculae (Fig. 4–19) or aryepiglottic folds.[28] Aryepiglottic fold cysts are usually filled with mucoid secretions, arising from the mucus-secreting glands of the saccule or appendix of the laryngeal ventricle.[28] Laryngoceles are expansions of the laryngeal ventricular apex or saccule into the submucosal portion of the anteroinferior aryepiglottic folds. They are filled with air or fluid, or both. Laryngoceles do not communicate with the pharynx.

MALIGNANT LESIONS

Double contrast radiographs of the pharynx can accurately define the intraluminal size, level, and extent of a mucosal lesion. The radiologic examination demonstrates regions of the pharynx (the valleculae, lower hypopharynx, and cricopharyngeus) that are difficult to visualize by indirect examination or during endoscopy.[29, 30] Although its accuracy is limited in the region of the palatine tonsil, the double contrast examination detects more than 95% of mucosal neoplasms in the pharynx below the level of the pharyngoepiglottic fold.[31]

In patients with known pharyngeal carcinoma, barium studies are also helpful for detecting separate, coexisting carcinomas of the pharynx or esophagus.

FIGURE 4–20

RADIOGRAPHIC FINDINGS IN PHARYNGEAL MALIGNANCY.
A frontal view of the pharynx demonstrates the radiographic
findings of malignancy: intraluminal mass, asymmetry and loss of
distensibility, and mucosal irregularity. A large, lobulated mass
replaces the normally smooth contour of the epiglottis *(open
arrow)*. Tumor extension into the left vallecula and
pharyngoepiglottic fold is indicated by flattening and lobulation
of the vallecular contour *(small arrows)*. Extension into the left
false vocal cord is indicated by mass effect and an irregular
mucosa of the left false cord *(arrowhead)*. Lobulation of the
contour and mucosal irregularity of the mucosa overlying the
muscular process of the arytenoid (a) can be seen. The left
hypopharyngeal wall is less distensible than the right. Note the
stasis of barium in the asymmetric left vallecula and the coating
of the laryngeal vestibule due to laryngeal penetration. (Reprinted
with permission from Rubesin, S.E., and Glick, S.N.: The tailored
double-contrast pharyngogram. Crit. Rev. Diagn. Imaging *28*:133,
1988. Copyright CRC Press, Inc., Boca Raton, FL.)

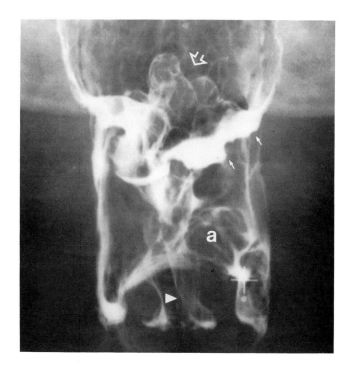

About 10% of the patients with squamous cell carcinomas of the head and neck develop a second primary
lesion,[32] and 1% develop synchronous or metachronous carcinomas of the esophagus.[33, 34]

The most important radiographic signs of pharyngeal carcinoma are (1) intraluminal mass, (2) loss of
distensibility, and (3) mucosal irregularity (Fig. 4–
20).[8, 25] An intraluminal mass may be depicted by
obliteration of the normal pharyngeal contour, barium-coated lines in an unusual location or shape, a
filling defect in the barium pool, or a superimposed
radiodensity. Loss of distensibility of a portion of the
pharynx may indicate direct invasion by infiltrative
tumor or neural damage. Tumors may have a lobulated, finely nodular, granular, or irregular mucosal
surface texture. Pharyngeal carcinomas may also impair pharyngeal motility or cause stasis, resulting in
laryngeal penetration or aspiration (see Fig. 4–20).
Soft palate tumors may cause reflux of contents from
the oropharynx into the nasopharynx (Fig. 4–21).[35]

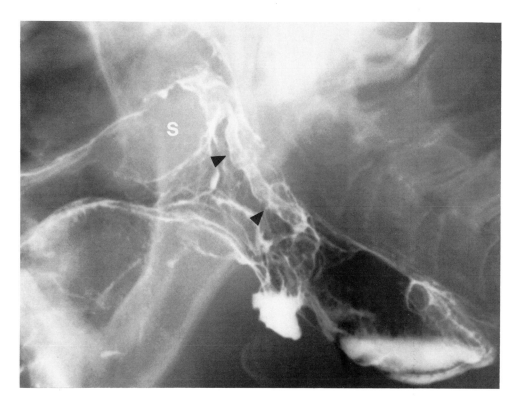

FIGURE 4–21

Soft palate and oropharyngeal
carcinoma causing nasal
regurgitation. A large tumor
involves the soft palate and the
posterolateral oropharyngeal
wall. The soft palate (S) is
enlarged with an irregular
contour. The posterior
pharyngeal wall has a lobulated
contour *(arrowheads)*. Irregular
lines and nodules in the region
of the tonsillar fossae also
indicate tumor spread.

Squamous cell carcinomas are by far the most common malignant tumor of the pharynx.[36] The overall 5-year survival rate is approximately 20%, a somewhat better prognosis than esophageal carcinoma.[37] Squamous cell carcinomas of the pharynx vary slightly in radiographic appearance and prognosis, depending on their location. Classification of tumors of the pharynx and larynx is confusing. Although the supraglottic laryngeal structures are part of the hypopharynx and are derived from pharyngobuccal an-

lage, supraglottic tumors confined by the aryepiglottic folds are classified as laryngeal carcinomas. Thus, tumors of the false vocal cords, laryngeal surface of the epiglottis (Fig. 4–22), aryepiglottic fold, arytenoid cartilage, and ventricles are defined as laryngeal. These supraglottic carcinomas are associated with approximately a 40% 5-year survival rate and often show early invasion of the pre-epiglottic space and lymph node metastasis.[25]

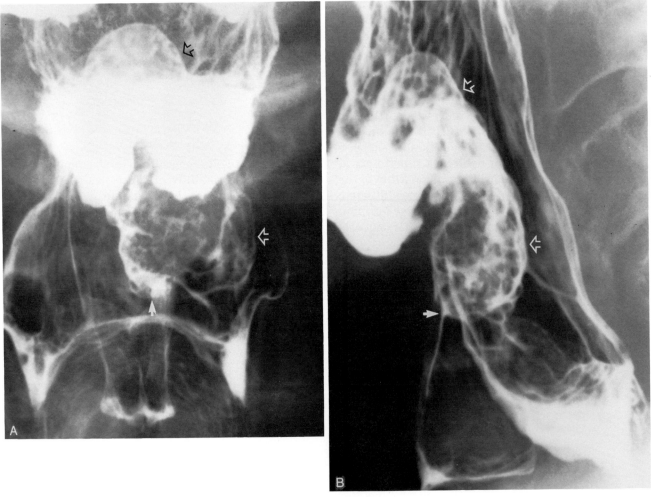

FIGURE 4–22

EPIGLOTTIC CARCINOMA. A frontal view (A) shows a nodular surface of the epiglottic tip and medial and lateral expansion of the left aryepiglottic fold. The lateral view (B) shows a mass (open arrows) involving the epiglottic tip and the superior portion of the anterior wall of the laryngeal vestibule (arrow). The anterior commissure is normal.

The palatine tonsil is the most common site of squamous cell carcinoma arising in the pharynx.[36] Bulky, exophytic tumors are easily detected radiographically. However, infiltrative tumors may be obscured by the nodular mucosa overlying the lymphoid tissue of the tonsillar fossa.

Carcinomas of the base of the tongue are usually clinically silent until they are advanced lesions with 70% lymph node metastasis. The 5-year survival rate approaches 15%.[38] Polypoid tumors project posteriorly from the base of the tongue (Fig. 4–23). Ulcerative tumors are seen as an irregular contrast collection extending anteriorly to disrupt the normal contour of the tongue.

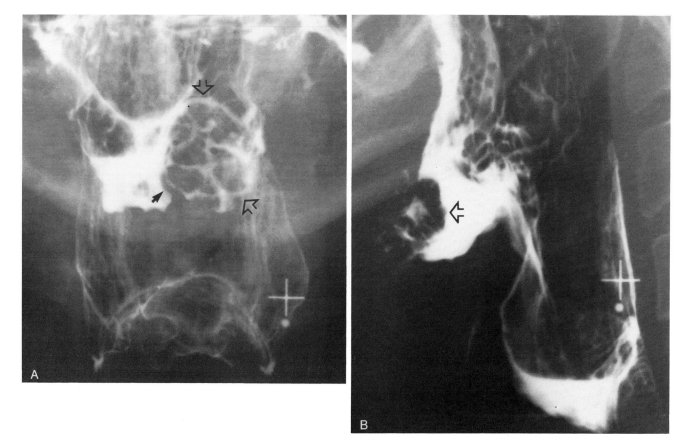

FIGURE 4–23

CARCINOMA OF THE BASE OF THE TONGUE. A, The frontal view shows obliteration of the normal contour of the left vallecula and lateral glossoepiglottic fold. Irregular nodular mucosa is seen in the region of the left vallecula (open arrows). The median glossoepiglottic fold is deviated to the right (solid arrow).

B, The lateral view shows a polypoid mass (open arrow) in the vallecula with barium tracks extending deep to the expected contour of the base of the tongue. (Reprinted with permission from Rubesin, S.E., and Glick, S.N.: The tailored double-contrast pharyngogram. Crit. Rev. Diagn. Imaging 28:133, 1988. Copyright CRC Press, Inc., Boca Raton, FL.)

Carcinomas of the piriform sinus metastasize early and are associated with 70% to 80% lymph node metastasis to the jugular chain at the time of diagnosis (Fig. 4–24).[37] Piriform sinus carcinomas are usually bulky and exophytic growths.

Posterior pharyngeal wall carcinomas are usually advanced when first seen, often presenting as a neck mass due to lymph node metastasis to the retropharyngeal or jugular chain. Posterior pharyngeal wall carcinomas have approximately a 20% 5-year survival rate.[25] These tumors are best seen on lateral films as large, fungating masses (Fig. 4–25).

Carcinomas arising in the region of the pharyngoesophageal segment (postcricoid carcinomas) are uncommon, except in Scandinavia. These tumors appear radiographically as annular, infiltrating lesions (Fig. 4–26). Postcricoid carcinomas may be difficult to detect while the pharyngoesophageal segment is constricted during suspended respiration or phonation. These lesions are best detected during swallowing, while a full-column of barium distends the pharyngoesophageal segment.

Instillation of intranasal barium may be helpful in discovering or defining nasopharyngeal carcinomas (Fig. 4–27).[39]

Lymphomas comprise 15% of oropharyngeal tumors and arise in the palatine tonsil, lingual tonsil, or lymphoid tissue distributed throughout the submucosa of the pharynx. These tumors are manifested radiographically by masses, lobulated contours, and variably surfaced nodular or smooth mucosa (Fig. 4–28).[9]

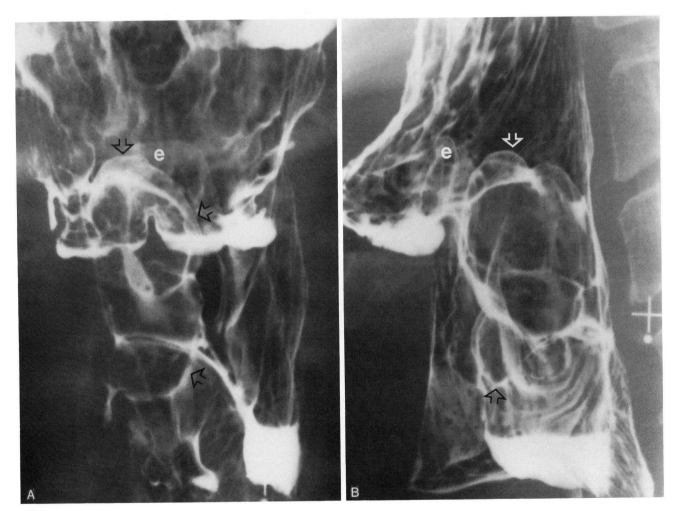

FIGURE 4–24

CARCINOMA OF THE HYPOPHARYNX. *A* and *B*, A large polypoid tumor (*arrows*) obliterates the right hypopharyngeal wall and invades the right aryepiglottic fold and laryngeal vestibule. The contours of the epiglottic tip (e) and valleculae are preserved. (Reprinted with permission from Rubesin, S.E., and Glick, S.N.: The tailored double-contrast pharyngogram. Crit. Rev. Diagn. Imaging 28:133, 1988. Copyright CRC Press, Inc., Boca Raton, FL.)

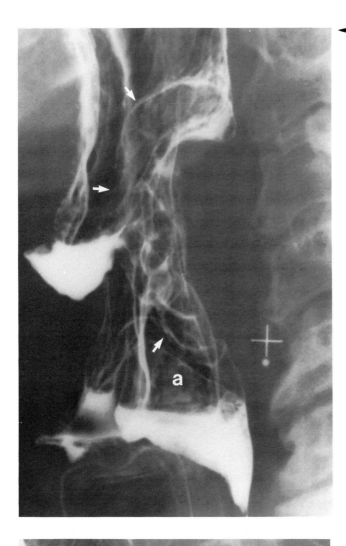

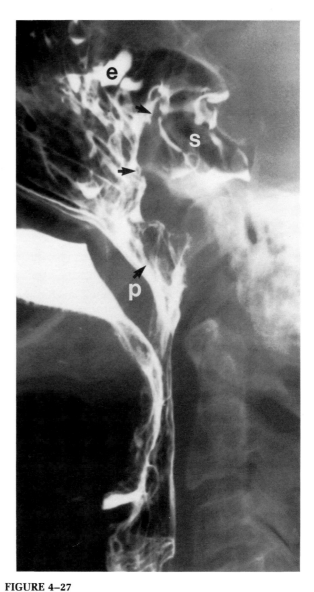

FIGURE 4–27

SQUAMOUS CELL CARCINOMA OF THE NASOPHARYNX. A large lobulated mass involves the posterior nasopharyngeal wall *(arrows)* and extends into the sphenoid sinus and posterior ethmoidal sinus. Opacification of the posterior ethmoidal sinus (e) and sphenoid sinus (s) is present. The soft palate is identified (p).

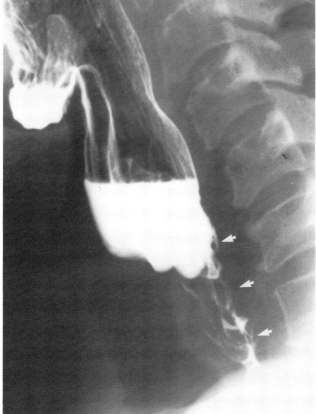

FIGURE 4–26

POSTCRICOID CARCINOMA. Lobulated mucosa and an irregular contour of the pharyngoesophageal segment are seen *(arrows)*. (From Levine, M.S., et al.: Update on esophageal radiology. AJR 155:993, 1990, with permission, © by American Roentgen Ray Society.)

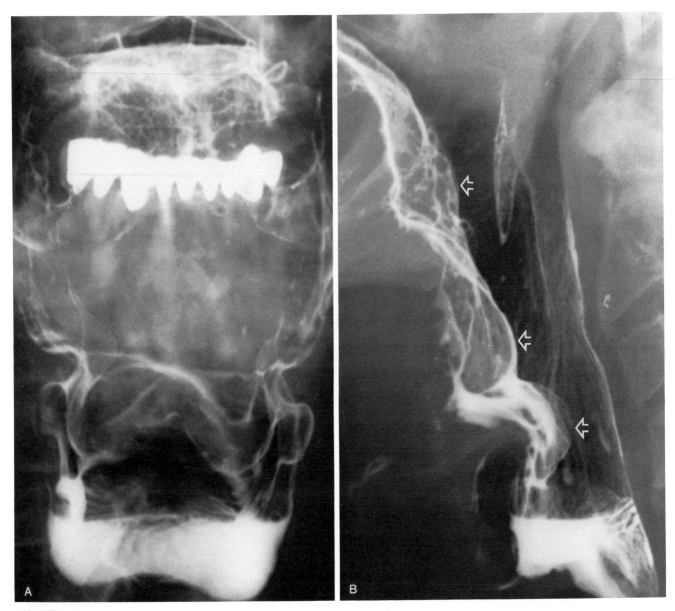

FIGURE 4–28

LYMPHOMA INVOLVING THE TONGUE AND EPIGLOTTIS. The frontal (A) and lateral (B) views of the pharynx show a relatively smooth-surfaced mass (arrows) involving the base of the tongue and epiglottis. The frontal view shows obliteration of the normal surface features of the base of the tongue, resulting in a nearly smooth surface due to the submucosal location of the tumor.

RADIATION CHANGES AND TRAUMA

Squamous cell carcinoma of the head and neck may be treated and cured with radiotherapy. However, radiation therapy may induce edema and fibrosis with resultant dysphagia, odynophagia, hoarseness, and aspiration.[40] Diffuse, symmetric swelling of the mucosa and submucosa of the pharynx occurs in the region of the radiation portal. Radiographically, smooth enlargement of the epiglottis may be seen.[25] Edema of the mucosa overlying the muscular processes of the arytenoid cartilages results in elevation of the mucosa over the cartilages. Arytenoid cartilage enlargement may be asymmetric with more enlargement occurring on the side of the tumor. The lumen of the laryngeal vestibule may be narrowed (Fig. 4–29). Dynamic examination may show diminished motility with one or more of the following signs: impairment of epiglottic tilt, paresis of the constrictor musculature, or diminished closure of the laryngeal vestibule.[40] Thus, diminished motility may result in laryngeal penetration or aspiration.

Contrast pharyngography may be helpful in evaluation of iatrogenic and other forms of trauma. Perforation of the pharynx usually occurs at the base of

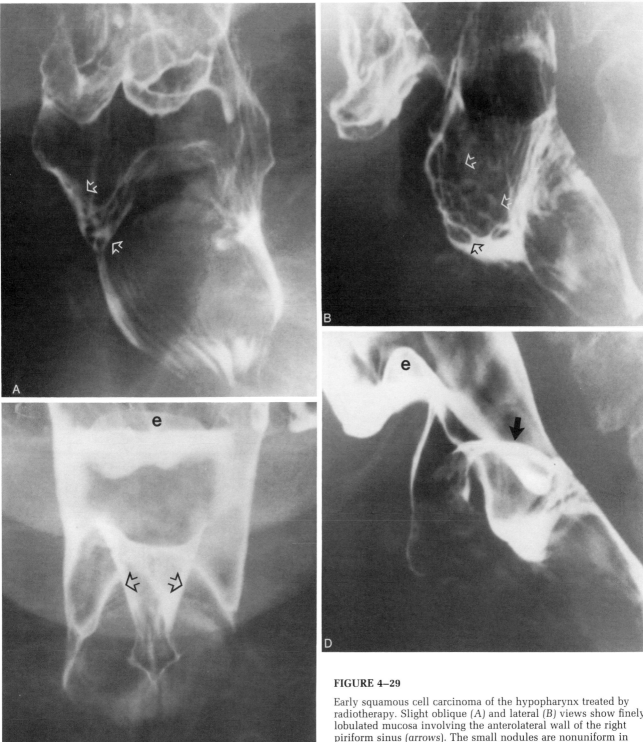

FIGURE 4–29

Early squamous cell carcinoma of the hypopharynx treated by radiotherapy. Slight oblique (A) and lateral (B) views show finely lobulated mucosa involving the anterolateral wall of the right piriform sinus (arrows). The small nodules are nonuniform in size, are irregularly shaped, and cause mild lobulation of the contour. Nine months following radiotherapy, the nodularity in the right piriform sinus has disappeared, and the mucosa is now smooth (C and D). The epiglottis (e) is enlarged, with a bulbous shape and a smooth surface. Pooling of barium can be seen in the valleculae. The valleculae also have a flattened, smooth contour. The mucosa overlying the muscular processes of the arytenoid cartilages (solid arrow in D) is elevated, though smooth. Laryngeal penetration has occurred. The laryngeal vestibule appears smooth and narrowed (open arrows in C). Thus, the squamous cell carcinoma has regressed, but changes from radiotherapy remain. (A and B, From Levine, M.S., et al.: Update on esophageal radiology. AJR 155:993, 1990, with permission, © by American Roentgen Ray Society.)

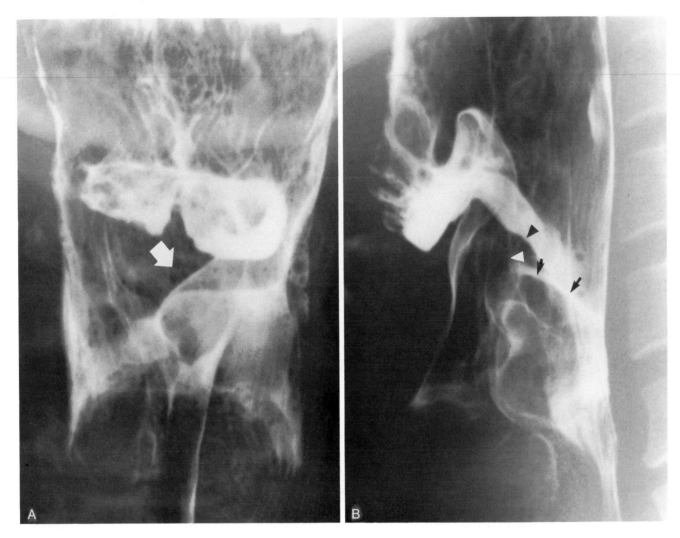

FIGURE 4–30

HEMATOMA FOLLOWING MOTOR VEHICLE ACCIDENT. Three days following a neck contusion, the patient complained of coughing. A frontal view *(A)* shows asymmetry and elevation of smooth mucosa overlying the muscular process of the left arytenoid cartilage *(arrow)*. The lateral view *(B)* shows asymmetry of the aryepiglottic folds *(arrowheads)*, elevation of mucosa overlying the muscular process of the left arytenoid cartilage *(arrows)*, and barium coating the laryngeal vestibule. A hematoma overlying the muscular process of the arytenoid cartilage and the left aryepiglottic fold was seen during endoscopy.

the piriform sinuses or in a Zenker's diverticulum. Thus, the region of the pharyngoesophageal segment must be examined carefully. Blunt trauma to the neck may result in a hematoma of the larynx or pharynx (Fig. 4–30). If laryngeal penetration is suspected, barium should be used to demonstrate a leak into the soft tissue of the neck. If no laryngeal penetration is suspected, a water-soluble contrast is used, followed by barium if no leak is seen.

POSTOPERATIVE CHANGES

Tumors of the larynx that extend into the laryngeal cartilages, extend more than 10 mm into the subepiglottic region, or cause vocal cord paralysis may be treated by total laryngectomy.[41, 42] Total laryngectomy

may also be performed when prior laryngeal conservation surgery has failed because of recurrent neoplasm or because of glottic insufficiency resulting in recurrent aspiration.

During laryngectomy, the hyoid bone, thyroid and cricoid cartilages, and epiglottis are removed. The aryepiglottic folds and piriform fossae are removed, resulting in a defect of the anterior wall of the hypopharynx. The constrictor muscles are incised, resulting in retraction of the thyropharyngeus and cricopharyngeus. A radical neck dissection may be performed at the same time for enlarged cervical lymph nodes or for piriform sinus tumors that show early nodal spread.[41]

Radiographically, the resultant neopharyngeal tube resembles an inverted cone with smooth mucosa (Fig. 4–31). The hyoid bone, epiglottis, aryepiglottic folds,

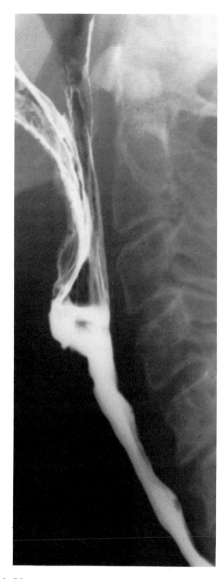

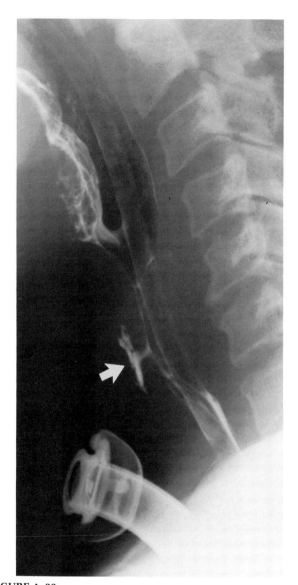

FIGURE 4–31

RADIOGRAPHIC CHANGES FOLLOWING TOTAL LARYNGECTOMY. The normal features of the pharynx are not apparent. The epiglottis, piriform fossae, and aryepiglottic folds are not seen. The hyoid bone is missing. The neopharynx appears as a relatively featureless tube. There is mild sacculation of the junction between the base of the tongue and neopharynx, and there is mild nasal regurgitation.

FIGURE 4–32

PHARYNGOCUTANEOUS FISTULA FOLLOWING SUPRAGLOTTIC LARYNGECTOMY. A lateral view shows a barium-filled tract along the junction line of the neopharyngeal tube (arrow).

and piriform sinuses are absent. The neopharyngeal tube has a 1- to 2.5-cm luminal diameter and is 0.5 to 1 cm anterior to the anterior margin of the C3-C5 vertebral bodies. Occasionally, there is sharp angulation or outpouching at the base of the tongue at the upper surgical line of closure. An abrupt transition to the cervical esophagus may be seen. A small cricopharyngeal impression may be noted. The pharynx should not be deviated from the midline more than approximately 0.5 cm.[41]

In the early postoperative period, the complications of laryngectomy include formation of fistula, abscess, and edema with obstruction. Late complications following laryngectomy include stricture for-

mation, dysphagia due to retracted constrictor muscles, and tumor recurrence.

Pharyngocutaneous Fistulae

Pharyngocutaneous fistulae occur in approximately 6% of patients following laryngectomy, usually in the immediate postoperative period.[41] If a pharyngocutaneous fistula occurs later, it may signify recurrent tumor. Fistulae usually develop along the anterior aspect of the neopharyngeal tube at the base of the tongue or near the tracheostomy (Fig. 4–32). Fistulae may extend onto the skin or end blindly in the soft tissues of the neck.

Benign Strictures

Luminal narrowing to a diameter of less than 5 mm is considered a postoperative stricture.[41] Benign strictures following laryngectomy appear (1) as short, web-like narrowings less than 5 mm in length at the upper or lower ends of the closure line or (2) as long, smooth, tapered symmetric narrowings greater than 3 cm in length involving the majority of the neopharynx (Fig. 4–33). Pharyngeal luminal narrowings of intermediate length (1 to 3 cm) are often due to recurrent tumor. Deviation of pharyngeal strictures from the midline is uncommon and usually indicates tumor recurrence. Short strictures usually represent a postoperative change. Long strictures are usually the result of radiotherapy or insufficient pharyngeal mucosa at the time of the surgical closure.

Despite the presence of a radiologic stricture, patients may not complain of dysphagia. Patients may compensate for pharyngeal narrowing by altering diet or chewing their food carefully.

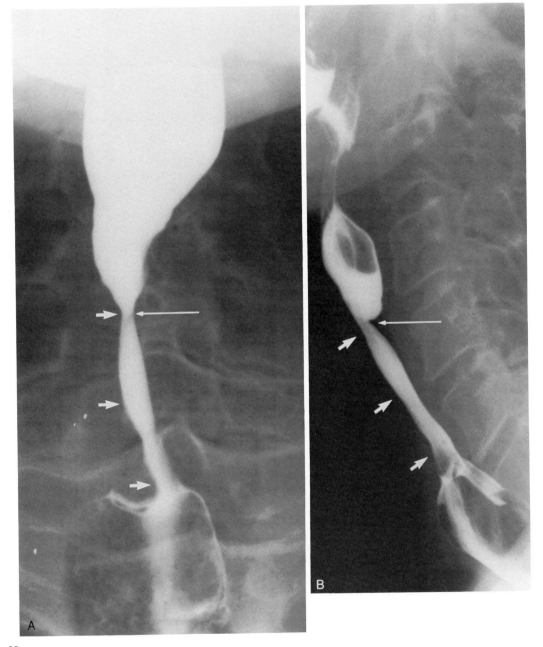

FIGURE 4–33

STRICTURE FOLLOWING TOTAL LARYNGECTOMY. A and B, A diffuse, smooth narrowing (*short arrows*) of most of the neopharyngeal tube can be seen. The luminal diameter measures less than 5 mm. A short web (*long arrow*) is present at the proximal margin of the stricture.

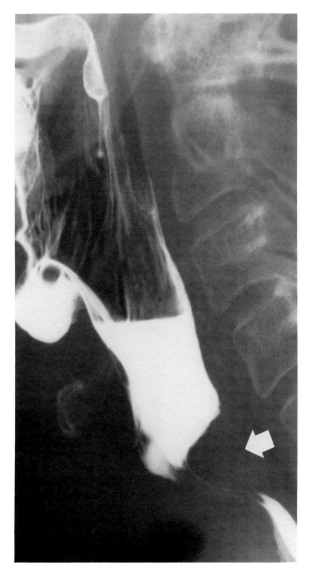

FIGURE 4-34

RETRACTED CRICOPHARYNGEUS MUSCLE FOLLOWING SUBTOTAL LARYNGECTOMY. Lateral views of the pharynx show a smooth, broad-based mass impression (*arrow*) with tapered edges at the pharyngoesophageal segment. This "mass" changed over time.

Retracted Cricopharyngeus

At the time of laryngectomy, the thyropharyngeus and cricopharyngeus are removed from their thyroid and cricoid cartilage attachments, respectively. These muscles retract toward the posterior pharyngeal wall. Innervation of the cricopharyngeus may be partially or completed destroyed. These retracted muscles, especially the retracted cricopharyngeus, may appear as an extrinsic mass impression on the posterior pharyngeal wall (Fig. 4-34) and may be confused with recurrent tumor. However, tumors remain fixed and have irregular contour, but the prominent cricopharyngeus causes a smooth impression that changes size, shape, and position with swallowing.[8]

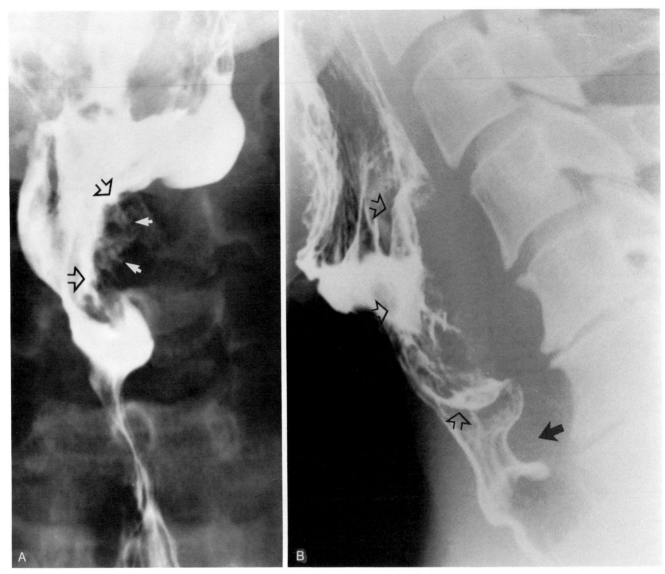

FIGURE 4–35

RECURRENT SQUAMOUS CELL CARCINOMA FOLLOWING LARYNGECTOMY. A frontal view (A) shows a focal mass (*open arrows*) that is 4 cm in length, has irregular mucosa (*white arrows*), and involves the left side of the neopharyngeal tube. The pharynx is mildly deviated to the right. The lateral view (B) shows lobulation of the posterior pharyngeal wall with increased thickness of the retropharyngeal space. This mass is superior to the smooth, 1-cm indentation of the cricopharyngeus (*black arrow*).

Recurrent Tumor

Tumor recurrence usually develops within the first 2 years following laryngectomy. The tumor is radiographically manifested as a focal mass that is larger than 1.5 to 2 cm and that does not change size or shape with swallowing (Fig. 4–35).[41] The mass deviates the pharynx more than 1 cm from the midline. The mass narrows the pharynx at the site of maximal deviation of the neopharyngeal tube. The mucosal surface is usually coarse or irregular. The posterior pharyngeal space may be widened, but this sign is not specific for tumor. Occasionally, fistulae into the soft tissues of the neck are seen. Thus, any mass measuring 1.5 to 2 cm that deviates the pharynx more than 1 cm from the midline should arouse suspicion of recurrent tumor.

REFERENCES

1. Jones, B., Kramer, S.S., and Donner, M.W.: Dynamic imaging of the pharynx. Gastrointest. Radiol. *10*:213, 1985.
2. DuBrul, E.L.: Sicher's Oral Anatomy, ed. 7. St. Louis, C.V. Mosby, 1980, p. 319.
3. Donner, M.W., Bosma, J.F., and Robertson, D.L.: Anatomy and physiology of the pharynx. Gastrointest. Radiol. *10*:196, 1985.
4. Ekberg, O., and Nylander, G.: Double contrast examination of the pharynx. Gastrointest. Radiol. *10*:263, 1985.
5. Rubesin, S.E., Jessurun, J., Robertson, D., et al.: Lines of the pharynx. Radiographics *7*:217, 1987.

6. Gromet, M., Homer, M.J., and Carter, B.L.: Lymphoid hyperplasia at the base of the tongue. Radiology 144:825, 1982.
7. Jones, B., Ravich, W.J., Donner, M.W., et al.: Pharyngoesophageal interrelationships: Observations and working concepts. Gastrointest. Radiol. 10:225, 1985.
8. Rubesin, S.E., and Glick, S.N.: The tailored double-contrast pharyngogram. CRC Crit. Rev. Diagn. Imaging 28:133, 1988.
9. Levine, M.S., and Rubesin, S.E.: Radiologic investigation of dysphagia. AJR 154:1157, 1990.
10. Jing, B.S.: Roentgen examination of the larynx and hypopharynx. Radiol. Clin. North Am. 8:361, 1970.
11. Jing, B.S.: The pharynx and larynx: Roentgenographic technique. Semin. Roentgenol. 9:259, 1974.
12. Rubesin, S.E., Jones, B., and Donner, M.W.: Contrast pharyngography: The importance of phonation. AJR 148:269, 1987.
13. Bachman, A.L., Seaman, W.B., and Macken, K.L.: Lateral pharyngeal diverticula. Radiology 91:774, 1968.
14. Rubesin, S.E., Jessurun, J., Robertson, D., et al.: Lines of the pharynx. Radiographics 7:217, 1987.
15. Ardran, G.M., Kemp, F.H., and Lund, W.S.: The aetiology of the posterior pharyngeal diverticulum: A cineradiographic study. J. Laryngol. Otol. 78:333, 1964.
16. Perott, J.W.: Anatomical aspects of hypopharyngeal diverticula. Aust. N. Z. J. Surg. 31:307, 1962.
17. Zaino, C., Jacobson, H.G., Lepow, H., and Ozturk, C.: The pharyngoesophageal sphincter. Radiology 89:639, 1967.
18. Ekberg, O., and Nylander, G.: Lateral diverticula from the pharyngo-esophageal junction area. Radiology 146:117, 1983.
19. Clements, J.L., Cox, G.W., Torres, W.E., and Weens, H.S.: Cervical esophageal webs—a roentgen-anatomic correlation. AJR 121:221, 1974.
20. Seaman, W.B.: The significance of webs in the hypopharynx and upper esophagus. Radiology 89:32, 1967.
21. Nosher, J.L., Campbell, W.L., and Seaman, W.B.: The clinical significance of cervical esophageal and hypopharyngeal webs. Radiology 117:45, 1975.
22. Ekberg, O., and Nylander, G.: Webs and web-like formations in the pharynx and cervical esophagus. Diagnostic Imaging 53:10, 1983.
23. Pitman, R.G., and Fraser, G.M.: The post-cricoid impression on the oesophagus. Clin. Radiol. 16:34, 1965.
24. Chisholm, M., Ardran, G.M., Callender, S.T., and Wright, R.: Iron deficiency and autoimmunity in post-cricoid webs. Q. J. Med. 40:421, 1971.
25. Balfe, D.M., and Heiken, J.P.: Contrast evaluation of structural lesions of the pharynx. Curr. Probl. Diagn. Radiol. 15:73, 1986.
26. Dodds, W.J., Logeman, J.A., and Stewart, E.T.: Radiologic assessment of abnormal oral and pharyngeal phases of swallowing. AJR 154:965, 1990.
27. Curtis, D.J., and Sepulveda, G.U.: Epiglottic motion: Video recording of muscular dysfunction. Radiology 148:473, 1983.
28. Bachman, A.L.: Benign, non-neoplastic conditions of the larynx and pharynx. Radiol. Clin. North Am. 16:273, 1978.
29. Levine, M.S., Rubesin, S.E., and Ott, D.J.: Update on esophageal radiology. AJR 155:993, 1990.
30. Seaman, W.B.: Contrast radiography in neoplastic disease of the larynx and pharynx. Semin. Roentgenol. 9:301, 1974.
31. Semenkovich, J.W., Balfe, D.M., Weyman, P.J., et al.: Barium pharyngography: Comparison of single and double contrast. AJR 144:715, 1985.
32. Wagonfeld, D.J.H., Harwood, A.R., Bryce, D.P., et al.: Secondary primary respiratory tract malignant neoplasms in supraglottic carcinoma. Arch. Otolaryngol. 107:135, 1981.
33. Goldstein, H.M., and Zornoza, J.: Association of squamous cell carcinoma of the head and neck with cancer of the esophagus. AJR 131:791, 1978.
34. Thompson, W.M., Oddson, T.A., Kelvin, F., et al.: Synchronous and metachronous squamous cell carcinoma of the head, neck, and esophagus. Gastrointest. Radiol. 3:123, 1978.
35. Rubesin, S.E., Jones, B., and Donner, M.W.: Radiology of the adult soft palate. Dysphagia 2:8, 1978.
36. Dockerty, M.D., Parkhill, E.M., Dahlin, D.C., et al.: Tumors of the Oral Cavity and Pharynx. Washington D.C., Armed Forces Institute of Pathology, 1968.
37. Silver, C.E.: Surgical management of neoplasms of the larynx, hypopharynx and cervical esophagus. Curr. Probl. Surg. 14:2, 1977.
38. Apter, A.J., Levine, M.S., and Glick, S.N.: Carcinomas of the base of the tongue: Diagnosis using double-contrast radiography of the pharynx. Radiology 151:123, 1984.
39. Rubesin, S.E., Rabischong, P., Bilaniuk, L.T., et al.: Contrast examination of the soft palate with cross-sectional correlation. Radiographics 8:641, 1988.
40. Ekberg, O., and Nylander, G.: Pharyngeal dysfunction after treatment for pharyngeal cancer with surgery and radiotherapy. Gastrointest. Radiol. 8:97, 1983.
41. Balfe, D.M., Koehler, R.E., Setzen, M., et al.: Barium examination of the esophagus after total laryngectomy. Radiology 143:501, 1982.
42. DiSantis, D.J., Balfe, D.M., Koehler, R.E., et al.: Barium examination of the pharynx after vertical hemilaryngectomy. AJR 141:335, 1983.

ESOPHAGUS

5

Marc S. Levine, M.D.
Igor Laufer, M.D.

TECHNIQUE

Double contrast views of the esophagus are obtained at the beginning of the routine upper gastrointestinal examination. In patients with esophageal symptoms, double contrast views of the esophagus are also obtained as part of the routine esophagram. After ingesting an effervescent agent, the patient gulps a high-density barium suspension in the upright, left posterior oblique position so that the esophagus is projected free of the spine. One 3-on-1 or two 2-on-1 spot radiographs of the upper and lower esophagus obtained in rapid succession usually provide excellent double contrast views of the distended esophagus (Fig. 5–1). If these views are inadequate, however, the examination of the stomach and duodenum should be completed before the esophagus is reexamined at the end of the study. At that time, other maneuvers may be attempted to improve the quality of the esophageal examination. The patient may be asked to pinch the nose with one hand while gulping barium to increase the amount of air swallowing. An additional dose of effervescent agent can also be given to improve gaseous distention of the esophagus. Bet-

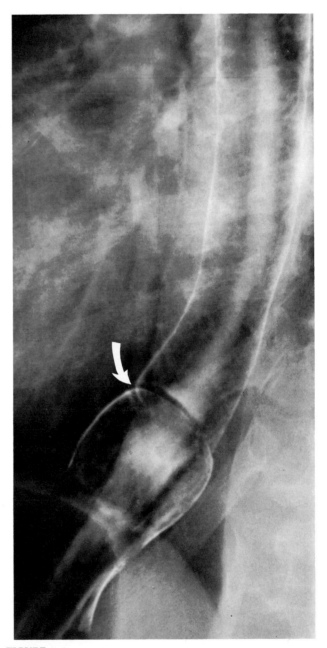

FIGURE 5–2

PRONE OBLIQUE POSITION. Double contrast view of hiatal hernia, lower esophageal ring *(arrow)*, and distal esophagus.

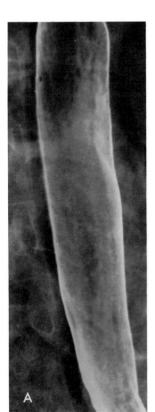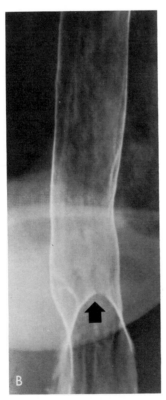

FIGURE 5–1

NORMAL ESOPHAGUS, UPRIGHT. *A,* Normal appearance of thoracic esophagus. Note how esophageal mucosa is smooth and featureless, and how mucosal folds have been completely effaced.

B, The distal esophagus with typical arch-shaped configuration *(arrow)* at gastroesophageal junction.

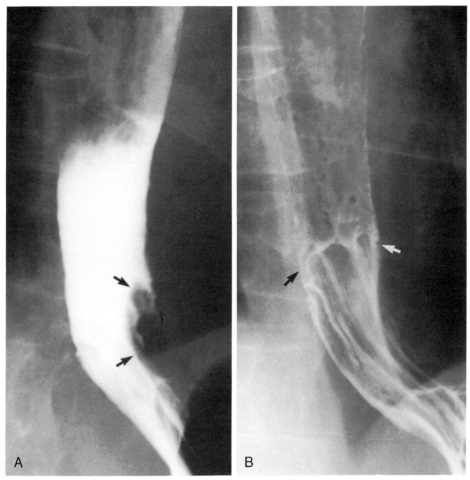

FIGURE 5–3

TUBE ESOPHAGRAM. *A,* Initial double contrast radiograph is suboptimal because of pooling of barium in distal esophagus. However, there is a suggestion of a polypoid lesion *(arrows)* near the gastroesophageal junction.

B, Tube esophagram shows that this apparent lesion resulted from prominent folds in a sliding hiatal hernia *(arrows)*. Note mucosal irregularity in distal esophagus due to reflux esophagitis. (From Levine, M.S., et al.: The tube esophagram: A technique for obtaining a detailed double-contrast examination of the esophagus. AJR *142*:293–298, 1984, with permission, © by American Roentgen Ray Society.)

ter double contrast views of the distal esophagus can sometimes be obtained with the patient in the prone oblique position, particularly if the lower esophageal sphincter is incompetent (Fig. 5–2).[1]

Paralysis of the esophagus by relaxant drugs may also facilitate the double contrast examination. Anticholinergic agents such as Buscopan (hyoscine *N*-butyl bromide) and Pro-Banthine (propantheline bromide) are effective in abolishing esophageal peristalsis. In contrast, glucagon relaxes the lower esophageal sphincter but does not affect esophageal peristalsis.[2] This drug therefore cannot be used to induce esophageal relaxation.

The greatest diagnostic difficulties usually occur in the distal esophagus, where poor distention or pooling of barium may obscure mucosal detail. When routine double contrast radiographs are inconclusive or when an equivocal abnormality is identified, a tube esophagram can be performed for a more detailed examination.[3] For this study, a small red rubber catheter is passed through the mouth into the proximal thoracic esophagus. The patient is instructed to swallow high-density barium as air is gently insufflated through the catheter. In this way, one can obtain more controlled double contrast views of the middle and distal esophagus in various projections to better delineate equivocal findings on the routine examination (Fig. 5–3).

NORMAL APPEARANCES

The fully distended esophagus normally has a smooth, featureless appearance on double contrast radiographs (see Fig. 5–1). During swallowing, the relaxed cardia produces a typical arch-shaped shadow at the gastroesophageal junction (see Fig. 5–1B). A small indentation is frequently seen on the anterior wall of the cervical esophagus (Fig. 5–4). This indentation is thought to be caused by a venous plexus and should not be mistaken for a cervical esophageal tumor or web (Fig. 5–5).[4] Typical indentations due to the aortic arch and left main bronchus may also be seen in the middle third of the esophagus (Fig. 5–6). In patients with a sliding hiatal hernia, a thin, zigzagging radiolucent line or "Z-line" demarcating the squamocolumnar junction is occasionally seen (Fig. 5–7).

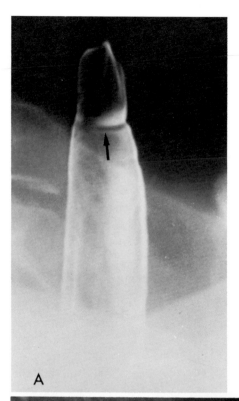

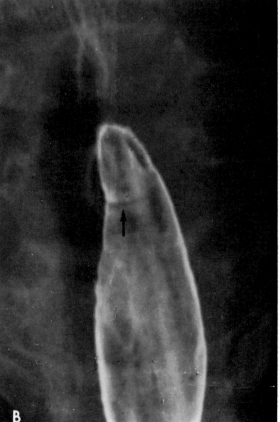

FIGURE 5–5

Cervical esophageal web (*arrows*) seen in lateral (*A*) and frontal (*B*) projections.

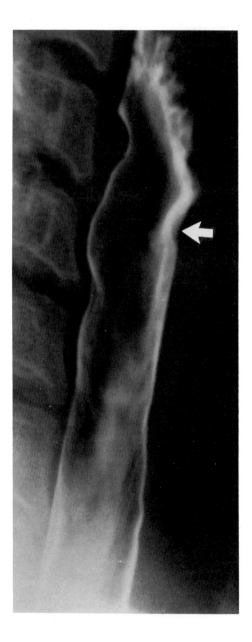

FIGURE 5–4

Normal cervical esophagus with anterior venous indentation (*arrow*). Note slight posterior impression from cervical osteophyte.

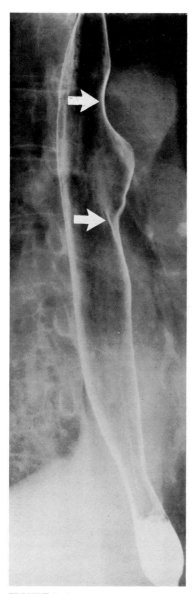

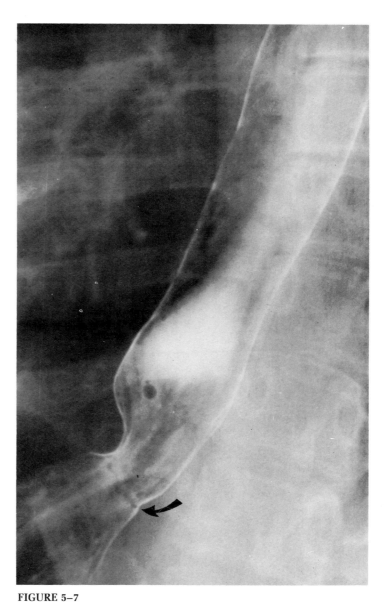

FIGURE 5–6

Normal impressions (*arrows*) due to aortic arch and left main bronchus.

FIGURE 5–7

Zigzagging radiolucent line or "Z-line" (*arrow*), probably representing the squamocolumnar junction.

As the esophagus collapses, the normal longitudinal folds become visible as thin, straight, parallel structures no more than several millimeters in width (Fig. 5–8). In some patients, fine transverse folds may also be demonstrated in the middle or distal esophagus (Fig. 5–9). These transverse folds were originally described as a normal feature of the feline esophagus.[5] However, they can also occur as a transient phenomenon in humans, due to contraction of the longitudinal fibers of the muscularis mucosae.[6] These delicate transverse folds are only 1 to 2 mm wide and extend completely across the esophagus without interruption.[7] Because the folds are transient, they may be seen on one spot film and disappear moments later (Fig. 5–10). Although its clinical significance is uncertain, this phenomenon has been observed with increased frequency in patients with gastroesophageal reflux.[7] Contraction of the muscularis mucosae could represent the earliest stage of a motor abnormality in the esophagus, either on an idiopathic basis or as a response to mild esophagitis. In any case, these transverse folds should be distinguished from the broad transverse bands seen in patients with nonpropulsive tertiary esophageal contractions (Fig. 5–11). They should also be differentiated from fixed transverse folds in the esophagus due to scarring from reflux esophagitis (see Fig. 5–34 and the later section, "Gastroesophageal Reflux Disease").

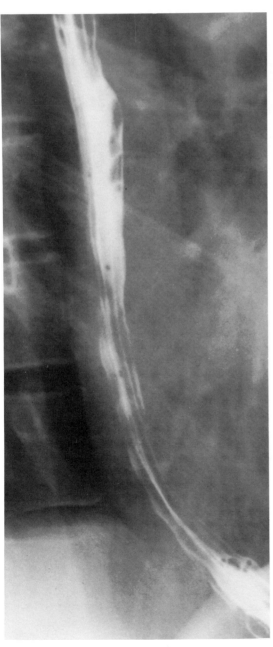

FIGURE 5–8

Normal longitudinal folds in partially collapsed esophagus.

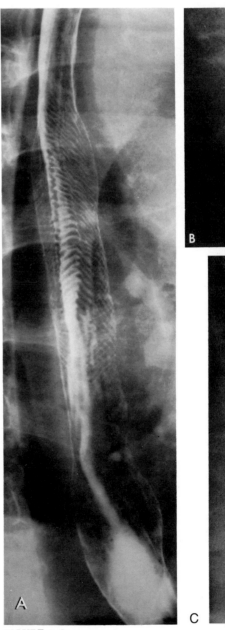
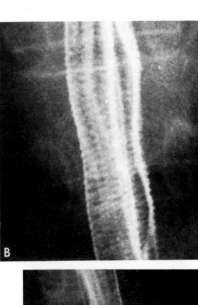
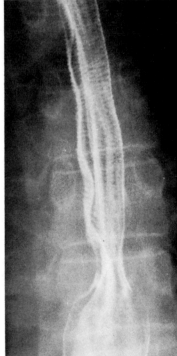

FIGURE 5–9

Three examples (A through C) of transverse folds in the esophagus. These folds are thought to result from contraction of the longitudinally oriented muscularis mucosae. (From Gohel, V.K., et al.: Transverse folds in the human esophagus. Radiology 128:303–308, 1978, with permission.)

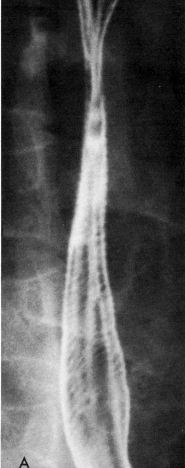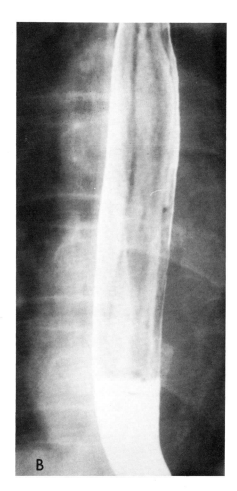

FIGURE 5–10

TRANSIENT NATURE OF TRANSVERSE FOLDS. *A,* Transverse folds are present in middle and distal esophagus.

B, Moments later, the folds are no longer visible.

FIGURE 5–11

Transverse bands due to contraction of muscularis propria. These bands are thicker than the transverse folds in Figures 5–9 and 5–10.

ARTIFACTS

Double contrast examinations of the esophagus may produce a variety of artifacts that simulate or obscure mucosal disease:[8]

1. *Localized noncoating* of a segment of the esophagus may suggest the presence of a tumor (Fig. 5–12A). With additional barium, however, the apparent abnormality disappears (Fig. 5–12B).

2. *"Kissing" artifact* in the esophagus due to incomplete distention with adherence of the anterior and posterior walls can also mimic the appearance of a mucosal or submucosal tumor on one or more films.

3. *Undissolved effervescent agent* may be seen as a transient finding in the normal esophagus (Fig. 5–13) or as a persistent finding in the presence of esophageal obstruction. Undissolved effervescent granules should not be mistaken for the nodular mucosa of *Candida* esophagitis.

4. *Gas bubbles* can usually be recognized as artifacts by their smooth, round appearance on double contrast radiographs. Occasionally, however, small air bubbles in the esophagus may simulate mucosal nodularity due to *Candida* esophagitis or superficial spreading carcinoma (Fig. 5–14).

5. *Barium precipitates* may be seen as small, white dots on the esophageal mucosa (Fig. 5–15A). These precipitates can be distinguished from superficial ulcers or erosions by the absence of edema, marginal irregularity, or associated motor abnormalities. These problems can be avoided by choosing a suitable high-density barium suspension for the double contrast examination and by insuring that the suspension is properly prepared.

6. A *pseudointraluminal diverticulum* may be seen in the esophagus when the barium column disintegrates, leaving a glob of barium surrounded by a thin, radiolucent halo (see Fig. 5–15B).[9] This artifact is caused by the interaction of barium with retained fluid and debris due to esophageal stasis in patients with strictures or motility disorders.

7. *Flow artifact* occurs when mucosal detail is obscured by a thick coating of high-density barium in the esophagus (Fig. 5–16A).[10] However, this problem can be minimized by slightly delaying exposure of the films and by asking the patient to take dry swallows after the barium bolus has been ingested (Fig. 5–16B).

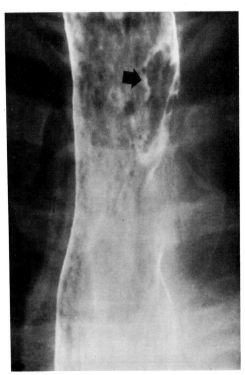

A

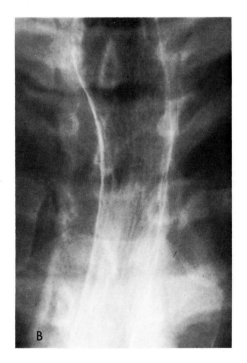

B

FIGURE 5–12

LOCALIZED NONCOATING IN ESOPHAGUS. *A,* Localized noncoating *(arrow)* simulating carcinoma.

    B, Additional view with improved coating shows that this area is normal.

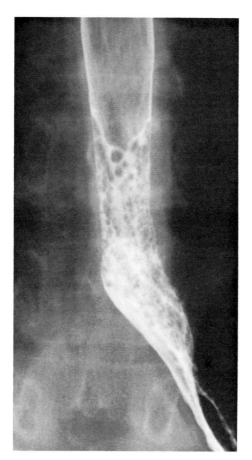

FIGURE 5–13

Undissolved effervescent granules in the distal esophagus.

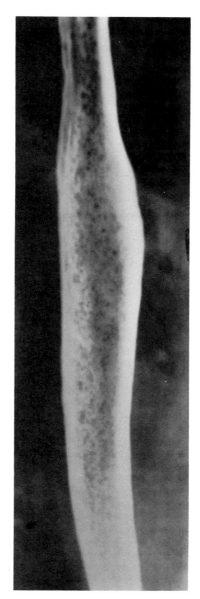

FIGURE 5–14

Gas bubbles throughout the esophagus, simulating diffuse mucosal nodularity.

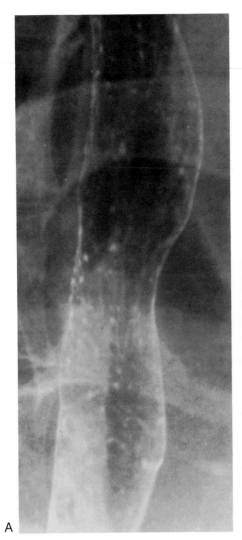

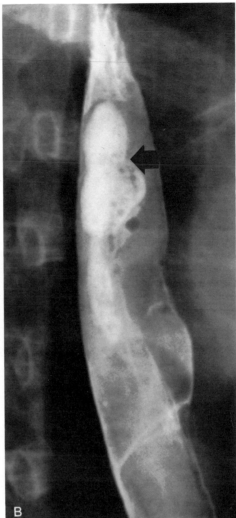

A

B

FIGURE 5–15

BARIUM-RELATED ARTIFACTS. *A,* Barium precipitates in esophagus.

B, Pseudointraluminal diverticulum *(arrow)* due to interaction of barium with retained fluid and debris in esophagus of a patient with a motility disorder. (*B,* From Levine, M.S.: Radiology of the Esophagus. Philadelphia, W.B. Saunders, 1989, p. 13.)

FIGURE 5–16

FLOW ARTIFACT IN ESOPHAGUS. *A,* Residual layer of high-density barium obscures mucosal detail in distal esophagus.

B, Repeat double contrast view moments later shows reflux esophagitis with mucosal nodularity and inflammatory esophagogastric polyp *(arrow)* not seen on earlier view. (From Levine, M.S., et al.: Double-contrast upper gastrointestinal examination: Technique and interpretation. Radiology *168:*593–602, 1988, with permission.)

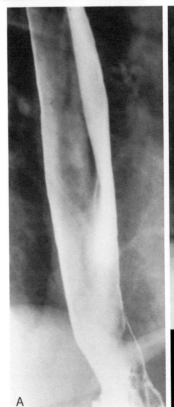

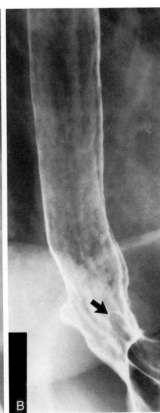

A

B

INFLAMMATORY CONDITIONS

Gastroesophageal Reflux Disease

Reflux Esophagitis

Reflux esophagitis is by far the most common inflammatory condition in the esophagus. Traditional signs of esophagitis revealed by single contrast barium studies include thickened folds, decreased distensibility, marginal irregularity or ulceration, and abnormal motility. However, these findings are difficult to evaluate and are frequently found only in patients with severe reflux disease. Double contrast examinations permit a more detailed assessment of the esophageal mucosa to detect superficial ulceration or other changes of mild or moderate esophagitis that cannot be detected by conventional barium studies. As a result, double contrast esophagography has a sensitivity approaching 90% in diagnosing reflux esophagitis.[11, 12]

Double contrast studies sometimes may demonstrate hiatal hernias and lower esophageal rings (see Fig. 5–2). However, single contrast esophagrams obtained with the patient in the prone position permit optimal distention of the distal esophagus and gastroesophageal junction, allowing demonstration of hernias, strictures, or rings that are not visible on the double contrast portion of the study (Fig. 5–17).[13] Thus, the routine esophagram should be performed as a biphasic examination that includes upright double contrast and prone single contrast views of the esophagus.

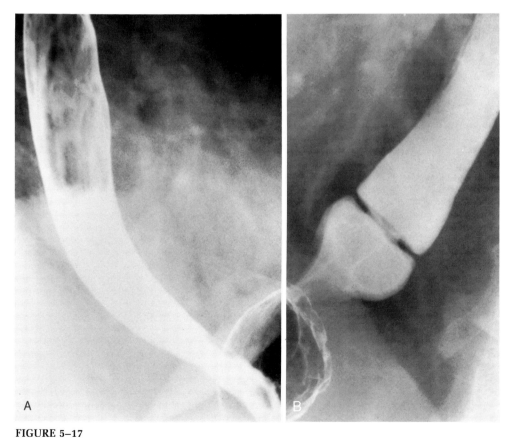

FIGURE 5–17

SCHATZKI RING ONLY SEEN ON PRONE SINGLE CONTRAST ESOPHAGRAM. *A*, Upright double contrast view of distal esophagus shows no evidence of lower esophageal ring.

B, However, prone single contrast view from same examination shows hiatal hernia with unequivocal Schatzki ring above hernia.

In the early stages of reflux esophagitis, edema and inflammation may be manifested by a finely nodular or granular appearance of the mucosa in the distal third or two thirds of the thoracic esophagus (Fig. 5–18).[14, 15] Other patients may have more coarse nodularity of the mucosa. Occasionally, severe reflux esophagitis may produce inflammatory exudates or pseudomembranes that are indistinguishable from the plaques of *Candida* esophagitis (Fig. 5–19A).[16] A single large pseudomembrane may also resemble a plaque-like carcinoma, particularly an adenocarcinoma arising in Barrett's esophagus (Fig. 5–19B).[16] However, pseudomembrane formation may be suggested by the presence of other discrete satellite lesions or by a change in the size or appearance of the lesion during the radiologic examination. When the radiographic findings are equivocal, endoscopy and biopsy may be required to rule out malignancy.

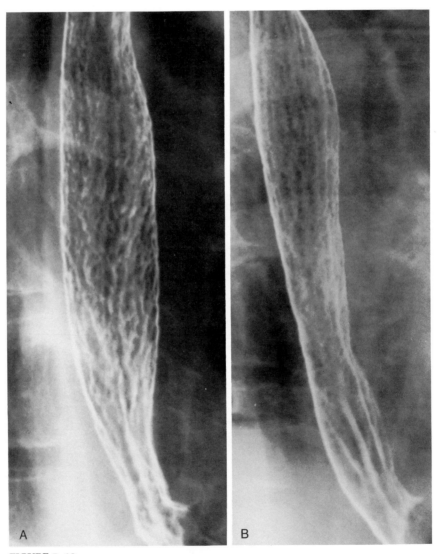

FIGURE 5–18

Two examples (A and B) of finely nodular or granular mucosa in distal half of esophagus due to reflux esophagitis. (From Levine, M.S.: Radiology of the Esophagus. Philadelphia, W.B. Saunders, 1989, p. 19.)

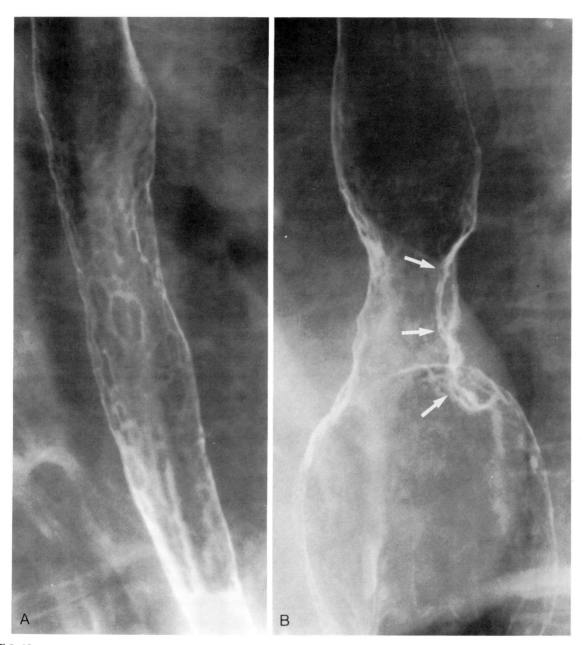

FIGURE 5–19

REFLUX ESOPHAGITIS WITH PSEUDOMEMBRANES. *A*, Multiple pseudomembranes in distal half of esophagus, mimicking the appearance of *Candida* esophagitis. (Courtesy of Howard Kessler, M.D., Philadelphia, Pennsylvania.)

B, Hiatal hernia and peptic stricture with large pseudomembrane *(arrows)* on one wall of stricture. A plaque-like carcinoma arising in Barrett's esophagus could produce a similar appearance. (From Levine, M.S., et al.: Pseudomembranes in reflux esophagitis. Radiology *159*:43–45, 1986, with permission.)

Reflux esophagitis may also be manifested by thickened longitudinal folds due to submucosal inflammation and edema. These thickened folds may have a smooth, lobulated, or scalloped configuration, occasionally mimicking the appearance of esophageal varices (Fig. 5–20). Other patients with reflux esophagitis may have a single prominent fold that arises in the gastric fundus and extends above the gastroesophageal junction as a polypoid protuberance in the distal esophagus (Fig. 5–21A; see Fig. 5–16B).[17, 18] Occasionally, these lesions may be seen in a hiatal hernia or in the stomach when the hernia is reduced (Fig. 5–

21B). These lesions are called "inflammatory" esophagogastric polyps and are thought to be a manifestation of chronic reflux esophagitis. Because these lesions have no malignant potential, endoscopic resection is unwarranted when typical inflammatory polyps are found on double contrast studies.

Shallow ulcers and erosions caused by reflux esophagitis may appear as one or more streaks or dots of barium in the distal esophagus at or near the gastroesophageal junction (Fig. 5–22).[19, 20] Some ulcers may be irregular, while others may have a linear configuration with their long axis perpendicular to

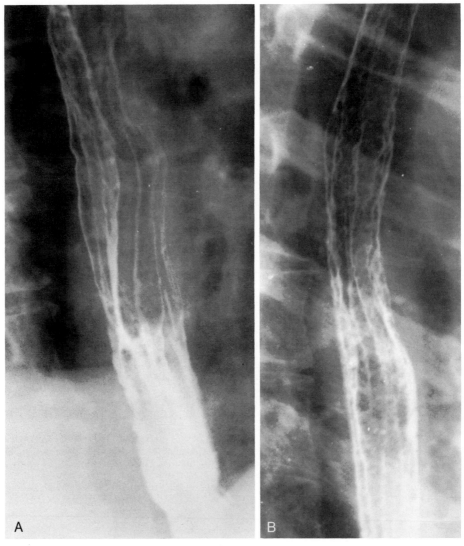

FIGURE 5–20

Two examples (A and B) of reflux esophagitis with thickened longitudinal folds. The folds in B are more serpiginous than those in A and could be mistaken for varices. (From Levine, M.S.: Radiology of the Esophagus. Philadelphia, W.B. Saunders, 1989, p. 25.)

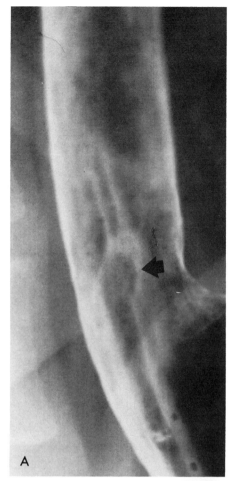

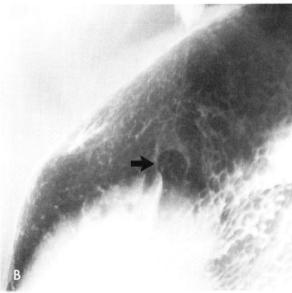

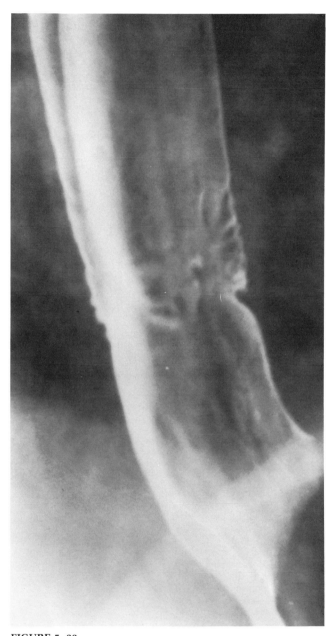

FIGURE 5–22

Reflux esophagitis with discrete, superficial ulcers in distal esophagus near the gastroesophageal junction. Note radiating folds and puckering of esophageal wall.

FIGURE 5–21

INFLAMMATORY ESOPHAGOGASTRIC POLYP. *A,* A prominent mucosal fold extends from the gastric fundus into the distal esophagus as a polypoid protuberance *(arrow).*

B, With the esophagus collapsed, the polypoid fold is visible within the stomach *(arrow).*

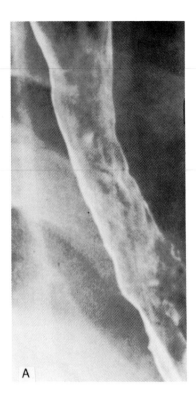

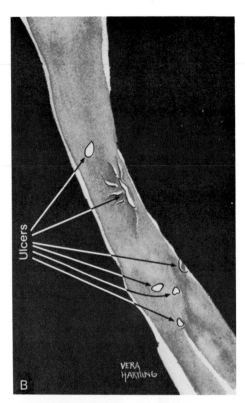

FIGURE 5–23

A and B, Reflux esophagitis with both linear and irregular shallow ulcers in middle and distal esophagus.

FIGURE 5–24

A and B, Reflux esophagitis with linear erosion in distal esophagus. Note radiating folds and retraction of adjacent esophageal wall. (Courtesy of Marc P. Banner, M.D., Philadelphia, Pennsylvania.)

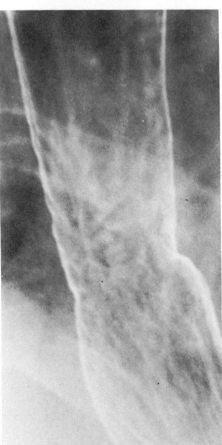

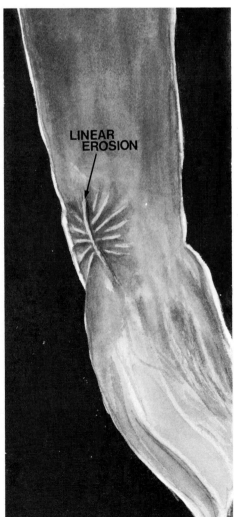

the gastroesophageal junction (Figs. 5–23 through 5–25). The ulcers may be surrounded by a radiolucent halo of edematous mucosa, and there may be fine radiating folds with slight retraction of the adjacent esophageal wall (Figs. 5–24 and 5–25). Occasionally, longitudinal ulcers may have a serpiginous or flowing appearance, with multiple transverse folds straddling the area of ulceration (Fig. 5–26).[21] Some patients may have relatively widespread ulceration involving the distal third or two thirds of the thoracic esophagus (Fig. 5–27). However, ulceration in reflux esophagitis

tends to occur as a continuous area of disease extending proximally from the gastroesophageal junction, so that the presence of superficial ulcers in the mid-esophagus with distal esophageal sparing should suggest another etiologic factor for the patient's esophagitis. With further progression, reflux esophagitis may be manifested by relatively large ulcer craters in the distal esophagus. These ulcers can be recognized en face but are best visualized when they are projected tangentially beyond the normal contour of the esophagus (Figs. 5–28 and 5–29).

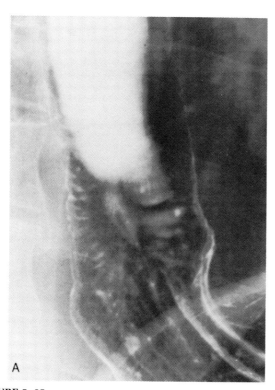
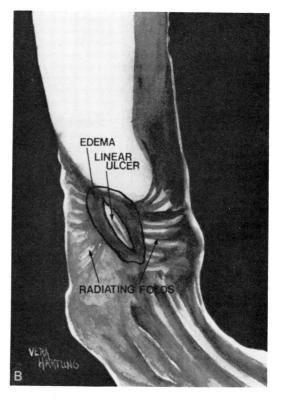

FIGURE 5–25

A and B, Reflux esophagitis with linear ulcer in distal esophagus. Note ulcer crater, surrounding edema, and radiating folds.

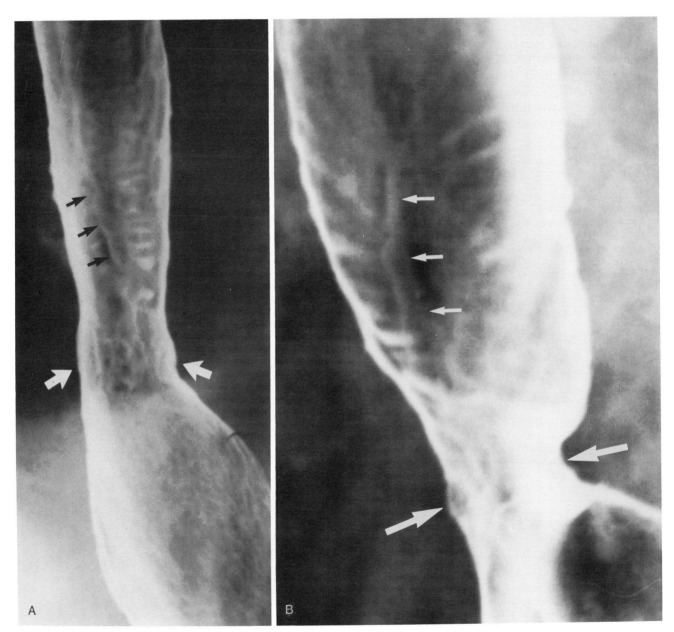

FIGURE 5–26

Two examples *(A and B)* of reflux esophagitis with serpiginous, longitudinally oriented ulcers *(small arrows)*. In both cases, note multiple transverse folds straddling ulcers and associated peptic strictures *(large arrows)*. *(A,* From Levine, M.S., and Goldstein, H.M.: Fixed transverse folds in the esophagus: A sign of reflux esophagitis. AJR 143:275–278, 1984, with permission, © by American Roentgen Ray Society. *B,* Courtesy of Harvey M. Goldstein, M. D., San Antonio, Texas.)

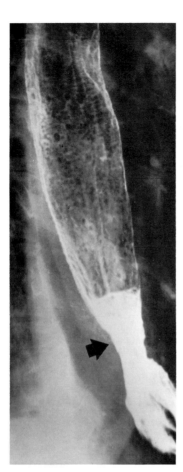

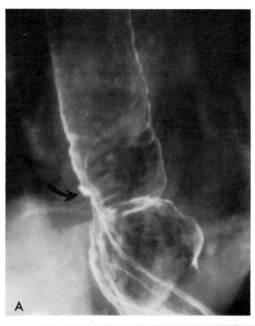

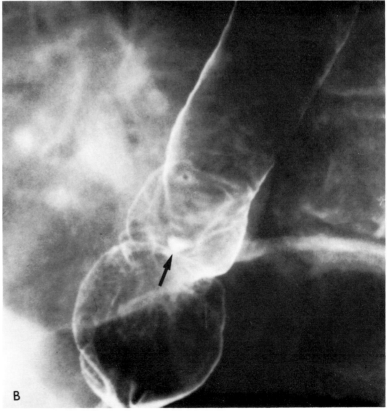

FIGURE 5–27

Reflux esophagitis with diffuse superficial ulceration of distal esophagus and associated peptic stricture *(arrow)* near gastroesophageal junction. (Courtesy of Henry I. Goldberg, M.D., San Francisco, California.)

FIGURE 5–28

Reflux esophagitis with discrete ulcer *(arrows)* in distal esophagus. *A,* Profile view. *B,* En face view.

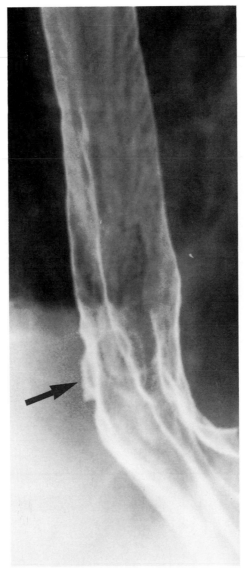

FIGURE 5–29

Reflux esophagitis with relatively large, flat ulcer *(arrow)* in distal esophagus. (From Levine, M.S.: Radiology of the Esophagus. Philadelphia, W.B. Saunders, 1989, p. 24.)

Peptic Scarring and Strictures

Healing of ulcers may be manifested by localized flattening or puckering of the distal esophagus at the site of the previous ulcer (Fig. 5–30). Further scarring from reflux esophagitis may lead to the development of circumferential peptic strictures, which classically appear as smooth, tapered areas of concentric narrowing in the distal esophagus above a sliding hiatal hernia (Fig. 5–31A). However, many strictures have an asymmetric appearance with puckering or deformity of one wall of the stricture due to asymmetric scarring from reflux esophagitis (Fig. 5–31B). As a result, a benign peptic stricture cannot always be differentiated radiographically from an infiltrating carcinoma, particularly an adenocarcinoma arising in Barrett's esophagus (see Chapter 6). Endoscopy therefore should be performed to rule out a malignant lesion when the radiographic findings are equivocal.

Peptic strictures occasionally may be associated with the development of focal outpouching or sacculation of the distal esophagus due to ballooning of the esophageal wall between areas of fibrosis (Fig. 5–32). The latter finding is particularly common in patients with scleroderma because of the severe esophagitis that occurs in these individuals (Fig. 5–

33). Scarring from reflux esophagitis may also be manifested by fixed transverse folds in the distal esophagus, producing a characteristic "stepladder" appearance due to pooling of barium between the folds (Fig. 5–34).[21] These transverse folds are usually 2 to 5 mm in width and do not extend more than halfway across the esophagus. They should be distinguished radiographically from the delicate transverse folds that are often observed as a transient finding on double contrast studies (see Figs. 5–9 and 5–10).

Esophageal intramural pseudodiverticulosis occasionally may be found in patients with peptic strictures (Fig. 5–35).[22] The pseudodiverticula represent dilated excretory ducts of deep mucous glands in the esophagus. They usually appear as 1- to 3-mm collec-

tions of barium projecting outside the esophageal lumen. Although the pseudodiverticula can be mistaken for ulcers, these structures often seem to be "floating" outside the esophagus without apparent communication with the lumen (Fig. 5–35), whereas true ulcers almost always communicate directly with the lumen. The majority of patients with esophageal intramural pseudodiverticulosis have associated reflux disease with localized pseudodiverticula in the region of a peptic stricture.[22] Thus, esophageal intramural pseudodiverticulosis probably represents a sequela of chronic reflux esophagitis, although the reason that so few patients with esophagitis develop this condition is unclear.

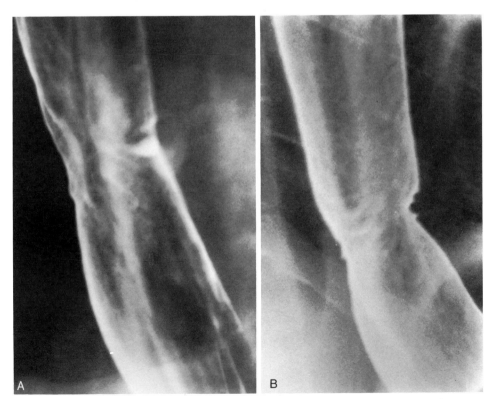

FIGURE 5–30

Two examples (A and B) of asymmetric puckering and retraction of distal esophagus, with radiating folds in this region due to scarring from reflux esophagitis.

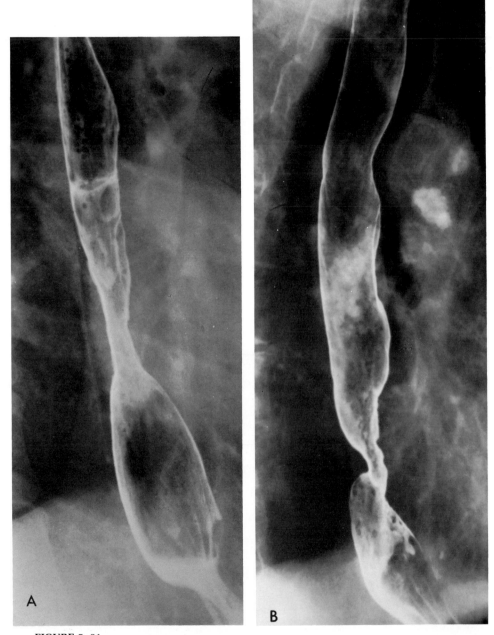

FIGURE 5–31

PEPTIC STRICTURES. *A*, Typical peptic stricture with concentric narrowing and smooth, tapered margins.

  B, Eccentric stricture with associated ulceration.

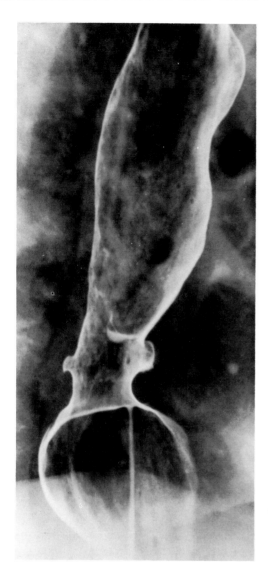

FIGURE 5-32

Peptic stricture with associated sacculations in distal esophagus. Note hiatal hernia below stricture.

FIGURE 5-33

Sacculated peptic stricture (arrows) in a patient with scleroderma.

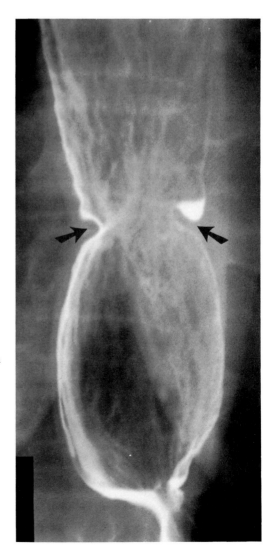

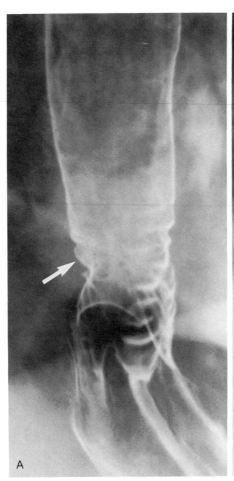
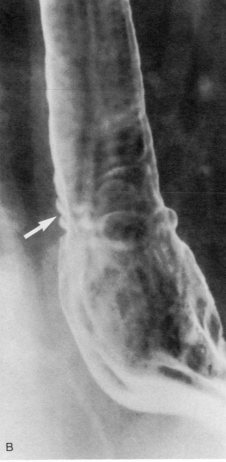

FIGURE 5–34

Two examples (A and B) of "stepladder" appearance with multiple transverse folds in distal esophagus due to scarring from reflux esophagitis. Note puckering of esophageal wall (arrows). (From Levine, M.S., and Goldstein, H.M.: Fixed transverse folds in the esophagus: A sign of reflux esophagitis. AJR 143:275–278, 1984, with permission, © by American Roentgen Ray Society.)

FIGURE 5–35

Two examples (A and B) of peptic strictures with localized esophageal intramural pseudodiverticulosis in region of stricture. Note how most pseudodiverticula, unlike ulcers, do not appear to communicate with esophageal lumen.

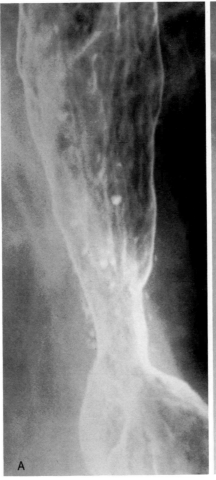
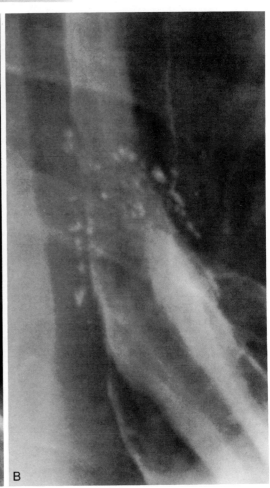

Barrett's Esophagus

Barrett's esophagus is a well-recognized entity in which there is progressive columnar metaplasia of the distal esophagus due to long-standing gastroesophageal reflux and reflux esophagitis. Barrett's esophagus is important because it is a premalignant condition associated with a significantly increased risk of the development of esophageal adenocarcinoma.

The classic radiologic features of Barrett's esopha-

gus consist of a high stricture or ulcer associated with a sliding hiatal hernia, gastroesophageal reflux, or both (Figs. 5–36 and 5–37).[23] However, recent studies have found that strictures are actually more common in the distal esophagus and that the majority of cases do not fit the classic description of a high stricture or ulcer.[24–26] A reticular mucosal pattern has also been described as a relatively specific sign of Barrett's esophagus on double contrast studies.[25] This reticular pattern is characterized by innumerable, tiny, barium-filled grooves or crevices on the esophageal mucosa,

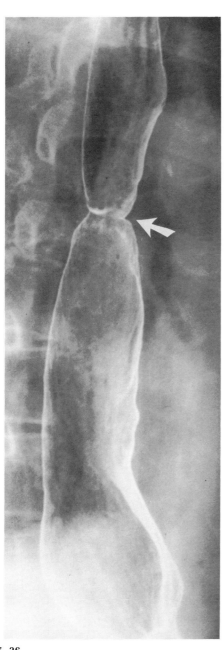

FIGURE 5–36

Barrett's esophagus with high stricture (arrow). (From Levine, M.S.: Radiology of the Esophagus. Philadelphia, W.B. Saunders, 1989, p. 40.)

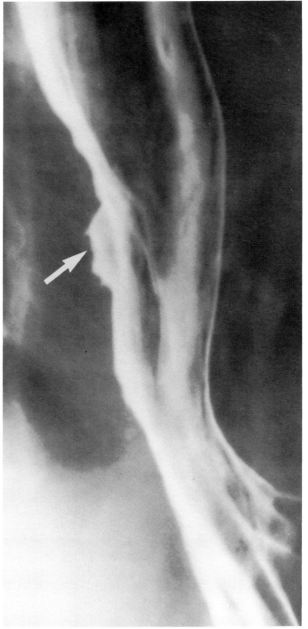

FIGURE 5–37

Barrett's esophagus with high ulcer (arrow). Note the relatively large ulcer crater at a greater distance from the gastroesophageal junction than would be expected for uncomplicated reflux esophagitis. (From Levine, M.S.: Radiology of the Esophagus. Philadelphia, W.B. Saunders, 1989, p. 41.)

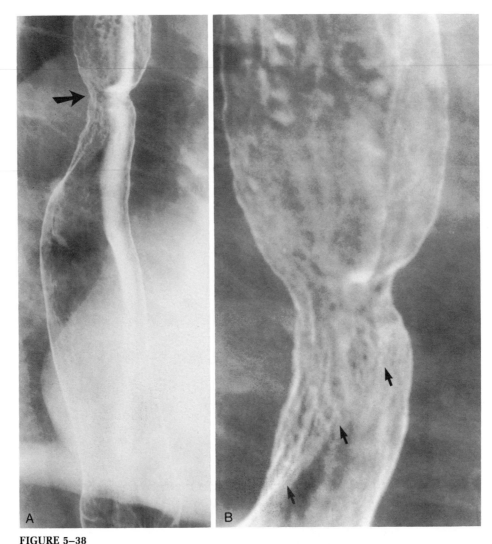

FIGURE 5–38

BARRETT'S ESOPHAGUS WITH HIGH STRICTURE AND RETICULAR MUCOSAL PATTERN.
A, Midesophageal stricture (arrow) with reticular pattern adjacent to distal aspect of stricture.
   B, Close-up view better delineates this delicate reticular pattern (arrows). (From Levine, M.S., et al.: Barrett esophagus: Reticular pattern of the mucosa. Radiology 147:663–667, 1983, with permission.)

often resembling the areae gastricae pattern found on double contrast studies of the stomach. In most cases, there is an associated stricture in the middle or, less frequently, distal esophagus, with the reticular pattern extending distally a short but variable distance from the stricture (Figs. 5–38 and 5–39). However, this finding has been observed in only a minority of patients with Barrett's esophagus.[25, 27] Other more common abnormalities in Barrett's esophagus, such as hiatal hernias, gastroesophageal reflux, reflux esophagitis, and peptic strictures, frequently occur in patients with uncomplicated reflux disease (Fig. 5–40). Thus, radiographic findings that are relatively

specific for Barrett's esophagus are not sensitive, and those that are sensitive are not specific. Many investigators therefore believe that esophagography has limited value as a screening examination for Barrett's esophagus and that endoscopy and biopsy are required to diagnose this condition.

Recently, however, Gilchrist and colleagues performed a blinded, retrospective study on 200 patients who underwent both double contrast esophagography and endoscopy because of severe reflux symptoms.[28] Patients were classified at high risk for Barrett's esophagus if the radiographs revealed a high stricture, high ulcer, or reticular mucosal pattern; at moderate risk if the radiographs revealed a distal stricture or reflux esophagitis; and at low risk if the esophagus appeared normal (i.e., if no esophagitis or strictures were noted). Using these radiologic criteria, the investigators found endoscopic proof of Barrett's esophagus in nine of 10 patients (90%) at high risk, in 12 of 73 patients (16%) at moderate risk, and in only one of 117 patients (less than 1%) at low risk for Barrett's esophagus. Although mild esophagitis can be missed radiographically, the data suggest that esophagitis severe enough to cause Barrett's esophagus can almost always be detected on technically adequate double contrast examinations. Thus, the major value of double contrast esophagography is its ability to classify patients with reflux symptoms into these various risk groups for Barrett's esophagus to determine the relative need for endoscopy and biopsy.

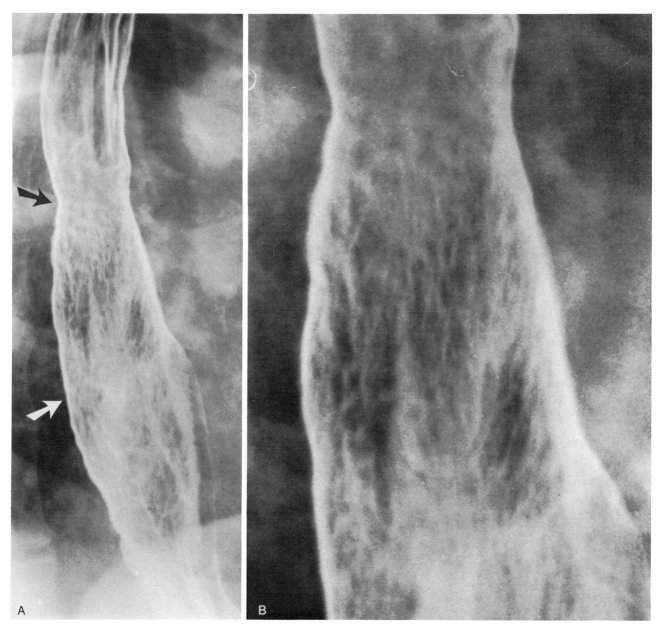

FIGURE 5–39

BARRETT'S ESOPHAGUS WITH HIGH STRICTURE AND RETICULAR MUCOSAL PATTERN. A, *Black arrow* indicates early stricture in midesophagus with reticular pattern extending distally to level of *white arrow*.

B, Close-up view better delineates this reticular pattern. (From Levine, M.S., et al.: Barrett esophagus: Reticular pattern of the mucosa. Radiology 147:663–667, 1983, with permission.)

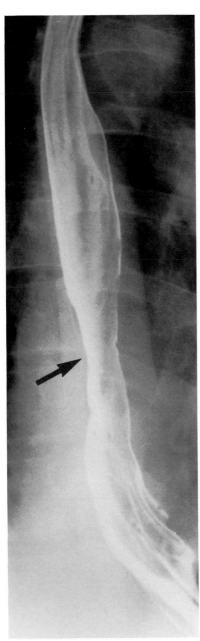

FIGURE 5–40

Barrett's esophagus with stricture (*arrow*) in distal esophagus above sliding hiatal hernia. An ordinary peptic stricture without Barrett's esophagus could produce identical findings. (From Gilchrist, A.M., et al.: Barrett's esophagus: Diagnosis by double-contrast esophagography. AJR *150*:97–102, 1988, with permission, © by American Roentgen Ray Society.)

Infections

Candida *Esophagitis*

Candida esophagitis is the most common infectious condition in the esophagus. It usually occurs as an opportunistic infection in patients who are immunocompromised as a result of underlying malignancy; other debilitating illnesses; treatment with radiation, steroids, or cytotoxic agents; or, most recently, acquired immunodeficiency syndrome (AIDS).[29–32] However, *Candida* esophagitis may also be caused by local esophageal stasis due to strictures, achalasia, or scleroderma.[33] Occasionally, *Candida* esophagitis may occur in otherwise healthy, "immunocompetent" individuals who have no underlying esophageal diseases.[34] The possibility of fungal infection therefore should not be excluded simply because the classic predisposing factors are not present in a particular patient.

Despite its frequency, the radiologic diagnosis of *Candida* esophagitis has been limited because it is a superficial disease with mucosal abnormalities that are difficult to detect with conventional single contrast barium studies. However, double contrast esophagography has a sensitivity of about 90% in diagnosing *Candida* esophagitis.[35, 36] The major advantage of this technique is its ability to demonstrate mucosal plaques that cannot easily be recognized by single contrast studies. As a result, only mild cases of *Candida* esophagitis are likely to be missed by the double contrast examination.

Candida esophagitis is first manifested radiographically by discrete plaque-like lesions corresponding to the characteristic white plaques seen during endoscopy. The plaques tend to be longitudinally oriented, appearing en face as linear or irregular filling defects with normal intervening mucosa (Fig. 5–41).[20, 35] Because these lesions have discrete borders, they may be etched in white by a thin layer of barium trapped between the edge of the plaque and the adjacent mucosa. Whether these mucosal plaques are localized or diffuse, their typical en face appearance should strongly suggest the diagnosis of *Candida* esophagitis.

In other patients, the esophagus may have a finely nodular or granular appearance due to mucosal edema and inflammation or actual tiny plaques on the mucosa (Fig. 5–42).[14, 37] When larger plaques are present, the lesions may coalesce, producing a distinctive "cobblestone" or "snakeskin" appearance (Fig. 5–43).[38] With further progression, the esophagus eventually may have a grossly irregular or "shaggy" contour due to multiple plaques, pseudomembranes, and ulcers (Fig. 5–44).[35, 37] Mucosal ulceration results primarily from sloughing of necrotic pseudomembranes in patients with advanced disease. Thus, ulceration in candidiasis is almost always associated with extensive plaque formation and rarely occurs on an otherwise normal background mucosa.

In recent years, the worsening AIDS epidemic has led to a much more fulminant form of *Candida* esophagitis. In one study, a shaggy esophagus was found in nearly 25% of AIDS patients with radio-graphically diagnosed *Candida* esophagitis.[37] Because this degree of esophagitis rarely occurs in other immunocompromised patients, the possibility of AIDS should be suspected when a shaggy esophagus is demonstrated by barium studies, particularly in high-risk patients.

Candida esophagitis occasionally may be associated with polypoid lesions in the esophagus due to coalescent masses of heaped-up necrotic debris and

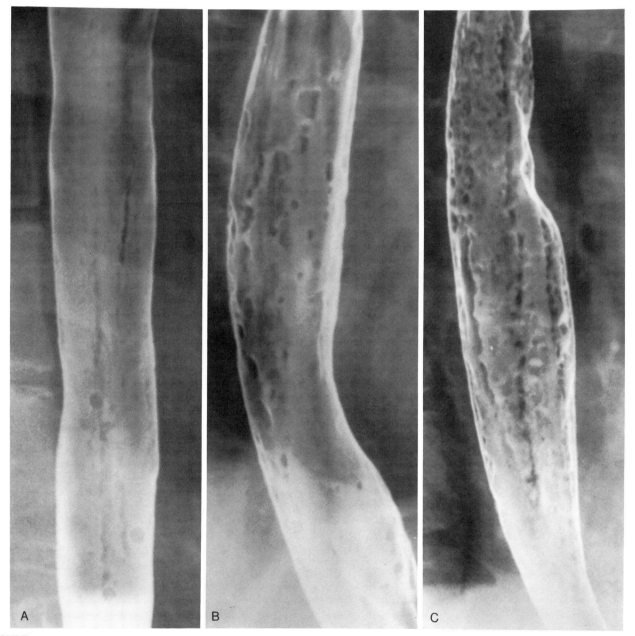

FIGURE 5–41

CANDIDA **ESOPHAGITIS WITH PLAQUES.** *A,* Several linear plaques seen in middle and distal esophagus are due to relatively early *Candida* esophagitis. (Note round filling defects due to air bubbles.)

B, More extensive plaque formation in another patient. Note irregular configuration of plaques.

C, More advanced case with numerous discrete, longitudinal plaques in esophagus. (From Levine, M.S., et al.: *Candida* esophagitis: Accuracy of radiographic diagnosis. Radiology *154*:581–587, 1985, with permission.)

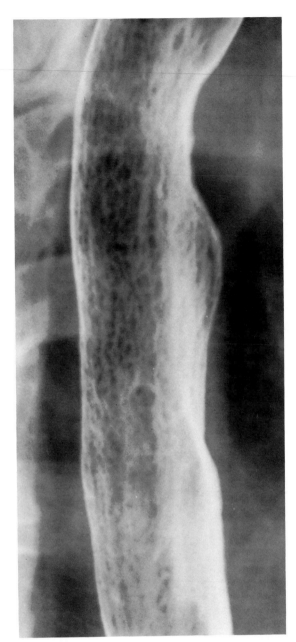

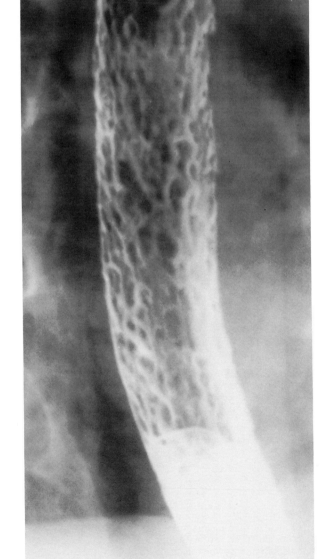

FIGURE 5–42

Candida esophagitis with finely nodular or granular mucosa due to tiny plaques in midesophagus.

FIGURE 5–43

Candida esophagitis with "cobblestone" or "snakeskin" appearance due to numerous coalescent plaques. (From Levine, M.S.: Radiology of the Esophagus. Philadelphia, W.B. Saunders, 1989, p. 54, with permission.)

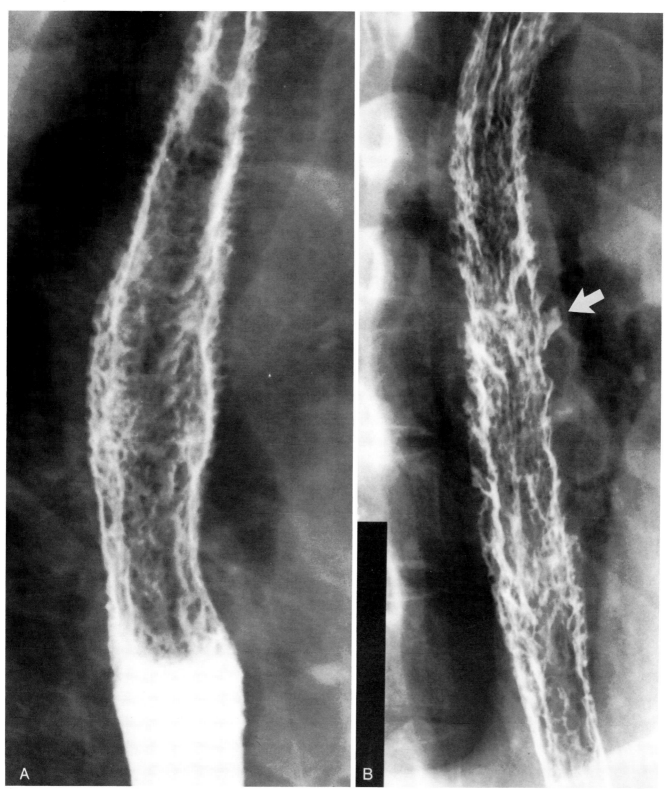

FIGURE 5–44

CANDIDA **ESOPHAGITIS WITH "SHAGGY" ESOPHAGUS.** *A,* Note grossly irregular esophageal contour due to numerous plaques and pseudomembranes. (From Levine, M.S., et al.: *Candida* esophagitis: Accuracy of radiographic diagnosis. Radiology 154:581–587, 1985, with permission.)

B, Shaggy esophagus in a patient with AIDS. Although this finding results primarily from trapping of barium between plaques, an area of relatively deep ulceration *(arrow)* can be seen. (From Levine, M.S., et al.: Opportunistic esophagitis in AIDS: Radiographic diagnosis. Radiology 165:815–820, 1987, with permission.)

fungal mycelia (i.e., fungus balls) (Fig. 5–45).[39] In patients with chronic esophageal stasis due to achalasia or scleroderma, *Candida* esophagitis may also be manifested by fine nodularity, polypoid folds, or a distinctive lacy appearance in the esophagus (Fig. 5–46).[33] *Candida* esophagitis usually responds quickly to treatment with ketoconazole or other antifungal agents, so that the findings may regress dramatically on repeat esophagrams within several days of treatment. Occasionally, severe *Candida* esophagitis may lead to the development of strictures that typically appear as long, tapered areas of narrowing in the middle or distal esophagus (Fig. 5–47).[40] Strictures are more likely to develop in patients who have chronic mucocutaneous candidiasis involving the nails, skin, mucous membranes, and esophagus.[41]

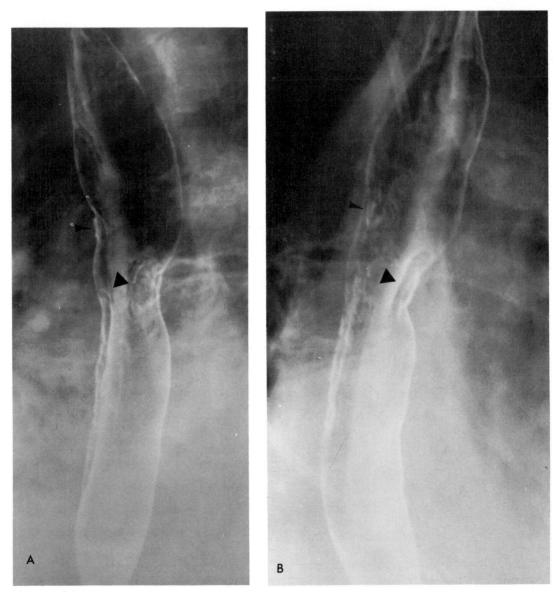

FIGURE 5–45

A and *B, Candida* esophagitis with a polypoid lesion *(wide arrowheads)* in midesophagus due to a fungus ball. Note ulceration more proximally *(narrow arrowheads)*.

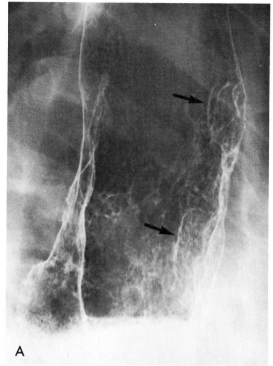

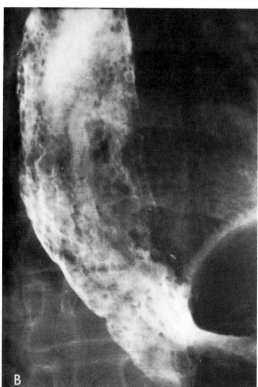

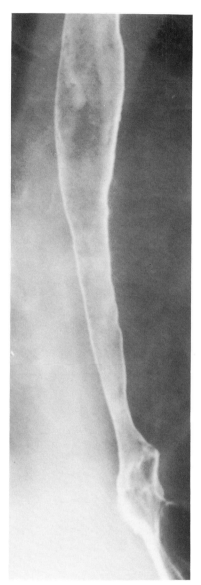

FIGURE 5–47

Long, tapered stricture involving middle and distal esophagus due to severe *Candida* esophagitis. (From Levine, M.S.: Radiology of the Esophagus. Philadelphia, W.B. Saunders, 1989, p. 56, with permission.)

FIGURE 5–46

CHRONIC CANDIDIASIS IN PATIENTS WITH ESOPHAGEAL STASIS. *A,* Note lacy appearance of mucosa with large plaques *(arrows)* in a patient with achalasia.

B, Note fine nodularity of the mucosa due to *Candida* esophagitis in another patient with scleroderma. Also note the dilated esophagus and patulous lower esophageal sphincter.

Herpes Esophagitis

Herpes simplex virus type 1 has been recognized as the second most frequent cause of opportunistic esophagitis in immunocompromised patients. Occasionally, however, an acute, transient form of herpes esophagitis may occur in otherwise healthy individuals who have no underlying immunologic problems.[42, 43] Patients with herpes esophagitis usually present with acute odynophagia or dysphagia, so that the clinical presentation is indistinguishable from that of *Candida* esophagitis. Although herpes esophagitis tends to be a self-limited disease, acyclovir, a potent antiviral agent, has been used successfully to treat these patients.

Vesicle formation, the earliest endoscopic finding in herpes esophagitis, has not been demonstrated by radiologic studies. However, the vesicles subsequently rupture to form discrete, superficial ulcers on the esophageal mucosa that can readily be visualized on double contrast radiographs. In one study, double contrast esophagrams revealed discrete ulcers without plaques in more than 50% of patients with endoscopically proved herpes esophagitis.[44] These ulcers may have a punctate, linear, or stellate configuration and are often surrounded by a radiolucent halo of edematous mucosa (Figs. 5–48 through 5–50).[44, 45] They may be clustered together or widely separated by intervening segments of normal mucosa. In the appropriate clinical setting, discrete ulcers on an otherwise normal background mucosa should strongly suggest herpes esophagitis, because ulcera-

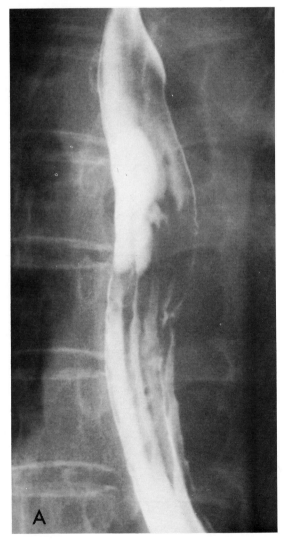
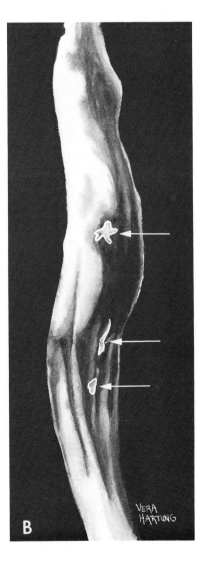

FIGURE 5–48

A and *B*, Herpes esophagitis with several shallow, widely separated ulcers (*arrows*) in midesophagus. Note stellate configuration of ulcers.

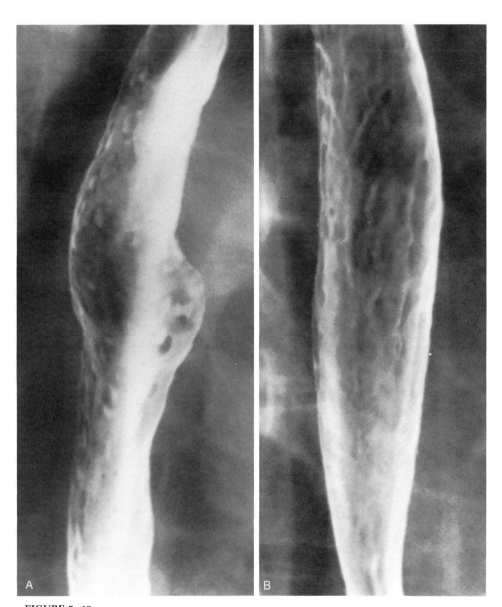

FIGURE 5–49

HERPES ESOPHAGITIS WITH DISCRETE ULCERS. *A,* Multiple superficial ulcers in midesophagus. Note halos of edematous mucosa surrounding ulcers.

B, Different patient with linear and serpiginous ulcers in midesophagus. (From Levine, M.S.: Radiology of the Esophagus. Philadelphia, W.B. Saunders, 1989, p. 62.)

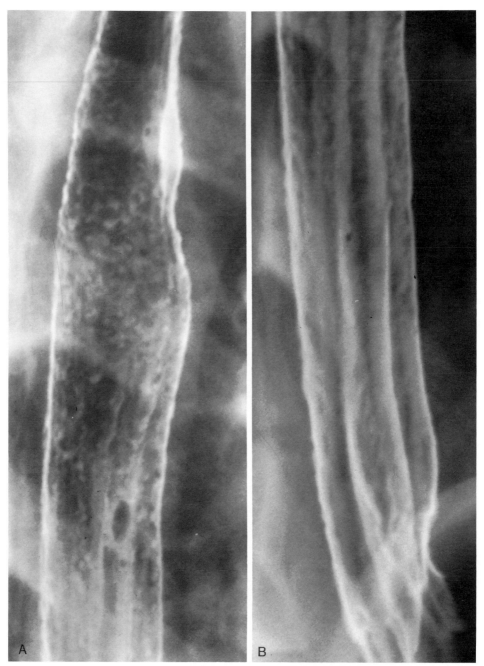

FIGURE 5–50

A and *B*, Herpes esophagitis with multiple tiny, superficial ulcers in midesophagus and scattered ulcers more distally. This patient was an otherwise healthy college student who presented with severe odynophagia. (From DeGaeta, L., et al.: Herpes esophagitis in an otherwise healthy patient. AJR *144*:1205–1206, 1985, with permission, © by American Roentgen Ray Society.)

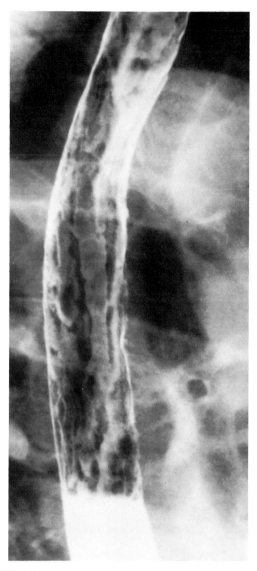

FIGURE 5–51

Advanced herpes esophagitis with multiple linear plaques indistinguishable from those of *Candida* esophagitis. (From Skucas, J., et al.: Herpes esophagitis: A case studied by air-contrast esophagography. AJR *128*:497–499, 1977, with permission, © by American Roentgen Ray Society.)

tion almost invariably occurs on a background of diffuse plaque formation in patients with candidiasis.[35, 37] However, more advanced herpes esophagitis may be manifested by extensive ulceration, plaque formation, or a combination of ulcers and plaques in the esophagus (Fig. 5–51).[44–46] Advanced herpes esophagitis therefore may be indistinguishable radiographically from *Candida* esophagitis.

The ability to distinguish fungal and viral esophagitis on double contrast radiographs is important in the treatment of all immunocompromised patients, but particularly in the treatment of patients with AIDS, as many gastroenterologists are reluctant to perform endoscopy on these individuals for fear of contaminating their endoscopic instruments or exposing themselves to the AIDS virus.[37] Recent data suggest that *Candida* esophagitis and herpes esophagitis can be accurately diagnosed in AIDS patients by their characteristic features on double contrast esophagrams, eliminating the need for endoscopic intervention in many cases (Fig. 5–52).[37] Nevertheless, endoscopy may be required for a definitive diagnosis if the radiographic findings are equivocal or if appropriate treatment with antifungal or antiviral agents fails to produce an adequate clinical response in these patients.

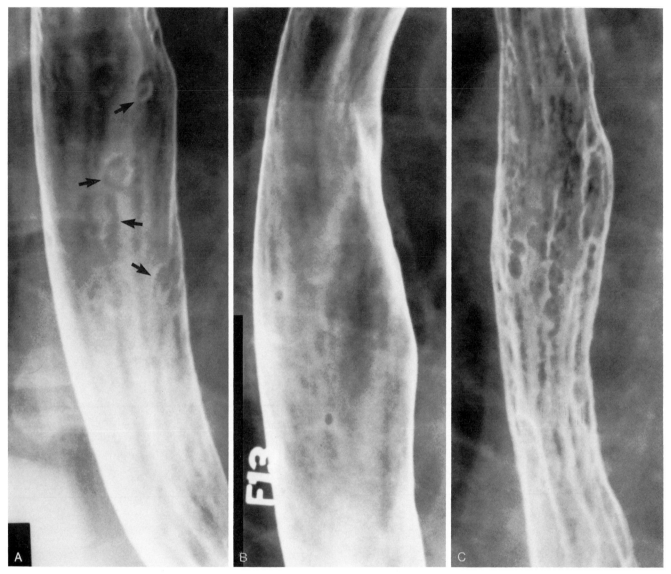

FIGURE 5-52

HERPES AND *CANDIDA* ESOPHAGITIS IN A PATIENT WITH AIDS. *A*, Initial esophagram shows discrete, superficial ulcers *(arrows)* in midesophagus without evidence of plaques. Note halos of edematous mucosa surrounding ulcers. These findings should strongly suggest herpes esophagitis.

B, Repeat esophagram obtained 2 weeks after treatment with intravenous acyclovir shows healing of ulcers with normal-appearing mucosa in this region. (Note air bubbles in esophagus.)

C, Third esophagram obtained 3 months later shows linear plaque-like lesions in esophagus that are compatible with *Candida* esophagitis. The patient had a dramatic clinical response to treatment with ketoconazole. (From Levine, M.S., et al.: Opportunistic esophagitis in AIDS: Radiographic diagnosis. Radiology 165:815–820, 1987, with permission.)

Cytomegalovirus Esophagitis

Cytomegalovirus (CMV) is another member of the herpes virus group that has recently been recognized as a cause of opportunistic esophagitis in patients with AIDS. Cytomegalovirus esophagitis may be manifested radiographically by discrete, superficial ulcers indistinguishable from those of herpes esophagitis (Fig. 5–53).[47] However, other patients may have one or more large, relatively flat ulcers in the middle or distal esophagus (Fig. 5–54).[37, 47] These ovoid or elongated ulcers may be surrounded by a radiolucent rim of edematous mucosa. Some of the ulcers may be several centimeters or greater in size. Because herpetic ulcers rarely become this large, the presence of one or more giant esophageal ulcers should strongly suggest CMV esophagitis in patients with AIDS. However, endoscopic brushings, biopsies, or cultures are required for a definitive diagnosis.

Recent reports indicate that giant esophageal ulcers sometimes may be caused directly by human immunodeficiency virus (HIV) without evidence of opportunistic infection by viral or fungal organisms.[48] Although these HIV-induced ulcers are indistinguishable radiographically from CMV ulcers in the esophagus, they may respond to treatment with steroids rather than antiviral agents. Thus, it is important to differentiate these entities in HIV-positive patients with esophageal ulcers.

Drug-Induced Esophagitis

Drug-induced esophagitis tends to involve the middle or upper esophagus with distal esophageal sparing.[49, 50] About half of the cases are caused by antibiotics, particularly tetracycline and doxycycline. Other oral medications implicated less frequently include potassium chloride, quinidine, and aspirin. These patients typically have a history of ingesting the medication with little or no water immediately before going to bed. Prolonged exposure to the tablets or capsules is thought to cause a focal contact esoph-

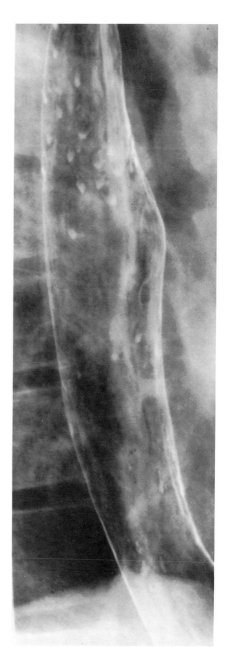

FIGURE 5–53

Probable CMV esophagitis with discrete, superficial ulcers separated by normal mucosa. Although endoscopic biopsies were negative for CMV, this patient had elevated CMV titers at the time of the barium study. (From Levine, M.S.: Radiology of the Esophagus. Philadelphia, W.B. Saunders, 1989, p. 66.)

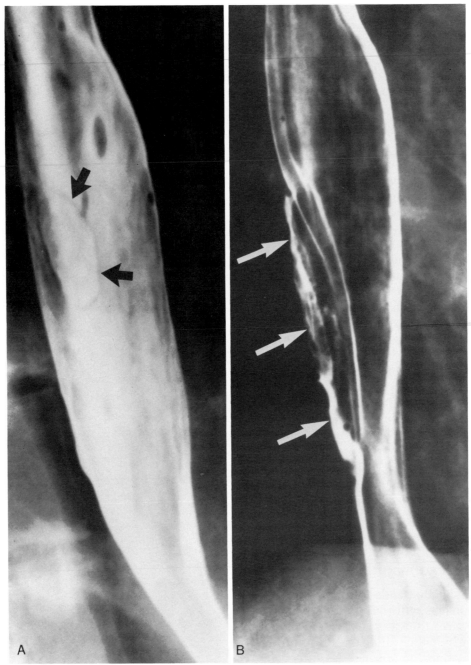

FIGURE 5–54

Two examples (A and B) of giant, relatively flat ulcers (arrows) in AIDS patients with CMV esophagitis. Note how ulcer is seen en face in A and in profile in B. (A, Courtesy of Kyunghee C. Cho, M.D., Bronx, New York. B, Courtesy of Patrick C. Freeny, M.D., Seattle, Washington.)

agitis, most frequently in the region of the aortic arch or left main bronchus. These patients often present with severe odynophagia.

Drug-induced esophagitis may be manifested by a solitary ulcer, by several discrete ulcers, or by a localized cluster of tiny ulcers distributed circumferentially on a normal background mucosa (Fig.

5–55).[49, 50] Although herpes esophagitis may produce identical radiographic findings, a history of recent drug ingestion should suggest the correct diagnosis. When esophageal ulcers are drug-induced, a repeat esophagram 7 to 10 days after withdrawal of the offending agent should show complete healing of the lesions.[49]

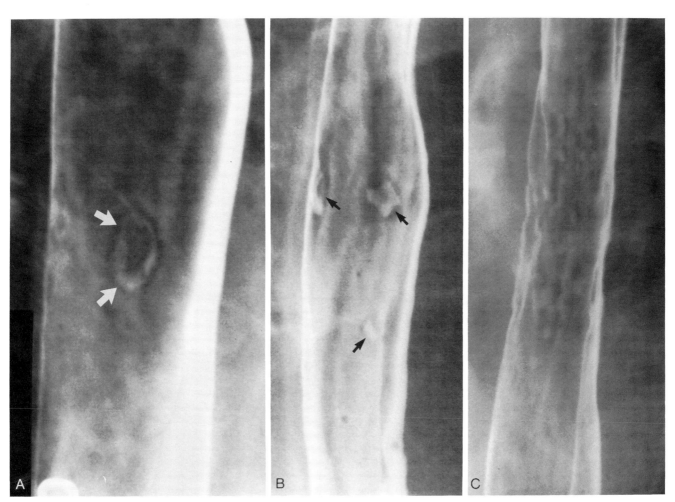

FIGURE 5–55

DRUG-INDUCED ESOPHAGITIS WITH SUPERFICIAL ULCERS. *A*, Solitary doxycycline-induced ulcer *(arrows)* in midesophagus. Note thin radiolucent halo surrounding ulcer.

B, Several discrete ulcers *(arrows)* in midesophagus due to tetracycline ingestion. Note stellate configuration of largest ulcer.

C, Doxycycline-induced esophagitis with multiple small, superficial ulcers clustered together in midesophagus. (From Levine, M.S.: Radiology of the Esophagus. Philadelphia, W.B. Saunders, 1989, p. 76.)

Other Types of Esophagitis

Nasogastric-Intubation Esophagitis

Nasogastric intubation occasionally may lead to the development of long strictures in the distal esophagus (Fig. 5–56). These patients probably have a severe form of reflux esophagitis induced by the tube.[51] The strictures are characterized by their tendency to progress rapidly in length and severity within a relatively short period.

Caustic Esophagitis

Long, ulcerated strictures may also be observed in patients who have ingested lye or other caustic agents. In severe cases, diffuse esophageal narrowing may reduce the thoracic esophagus to a thin, filiform structure (Fig. 5–57). Long-standing lye strictures apparently predispose patients to the development of esophageal carcinoma.[52] Thus, any mucosal irregularity in a chronic lye stricture should raise the possibility of carcinoma (Fig. 5–58).

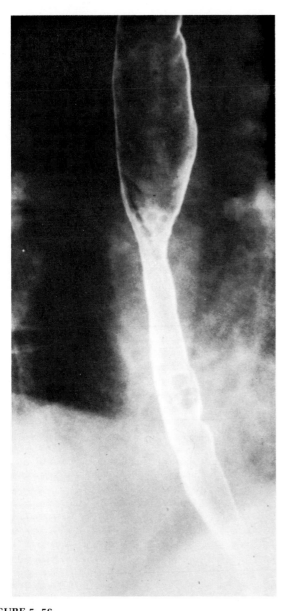

FIGURE 5–56

Long stricture in distal esophagus due to prolonged nasogastric intubation.

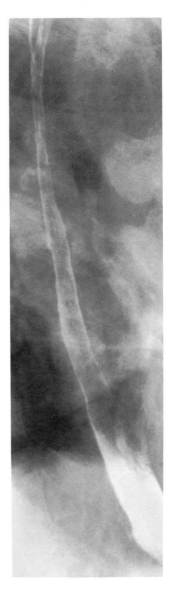

FIGURE 5–57

Lye stricture with diffuse narrowing of thoracic esophagus. This appearance should suggest caustic injury, as other conditions rarely cause such extensive esophageal narrowing.

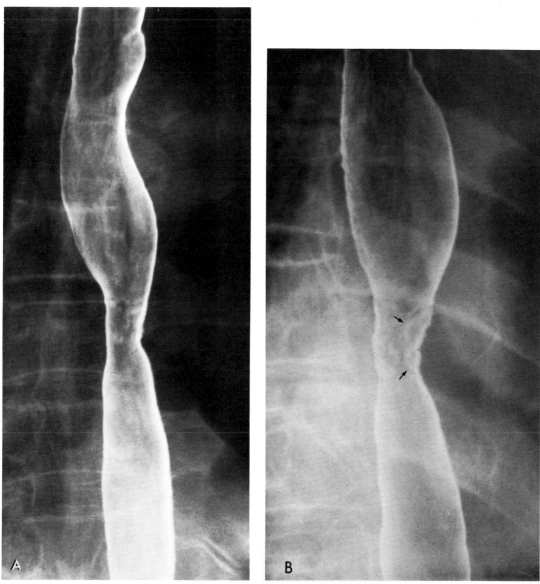

FIGURE 5–58

A and *B*, Carcinoma developing at the site of a lye stricture in a 70-year-old man who had ingested lye at the age of 4 years. Note focal stricture in midesophagus with superficial ulceration and nodularity of mucosa *(arrows)* in region of stricture. Endoscopic brushings and biopsies revealed squamous cell carcinoma, but the patient refused surgery.

Radiation Esophagitis

Radiation therapy to the chest or mediastinum may cause severe esophagitis and strictures when the dose to the esophagus approaches 5000 to 6000 rads.[53] Radiation strictures are frequently seen following successful treatment of esophageal carcinoma. They typically appear as smooth, tapered areas of narrowing within a pre-existing radiation portal (Fig. 5–59).

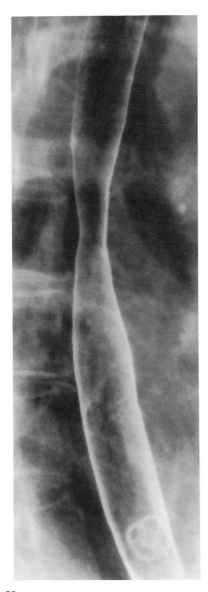

FIGURE 5–59

Smooth, tapered radiation stricture in midesophagus following successful irradiation of esophageal carcinoma.

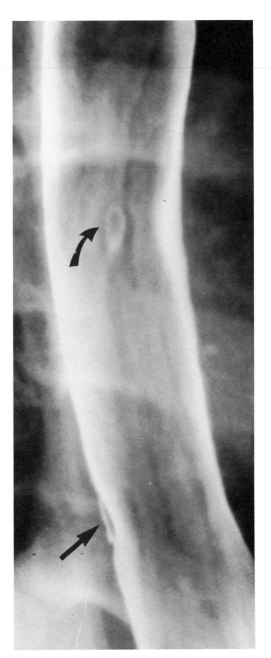

FIGURE 5–60

Esophageal Crohn's disease with discrete "aphthous" ulcers seen en face (curved arrow) and in profile (straight arrow). (From Gohel, V., et al.: Aphthous ulcers in the esophagus with Crohn's disease. AJR 137:872, 1981, with permission.)

Miscellaneous

Other inflammatory diseases, such as Crohn's disease,[54, 55] benign mucous membrane pemphigoid,[56] and epidermolysis bullosa dystrophica,[57] may also involve the esophagus. Rarely, esophageal Crohn's disease may be manifested by discrete "aphthous" ulcers similar to those found in granulomatous colitis (Fig. 5–60).[54, 55] However, these patients almost always have advanced Crohn's disease in the small bowel or colon.

Differential Diagnosis of Esophagitis

Nodularity

Mucosal nodularity may be a feature of reflux esophagitis or infectious esophagitis. However, the nodules of reflux esophagitis tend to have poorly defined borders that fade peripherally into the adjacent mucosa, whereas the plaque-like lesions of *Candida* esophagitis usually have discrete borders separated by normal mucosa. Mucosal nodularity may also be caused by glycogenic acanthosis, a benign, degenerative condition in which cellular glycogen accumulates in the squamous epithelial lining of the esophagus. Double contrast esophagrams may reveal nodules or plaques indistinguishable from those of reflux or *Candida* esophagitis (Fig. 5–61; see Chapter 6).[58] However, patients with glycogenic acanthosis are almost always asymptomatic. Occasionally, a superficial spreading carcinoma, or even an advanced car-

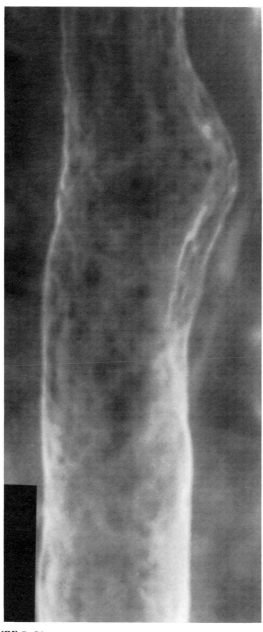

FIGURE 5–61

GLYCOGENIC ACANTHOSIS WITH MUCOSAL NODULARITY.
Reflux esophagitis or *Candida* esophagitis could produce similar findings, but this patient was asymptomatic.

cinoma, may cause localized or diffuse nodularity of the mucosa (Fig. 5–62; see Chapter 6).[59]

Ulceration

Mucosal ulceration may be simulated by transverse folds seen in profile (see Figs. 5–9 and 5–10). Scarring from reflux esophagitis may produce one or more sacculations or outpouchings near the gastroesophageal junction that can also be mistaken for ulcers (see Figs. 5–32 and 5–33). However, these sacculations tend to have a more rounded configuration and are not associated with radiating folds or surrounding mounds of edema. Also, unlike ulcers, sacculations tend to change in size and shape during the fluoroscopic examination. Esophageal intramural pseudodiverticulosis is another cause of barium projections that must be differentiated from ulcers (see Fig. 5–35). As indicated earlier, these pseudodiverticula often do not appear to communicate with the esophageal lumen when viewed in profile.[22]

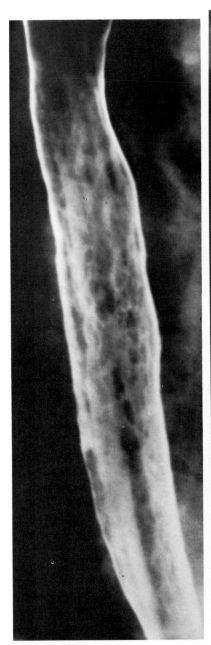 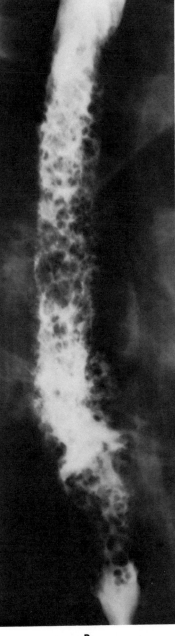

A   B

FIGURE 5–62

ESOPHAGEAL CARCINOMA WITH NODULAR MUCOSA. *A,* Diffuse mucosal nodularity due to superficial spreading carcinoma. (Courtesy of Akiyoshi Yamada, M.D., Tokyo, Japan.)

B, Diffuse mucosal nodularity due to advanced esophageal carcinoma. (Courtesy of Hans Herlinger, M.D., Philadelphia, Pennsylvania.)

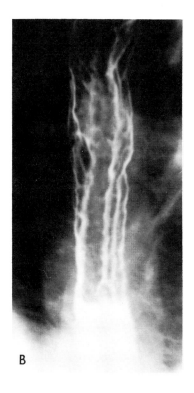

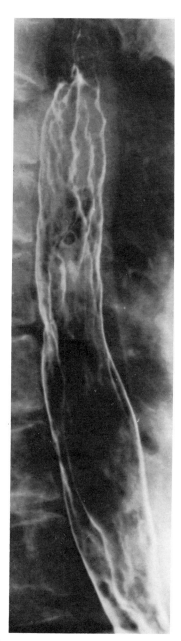

Abnormal Mucosal Folds

Esophageal varices may resemble the enlarged folds of chronic esophagitis (Fig. 5–63). However, varices tend to be more tortuous or serpiginous and can be effaced to a greater degree or even obliterated by esophageal distention, peristalsis, or Valsalva maneuvers. Occasionally, "varicoid" carcinomas may also be manifested by thickened, tortuous longitudinal folds due to submucosal spread of tumor (Fig. 5–64; see Chapter 6).[60, 61]

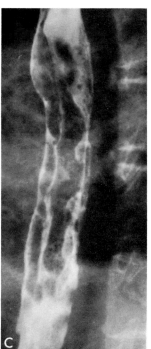

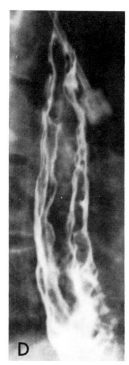

FIGURE 5–63

Four examples (A through D) of esophageal varices, with thickened longitudinal folds resembling those in patients with esophagitis. However, varices tend to have a more scalloped appearance.

FIGURE 5–64

"Varicoid" carcinoma with thickened, tortuous folds, mimicking the appearance of esophageal varices. (Courtesy of Akiyoshi Yamada, M.D., Tokyo, Japan.)

REFERENCES

1. Cassel, D.M., Anderson, M.F., and Zboralske, F.F.: Double-contrast esophagrams: The prone technique. Radiology 139:737, 1981.
2. Hogan, W.J., Dodds, W.J., Hoke, S.E., et al.: Effect of glucagon on esophageal motor function. Gastroenterology 69:160, 1975.
3. Levine, M.S., Kressel, H.Y., Laufer, I., et al.: The tube esophagram: A technique for obtaining a detailed double-contrast examination of the esophagus. AJR 142:293, 1984.
4. Friedland, G.W., and Filly, R.: The post-cricoid impression masquerading as an esophageal tumor. Am. J. Dig. Dis. 20:287, 1985.
5. Goldberg, H.I., Dodds, W.J., and Jenis, E.H.: Experimental esophagitis: Roentgenographic findings after insufflation of tantalum powder. AJR 110:288, 1970.
6. Gohel, V.K., Edell, S.L., Laufer, I., et al.: Transverse folds in the human esophagus. Radiology 128:303, 1978.
7. Williams, S.M., Harned, R.K., Kaplan, P., et al.: Transverse striations of the esophagus: Association with gastroesophageal reflux. Radiology 146:25, 1983.
8. Gohel, V.K., Kressel, H.Y., and Laufer, I.: Double-contrast artifacts. Gastrointest. Radiol. 3:139, 1978.
9. Cho, S.R., Henry, D.A., Shaw, C.I., et al.: Vanishing intraluminal diverticulum of the esophagus. Gastrointest. Radiol. 7:315, 1982.
10. Maglinte, D.D.T., Lappas, J.C., Chernish, S.M., et al.: Flow artifacts in double-contrast esophagography. Radiology 157:535, 1985.
11. Creteur, V., Thoeni, R.F., Federle, M.P., et al.: The role of single and double-contrast radiography in the diagnosis of reflux esophagitis. Radiology 147:71, 1983.
12. Graziani, L., De Nigris, E., Pesaresi, A., et al.: Reflux esophagitis: Radiologic-endoscopic correlation in 39 symptomatic cases. Gastrointest. Radiol. 8:1, 1983.
13. Chen, Y.M., Ott, D.J., Gelfand, D.W., et al.: Multiphasic examination of the esophagogastric region for strictures, rings, and hiatal hernia: Evaluation of the individual techniques. Gastrointest. Radiol. 10:311, 1985.
14. Kressel, H.Y., Glick, S.N., Laufer, I., et al.: Radiologic features of esophagitis. Gastrointest. Radiol. 6:103, 1981.
15. Graziani, L., Bearzi, I., Romagnoli, A., et al.: Significance of diffuse granularity and nodularity of the esophageal mucosa at double-contrast radiography. Gastrointest. Radiol. 10:1, 1985.
16. Levine, M.S., Cajade, A.G., Herlinger, H., et al.: Pseudomembranes in reflux esophagitis. Radiology 159:43, 1986.
17. Bleshman, M.H., Banner, M.P., Johnson, R.C., et al.: The inflammatory esophagogastric polyp and fold. Radiology 128:589, 1978.
18. Styles, R.A., Gibb, S.P., Tarshis, A., et al.: Esophagogastric polyps: Radiographic and endoscopic findings. Radiology 154:307, 1985.
19. Laufer, I.: Radiology of esophagitis. Radiol. Clin. North Am. 20:687, 1982.
20. Levine, M.S.: Radiology of the Esophagus. Philadelphia, W.B. Saunders, 1989.
21. Levine, M.S., and Goldstein, H.M.: Fixed transverse folds in the esophagus: A sign of reflux esophagitis. AJR 143:275, 1984.
22. Levine, M.S., Moolten, D.N., Herlinger, H., et al.: Esophageal intramural pseudodiverticulosis: A reevaluation. AJR 147:1165, 1986.
23. Robbins, A.H., Hermos, J.A., Schimmel, E.M., et al.: The columnar-lined esophagus: Analysis of 26 cases. Radiology 123:1, 1977.
24. Robbins, A.H., Vincent, M.E., Saini, M., et al.: Revised radiologic concepts of Barrett's esophagus. Gastrointest. Radiol. 3:377, 1978.
25. Levine, M.S., Kressel, H.Y., Caroline, D.F., et al.: Barrett esophagus: Reticular pattern of the mucosa. Radiology 147:663, 1983.
26. Agha, F.P.: Radiologic diagnosis of Barrett's esophagus: Critical analysis of 65 cases. Gastrointest. Radiol. 11:123, 1986.
27. Chernin, M.M., Amberg, J.R., Kogan, F.J., et al.: Efficacy of radiologic studies in the detection of Barrett's esophagus. AJR 147:257, 1986.
28. Gilchrist, A.M., Levine, M.S., Carr, R.F., et al.: Barrett's esophagus: Diagnosis by double-contrast esophagography. AJR 150:97, 1988.
29. Sheft, D.J., and Shrago, G.: Esophageal moniliasis: The spectrum of the disease. JAMA 213:1859, 1970.
30. Eras, P., Goldstein, M.J., and Sherlock, P.: Candida infection of the gastrointestinal tract. Medicine (Baltimore) 51:367, 1972.
31. Wall, S.D., Ominsky, S., Altman, D.F., et al.: Multifocal abnormalities of the gastrointestinal tract in AIDS. AJR 146:1, 1986.
32. Frager, D.H., Frager, J.D., Brandt, L.J., et al.: Gastrointestinal complications of AIDS: Radiological features. Radiology 158:597, 1986.
33. Gefter, W.B., Laufer, I., Edell, S., et al.: Candidiasis in the obstructed esophagus. Radiology 138:25, 1981.
34. Kodsi, B.E., Wickremesinghe, P.C., Kozinn, P.J., et al.: Candida esophagitis. Gastroenterology 71:715, 1976.
35. Levine, M.S., Macones, A.J., Jr., and Laufer, I.: Candida esophagitis: Accuracy of radiographic diagnosis. Radiology 154:581, 1985.
36. Vahey, T.N., Maglinte, D.D.T., and Chernish, S.M.: State-of-the-art barium examination in opportunistic esophagitis. Dig. Dis. Sci. 31:1192, 1986.
37. Levine, M.S., Woldenberg, R., Herlinger, H., and Laufer, I.: Opportunistic esophagitis in AIDS: Radiographic diagnosis. Radiology 165:815, 1987.
38. Goldberg, H.I., and Dodds, W.J.: Cobblestone esophagus due to monilial infection. AJR 104:608, 1968.
39. Ho, C.S., Cullen, J.B., and Gray, R.R.: An unusual manifestation of esophageal moniliasis. Radiology 123:287, 1977.
40. Agha, F.P.: Candidiasis-induced esophageal strictures. Gastrointest. Radiol. 9:283, 1984.
41. Rohrmann, C.A., and Kidd, R.: Chronic mucocutaneous candidiasis: Radiologic abnormalities in the esophagus. AJR 130:473, 1978.
42. Deschmukh, M., Shah, R., and McCallum, R.W.: Experience with herpes esophagitis in otherwise healthy patients. Am. J. Gastroenterol. 79:173, 1984.
43. DeGaeta, L., Levine, M.S., Guglielmi, G.E., et al.: Herpes esophagitis in an otherwise healthy patient. AJR 144:1205, 1985.
44. Levine, M.S., Loevner, L.A., Saul, S.H., et al.: Herpes esophagitis: Sensitivity of double-contrast esophagography. AJR 151:57, 1988.
45. Levine, M.S., Laufer, I., Kressel, H.Y., et al.: Herpes esophagitis. AJR 136:863, 1981.
46. Skucas, J., Schrank, W.W., Meyer, P.C., et al.: Herpes esophagitis: A case studied by air-contrast esophagography. AJR 128:497, 1977.
47. Balthazar, E.J., Megibow, A.J., Hulnick, D., et al.: Cytomegalovirus esophagitis in AIDS: Radiographic features in 16 patients. AJR 149:919, 1987.
48. Rabeneck, L., Popovic, M., Gartner, S., et al.: Acute HIV infection presenting with painful swallowing and esophageal ulcers. JAMA 263:2318, 1990.
49. Creteur, V., Laufer, I., Kressel, H.Y., et al.: Drug-induced esophagitis detected by double contrast radiography. Radiology 147:365, 1983.
50. Bova, J.G., Dutton, N.E., Goldstein, H.M., et al.: Medication-induced esophagitis: Diagnosis by double-contrast esophagography. AJR 148:731, 1987.
51. Graham, J., Barnes, M., and Rubenstein, A.S.: The nasogastric tube as a cause of esophagitis and stricture. Am. J. Surg. 98:116, 1959.
52. Appleqvist, P., and Salmo, M.: Lye corrosion carcinoma of the esophagus: A review of 63 cases. Cancer 45:2655, 1980.
53. Lepke, R.A., and Libshitz, H.I.: Radiation-induced injury of the esophagus. Radiology 148:375, 1983.
54. Gohel, V., Long, B.W., and Richter, G.: Aphthous ulcers in the esophagus with Crohn colitis. AJR 137:872, 1981.
55. Degryse, H.R.M., and De Schepper, A.M.: Aphthoid esophageal

ulcers in Crohn's disease of ileum and colon. Gastrointest. Radiol. *9*:197, 1984.

56. Agha, F.P., and Raji, M.R.: Esophageal involvement in pemphigoid: Clinical and roentgen manifestations. Gastrointest. Radiol. *7*:109, 1982.

57. Agha, F.P., Francis, I.R., and Ellis, C.N.: Esophageal involvement in epidermolysis bullosa dystrophica: Clinical and roentgenographic manifestations. Gastrointest. Radiol. *8*:111, 1983.

58. Glick, S.N., Teplick, S.K., Goldstein, J., et al.: Glycogenic acanthosis of the esophagus. AJR *139*:683, 1982.

59. Itai, Y., Kogure, T., Okuyama, Y., et al.: Diffuse finely nodular lesions of the esophagus. AJR *128*:563, 1977.

60. Lawson, T.L., Dodds, W.J., and Sheft, D.J.: Carcinoma of the esophagus simulating varices. AJR *107*:83, 1969.

61. Yates, C.W., LeVine, M.A., and Jensen, K.M.: Varicoid carcinoma of the esophagus. Radiology *122*:605, 1977.

TUMORS OF THE ESOPHAGUS

Marc S. Levine, M.D.
Igor Laufer, M.D.
Akiyoshi Yamada, M.D.

6

BENIGN TUMORS

Benign tumors of the esophagus are relatively uncommon. The vast majority are small, asymptomatic lesions that are discovered as incidental findings on radiologic or endoscopic examinations. Occasionally, however, these tumors may cause dysphagia or gastrointestinal bleeding. Depending on their site of origin, benign tumors may be classified as mucosal or submucosal lesions that have typical radiologic features.

Mucosal Lesions

Squamous papillomas are the most frequent benign mucosal tumors in the esophagus. These lesions appear as coral-like excrescences containing a central fibrovascular core with multiple finger-like projections covered by hyperplastic squamous epithelium.[1] Papillomas are difficult to detect on conventional single contrast barium studies because of the small size of the lesions. However, they are often recognized on double contrast studies as sessile, smooth or slightly lobulated polyps less than 1 cm in size (Fig. 6–1).[2] Some papillomas may produce a ring shadow similar to that of colonic polyps on double contrast barium enemas due to barium trapped between the edge of the lesion and the adjacent mucosa (Fig. 6–1A). Because early esophageal cancers may also appear as small polypoid lesions, endoscopy and biopsy should be performed to differentiate a squamous papilloma from an early carcinoma.

Multiple benign mucosal elevations are frequently found in the esophagus in patients with glycogenic acanthosis, a benign condition of unknown etiology

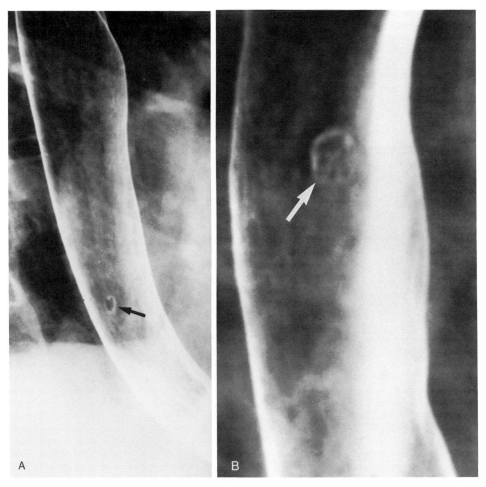

FIGURE 6–1

SQUAMOUS PAPILLOMAS. *A*, Small papilloma in distal esophagus appears as ring shadow *(arrow)* because of barium trapped between edge of polyp and adjacent esophageal wall. (From Montesi, A., et al.: Small benign tumors of the esophagus: Radiological diagnosis with double-contrast examination. Gastrointest. Radiol. 8:207, 1983, with permission.)

B, Larger, more lobulated papilloma *(arrow)* in another patient. Early esophageal cancer could produce a similar appearance. (Courtesy of Harry Allen III, M.D., Norfolk, Virginia.)

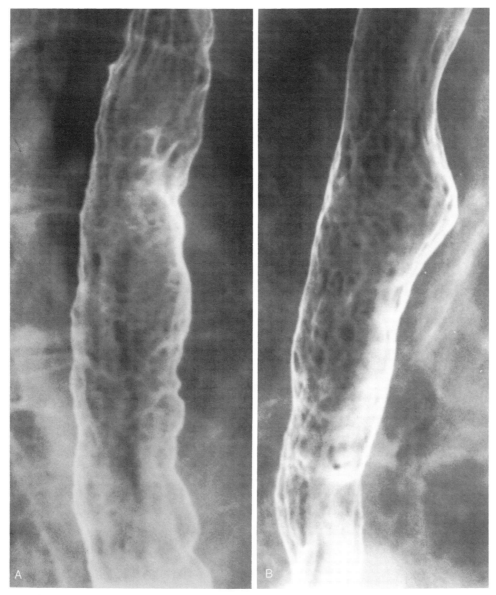

FIGURE 6–2

Two examples (A and B) of glycogenic acanthosis manifested by multiple small plaques and nodules in midesophagus. Although *Candida* esophagitis could produce similar findings, patients with glycogenic acanthosis are almost always asymptomatic. (From Levine, M.S.: Radiology of the Esophagus. Philadelphia, W.B. Saunders, 1989, p. 118.)

in which there is accumulation of cytoplasmic glycogen in the squamous epithelial cells lining the esophagus.[3] Glycogenic acanthosis is a degenerative condition, predominantly occurring in middle-aged or elderly individuals. It usually is manifested on double contrast studies by multiple small nodules or plaques in the middle or distal esophagus (Fig. 6–2).[4–6] *Candida* or reflux esophagitis may produce similar findings. However, patients with glycogenic acanthosis are almost always asymptomatic, so that the clinical history is extremely helpful for differentiating these conditions.

Esophageal papillomatosis, leukoplakia, and acanthosis nigricans are other rare causes of multiple small nodules or plaques in the esophagus.[7–9] The diagnosis of esophageal papillomatosis may be suggested on double contrast studies by the presence of multiple, discrete, wart-like excrescences on the esophageal mucosa (Fig. 6–3). Even when multiple papillomas are present, however, these lesions rarely cause obstruction.

Submucosal Lesions

The vast majority of benign submucosal tumors in the esophagus are leiomyomas.[10] Histologically, these lesions consist of intersecting bands of smooth muscle and fibrous tissue surrounded by a well-defined capsule. Leiomyomas are frequently found in the middle or distal third of the esophagus, but they are much less common in the proximal third because of the presence of striated rather than smooth muscle in the esophagus above the level of the aortic arch. Most patients with esophageal leiomyomas are asymptomatic. However, lesions that are unusually large may

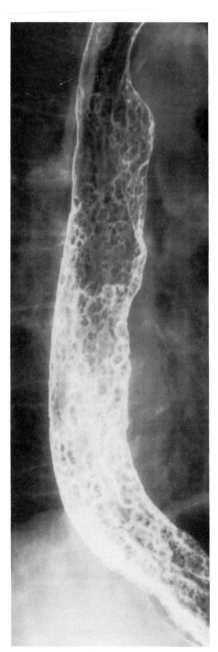

FIGURE 6–3

Esophageal papillomatosis with innumerable papillomas, appearing as wart-like excrescences on esophageal mucosa. Despite the dramatic radiographic findings, this patient had no esophageal symptoms. (Courtesy of Harvey M. Goldstein, M.D., San Antonio, Texas.)

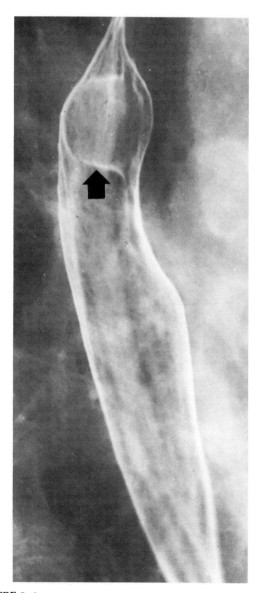

FIGURE 6–4

LEIOMYOMA. Note typical submucosal appearance of tumor (*arrow*) with smooth, stretched mucosa over lesion.

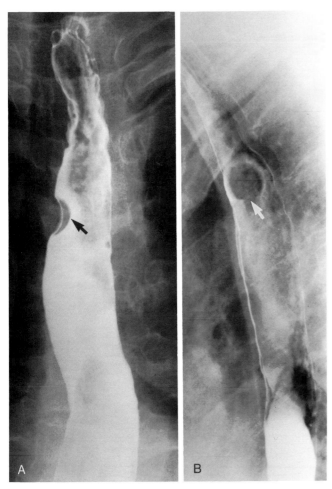

FIGURE 6–5

LEIOMYOMA. *A,* Tangential view shows characteristic features of submucosal mass *(arrow)* with smooth surface and slightly obtuse angle between edge of lesion and adjacent esophageal wall.

   B, En face view shows well-defined, ovoid filling defect *(arrow)* in esophagus.

cause dysphagia. Unlike smooth muscle tumors elsewhere in the gastrointestinal tract, esophageal leiomyomas almost never undergo sarcomatous degeneration.[11]

   Leiomyomas usually appear radiographically as discrete submucosal masses in the esophagus (Figs. 6–4 through 6–6). When viewed in profile, the lesions have a smooth surface that is etched in white, and their upper and lower borders form either abrupt right angles or slightly obtuse angles with the adjacent esophageal wall (Figs. 6–5A and 6–6A). When viewed en face, the lesions may cause apparent widening of the esophageal lumen as barium flows around the lateral borders of the tumor (Fig. 6–6B). Unlike leiomyomas in the stomach, esophageal leiomyomas are

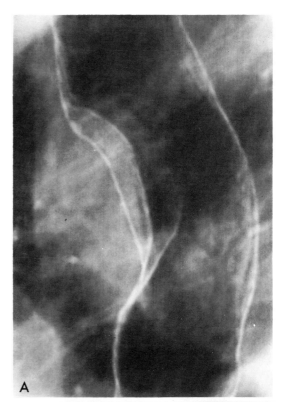

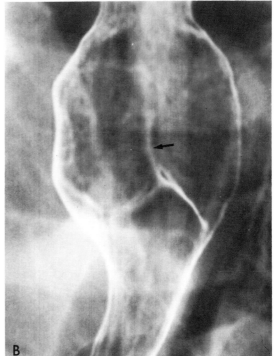

FIGURE 6–6

LEIOMYOMA. *A,* Tangential view shows large submucosal mass in esophagus.

   B, En face view shows widening of esophageal lumen with smooth mucosal surface and central furrow *(arrow).* (Courtesy of Marc P. Banner, M.D., Philadelphia, Pennsylvania.)

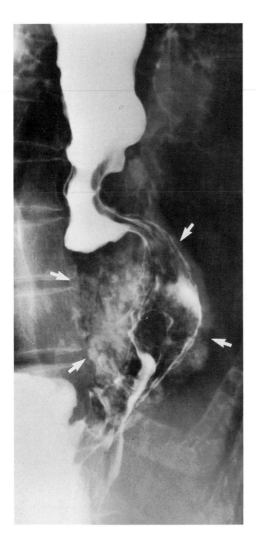

FIGURE 6–7

CALCIFIED LEIOMYOMA. Note large mass (*arrows*) in distal esophagus, with amorphous calcification in lesion.

FIGURE 6–8

IDIOPATHIC ESOPHAGEAL VARIX. *A*, View of partially collapsed esophagus shows solitary submucosal mass (*arrow*) indistinguishable from leiomyoma or other intramural lesion.

B, Repeat double contrast view, however, shows obliteration of varix with greater esophageal distention. (From Trenkner, S.W., et al.: Idiopathic esophageal varix. AJR *141*:43–44, 1983, with permission, © by American Roentgen Ray Society.)

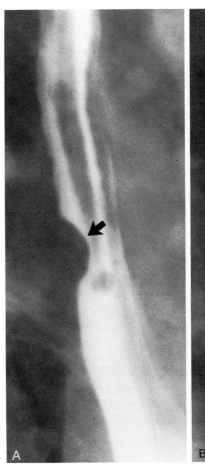
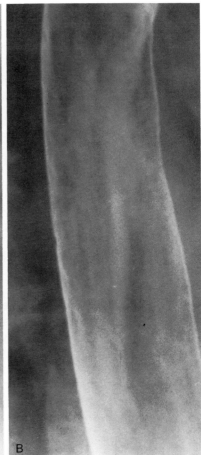

almost never ulcerated. Rarely, these tumors may contain areas of calcification (Fig. 6–7).[12]

Although most submucosal masses in the esophagus are leiomyomas, other intramural lesions such as fibromas, neurofibromas, lipomas, hemangiomas, granular cell tumors, and duplication or retention cysts may produce identical radiographic findings.[13–16] Rarely, an isolated esophageal varix may also resemble a submucosal mass (Fig. 6–8A), but effacement or obliteration of the lesion by esophageal distention should suggest its vascular origin (Fig. 6–8B).[17] When multiple submucosal masses are present in the esophagus, the differential diagnosis should include not only multiple leiomyomas but also multiple neurofibromas, esophageal retention cysts (i.e., esophagitis cystica), hematogenous metastases from malignant melanoma, and leukemic or lymphomatous deposits in the esophagus (see Fig. 6–36).

Fibrovascular polyps are uncommon benign submucosal tumors in the esophagus that consist of fibrovascular and adipose tissue covered by normal squamous epithelium.[18] They almost always arise in the cervical esophagus, gradually forming a pedicle and elongating distally into the thoracic esophagus as a result of the constant traction of esophageal peristalsis. These pedunculated masses are dangerous because they may be regurgitated into the oropharynx, causing laryngeal obstruction and sudden death.[19] Fibrovascular polyps appear radiographically as smooth, sausage-shaped masses extending into the middle or distal esophagus (Fig. 6–9).[18] A discrete pedicle occasionally may be detected in the cervical esophagus at the site of origin of the tumor.

ESOPHAGEAL CARCINOMA

Esophageal carcinoma is a deadly disease with 5-year survival rates of less than 10%. Unfortunately, most patients with esophageal cancer develop dysphagia only after the tumor has invaded periesophageal lymphatics or other mediastinal structures, so that they usually have advanced, unresectable lesions at the time of clinical presentation. About 80% to 90% of these tumors are squamous cell carcinomas, and the remaining 10% to 20% are adenocarcinomas arising in Barrett's mucosa.[20, 21] Although the major risk factors for squamous cell carcinoma are tobacco and alcohol,[22] other conditions associated with an increased risk of the development of esophageal cancer include achalasia,[23] lye strictures,[24] head and neck tumors,[25] celiac disease,[26] Plummer-Vinson syndrome,[27] and tylosis.[28] Some investigators advocate routine screening of patients with these conditions to allow detection of a superimposed carcinoma at the

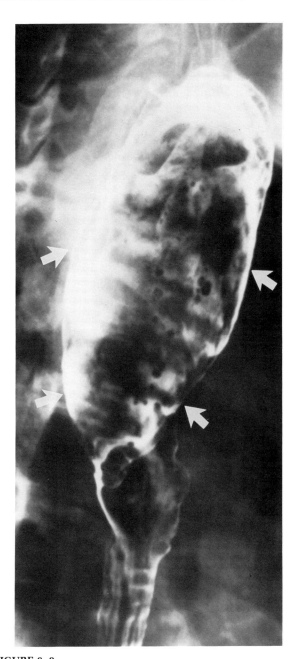

FIGURE 6–9

GIANT FIBROVASCULAR POLYP. Note smooth, sausage-shaped mass (*arrows*) that expands lumen of upper esophagus. (Courtesy of Duane Mezwa, M.D., Royal Oak, Michigan.)

earliest possible stage (see the next section, "Early Esophageal Cancer").

Unlike squamous cell carcinoma, esophageal adenocarcinoma virtually always arises on a background of Barrett's mucosa in the esophagus. The reported prevalence of adenocarcinoma in patients with Barrett's esophagus is about 15%.[29] Adenocarcinoma apparently evolves through a sequence of progressively severe epithelial dysplasia in areas of pre-existing columnar metaplasia. These dysplastic or early carcinomatous changes can be recognized by endoscopic biopsy or cytology. As a result, many investigators advocate routine endoscopic surveillance of patients with Barrett's esophagus for early detection of cancer.

Early Esophageal Cancer

Various terms have been used to describe the earliest diagnosable form of esophageal cancer. *Early esophageal cancer* is defined histologically as cancer limited to the mucosa or submucosa without lymph node metastases.[30] Unlike advanced carcinoma, early esophageal cancer is a readily curable lesion with 5-year survival rates approaching 90%.[31] So far, most cases have been found in parts of Northern China, where the high incidence of esophageal cancer has led to mass screening of the adult population to detect these lesions at the earliest possible stage. *Superficial esophageal cancer* is also confined to the mucosa or submucosa, but unlike early esophageal cancer, lymph node metastases may be present in this disease.[30] *Small esophageal cancer* is another term used to describe tumors less than 3.5 cm in size, regardless

of the depth of invasion or the presence or absence of lymph node metastases.[32] Thus, some small or superficial esophageal cancers may be "early" lesions histologically, but others may have invaded regional lymph nodes with a prognosis comparable to that of advanced esophageal carcinoma. Although these distinctions are made on pathologic criteria, lesions that are small or superficial are more likely to be early cancers with the greatest possibility for cure.

The diagnosis of esophageal cancer is usually limited by the late onset of symptoms in patients with this disease. However, some patients do experience dysphagia or upper gastrointestinal bleeding while the tumor is still at an early stage. At Tokyo Women's Medical College, about 70% of patients with early esophageal cancer have symptoms suggestive of esophageal disease. Patients with early adenocarcinoma arising in Barrett's mucosa may also seek medical attention because of their underlying reflux disease, so that early esophageal cancer may be detected fortuitously in patients with reflux symptoms.[33] Finally, early esophageal cancer may be diagnosed on radiologic or endoscopic examinations performed as screening studies in asymptomatic patients with Bar-

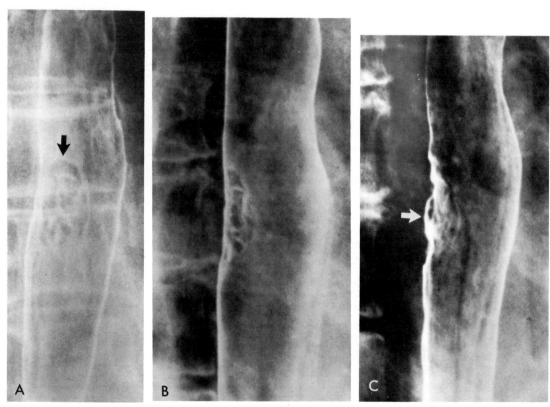

FIGURE 6–10

ULCERATED, PLAQUE-LIKE CARCINOMA SEEN IN MULTIPLE PROJECTIONS. *A,* En face view shows poorly defined filling defect (*arrow*) in midesophagus.
   B, Oblique view better delineates irregular surface of lesion.
   C, Profile view shows plaque-like nature of lesion with central area of ulceration (*arrow*).

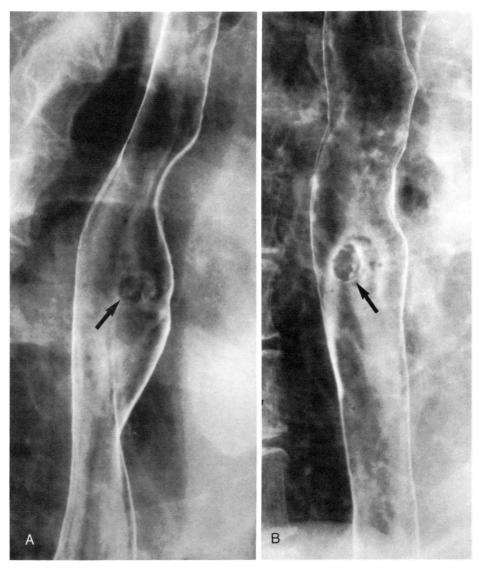

FIGURE 6–11

Two examples (A and B) of small esophageal cancers appearing as sessile, slightly lobulated polyps (arrows) in midesophagus. Note resemblance to squamous papilloma in Figure 6–1B.

rett's esophagus, achalasia, lye strictures, or other conditions that predispose patients to the development of esophageal carcinoma.

Double contrast esophagography has been widely advocated as the best radiologic technique for diagnosing early esophageal cancer. At Tokyo Women's Medical College, about 75% of these lesions are detected on double contrast studies. However, the higher sensitivity of this technique has resulted in a lower specificity, as more subtle lesions are identified and are suspected of representing cancer.[34] Nevertheless, it is probably best to accept a certain percentage of false-positive findings to avoid missing early can-

cers. The possibility of esophageal carcinoma should therefore be considered for any lesion that does not have a classically benign appearance. Although some benign lesions may be erroneously suspected of harboring malignancy, scrupulous endoscopic follow-up should clarify the diagnosis and lead to earlier detection of esophageal cancer.

In their early stages, esophageal cancers classically appear on double contrast radiographs as small, protruded lesions less than 3.5 cm in diameter.[33–35] They may be plaque-like lesions (often containing central ulceration) (Fig. 6–10) or flat, sessile polyps with a smooth or slightly lobulated contour (Fig. 6–11).

Other superficial tumors may cause focal irregularity, nodularity, or ulceration of the mucosa without a discrete lesion (Fig. 6–12).[36, 37] In patients with Barrett's esophagus, the earliest manifestation of a developing adenocarcinoma may be a localized area of wall flattening or stiffening in a pre-existing peptic stricture (Fig. 6–13).[33]

Because small or superficial tumors may produce relatively subtle radiographic findings, double contrast views should be obtained in multiple projections to evaluate a possible lesion both en face and in profile. Tangential views are particularly helpful for assessing the degree of intraluminal protrusion and the presence of associated ulceration (see Fig. 6–10). When the initial double contrast views are equivocal, a tube esophagram occasionally may be performed to confirm the presence of a lesion and to define its full extent (see Chapter 5).

Superficial spreading carcinoma is another potentially curable form of esophageal cancer that extends longitudinally in the esophageal wall without invading beyond the mucosa or submucosa. These lesions are manifested radiographically by tiny, coalescent nodules or plaques, causing nodularity or granularity of the mucosa (Fig. 6–14).[8, 33, 36, 37] Less frequently, an erosive form of superficial spreading cancer may be associated with shallow areas of ulceration (Fig. 6–15). The findings are often quite subtle, so that opti-

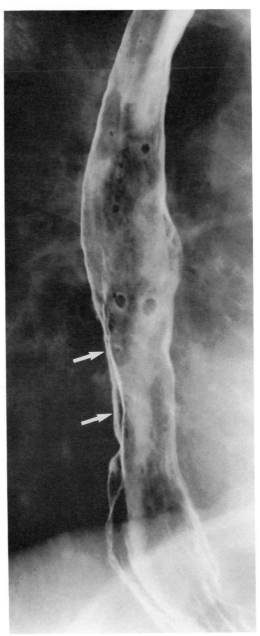

FIGURE 6–13

EARLY ADENOCARCINOMA IN BARRETT'S ESOPHAGUS. Relatively long peptic stricture is present in distal esophagus with slight flattening of one wall of stricture (*arrows*). (Note air bubbles in esophagus.) At surgery, this patient had carcinoma in situ within Barrett's mucosa.

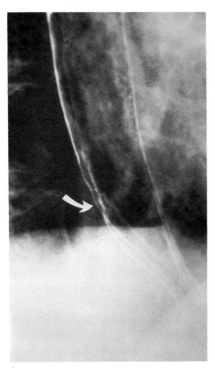

FIGURE 6–12

Superficial esophageal carcinoma with focal irregularity of esophageal wall due to shallow ulceration (*arrow*).

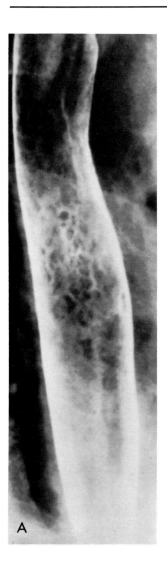
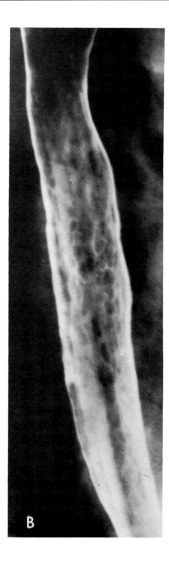

FIGURE 6–14

Two examples (A and B) of superficial spreading carcinoma. In both cases, note coarse, granular appearance of mucosa due to tiny mucosal elevations.

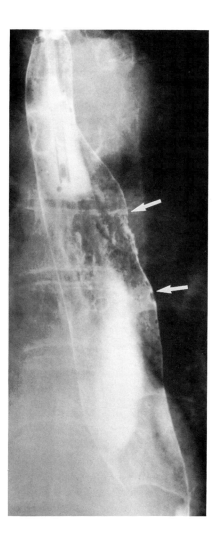

FIGURE 6–15

Erosive form of superficial spreading carcinoma with shallow, irregular areas of ulceration demarcated superiorly and inferiorly by *arrows*.

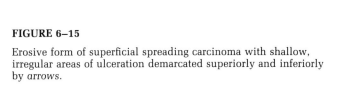

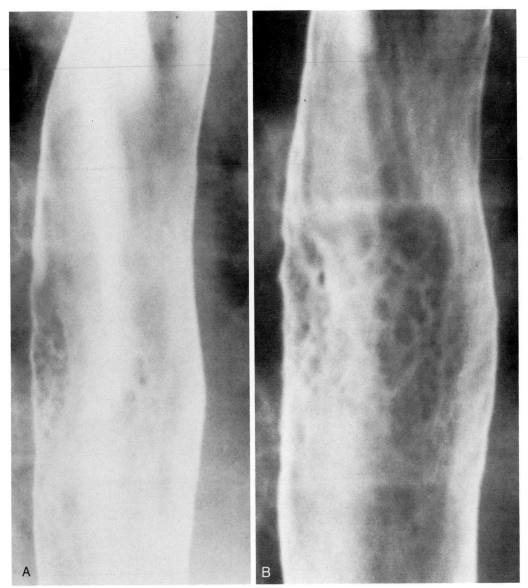

FIGURE 6–16

SUPERFICIAL SPREADING CARCINOMA–IMPORTANCE OF TECHNIQUE. *A,* Initial view shows barely discernible abnormality in midesophagus. Unfortunately, details of lesion are obscured by thick coating of high-density barium in esophagus—a phenomenon known as "flow artifact."

B, Repeat view moments later reveals coalescent plaques and nodules due to superficial spreading carcinoma. This case shows how demonstration of these lesions requires optimal radiographic technique.

mal radiographic technique is needed to demonstrate these lesions (Fig. 6–16).

Superficial spreading carcinoma occasionally can be mistaken for a localized area of *Candida* esophagitis. However, the plaque-like defects of candidiasis tend to be discrete lesions with sharp borders and normal intervening mucosa (Fig. 6–17),[38] whereas the nodules or plaques of superficial spreading carcinoma tend to coalesce, producing a continuous area of disease. Other considerations in the differential diagnosis include glycogenic acanthosis, esophageal papillomatosis, and leukoplakia.[4–8] However, these other conditions also tend to be manifested by discrete lesions rather than by a continuous area of mucosal disease. Finally, superficial spreading carcinoma may produce a reticulonodular appearance that closely resembles the reticular pattern of Barrett's mucosa (see Chapter 5). However, patients with Barrett's esophagus usually have a midesophageal stricture, with the reticular pattern extending distally a short but variable distance from the stricture (Fig. 6–18).[39]

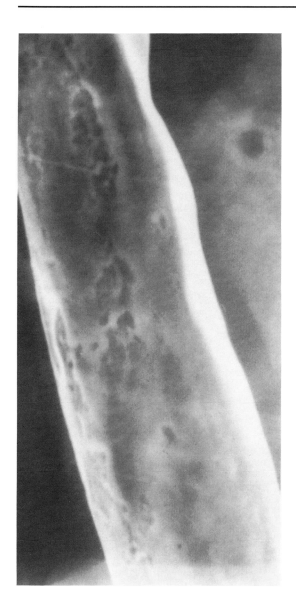

FIGURE 6–17

***CANDIDA* ESOPHAGITIS WITH MULTIPLE PLAQUES IN MIDESOPHAGUS.** Although this appearance could be mistaken for that of a superficial spreading carcinoma, note how the plaque-like defects of candidiasis are discrete lesions with normal intervening mucosa.

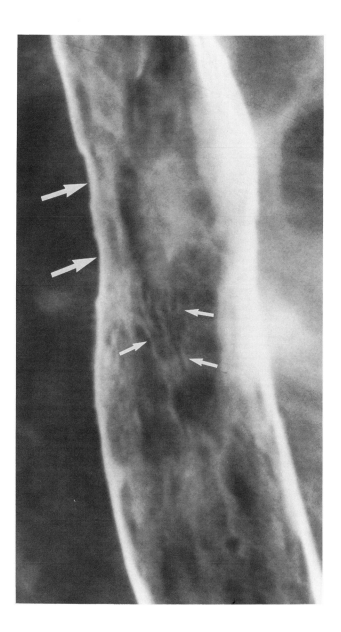

FIGURE 6–18

Barrett's esophagus with early stricture in midesophagus, manifested by slight flattening of esophageal wall *(large arrows).* A delicate reticular pattern adjacent to distal aspect of stricture *(small arrows)* could be mistaken for superficial spreading carcinoma. However, the typical appearance and location of reticular pattern adjacent to stricture should suggest Barrett's mucosa. (From Levine, M.S., et al.: Barrett esophagus: Reticular pattern of the mucosa. Radiology *147:*663–667, 1983, with permission.)

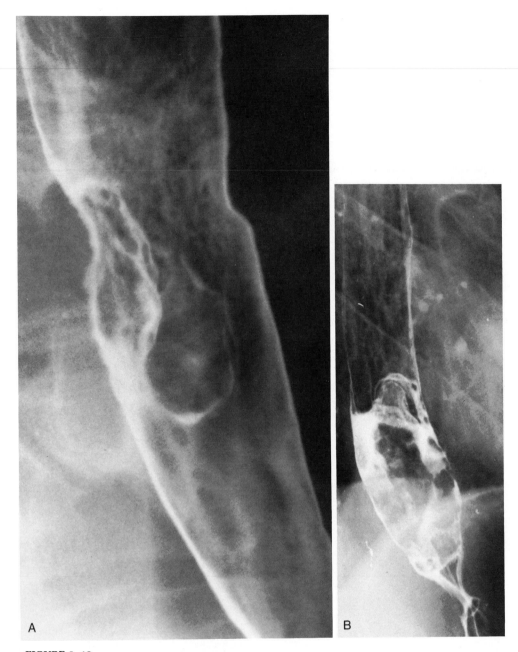

FIGURE 6–19

Two examples (A and B) of early esophageal cancers appearing as relatively large polypoid masses indistinguishable from advanced carcinomas. (A, From Levine, M.S.: Radiology of the Esophagus. Philadelphia, W.B. Saunders, 1989, p. 139.)

While early esophageal cancers are generally thought to be small lesions, some early cancers may appear as relatively large intraluminal masses greater than 3.5 cm in diameter (Fig. 6–19). Such polypoid lesions may be indistinguishable radiographically from advanced carcinomas.[33] Thus, early esophageal cancers are not necessarily small cancers, as they may undergo considerable intraluminal or intramural growth and still be classified histologically as early lesions.

Advanced Carcinoma

Advanced esophageal carcinomas (whether squamous cell carcinomas or adenocarcinomas) usually appear radiographically as infiltrating, polypoid, ulcerative, or varicoid lesions.[40] *Infiltrating* carcinomas are classically manifested by irregular narrowing and constriction of the lumen with nodular or ulcerated mucosa and abrupt, well-defined proximal and distal borders (Fig. 6–20). *Polypoid* carcinomas appear as

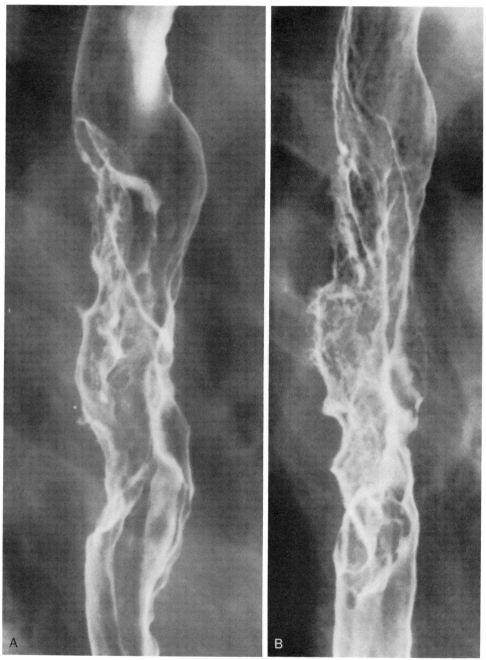

FIGURE 6–20

Infiltrating esophageal carcinomas (*A* and *B*) with irregular narrowing of lumen, ulceration, and relatively abrupt proximal and distal borders. (From Levine, M.S.: Radiology of the Esophagus. Philadelphia, W.B. Saunders, 1989, p. 141.)

lobulated or fungating intraluminal masses, usually greater than 3.5 cm in size (Fig. 6–21). *Ulcerative* carcinomas are relatively flat lesions in which the bulk of the tumor is replaced by ulceration. When viewed in profile, these lesions appear as irregular, meniscoid ulcers surrounded by a radiolucent rim of tumor (Fig. 6–22).[41] Finally, *varicoid* carcinomas are those in which submucosal spread of tumor produces thickened, tortuous longitudinal folds, mimicking the appearance of esophageal varices (Fig. 6–23).[42, 43] However, these lesions have a rigid, fixed configuration at fluoroscopy, whereas true varices tend to change in size and shape with peristalsis, respiration, and Valsalva maneuvers. Varicoid tumors are also manifested by a relatively abrupt demarcation between the involved segment and the adjacent normal

mucosa and often spare the distal esophagus. Thus, it usually is possible to differentiate varicoid tumors from varices on radiologic criteria.

Although advanced esophageal carcinomas may be classified by their predominant morphologic features, infiltrating lesions often have polypoid or ulcerated components (Fig. 6–24*A* and *B*), and polypoid lesions often have large areas of ulceration (see Fig. 24*C*). Thus, many lesions have mixed radiographic patterns, so that there is considerable overlap in the classification of these tumors.

Esophageal adenocarcinomas arising in Barrett's mucosa usually cannot be distinguished radiographically from squamous cell carcinomas. However, squamous cell carcinomas tend to involve the upper or middle third of the esophagus, whereas adenocar-

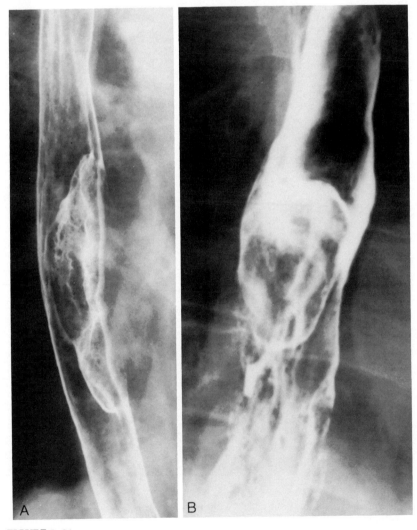

FIGURE 6–21

Polypoid carcinomas (*A* and *B*) appearing as lobulated intraluminal masses in esophagus. (*A*, From Collins, S.M., et al.: Small-bowel malabsorption and gastrointestinal malignancy. Radiology 126:603–609, 1978, with permission. *B*, From Levine, M.S.: Radiology of the Esophagus. Philadelphia, W.B. Saunders, 1989, p. 143.)

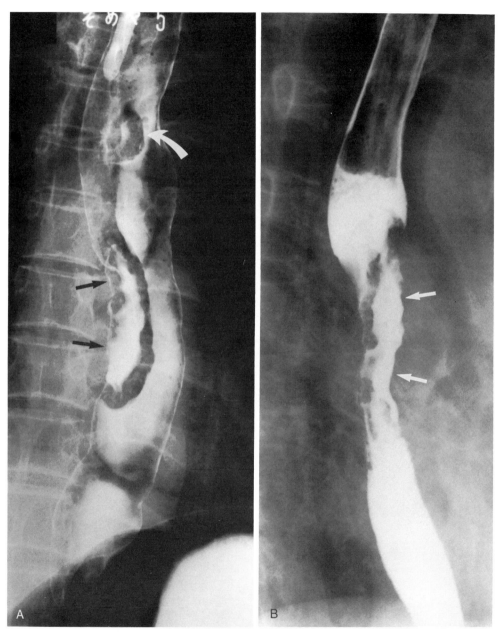

FIGURE 6–22

Ulcerative carcinomas (A and B) with large, meniscoid ulcers (straight arrows) and radiolucent rim of tumor adjacent to ulcers. Note discrete lymphatic metastasis with central ulceration (curved arrow) seen proximally in esophagus in A.

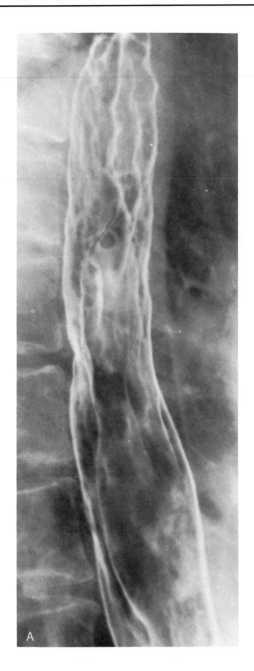

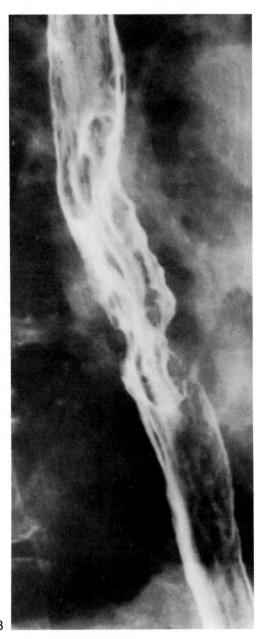

FIGURE 6–23

Varicoid carcinomas (*A* and *B*) in midesophagus with thickened, tortuous folds due to submucosal spread of tumor. These lesions could be mistaken for esophageal varices.

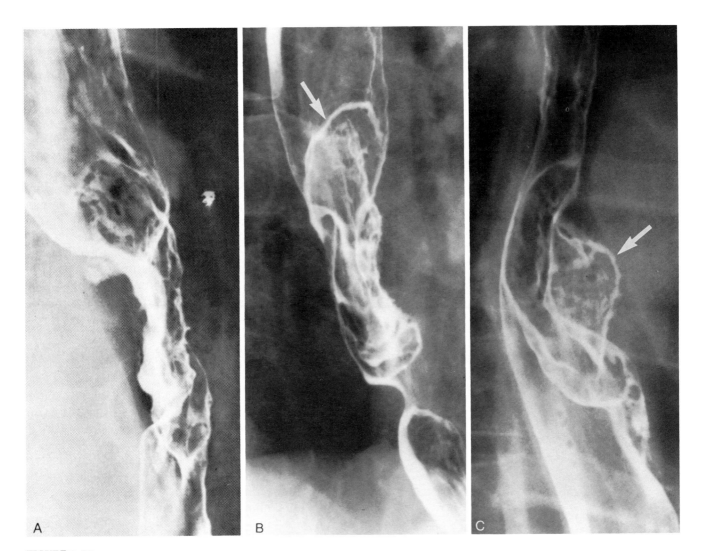

FIGURE 6–24

MIXED RADIOGRAPHIC PATTERNS IN ADVANCED ESOPHAGEAL CARCINOMA. *A*, Polypoid, infiltrating, and ulcerating carcinoma.
  B, Infiltrating carcinoma with polypoid superior component *(arrow)*.
  C, Polypoid carcinoma with large area of ulceration *(arrow)*.

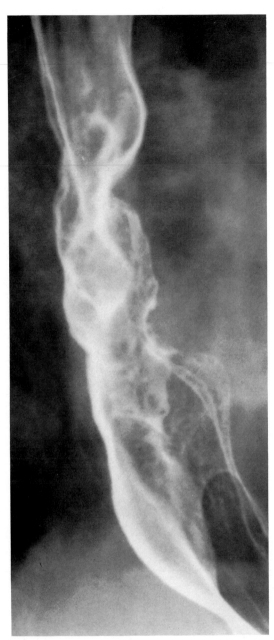

FIGURE 6–25

INFILTRATING ESOPHAGEAL CARCINOMA ARISING IN BARRETT'S MUCOSA. Note how lesion is located in distal esophagus above hiatal hernia. (From Levine, M.S.: Radiology of the Esophagus. Philadelphia, W.B. Saunders, 1989, p. 155.)

cinomas are predominantly located in the distal third (Fig. 6–25). Unlike squamous cell carcinomas, esophageal adenocarcinomas also have a marked tendency to invade the gastric cardia or fundus.[20, 21, 44] In the past, these tumors at the gastroesophageal junction have almost always been classified as primary gastric

carcinomas secondarily invading the lower end of the esophagus (see Chapter 8). However, recent data indicate that as many as 50% of adenocarcinomas at the gastroesophageal junction are Barrett's carcinomas invading the stomach.[20] Gastric involvement may be manifested radiographically by a polypoid or ulcerated mass in the fundus. In other patients, these tumors may cause obliteration of the normal anatomic landmarks at the cardia and irregular areas of ulceration without a discrete lesion (Fig. 6–26).[20] The findings may be quite subtle, so that optimal double contrast views of the gastric cardia and fundus are required to determine the full extent of tumor in this region.

Dissemination of esophageal carcinoma via the rich submucosal lymphatic channels in the esophagus may also result in discrete implants adjacent to or remote from the primary tumor. These lymphatic metastases may appear radiographically as polypoid, plaque-like, or ulcerated lesions that are separated from the main tumor by normal intervening mucosa (Fig. 6–27; see Fig. 6–22A).[45] In other patients, tumor emboli from squamous cell carcinoma may spread subdiaphragmatically to the gastric fundus via submucosal esophageal lymphatics. These squamous cell metastases to the stomach usually appear as large submucosal masses, often containing central areas of ulceration (Fig. 6–28).[46] Because the appropriate treatment for esophageal cancer depends on accurate staging of the tumor, the gastric cardia and fundus should be carefully examined in all patients with esophageal cancer to rule out unsuspected metastases to the stomach.

Once a lesion has been detected on double contrast studies, the presence of tumor can usually be confirmed at endoscopy. When biopsies and brushings are obtained, endoscopy has a sensitivity of more than 95% in diagnosing esophageal carcinoma.[47, 48] Nevertheless, negative endoscopic biopsies should not exclude the possibility of esophageal cancer if the radiographic findings are highly suggestive of tumor. In some cases, repeat radiologic or endoscopic examinations, or even surgery, may be necessary to establish the diagnosis.

Computed tomography, magnetic resonance imaging, and, most recently, endoscopic sonography have been used for preoperative staging of esophageal carcinoma.[49–51] Important prognostic features that can be assessed with these imaging techniques include the depth of esophageal wall invasion and the presence or absence of lymph node metastases or other metastatic lesions in the mediastinum. Even with these cross-sectional studies, however, it is difficult to detect lymph node metastases that are less than 1 cm in size.

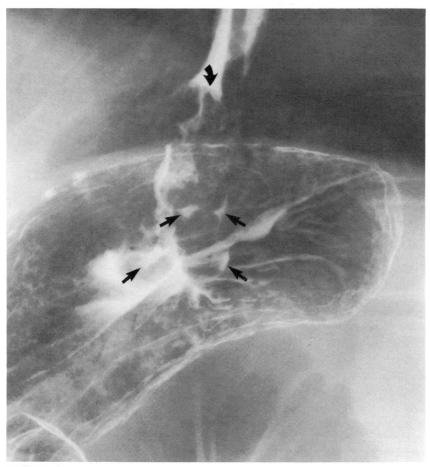

FIGURE 6–26

BARRETT'S ESOPHAGUS WITH ADENOCARCINOMA INVADING THE STOMACH.
Double contrast view of fundus shows obliteration of normal anatomic landmarks at
cardia with irregular areas of ulceration *(straight arrows)*. Note polypoid tumor in
distal esophagus *(curved arrow)*. (From Levine, M.S., et al.: Adenocarcinoma of the
esophagus: Relationship to Barrett mucosa. Radiology *150*:305–309, 1984, with
permission.)

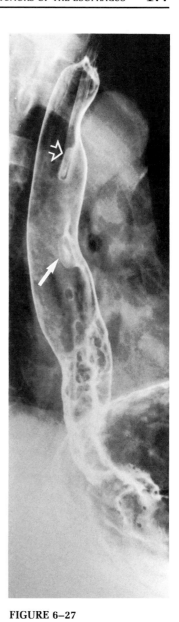

FIGURE 6–27

**ADVANCED ESOPHAGEAL
CARCINOMA WITH
LYMPHATIC METASTASIS.**
Note varicoid appearance of
tumor in distal esophagus with
discrete metastatic implant *(solid
arrow)* separated from main
lesion by normal intervening
mucosa. (This study was
performed as a tube *[open arrow]*
esophagram.)

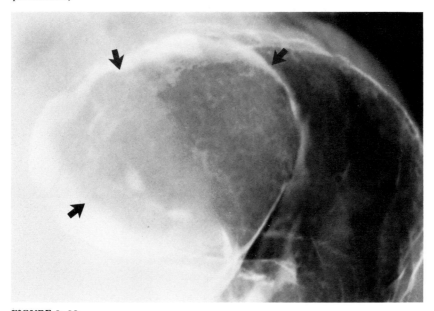

FIGURE 6–28

SQUAMOUS CELL METASTASIS TO STOMACH FROM ESOPHAGEAL CARCINOMA. Note giant submucosal
mass *(arrows)* in gastric fundus. (From Glick, S.N., et al.: Squamous cell metastases to the gastric cardia.
Gastrointest. Radiol. *10*:339, 1985, with permission.)

Associated Conditions

Achalasia is a premalignant condition in the esophagus associated with a significantly increased risk of the development of esophageal carcinoma.[23] Because the esophagus is already dilated, these tumors often reach an enormous size before causing dysphagia. As a result, the lesions are usually discovered as bulky intraluminal masses, most frequently in the middle or upper esophagus (Fig. 6–29).[52] Because these tumors can be obscured by retained fluid and debris, esophageal lavage with a soft rubber catheter may be necessary to cleanse the esophagus before performing the double contrast examination. With adequate preparation, a superimposed carcinoma can be demonstrated even in patients who have a massively dilated esophagus due to long-standing achalasia.

Patients with chronic lye strictures are also at increased risk for developing esophageal cancer.[24] It has been postulated that chronic inflammation and scarring from caustic ingestion are predisposing factors in the development of esophageal carcinoma. These lesions have a much better prognosis than other esophageal cancers, probably because of dense scar tissue surrounding the tumor, which prevents early invasion of adjacent mediastinal structures.[24] Any change in swallowing function in patients with chronic lye strictures should therefore lead to further investigation to detect this complication. The development of cancer may be manifested radiographically by increasing stenosis, mass effect, nodularity, or ulceration within a pre-existing lye stricture (Fig. 6–30). These lesions may be relatively subtle, so that any change in the appearance of a chronic lye stricture should be evaluated endoscopically to rule out a superimposed carcinoma.

Post-treatment Studies

Double contrast studies can be performed following palliative or, less frequently, curative radiotherapy for esophageal carcinoma. In general, squamous cell carcinomas of the esophagus are more radiosensitive than adenocarcinomas. Regression of tumor after radiotherapy is manifested by a decrease in the size or bulk of the lesion as compared with pretreatment studies. If the tumor regresses completely, follow-up barium studies may reveal a normal esophagus or a smooth, tapered stricture with a benign appearance at the site of the previous lesion (Figs. 6–31 and 6–32).[53] However, the latter patients often die from distant metastases, so that disappearance of the cancer on radiologic or endoscopic examinations does not necessarily indicate a cure. Recurrent dysphagia following radiotherapy may result not only from re-

Text continued on page 183

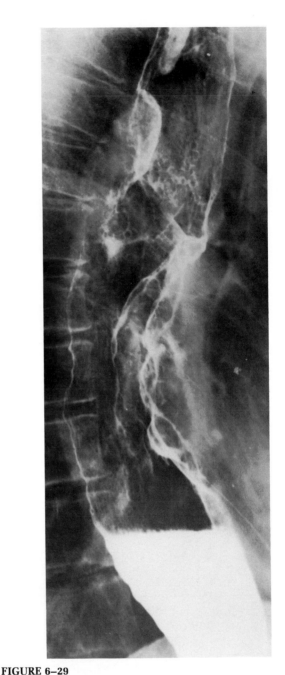

FIGURE 6–29

Advanced esophageal carcinoma in a patient with long-standing achalasia. Note barium level in distal esophagus below tumor.

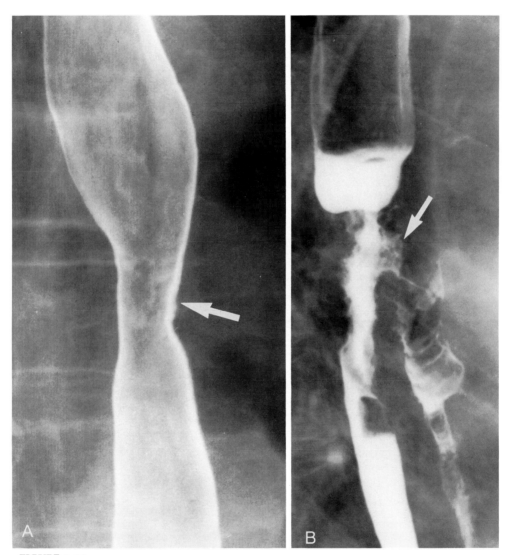

FIGURE 6–30

ESOPHAGEAL CARCINOMA IN LYE STRICTURE. *A,* Initial double contrast study shows focal stricture *(arrow)* in midesophagus due to previous lye ingestion. Note superficial ulceration and nodularity of mucosa in region of stricture. The patient refused surgery at this time.

   B, Repeat study 2 years later shows advanced esophageal carcinoma at site of previous stricture with esophagobronchial fistula *(arrow).* (From Levine, M.S.: Radiology of the Esophagus. Philadelphia, W.B. Saunders, 1989, p. 150.)

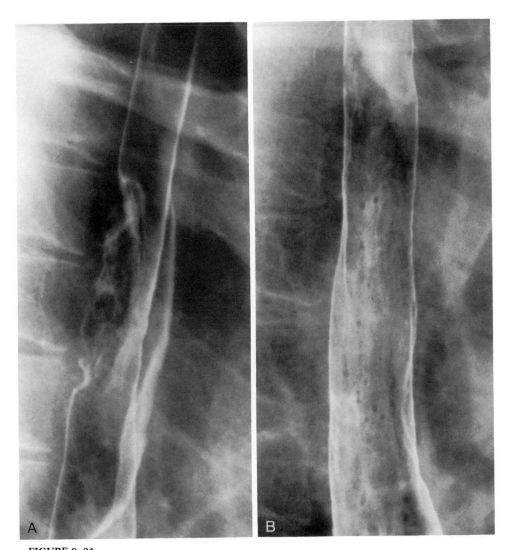

FIGURE 6–31

TOTAL REGRESSION OF ESOPHAGEAL CARCINOMA AFTER RADIATION THERAPY.
  A, Polypoid carcinoma in upper esophagus.
  B, Normal appearance of esophagus without evidence of residual tumor 2 years after radiation therapy. (From Levine, M.S., et al.: Radiation therapy of esophageal carcinoma: Correlation of clinical and radiographic findings. Gastrointest. Radiol. *12:*99, 1987, with permission.)

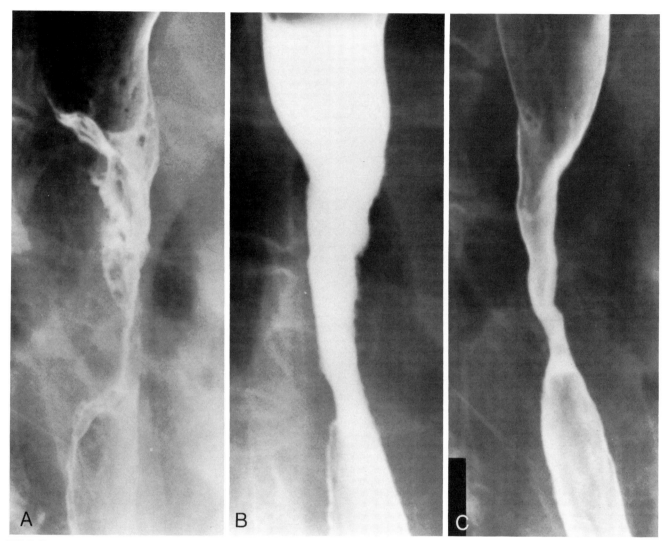

FIGURE 6–32

TOTAL REGRESSION OF ESOPHAGEAL CARCINOMA AFTER RADIATION THERAPY WITH BENIGN RESIDUAL STRICTURE. *A,*
Infiltrating carcinoma in midesophagus.

B, Partial regression of tumor with residual areas of ulceration 4 months after radiation therapy.

C, Total regression of tumor with smooth, tapered stricture in this region 6 months after radiation therapy. (From Levine, M.S.:
Radiology of the Esophagus. Philadelphia, W.B. Saunders, 1989, p. 164.)

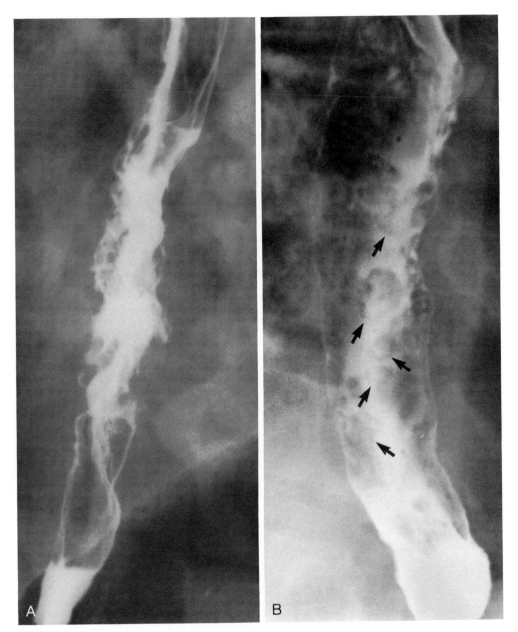

FIGURE 6–33

HERPES ESOPHAGITIS AFTER RADIATION THERAPY FOR ESOPHAGEAL CARCINOMA.
    A, Infiltrating carcinoma in distal esophagus.
    B, Repeat esophagram, obtained to evaluate recurrent dysphagia 18 months after radiation therapy, shows regression of tumor. However, note discrete ulcers with surrounding halos of edematous mucosa *(arrows)* due to herpes esophagitis. (From Levine, M.S., et al.: Radiation therapy of esophageal carcinoma: Correlation of clinical and radiographic findings. Gastrointest. Radiol. *12*:99, 1987, with permission.)

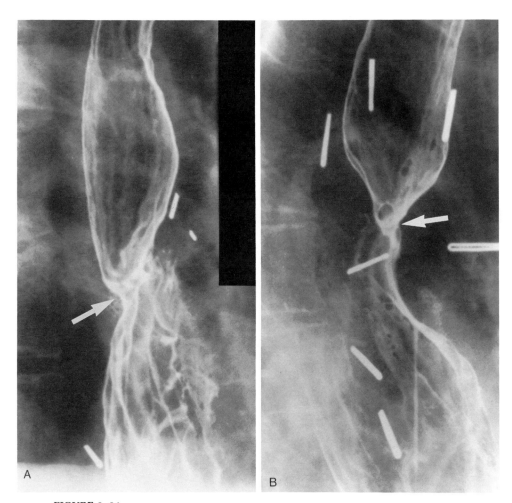

FIGURE 6–34

APPEARANCES FOLLOWING ESOPHAGOGASTRECTOMY. *A*, Normal postoperative
appearance of esophagogastric anastomosis *(arrow)*.
    B, Benign anastomotic stricture *(arrow)* in another patient.

current tumor but also from benign radiation strictures, fistulas, or opportunistic esophageal infection
(e.g., *Candida* or herpes esophagitis) (Fig. 6–33).
Thus, double contrast studies are particularly helpful
for differentiating recurrent carcinoma from other
esophageal complications in these patients.[53]

Double contrast studies can also be used to evaluate
patients who have undergone surgical resection of

esophageal carcinoma. The most frequently performed operation is an esophagogastrectomy and gastric pull-through. With double contrast technique, it
usually is possible to demonstrate the normal anatomy of the esophagogastric anastomosis and intratho-
racic stomach (Fig. 6–34A), so that anastomotic strictures or recurrent tumor can be detected (Fig. 6–
34B).[54]

METASTATIC DISEASE

Metastases to the esophagus can result from direct invasion by primary malignant tumors of the stomach, pharynx, or lung; from contiguous involvement by tumor-containing lymph nodes in the mediastinum; or from hematogenous metastases.[55] Direct extension of tumor from the adjacent lung or mediastinum may cause extensive mass effect, tethered folds, nodularity, ulceration, or in advanced cases, circumferential narrowing of the esophagus (Fig. 6–35). True blood-borne or hematogenous metastases are most frequently caused by carcinoma of the breast. They usually appear as short, eccentric strictures in the midesophagus.[55] Occasionally, carcinoma of the breast can metastasize to the esophagus many years after treatment of the original lesion.

LYMPHOMA

Both non-Hodgkin's and, less frequently, Hodgkin's lymphoma may involve the esophagus. These patients almost always have generalized lymphoma with direct invasion of the esophagus by lymphomatous nodes in the mediastinum, contiguous spread of lymphoma from the gastric fundus, or synchronous development of lymphoma in the wall of the esophagus. Esophageal lymphoma may demonstrate a spectrum of findings, including submucosal masses, enlarged folds, polypoid lesions, and strictures.[56] Occasionally, the esophagus may have a diffusely nodular appearance due to innumerable tiny, submucosal nodules extending from the thoracic inlet to the gastroesophageal junction (Fig. 6–36).[57] Other rare causes of submucosal nodules include leukemic infiltrates, he-

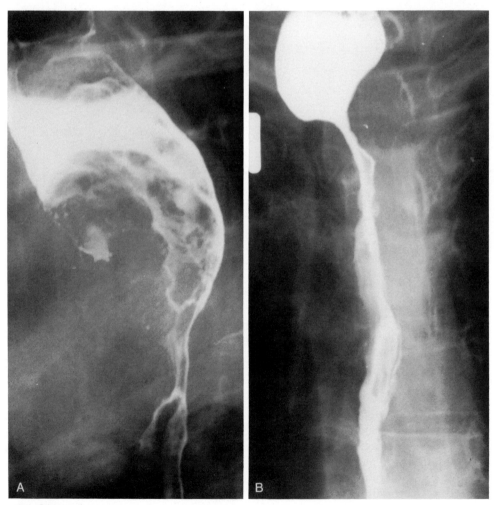

FIGURE 6–35

CARCINOMA OF LUNG INVADING ESOPHAGUS. *A,* Eccentric mass effect and narrowing of esophagus with irregular areas of ulceration due to direct invasion by mediastinal tumor. (From Levine, M.S.: Radiology of the Esophagus. Philadelphia, W.B. Saunders, 1989, p. 171.)

B, Another patient with a long segment of irregular narrowing in upper thoracic esophagus due to circumferential involvement by metastatic tumor in the mediastinum. (Courtesy of Robert Goren, M.D., Philadelphia, Pennsylvania.)

matogenous metastases, esophageal retention cysts, and multiple leiomyomas, but the lesions tend to be larger and less numerous in these conditions.

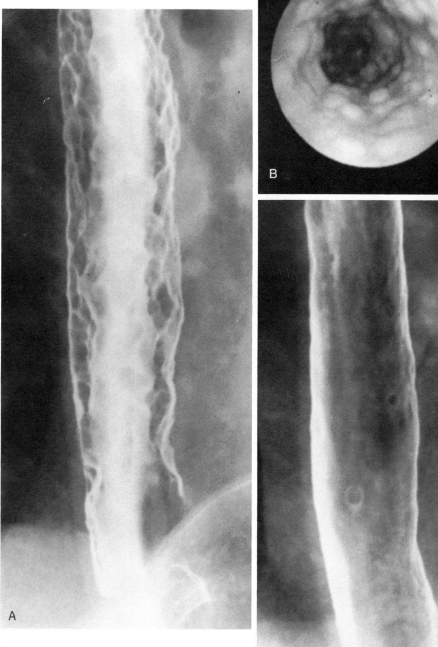

FIGURE 6–36

NON-HODGKIN'S LYMPHOMA INVOLVING ESOPHAGUS.
A, Initial esophagram shows innumerable small submucosal-appearing defects in thoracic esophagus. Note resemblance to varices.

   B, Endoscopic photograph reveals multiple, discrete submucosal nodules.

   C, Repeat esophagram 2 months after chemotherapy shows virtually complete regression of lesions seen on earlier study. (Note air bubbles in esophagus.) (From Levine, M.S., et al.: Diffuse nodularity in esophageal lymphoma. AJR *145:*1218–1220, 1985, with permission, © by American Roentgen Ray Society.)

OTHER MALIGNANT TUMORS

Polypoid malignant tumors of the esophagus containing both carcinomatous and sarcomatous elements are rare. In the past, these lesions have been called carcinosarcomas or pseudosarcomas. However, they are now classified as spindle cell carcinomas, as they are thought to represent carcinomas that have undergone varying degrees of spindle cell metaplasia.[58] Spindle cell carcinomas typically appear radiographically as polypoid intraluminal masses that expand the esophageal lumen without causing obstruction (Fig. 6–37).[58, 59] Other esophageal neoplasms may produce similar findings, however, so that spindle

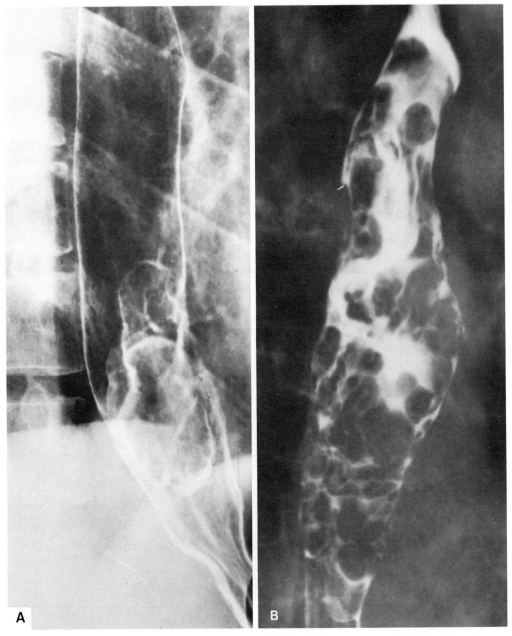

A

B

FIGURE 6–37

TWO EXAMPLES OF SPINDLE CELL CARCINOMA. *A*, Polypoid intraluminal mass in distal esophagus.
B, More extensive intraluminal mass that locally expands esophagus without causing obstruction. Note scalloped borders of lesion.

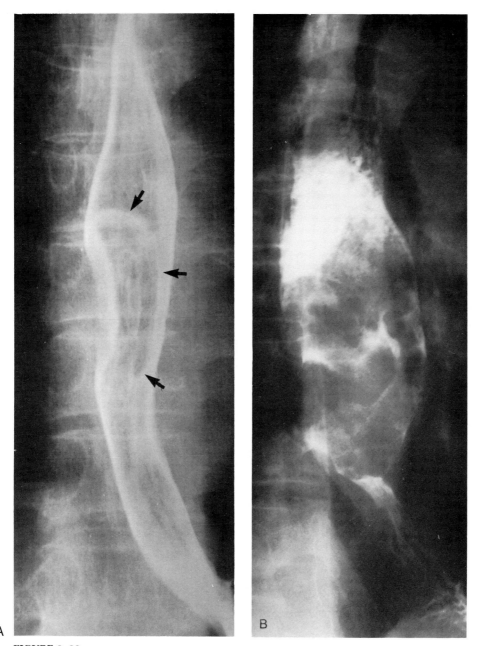

A

B

FIGURE 6–38

LEIOMYOSARCOMAS. *A*, Note large intramural tumor (*arrows*) in midesophagus. The appearance is indistinguishable from that of other submucosal lesions.

B, More advanced lesion appearing as bulky intraluminal mass in distal esophagus. (*B*, Courtesy of William M. Thompson, M.D., Minneapolis, Minnesota.)

cell carcinomas can only be diagnosed definitively on histologic grounds.

Leiomyosarcomas and melanosarcomas are other rare sarcomatous lesions in the esophagus that typically appear radiographically as bulky intraluminal masses (Fig. 6–38).[60, 61] Recently, esophageal involvement by Kaposi's sarcoma has also been recognized with increased frequency in patients with AIDS. These tumors are characterized by multiple submucosal masses or by a single polypoid or infiltrating lesion in the esophagus (Fig. 6–39).[62, 63] Double contrast studies are particularly helpful for differentiating opportunistic esophagitis from Kaposi's sarcoma involving the esophagus in patients with AIDS.

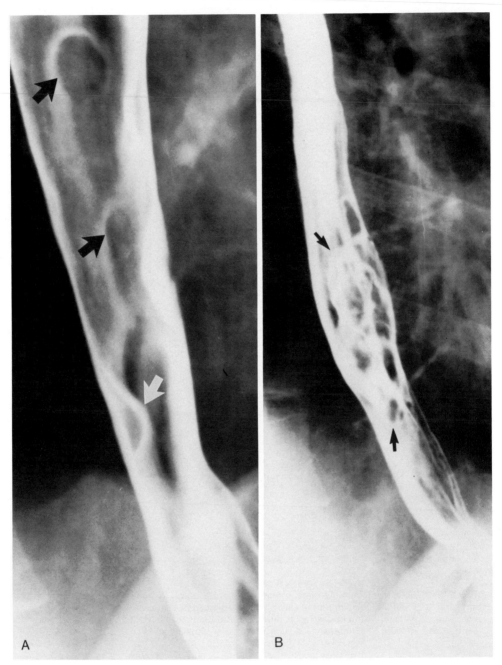

FIGURE 6–39

KAPOSI'S SARCOMA INVOLVING ESOPHAGUS. *A,* Several discrete submucosal masses *(arrows)* are present in esophagus in AIDS patient with Kaposi's sarcoma. (Courtesy of Robert Goren, M.D., Philadelphia, Pennsylvania.)

B, Another patient with Kaposi's sarcoma manifested by large polypoid mass *(arrows)* in distal esophagus. (From Rose, H.S., et al.: Alimentary tract involvement in Kaposi sarcoma: Radiographic and endoscopic findings in 25 homosexual men. AJR 139:661–666, 1982, with permission, © by American Roentgen Ray Society.)

REFERENCES

1. Miller, B.J., Murphy, F., and Lukie, B.E.: Squamous cell papilloma of esophagus. Can. J. Surg. 21:538, 1978.
2. Montesi, A., Alessandro, P., Graziani, L., et al.: Small benign tumors of the esophagus: Radiological diagnosis with double-contrast examination. Gastrointest. Radiol. 8:207, 1983.
3. Rywlin, A.M., and Ortega, R.: Glycogenic acanthosis of the esophagus. Arch. Pathol. 90:439, 1970.
4. Berliner, L., Redmond, P., Horowitz, L., et al.: Glycogen plaques (glycogenic acanthosis) of the esophagus. Radiology 141:607, 1981.
5. Glick, S.N., Teplick, S.K., Goldstein, J., et al.: Glycogenic acanthosis of the esophagus. AJR 139:683, 1982.
6. Ghahremani, G.G., and Rushovich, A.M.: Glycogenic acanthosis of the esophagus: Radiographic and pathologic features. Gastrointest. Radiol. 9:93, 1984.
7. Nuwayhid, N.S., Ballard, E.T., and Cotton, R.: Esophageal papillomatosis. Ann. Otol. Rhinol. Laryngol. 86:623, 1977.
8. Itai, Y., Kogure, T., Okiyama, Y., et al.: Diffuse finely nodular lesions of the esophagus. AJR 128:563, 1977.
9. Itai, Y., Kogure, T., Okiyama, Y., et al.: Radiological manifestations of oesophageal involvement in acanthosis nigricans. Br. J. Radiol. 49:592, 1976.
10. Plachta, A.: Benign tumors of the esophagus: Review of literature and report of 99 cases. Am. J. Gastroenterol. 38:639, 1962.
11. Glanz, I., and Grunebaum, M.: The radiological approach to leiomyoma of the oesophagus with a long-term follow-up. Clin. Radiol. 28:197, 1977.
12. Gutman, E.: Posterior mediastinal calcification due to esophageal leiomyoma. Gastroenterology 63:665, 1972.
13. Nora, P.F.: Lipoma of the esophagus. Am. J. Surg. 108:353, 1964.
14. Govoni, A.F.: Hemangiomas of the esophagus. Gastrointest. Radiol. 7:113, 1982.
15. Rubesin, S.E., Herlinger, H., and Sigal, H.: Granular cell tumors of the esophagus. Gastrointest. Radiol. 10:11, 1985.
16. Farman, J., Rosen, Y., Dallemand, S., et al.: Esophagitis cystica: Lower esophageal retention cysts. AJR 128:495, 1977.
17. Trenkner, S.W., Levine, M.S., Laufer, I., et al.: Idiopathic esophageal varix. AJR 141:43, 1983.
18. Carter, M.M., and Kulkarni, M.V.: Giant fibrovascular polyp of the esophagus. Gastrointest. Radiol. 9:301, 1984.
19. Cochet, B., Hohl, P., Sans, M., et al.: Asphyxia caused by laryngeal impaction of an esophageal polyp. Arch. Otolaryngol. 106:176, 1980.
20. Levine, M.S., Caroline, D., Thompson, J.J., et al.: Adenocarcinoma of the esophagus: Relationship to Barrett mucosa. Radiology 150:305, 1984.
21. Agha, F.P.: Barrett carcinoma of the esophagus: Clinical and radiographic analysis of 34 cases. AJR 145:41, 1985.
22. Wynder, E.L., and Mabuchi, K.: Cancer of the esophagus: Etiological and environmental factors. JAMA 226:1546, 1973.
23. Carter, R., and Brewer, L.A.: Achalasia and esophageal carcinoma. Am. J. Surg. 130:114, 1975.
24. Appleqvist, P., and Salmo, M.: Lye corrosion carcinoma of the esophagus: A review of 63 cases. Cancer 45:2655, 1980.
25. Goldstein, H.M., and Zornoza, J.: Association of squamous cell carcinoma of the head and neck with cancer of the esophagus. AJR 131:791, 1978.
26. Collins, S.M., Hamilton, J.D., Lewis, T.D., and Laufer, I.: Small-bowel malabsorption and gastrointestinal malignancy. Radiology 126:603, 1978.
27. Chisholm, M.: The association between webs, iron and postcricoid carcinoma. Postgrad. Med. J. 50:215, 1974.
28. Harper, P.S., Harper, R.M.J., and Howel-Evans, A.W.: Carcinoma of the oesophagus with tylosis. Q.J. Med. 39:317, 1970.
29. Levine, M.S.: Barrett's esophagus: A radiologic diagnosis? AJR 151:433, 1988.
30. Japanese Society for Esophageal Diseases: Guidelines for the clinical and pathologic studies on carcinoma of the esophagus. Jpn. J. Surg. 6:69, 1976.
31. Guojun, H., Lingfang, S., Dawei, Z., et al.: Diagnosis and surgical treatment of early esophageal carcinoma. Chin. Med. J. [Engl.] 94:229, 1981.
32. Zornoza, J., and Lindell, M.M.: Radiologic evaluation of small esophageal carcinoma. Gastrointest. Radiol. 5:107, 1980.
33. Levine, M.S., Dillon, E.C., Saul, S.H., et al.: Early esophageal cancer. AJR 146:507, 1986.
34. Moss, A.A., Koehler, R.E., and Margulis, A.R.: Initial accuracy of esophagograms in detection of small esophageal carcinoma. AJR 127:909, 1976.
35. Koehler, R.E., Moss, A.A., and Margulis, A.R.: Early radiographic manifestations of carcinoma of the esophagus. Radiology 119:1, 1976.
36. Itai, Y., Kogure, T., Okiyama, Y., et al.: Superficial esophageal carcinoma: Radiological findings in double-contrast studies. Radiology 126:597, 1978.
37. Sato, T., Sakai, Y., Kajita, A., et al.: Radiographic microstructures of early esophageal carcinoma: Correlation of specimen radiography with pathologic findings and clinical radiography. Gastrointest. Radiol. 11:12, 1986.
38. Levine, M.S., Macones, A.J., and Laufer, I.: Candida esophagitis: Accuracy of radiographic diagnosis. Radiology 154:581, 1985.
39. Levine, M.S., Kressel, H.Y., Caroline, D.F., et al.: Barrett esophagus: Reticular pattern of the mucosa. Radiology 147:663, 1983.
40. Goldstein, H.M., Zornoza, J., and Hopens, T.: Intrinsic diseases of the adult esophagus: Benign and malignant tumors. Semin. Roentgenol. 16:183, 1981.
41. Gloyna, R.E., Zornoza, J., and Goldstein, H.M.: Primary ulcerative carcinoma of the esophagus. AJR 129:599, 1977.
42. Lawson, T.L., Dodds, W.J., and Sheft, D.J.: Carcinoma of the esophagus simulating varices. AJR 107:83, 1969.
43. Yates, C.W., LeVine, M.A., and Jensen, K.M.: Varicoid carcinoma of the esophagus. Radiology 122:605, 1977.
44. Keen, S.J., Dodd, G.D., and Smith, J.L.: Adenocarcinoma arising in Barrett's esophagus: Pathologic and radiologic features. Mt. Sinai J. Med. 51:442, 1984.
45. Steiner, H., Lammer, J., and Hackl, A.: Lymphatic metastases to the esophagus. Gastrointest. Radiol. 9:1, 1984.
46. Glick, S.N., Teplick, S.K., Levine, M.S., et al.: Gastric cardia metastasis in esophageal carcinoma. Radiology 160:627, 1986.
47. Sherlock, P., Ehrlich, A.N., and Winawer, S.J.: Diagnosis of gastrointestinal cancer: Current status and recent progress. Gastroenterology 63:672, 1972.
48. Bemvenuti, G.A., Hattori, K., Levin, B., et al.: Endoscopic sampling for tissue diagnosis in GI malignancy. Gastrointest. Endosc. 21:159, 1975.
49. Thompson, W.M., Halvorsen, R.A., Foster, W.L., et al.: Computed tomography for staging esophageal and gastroesophageal cancer: Reevaluation. AJR 141:951, 1983.
50. Petrillo, R., Balzarini, L., Bidoli, P., et al.: Esophageal squamous cell carcinoma: MRI evaluation of the mediastinum. Gastrointest. Radiol. 15:275, 1990.
51. Vilgrain, V., Mompoint, D., Palazzo, L., et al.: Staging of esophageal carcinoma: Comparison of results with endoscopic sonography and CT. AJR 155:277, 1990.
52. Hankins, J.R., and McLaughlin, J.S.: The association of carcinoma of the esophagus with achalasia. J. Thorac. Cardiovasc. Surg. 69:355, 1975.
53. Levine, M.S., Langer, J., Laufer, I., et al.: Radiation therapy of esophageal carcinoma: Correlation of clinical and radiographic findings. Gastrointest. Radiol. 12:99, 1987.
54. Owen, J.W., Balfe, D.M., Koehler, R.E., et al.: Radiologic evaluation of complications after esophagogastrectomy. AJR 140:1163, 1983.
55. Anderson, M.F., and Harell, G.S.: Secondary esophageal tumors. AJR 135:1243, 1980.
56. Carnovale, R.L., Goldstein, H.M., Zornoza, J., et al.: Radiologic manifestations of esophageal lymphoma. AJR 128:751, 1977.

57. Levine, M.S., Sunshine, A.G., Reynolds, J.C., et al.: Diffuse nodularity in esophageal lymphoma. AJR 145:1218, 1985.

58. Agha, F.P., and Keren, D.F.: Spindle-cell squamous carcinoma of the esophagus: A tumor with biphasic morphology. AJR 145:541, 1985.

59. Olmsted, W.W., Lichtenstein, J.E., and Hyams, V.J.: Polypoid epithelial malignancies of the esophagus. AJR 140:921, 1983.

60. Wolfel, D.A.: Leiomyosarcoma of the esophagus. AJR 89:127, 1963.

61. Hendricks, G.L., Barnes, W.T., and Suter, H.J.: Primary malignant melanoma of the esophagus. Am. Surg. 40:468, 1974.

62. Rose, H.S., Balthazar, E.J., Megibow, A.J., et al.: Alimentary tract involvement in Kaposi sarcoma: Radiographic and endoscopic findings in 25 homosexual men. AJR 139:661, 1982.

63. Umerah, B.C.: Kaposi sarcoma of the oesophagus. Br. J. Radiol. 53:807, 1980.

STOMACH

7

Marc S. Levine, M.D.
Igor Laufer, M.D.

NORMAL APPEARANCES

The normal appearance of the stomach is familiar to all physicians. The double contrast examination provides additional detail, however, about the anatomic structure of the stomach, including (1) the surface pattern, (2) the cardia, and (3) compression by adjacent structures.

Surface Pattern

While single contrast barium studies of the stomach rely heavily on analysis of the rugal fold pattern, gastric distention effaces the normal rugal folds on double contrast studies. Abnormal folds, such as those associated with a healing gastric ulcer or early gastric cancer, may be stiffer than normal and therefore tend to resist effacement. As a result, they may become particularly prominent when the surrounding normal folds are flattened.

When adequate mucosal coating and gaseous distention of the stomach have been achieved, the surface pattern or areae gastricae can be seen (Fig. 7–1).[1] The frequency of visualization of the normal areae gastricae depends not only on radiographic technique but also on the amount and viscosity of mucus in the stomach. With high-density barium suspensions, the areae gastricae can be detected on routine double contrast studies in about 70% of patients.[2] This surface pattern is observed most frequently in the antrum or body of the stomach (Fig. 7–1A), but it can also be seen in the fundus (Fig. 7–1B). Areae gastricae are easier to visualize on barium studies than on endoscopy, presumably because of the thin layer of mucus

that obscures these tiny crevices in the mucosa on endoscopic examinations. However, the normal surface pattern of the stomach can be well demonstrated on scanning electron micrographs (Fig. 7–2).

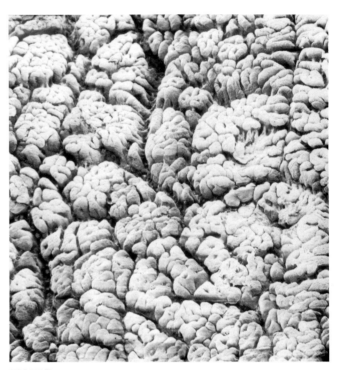

FIGURE 7–2

Scanning electron micrograph showing normal surface pattern of stomach. Innumerable gastric sulci account for reticular appearance seen on radiographs. The tiny black dots represent openings of gastric pits. (Magnification, × 20.) (Courtesy of Gerald D. Dodd, M.D., and J.D. Anderson, M.D., Houston, Texas, and Harvey M. Goldstein, M.D., San Antonio, Texas.)

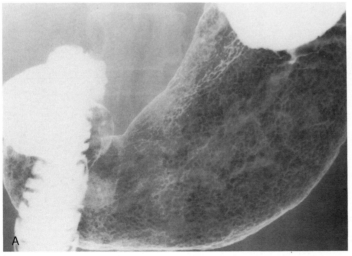
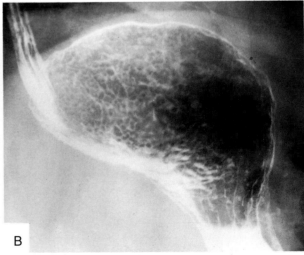

FIGURE 7–1

NORMAL SURFACE PATTERN OF STOMACH. *A,* Areae gastricae in antrum and body.
   B, Areae gastricae in fundus.

Variations in the size and appearance of the areae gastricae are sometimes seen on double contrast studies. It has been postulated that the size of the areae gastricae depends on parietal cell mass.[1] As a result, hypersecretory states or duodenal ulcers may be associated with enlarged areae gastricae, particularly in the upper body and fundus of the stomach (Fig. 7–3).[3, 4] Focal enlargement or distortion of the areae gastricae may also be a manifestation of nonspecific inflammation, intestinal metaplasia (Fig. 7–4), or even mucosal spread of cancer (Fig. 7–5).[5] Conversely, patients with atrophic gastritis tend to have small or

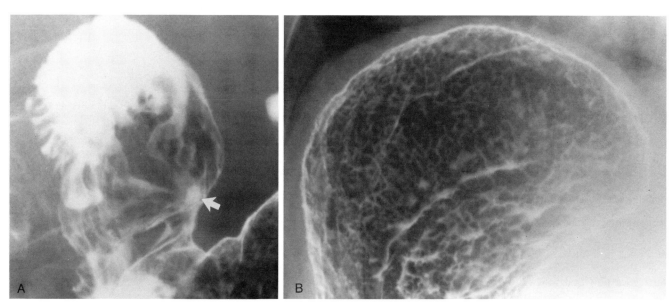

FIGURE 7–3

DUODENAL ULCER WITH ENLARGED AREAE GASTRICAE IN FUNDUS. *A,* Small ulcer *(arrow)* at base of duodenal bulb. *B,* Enlarged areae gastricae in fundus, probably secondary to hypersecretion of acid associated with peptic ulcer.

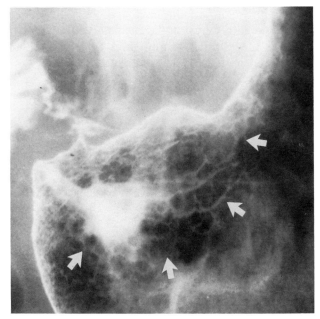

FIGURE 7–4

Intestinal metaplasia in antrum, causing focal irregularity and enlargement of areae gastricae *(arrows).*

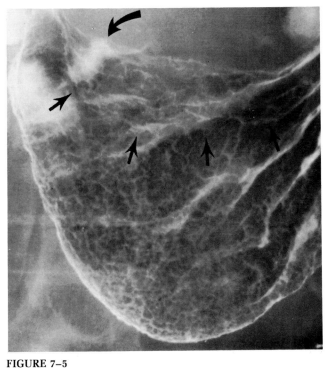

FIGURE 7–5

Ulcerated carcinoma *(curved arrow)* on lesser curvature of antrum. Note enlarged, distorted areae gastricae *(straight arrows)* in adjacent stomach due to mucosal spread of tumor.

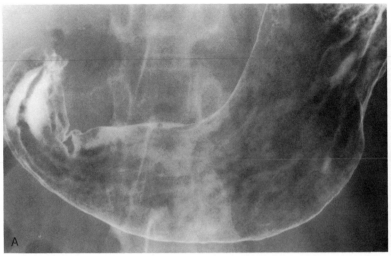

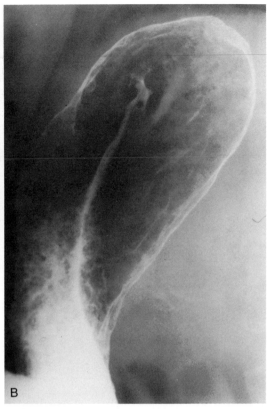

FIGURE 7–6

A and *B*, Atrophic gastritis with tiny, barely discernible areae gastricae in stomach. Note decreased distensibility and paucity of mucosal folds in antrum, body, and fundus. (From Levine, M.S., et al.: Atrophic gastritis in pernicious anemia: Diagnosis by double-contrast radiography. Gastrointest. Radiol. 14:215, 1989, with permission.)

absent areae gastricae (Fig. 7–6), presumably because of achlorhydria and the loss of parietal cells that occur in these individuals.[6] However, other investigators have found no correlation between the size of the areae gastricae and the presence or absence of superficial or atrophic gastritis.[7] As a result, it is generally difficult to diagnose abnormalities on the basis of the areae gastricae. When there is a striking focal alteration, however, endoscopic biopsies should be performed to rule out an early gastric cancer.

Occasionally, fine transverse folds or striae may also be seen in the gastric antrum (Fig. 7–7).[8, 9] Unlike transverse folds in the esophagus, which occur as a transient phenomenon, these gastric folds are more persistent. Some patients have associated antral gastritis.[9] The pathophysiologic basis and clinical significance of these folds are uncertain, however, and we tend to consider them a normal variant.

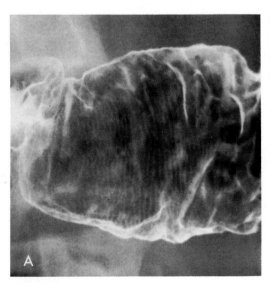

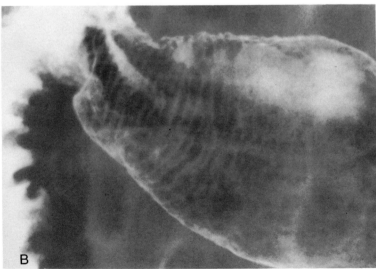

FIGURE 7–7

Two examples (*A* and *B*) of fine transverse folds or striae in antrum, probably occurring as a normal variant.

Cardia

The gastric cardia and fundus are particularly well demonstrated by double contrast technique.[10, 11] The radiographic appearance of the cardia on double contrast studies depends on how firmly it is anchored by the surrounding phrenoesophageal membrane to the esophageal hiatus of the diaphragm. When the cardia is well anchored, protrusion of the distal esophagus into the fundus produces a circular elevation containing four or five stellate folds that radiate to a central point at the gastroesophageal junction (the cardiac "rosette") (Fig. 7–8A).[10, 11] The circular elevation may be etched in white or may appear as a filling defect in the surrounding barium pool, depending on the amount of barium in the fundus. This elevation is demarcated from the adjacent fundus by a "hooding" fold that surrounds it laterally and superiorly. In the past, this hooding fold has been called the "sign of the burnous" because of its resemblance to the cloak-like garment worn by Arabs and Moors.[12] Several longitudinal folds characteristically extend inferiorly from the cardiac rosette along the posterior wall and lesser curvature.

When the cardia is less firmly anchored, an esophageal rosette may be visible without an associated protrusion or circular elevation (see Fig. 7–8B).[11] With further ligamentous laxity, the rosette may also vanish, and the cardia may be recognized by only a single crescentic line that crosses the area of the esophageal orifice (see Fig. 7–8C).[11] Finally, severe ligamentous

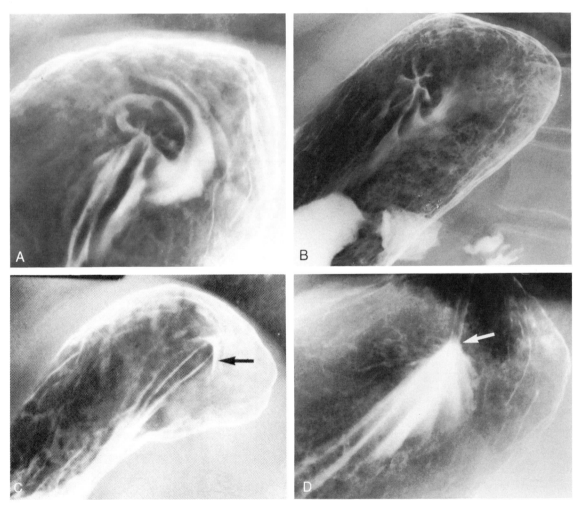

FIGURE 7–8

NORMAL CARDIA AND ITS VARIATIONS. *A,* Well-anchored cardia appearing as circular elevation with centrally radiating folds (the cardiac "rosette").

B, Stellate folds without surrounding elevation due to laxity of ligamentous attachments.

C, Further weakening of ligaments with obliteration of cardiac rosette. Note crescentic line *(arrow)* that crosses area of esophageal orifice.

D, Severe ligamentous laxity with gastric folds in small hiatal hernia converging superiorly *(arrow)* above esophageal hiatus of diaphragm.

laxity may lead to the formation of a hiatal hernia, so that no cardiac structure is identified below the diaphragm (see Fig. 7–8D).

Radiologists should be familiar with the range of appearances of the cardia to avoid mistaking the normal anatomic landmarks in this region for ulcers or mass lesions. At the same time, abnormalities at the cardia may be manifested by relatively subtle findings. For example, an ulcer adjacent to the cardia can be mistaken for the esophageal orifice (Fig. 7–9A). Carcinoma of the cardia may cause distortion or obliteration of the cardiac rosette without a discrete mass (Fig. 7–9B; see Chapter 8). Finally, gastric varices may be manifested by enlarged, scalloped folds adjacent to the cardia (Fig. 7–9C and D). Thus, radiologic evaluation of the cardia requires meticulous attention to anatomic detail in this region.

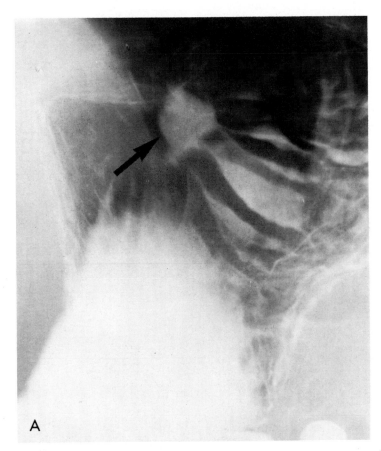

A

FIGURE 7–9

ABNORMALITIES AROUND CARDIA. *A*, Gastric ulcer *(arrow)* adjacent to cardia. Note how radiating folds are longer and more prominent than normal stellate folds in cardiac rosette.

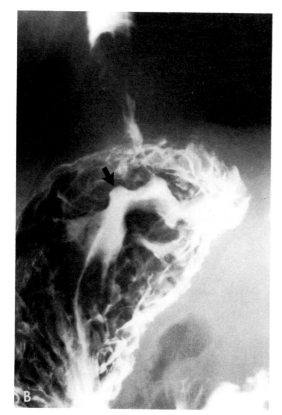

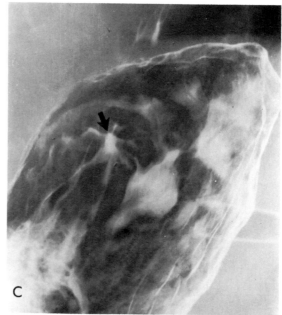

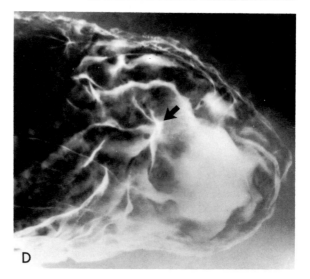

FIGURE 7–9 *Continued*

B, Carcinoma of cardia with obliteration of
normal cardiac structures and associated ulceration
(arrow). Note how tumor extends into distal
esophagus.

C and *D*, Two examples of gastric varices with
enlarged, lobulated folds adjacent to cardia. The
central button of cardiac rosette is indicated by
arrows.

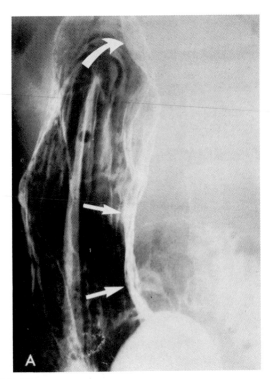
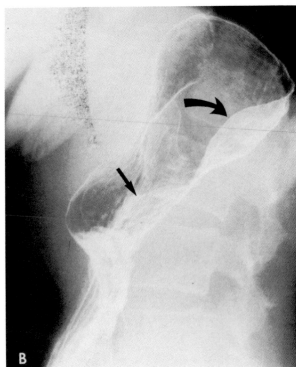

FIGURE 7–10

NORMAL RETROGASTRIC IMPRESSIONS. *A,* Subtle impressions on posterior wall of stomach from normal retrogastric structures such as pancreas *(straight arrows)* and spleen *(curved arrow).*

B, In thin patients, these impressions from pancreas *(straight arrow)* and spleen *(curved arrow)* may become more prominent but are still normal.

Extrinsic Impressions

The double contrast examination results in considerable distention of the stomach, particularly when a hypotonic agent is employed. As a result, neighboring structures may produce a variety of extrinsic impressions on the distended stomach. On lateral views, the posterior wall of the stomach may be compressed by normal retrogastric structures such as the pancreas and spleen (Fig. 7–10A). This finding may be particularly prominent in thin patients (see Fig. 7–10B). Although impressions caused by the liver are usually quite subtle, enlargement of the left lobe of the liver or anomalous lobulation of the liver may produce an extrinsic impression on the lesser curvature of the gastric body, mimicking the appearance of an intramural gastric lesion (Fig. 7–11). A gas- or stool-filled splenic flexure of the colon may also cause an impression on the posterolateral wall of the upper stomach.

Retrogastric masses can be recognized en face by an ill-defined translucency in the stomach (Fig. 7–12A), or on oblique views by a double contour seen through the gas-filled stomach, with one line representing the edge of the mass. However, lateral views are best for showing these extrinsic impressions on the posterior gastric wall in profile (Fig. 7–12B). If an abnormal extrinsic mass lesion is suspected on double contrast studies, computed tomography (CT) may be helpful for determining the origin, extent, and nature of the lesion (Fig. 7–12C).

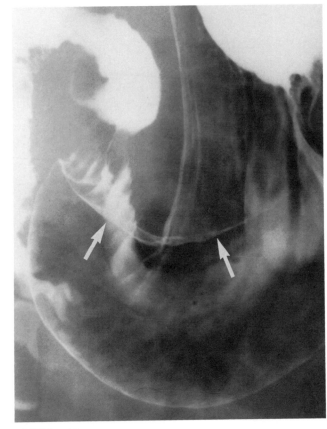

FIGURE 7–11

Enlarged left lobe of liver causing smooth extrinsic impression *(arrows)* on superior border of antrum. This appearance could be mistaken for an intramural mass.

198

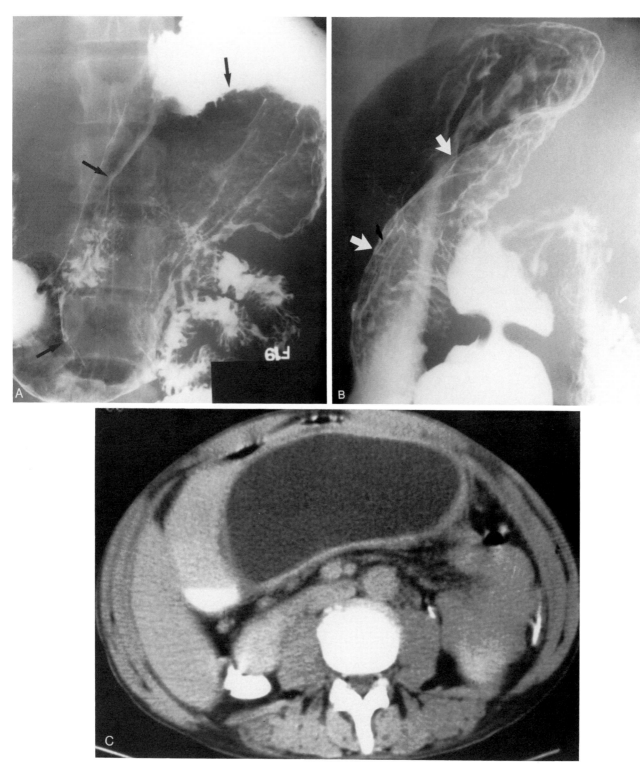

FIGURE 7–12

ABNORMAL RETROGASTRIC MASS. *A,* Supine film shows ill-defined translucency *(arrows)* suggestive of extrinsic mass lesion compressing stomach.

B, Lateral film confirms presence of large retrogastric mass causing extrinsic impression *(arrows)* on posterior gastric wall.

C, Computed tomography (CT) scan shows giant pancreatic pseudocyst compressing and displacing stomach.

Mucosal Folds

The rugal folds in the antrum should be completely effaced on routine double contrast studies. Persistence of the folds despite adequate distention should suggest antral gastritis, particularly if the folds have a scalloped or irregular appearance (Fig. 7–13). Rarely, other causes of thickened, lobulated antral folds, such as arteriovenous malformations, may be encountered (Fig. 7–14).[13]

The rugal folds in the body and fundus of the stomach are more difficult to evaluate on double contrast studies. Even with optimal gaseous distention, the folds are often visible as persistent structures, particularly along the greater curvature. However, the folds should have a relatively smooth, straight contour in the normal stomach. In contrast,

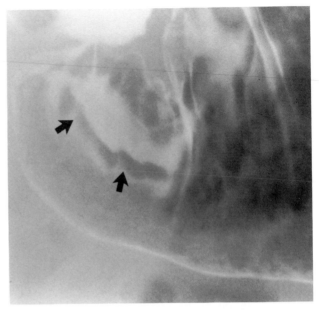

FIGURE 7–13

Antral gastritis with thickened, scalloped fold (*arrows*) in antrum.

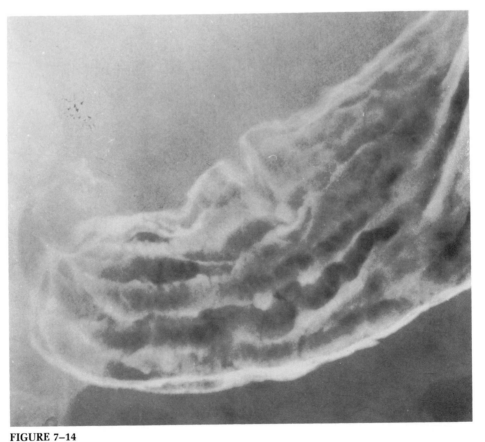

FIGURE 7–14

Arteriovenous malformation with thickened, tortuous folds in antrum. (From Lewis, T.D., et al.: Arteriovenous malformation of the stomach: Radiologic and endoscopic features. Am. J. Dig. Dis. *23*:467, 1978, with permission.)

folds that are unusually thickened and lobulated should arouse suspicion of hypertrophic gastritis (Fig. 7–15A), Ménétrier's disease (Fig. 7–15B), lymphoma (Fig. 7–15C), or even a submucosally infiltrating adenocarcinoma (Fig. 7–15D). Occasionally, folds in the upper body or fundus of the stomach may appear abnormal because of inadequate gaseous distention, erroneously suggesting an infiltrating process (Fig. 7–16A). In such cases, administration of additional effervescent agent to increase gastric distention should allow demonstration of these folds as normal (Fig. 7–16B).

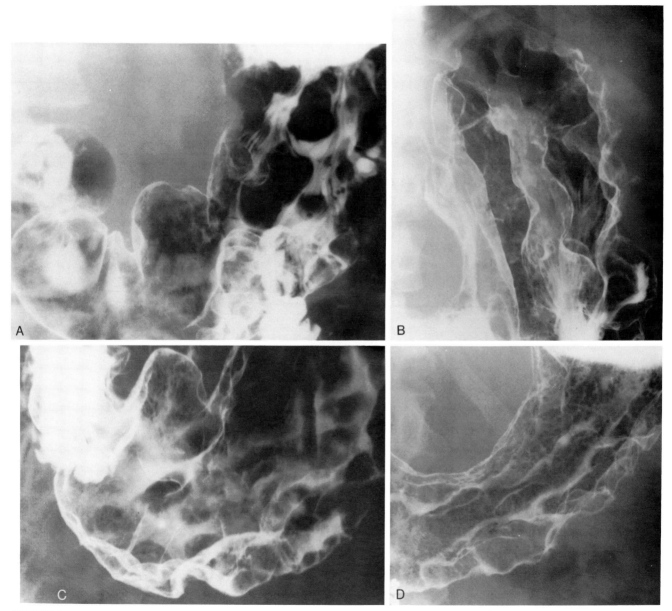

FIGURE 7–15

OTHER CAUSES OF THICKENED FOLDS IN STOMACH. A, Thickened, lobulated folds in body due to hypertrophic gastritis.
  B, Grossly thickened folds in fundus due to Ménétrier's disease.
  C, Thickened, polypoid folds in antrum and body due to lymphoma. Note how stomach retains its normal distensibility.
  D, Thickened, irregular folds in body due to gastric carcinoma. Unlike lymphoma, infiltrating carcinomas typically limit gastric distensibility, as in this case. (D, From Levine, M.S., et al.: Scirrhous carcinoma of the stomach: Radiologic and endoscopic diagnosis. Radiology 175:151–154, 1990, with permission.)

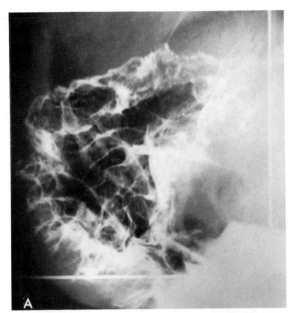

FIGURE 7–16

IMPORTANCE OF DISTENTION FOR EVALUATING GASTRIC FOLDS. *A*, Right lateral view of fundus shows apparently thickened, irregular folds in proximal portion of stomach, suggesting diffuse infiltration by tumor.

B, With further distention, the folds are seen to straighten, and there is no evidence of tumor.

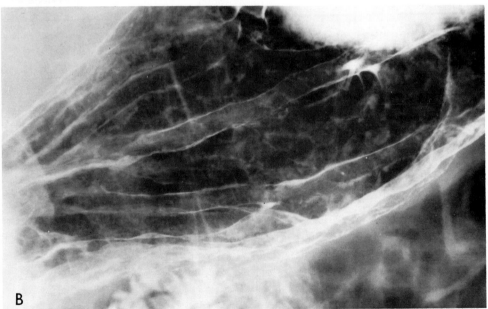

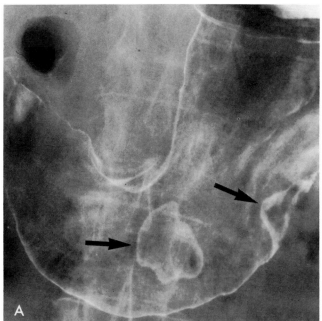

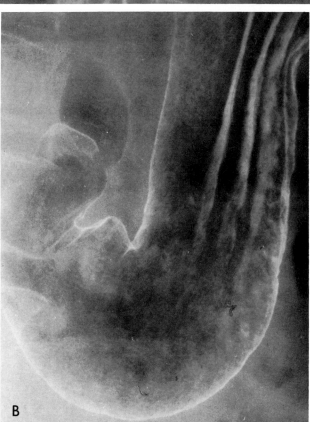

ARTIFACTS

The general nature of double contrast artifacts has been discussed in Chapter 2. Some of the major artifacts that can simulate disease in the stomach are listed in the following:[14]

1. *"Kissing" artifacts* due to underdistention of the stomach with adherence of the anterior and posterior walls can mimic the appearance of mucosal or submucosal masses (Fig. 7–17).

2. *Undissolved effervescent agent* or *gas bubbles* in the stomach can also be mistaken for polypoid lesions.

3. *Barium precipitates* may appear as tiny, white dots on the gastric mucosa that resemble gastric erosions (see the next section, "Erosive Gastritis") (Fig. 7–18).

FIGURE 7–17

"KISSING" ARTIFACTS SIMULATING GASTRIC LESIONS. *A,* In supine position, anterior and posterior walls are adherent *(arrows).* The resulting artifacts could be mistaken for polypoid lesions in stomach.

B, With further distention, the walls are separated, and these artifacts disappear. (From Laufer, I.: A simple method for routine double-contrast study of the upper gastrointestinal tract. Radiology 117:513–518, 1975, with permission.)

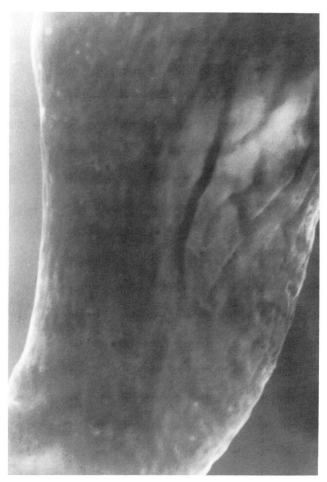

FIGURE 7–18

Barium precipitates simulating gastric erosions. Unlike gastric erosions, however, the precipitates are sharp and distinct and have no surrounding radiolucent halos.

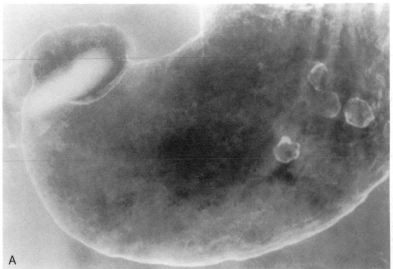

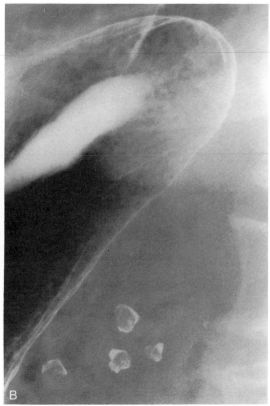

FIGURE 7–19

SEE-THROUGH ARTIFACTS SIMULATING GASTRIC POLYPS. *A,* Supine view shows multiple ring shadows in gastric body that could represent anterior wall polyps etched in white.

B, Lateral view shows barium-filled colonic diverticula behind stomach.

4. *See-through artifacts* due to overlying structures such as calcified vessels or barium-filled duodenal or colonic diverticula can simulate polyps or ulcers in a particular projection (Fig. 7–19).

5. *Stalactites* or droplets of barium suspended from folds on the anterior wall of the stomach can also be mistaken for ulcers (Fig. 7–20).

The transient nature of these various artifacts usually can be recognized during fluoroscopy by turning the patient into different positions or, if necessary, by obtaining additional views of the stomach after reviewing the films.

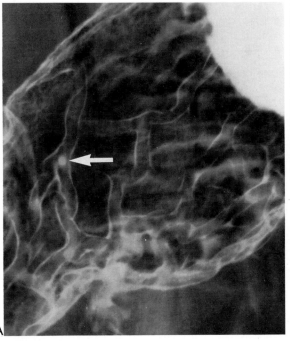

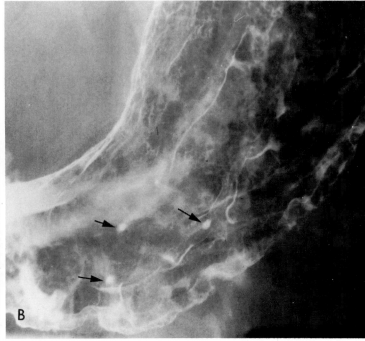

FIGURE 7–20

STALACTITE PHENOMENON. *A,* Small, rounded density *(arrow)* overlying anterior wall fold. This hanging droplet of barium or stalactite could be mistaken for a tiny ulcer.

B, Multiple stalactites *(arrows).*

EROSIVE GASTRITIS

Erosions are defined histologically as epithelial defects that do not penetrate beyond the muscularis mucosae. In approximately 50% of patients with erosive gastritis, there are no apparent predisposing factors.[15] However, known causes include alcohol, aspirin, other nonsteroidal anti-inflammatory drugs, steroids, stress, trauma, burns, Crohn's disease, and viral or fungal infection.[16-19] Patients with erosive gastritis may have vague dyspepsia, ulcer-like symptoms, or, less frequently, upper gastrointestinal bleeding.[20] However, some patients with this condition are asymptomatic. Thus, it may be difficult to establish the clinical significance of gastric erosions demonstrated on radiologic or endoscopic examination.

Although gastric erosions are frequently seen at endoscopy, they have been diagnosed only rarely on single contrast barium studies. By comparison, erosive gastritis has become a relatively frequent finding on double contrast studies, with an overall incidence of 0.5% to 20%.[21-26] Two types of erosions may be identified. The most common type is the complete or "varioliform" erosion, in which a punctate or slit-like collection of barium representing the epithelial defect is surrounded by a radiolucent halo of edematous, elevated mucosa.[15, 23, 25] Varioliform erosions typically occur in the gastric antrum and are often aligned on rugal folds (Fig. 7–21).[20, 23, 25] Because they are shallow lesions, erosions on the dependent or posterior wall may be better delineated by using flow technique to manipulate a thin layer of barium over the mucosal surface (Fig. 7–22).[27] In some patients, erosive gastritis may be manifested only by scalloped or nodular antral folds. Depending on the quality of the mucosal coating, erosions may be faintly seen on the crests of the folds (Fig. 7–23A). These scalloped antral folds may persist after the erosions have healed (Fig. 7–23B). Occasionally, residual epithelial nodules may also be detected at the site of the healed erosions. These hyperplastic nodules or polyps are thought to represent the sequelae of chronic erosive gastritis.[20, 28] In other patients, erosions may persist for years, even in the absence of clinical symptoms.[29]

Incomplete or "flat" erosions are epithelial defects without elevation of the surrounding mucosa. They appear radiographically as linear streaks or dots of barium (Fig. 7–24).[15, 26] As a result, they are much more difficult to detect than are varioliform erosions, and they account for less than 5% of all erosions seen on double contrast studies.[26] Occasionally, incomplete erosions may be associated with slight flattening or deformity of the adjacent gastric wall (Fig. 7–24B).

Although no etiologic significance is usually attributed to the shape or location of gastric erosions seen on double contrast studies, aspirin and other nonsteroidal anti-inflammatory drugs may produce distinctive linear or serpiginous erosions that tend to be clustered in the body of the stomach, on or near the greater curvature (Fig. 7–25).[30] It has been postulated that these erosions result from localized mucosal injury that occurs as the dissolving tablets collect by gravity in the dependent portion of the stomach. Other patients receiving nonsteroidal anti-inflammatory drugs may have linear erosions in the antrum (Fig. 7–26). Detection of these lesions therefore should lead to careful questioning of the patient about the possibility of the use of nonsteroidal anti-inflammatory drugs. If recent ingestion of these drugs is confirmed in symptomatic patients, withdrawal of the offending agent often produces a rapid clinical response.[30]

Other conditions may also be manifested by erosive gastritis. In some patients, gastric erosions are seen as an early sign of Crohn's disease with multiple "aphthous ulcers" in the stomach (Fig. 7–27).[17, 18] This topic is discussed in more detail in Chapter 17. Severe erosive gastritis or ulceration may also result from opportunistic infection by cytomegalovirus in patients with AIDS.[31] Rarely, one or more shallow ulcers may develop as a complication of endoscopic heater-probe therapy or of other iatrogenic trauma (Fig. 7–28).[32]

Gastric erosions must be differentiated on double contrast studies from barium precipitates in the stomach (see Fig. 7–18).[14] However, barium precipitates are sharp, crisp, and well defined. They do not have a radiolucent halo, and when viewed in profile, they appear as small clumps of barium on the mucosal surface rather than as projections of barium beyond the gastric contour.

Text continued on page 210

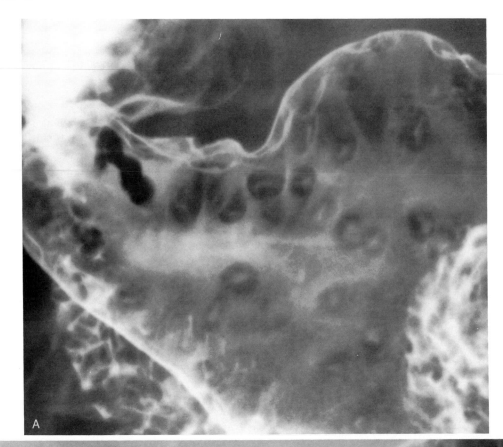

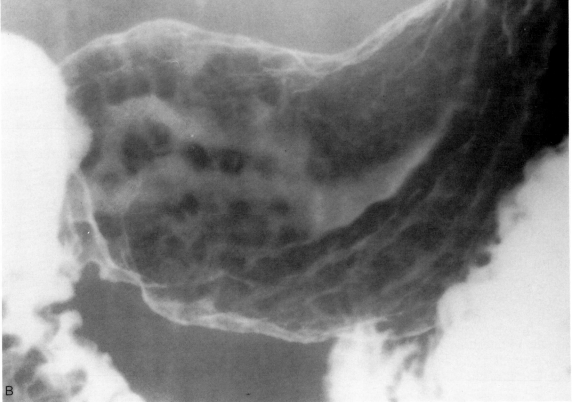

FIGURE 7–21

Two examples (A and B) of varioliform erosions in antrum with central barium collections surrounded by radiolucent halos of edematous mucosa. In B, note how erosions are aligned on rugal folds.

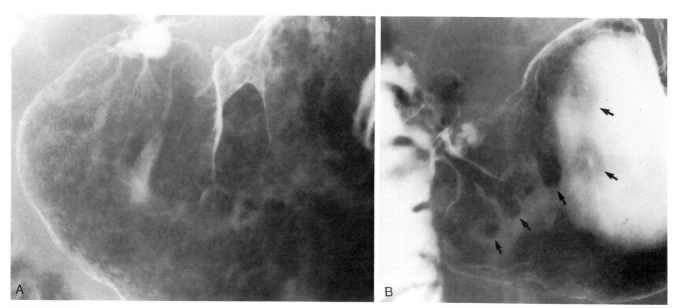

FIGURE 7–22

VALUE OF FLOW TECHNIQUE FOR DEMONSTRATING GASTRIC EROSIONS. *A,* Initial view of antrum shows irregular, nodular mucosa without discrete lesions.

B, Flow technique shows varioliform erosions as circular filling defects *(arrows)* in barium pool due to mound of edema surrounding central part of erosion. Even in retrospect, these lesions are barely discernible on earlier view. (From Kikuchi, Y., et al.: Value of flow technique for double-contrast examination of the stomach. AJR *147*:1183–1184, 1986, with permission, © by American Roentgen Ray Society.)

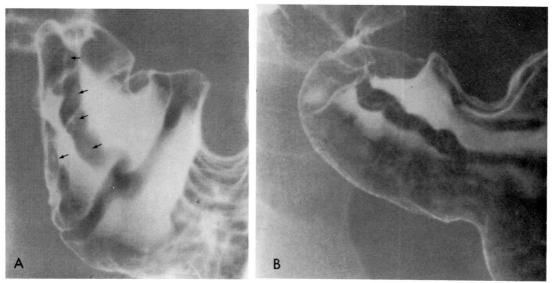

FIGURE 7–23

EROSIVE GASTRITIS WITH SCALLOPED FOLDS. *A,* Scalloped antral folds with erosions *(arrows)* faintly seen on crests of folds.

B, Persistent scalloped fold after erosions have healed.

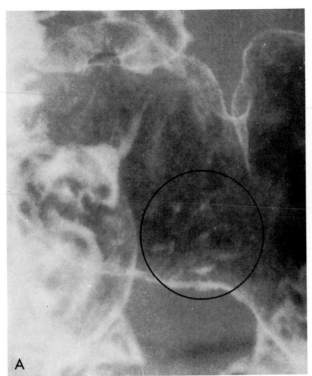

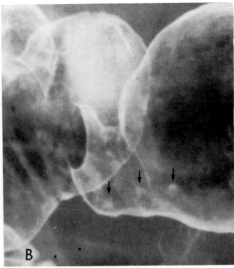

FIGURE 7–24

INCOMPLETE EROSIONS. *A,* Linear streaks and dots of barium in antrum *(inside circle)* due to incomplete erosions.

B, Another patient with incomplete erosions *(arrows)* in antrum. Note associated flattening of adjacent greater curvature.

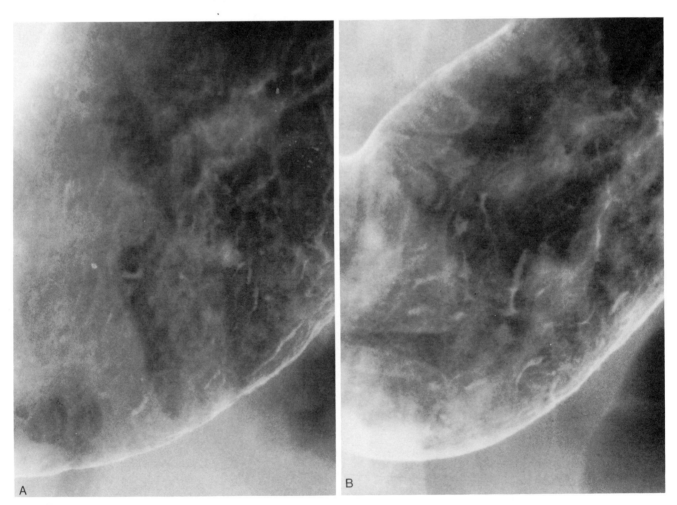

FIGURE 7–25

Two examples (*A* and *B*) of distinctive linear and serpiginous erosions in body of stomach near greater curvature due to aspirin in *A* and indomethacin in *B*. (From Levine, M.S., et al.: Serpiginous gastric erosions caused by aspirin and other nonsteroidal antiinflammatory drugs. AJR 146:31–34, 1986, with permission, © by American Roentgen Ray Society.)

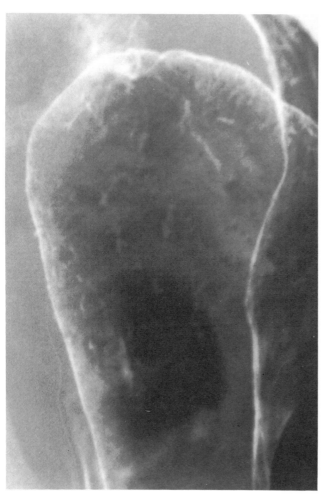

FIGURE 7–26

Numerous linear erosions in antrum due to naproxen, a nonsteroidal anti-inflammatory drug. (From Levine, M.S., et al.: Serpiginous gastric erosions caused by aspirin and other nonsteroidal antiinflammatory drugs. AJR 146:31–34, 1986, with permission, © by American Roentgen Ray Society.)

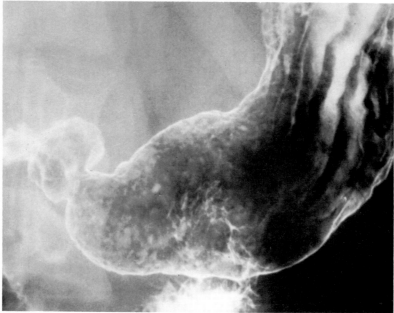

FIGURE 7–27

Erosive gastritis with multiple aphthous ulcers in antrum due to Crohn's disease involving stomach. Note duodenal ulcer. This patient had typical changes of Crohn's disease in terminal ileum. Subsequent endoscopy confirmed presence of superficial gastric erosions, and biopsies revealed noncaseating granulomas. (From Laufer, I., et al.: Multiple superficial gastric erosions due to Crohn's disease of the stomach: Radiologic and endoscopic diagnosis. Br. J. Radiol. 49:726–728, 1976, with permission.)

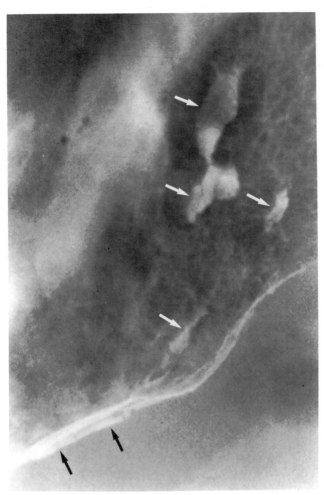

FIGURE 7–28

Heater probe ulcers in stomach. Note shallow, irregular ulcers (*white arrows*) on posterior wall and flat ulcer (*black arrows*) on greater curvature. (From Rumerman, J., et al.: Gastric ulceration caused by heater probe coagulation. Gastrointest. Radiol. *13*:200, 1988, with permission.)

GASTRIC ULCERS

The radiologic diagnosis of gastric ulcers is important not only because of the frequent occurrence of ulcer symptoms or complications but also because a small percentage of these lesions are found to be malignant. The double contrast examination permits not only detection of small ulcers but also assessment of the en face appearance of the surrounding gastric mucosa for more accurate differentiation between benign and malignant ulcers. As a result, gastric ulcers that have an unequivocally benign appearance on double contrast studies can be followed radiographically until healing without the need for endoscopic intervention.

Technical Points

Mucosal Coating

In the search for gastric ulcers, adequate mucosal coating is critical. In the absence of adequate coating, small or even large ulcers can easily be overlooked (Fig. 7–29). Mucosal coating is adequate when a uniform white line is visible along the contour of the stomach. The normal areae gastricae should also be visualized in the majority of patients.

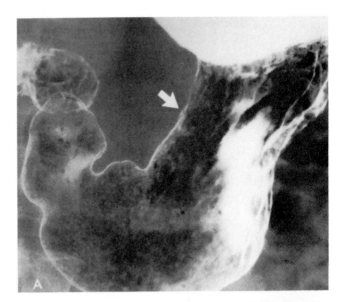

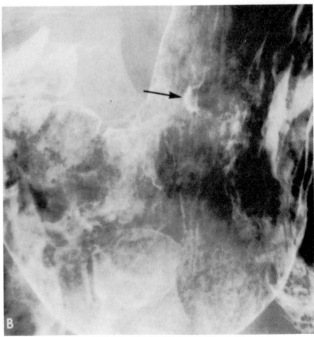

FIGURE 7–29

DANGER OF POOR COATING. A, Supine film shows no definite abnormality in stomach. However, note area of incomplete coating (*arrow*) near lesser curvature.

B, With improved coating, semilunar shadow of ulcer crater (*arrow*) is clearly seen.

Distention

Gastric distention is important because overlying mucosal folds may obscure small ulcers, and small collections of barium trapped between folds may simulate ulcers. The stomach therefore must be distended sufficiently to efface the normal mucosal folds. This technique improves our ability to detect ulcers and also accentuates abnormal folds or areas of decreased distensibility in relation to ulcers (Fig. 7–30).

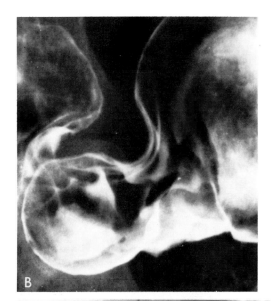

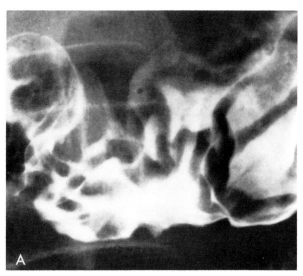

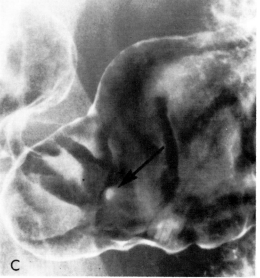

FIGURE 7–30

IMPORTANCE OF GASTRIC DISTENTION. *A,* With antrum collapsed, no diagnosis is possible.

B, With partial distention of antrum, ulcer is recognizable only in retrospect.

C, With further distention, small ulcer crater *(arrow)* and its radiating folds are now clearly visible. (From Laufer, I., et al.: The diagnostic accuracy of barium studies of the stomach and duodenum—correlation with endoscopy. Radiology 115:569–579, 1975, with permission.)

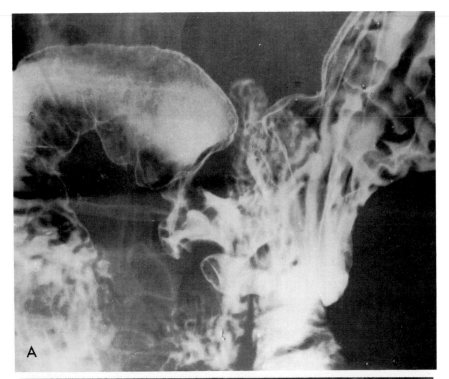

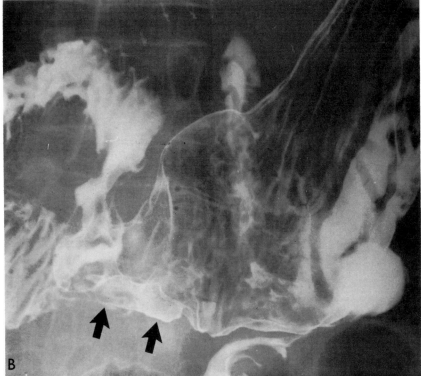

FIGURE 7–31

IMPORTANCE OF PROJECTION. *A*, Small bowel loops overlap greater curvature of antrum in left posterior oblique projection, obscuring this region.

B, Overlapping loops are thrown clear of greater curvature in supine projection, and large greater curvature ulcer *(arrows)* is now seen.

Positioning

An adequate number of views must be obtained to show each area of the stomach clearly. It is particularly important to obtain multiple projections because a peristaltic wave may conceal a small ulcer, and overlapping loops of small bowel may obscure surface detail on a single radiograph (Fig. 7–31). In addition, the duodenal bulb may overlap the distal antrum and pyloric channel, so that small degrees of rotation may demonstrate lesions that are hidden in other projections. Ulcers high on the lesser curvature of the stomach may also be difficult to detect in profile because of prominent rugal folds that are normally found in this area. En face views of the proximal stomach with the patient turned to the right and barium drained out of the fundus are particularly important for evaluating this area (Fig. 7–32).

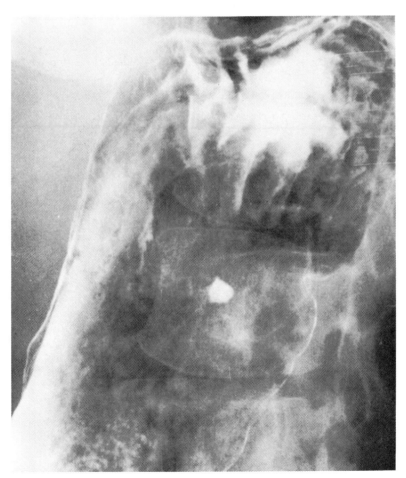

FIGURE 7–32

High lesser curvature ulcer seen en face in right posterior oblique projection.

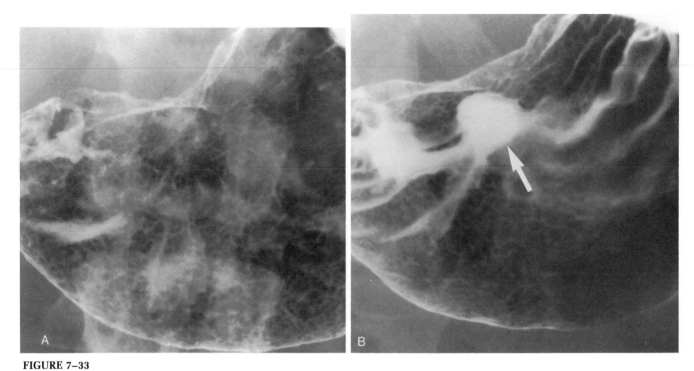

FIGURE 7–33

IMPORTANCE OF FLOW TECHNIQUE. *A,* Supine film shows no evidence of ulcer, even in retrospect.

B, With flow technique, ulcer *(arrow)* is now seen on posterior wall of antrum. Note folds radiating to edge of crater.

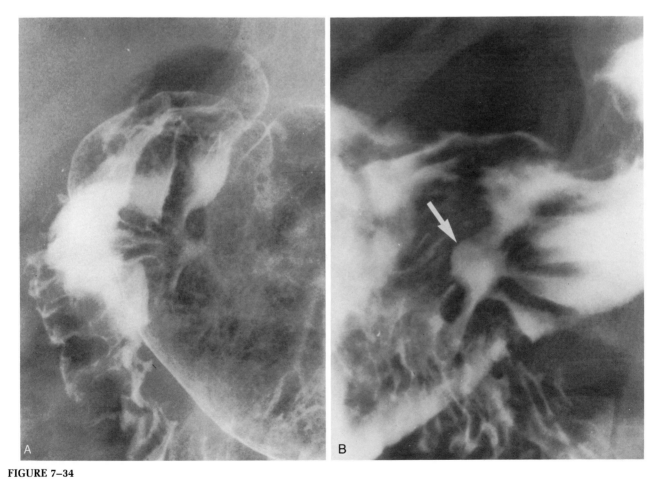

FIGURE 7–34

IMPORTANCE OF PRONE COMPRESSION FOR ANTERIOR WALL ULCERS. *A,* Supine film shows abnormal folds in antrum without definite ulcer.

B, Prone compression film results in filling of anterior wall ulcer *(arrow).* Note folds radiating to ulcer crater.

Flow Technique

Flow technique can be used to better delineate ulcers on the posterior wall or lesser curvature (Fig. 7–33).[27] Slow rotation of the patient from side to side allows manipulation of the barium pool across the dependent surface of the stomach. This technique is particularly helpful for demonstrating ulcers high on the lesser curvature near the gastric cardia.[27]

Compression Study

Because of the effects of gravity, ulcers on the nondependent or anterior wall of the stomach do not fill with barium on double contrast radiographs obtained in the usual supine or oblique projections (Fig. 7–34A). Prone compression views of the gastric antrum and body therefore should be obtained routinely to demonstrate ulcers on the anterior wall (Fig. 7–34B).

Recognition of Gastric Ulcers

The presence of a gastric ulcer may be suggested on conventional single contrast barium studies by secondary signs such as radiating folds, edema, or spasm. However, a definitive diagnosis of a gastric ulcer requires demonstration of a barium collection representing the ulcer crater. Ideally, the ulcer should be visualized both en face and in profile.

The appearance of a gastric ulcer on double contrast studies depends on whether it is located on the dependent or nondependent wall of the stomach. An ulcer on the dependent or posterior wall may fill with barium, producing the conventional appearance of an ulcer crater (Fig. 7–35). However, shallow ulcers on the dependent wall may be coated by only a thin layer of barium, producing a ring shadow (Fig. 7–36A). In such cases, the use of flow technique to

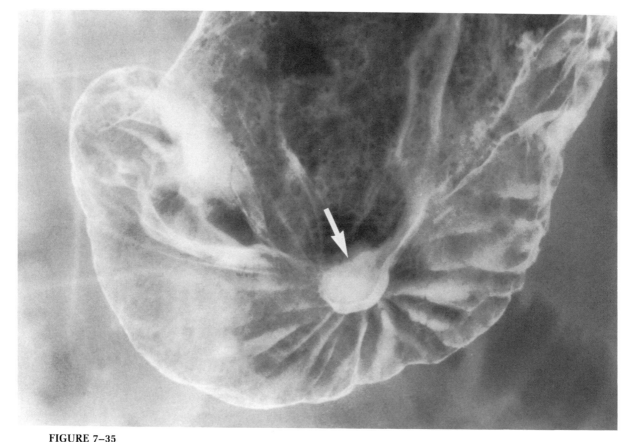

FIGURE 7–35

Posterior wall ulcer (arrow) filling with barium on supine film. Note spectacular folds radiating to edge of crater.

manipulate the barium pool over the surface of the ulcer should result in filling of the crater (Fig. 7–36B).[27]

An ulcer on the nondependent or anterior wall of the stomach may also appear as a ring shadow due to barium coating the rim of the unfilled ulcer crater tangential to the central beam of the x-ray (Fig. 7–37A).[33] The ulcer may be manifested by a partial or incomplete ring shadow if one wall is sloping and the other is vertical in relation to the x-ray beam (Fig. 7–38A). In such patients, the ulcer may be demonstrated by visualizing the crater in profile or by turning the patient 180 degrees to the prone position, so that the ulcer is located on the dependent wall and fills with barium (Figs. 7–37B and 7–38B). Occasionally, when the base of a nondependent ulcer is broader than the neck, a double ring shadow may be seen (Fig. 7–39).

A ring shadow therefore must be recognized as an important sign of an ulcer. This ring shadow may represent (a) a shallow, dependent wall ulcer coated with barium (see Fig. 7–36), (b) a nondependent wall ulcer coated with barium (see Figs. 7–37 through 7–39), or (c) a dependent wall ulcer containing a filling

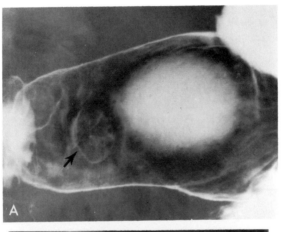

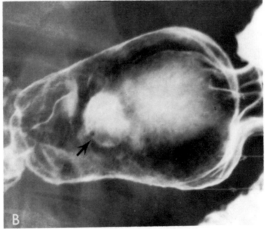

FIGURE 7–36

RING SHADOW DUE TO SHALLOW POSTERIOR WALL ULCER. *A,* Supine film shows ring shadow *(arrow)* due to barium coating rim of unfilled ulcer crater on posterior wall of antrum.

B, Use of flow technique to manipulate barium pool over surface of ulcer shows filling of crater *(arrow).*

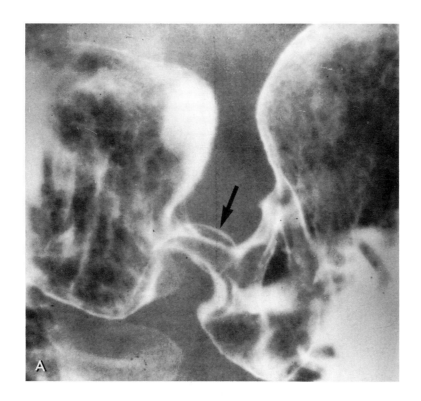

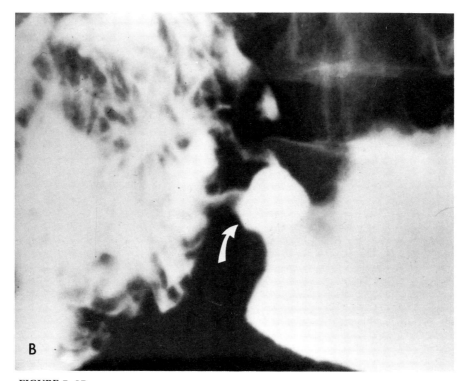

FIGURE 7–37

RING SHADOW DUE TO ANTERIOR WALL ULCER. *A,* Supine film shows ring shadow *(arrow)* in pyloric channel.

B, Prone film shows anterior wall ulcer *(arrow)* filling with barium.

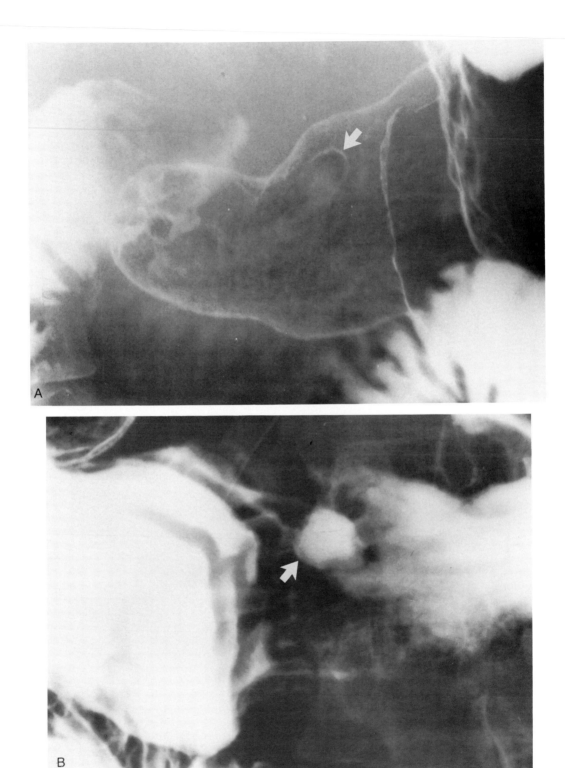

FIGURE 7–38

PARTIAL RING SHADOW DUE TO ANTERIOR WALL ULCER. *A,* Supine film shows partial ring shadow *(arrow)* in antrum. *B,* Prone compression film shows anterior wall ulcer *(arrow)* filling with barium.

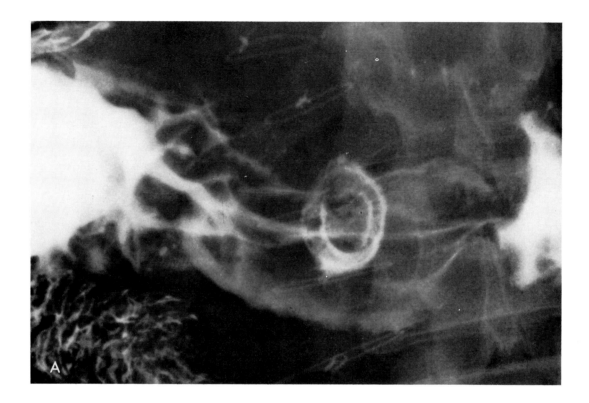

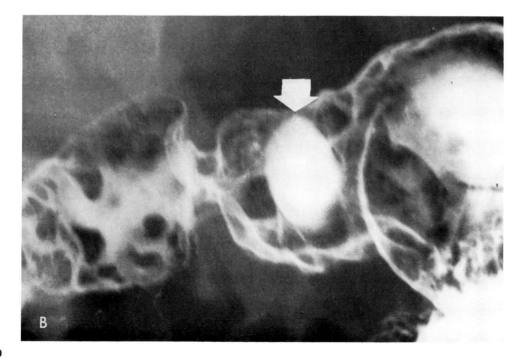

FIGURE 7–39

A, Double ring shadow due to empty ulcer crater on posterior wall with patient in prone position. This appearance occurs because base of nondependent ulcer is wider than neck.
B, Posterior wall ulcer *(arrow)* fills with barium in supine position.

defect such as a blood clot at its base (Fig. 7–40). Use of flow technique and prone compression views to supplement the routine double contrast study should allow differentiation of these lesions in most patients.

An ulcer crater may have several other appearances on double contrast studies. When an ulcer is seen obliquely but not quite in profile, it may be manifested by only a crescentic or semilunar line (Fig. 7–41A). When the patient is rotated under fluoroscopic control, the lesion can usually be demonstrated to represent a projecting ulcer crater (Fig. 7–41B). In elderly or debilitated patients who are unable to turn 360 degrees, an uncoated ulcer crater may be manifested by a collection of gas outside the contour of the stomach before entry of barium (Fig. 7–42).

Radiologists must also be aware of the various artifacts of the double contrast examination that may simulate gastric ulcers (see Chapter 2).[14] These artifacts include the stalactite phenomenon (see Fig. 7–20); the see-through effect, in which an overlying colonic or small bowel diverticulum can mimic the appearance of a gastric ulcer (Fig. 7–43); and patchy coating due to mucus in the stomach, which can

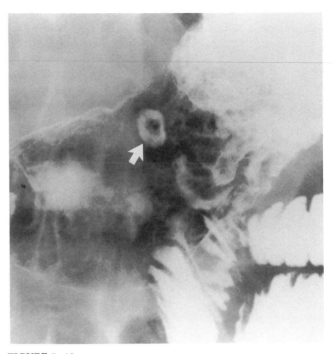

FIGURE 7–40

Ring shadow (arrow) due to blood clot at base of posterior wall ulcer in body of stomach.

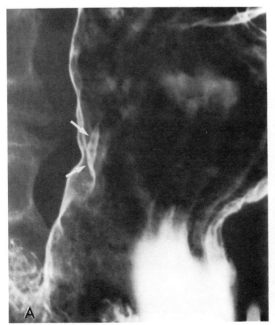

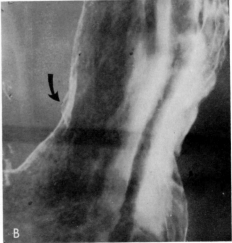

FIGURE 7–41

A, Ulcer crater, not quite seen in profile, is manifested by crescentic line (arrows).
B, With slight rotation of patient, projecting ulcer (arrow) is clearly seen.

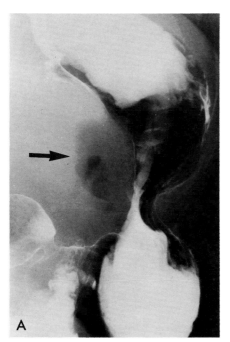

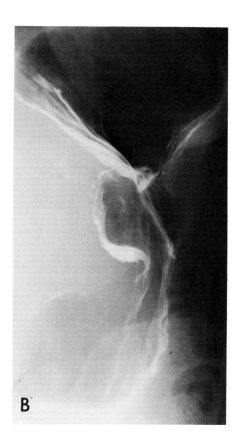

FIGURE 7–42

UNCOATED ULCER FILLING WITH GAS. *A,* Early film from double contrast study shows large gas collection *(arrow)* adjacent to lesser curvature.

B, With additional turning of patient, barium-coated ulcer crater is seen on lesser curvature.

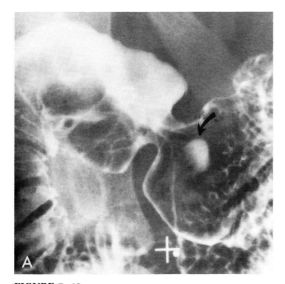

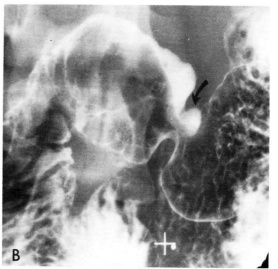

FIGURE 7–43

A and *B,* Duodenal diverticulum *(arrows)* simulating antral ulcer.

simulate a shallow, irregular ulcer. Normal anatomic structures can also mimic the appearance of ulcers. Radiating folds are usually seen at the gastric cardia (the cardiac rosette) (see Fig. 7–8).[10, 11] If the cardia is slightly open, it may collect a drop of barium, erroneously suggesting an ulcer. Similarly, the normal pylorus may be seen en face, particularly in the right posterior oblique projection. The pyloric channel may appear as a ring shadow with radiating folds, or a drop of barium may be trapped in the pyloric channel, resembling a shallow ulcer (Fig. 7–44). However, familiarity with the normal double contrast appearance of the cardia and pylorus should prevent confusion in these areas.

Features of Gastric Ulcers

Shape

Radiologists are accustomed to looking for a circular collection of barium as a sign of a gastric ulcer. With double contrast techniques, however, linear ulcers can be demonstrated (Fig. 7–45).[34–36] Linear ulcers often occur in the healing phase of larger ulcers.[36] Ulcer craters may have other unusual forms, appearing as rod-shaped, rectangular, serpiginous, or flame-shaped lesions (Figs. 7–46 and 7–47). Radiologists therefore should be aware that barium collections of unusual shape may represent ulcer craters.

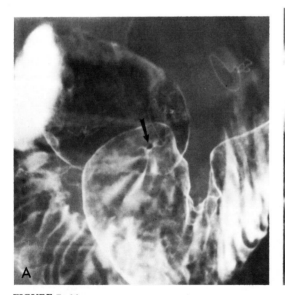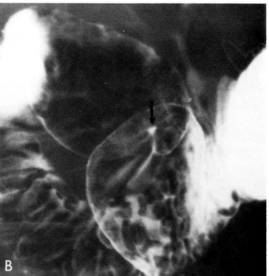

FIGURE 7–44

A and *B*, Normal pyloric channel (*arrows*) simulating tiny ulcer.

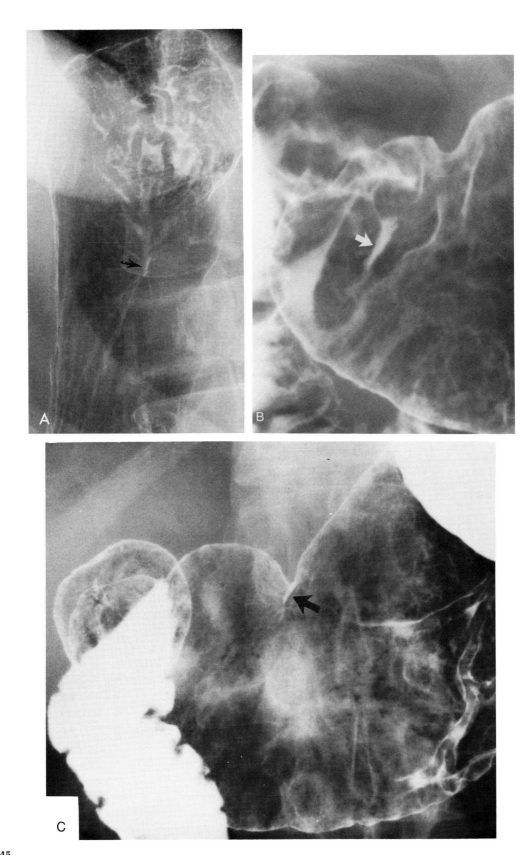

FIGURE 7–45

Three examples (A to C) of linear ulcers (arrows) in fundus (A), antrum (B), and body (C). Note large mound of edema surrounding ulcer in B. (A, From Laufer, I.: An assessment of the accuracy of double contrast gastroduodenal radiology. Gastroenterology 71:874, 1976, with permission. C, Courtesy of Hans Herlinger, M.D., Philadelphia, Pennsylvania.)

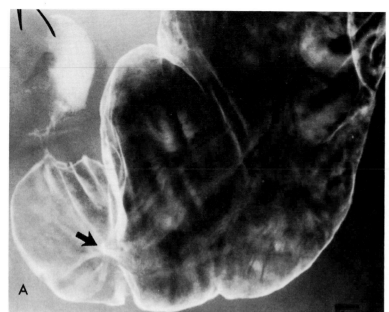

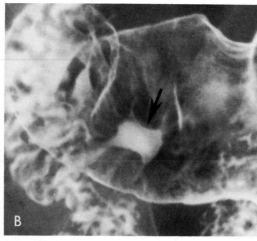

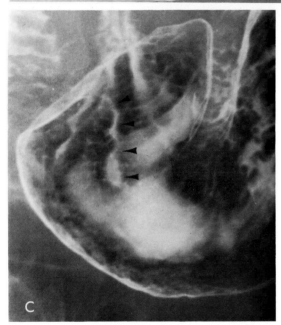

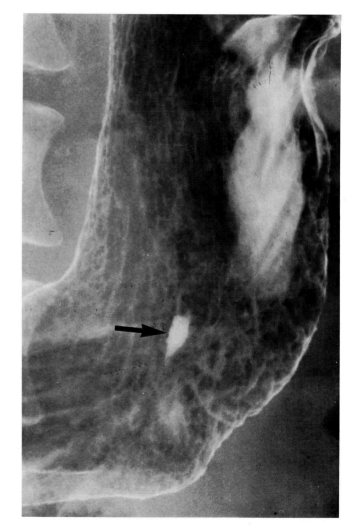

FIGURE 7–46

GASTRIC ULCERS OF DIFFERENT SHAPES. *A*, Rod-shaped ulcer *(arrow)*.
    B, Rectangular ulcer *(arrow)*.
    C, Serpiginous ulcer *(arrowheads)*.

FIGURE 7–47

Flame-shaped ulcer *(arrow)* on posterior gastric wall. Note slight retraction of greater curvature due to scarring. Also note enlarged areae gastricae due to inflammation of mucosa adjacent to ulcer. (From Laufer, I.: An assessment of the accuracy of double contrast gastroduodenal radiology. Gastroenterology 71:874, 1976, with permission.)

Size

Gastric ulcers may be of any size, and it is now accepted that the size of the ulcer has no relationship to the presence of carcinoma. However, a major advantage of the double contrast technique is its ability to distend the stomach and efface the normal mucosal folds to demonstrate small ulcers (Figs. 7–48 through 7–50). As a result, the majority of gastric ulcers diagnosed on double contrast studies are less than 1 cm in size.[36] The increasing prevalence of small ulcers may also be related to the aggressive medical treatment these patients often receive before undergoing radiologic investigations.

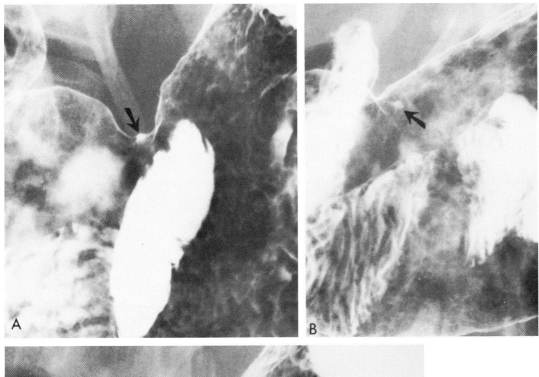

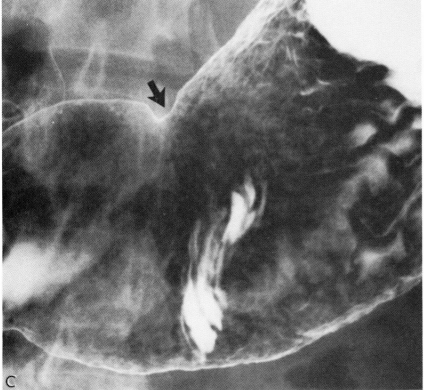

FIGURE 7–48

Small lesser curvature ulcer (*arrows*) seen in profile (*A*) and en face (*B*). After ulcer healing, there is a short, flat scar (*arrow*) on lesser curvature (*C*).

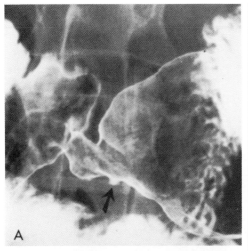

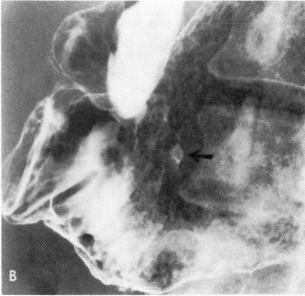

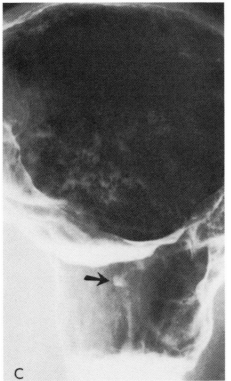

FIGURE 7–49

**VARIETY OF SMALL GASTRIC
ULCERS.** *A,* Greater curvature antral
ulcer *(arrow).*

B, Posterior wall antral ulcer
(arrow).

C, Posterior wall ulcer *(arrow)* high
in body of stomach.

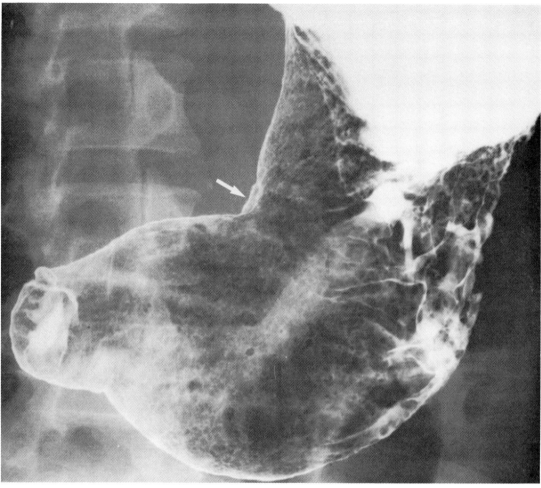

FIGURE 7–50

Broad, shallow ulcer *(arrow)* on lesser curvature at angle of stomach.

Location

Most gastric ulcers are located on the lesser curvature or posterior wall of the antrum or body of the stomach.[36–39] Ulcers on the lesser curvature typically project beyond the adjacent gastric contour and may be associated with smooth, symmetric mucosal folds that radiate to the edge of the crater (Fig. 7–51). Fewer than 15% of gastric ulcers are located on the anterior wall or greater curvature.[36, 37, 39] In younger patients, ulcers tend to occur in the distal part of the stomach (Fig. 7–52), whereas in older patients, they tend to be located more proximally in the stomach, particularly on the lesser curvature (Fig. 7–53).[40, 41] The latter ulcers have been described as "geriatric ulcers."[40] Thus, the distribution of gastric ulcers is influenced by the age of the patients being studied.

Benign greater curvature ulcers are almost always located in the distal half of the stomach (Figs. 7–54 through 7–57).[36, 42, 43] The vast majority are caused by ingestion of aspirin or other nonsteroidal anti-inflammatory drugs.[36, 43] The dissolving aspirin tablets presumably collect by gravity on the greater curvature, causing localized ulceration. This phenomenon may also explain why aspirin-induced erosions are frequently located near the greater curvature (see Fig. 7–25 and the earlier section, "Erosive Gastritis").[30]

Unlike benign ulcers on the lesser curvature, greater curvature ulcers often appear to have an intraluminal location and may be associated with considerable mass effect and thickened, irregular folds as a result of marked edema and inflammation surrounding the ulcer (see Figs. 7–55 and 7–56).[36, 44] Because of these morphologic features, endoscopy and biopsy may be required for some greater curvature ulcers despite a history of aspirin ingestion. When these greater curvature ulcers heal, they also tend to result

Text continued on page 233

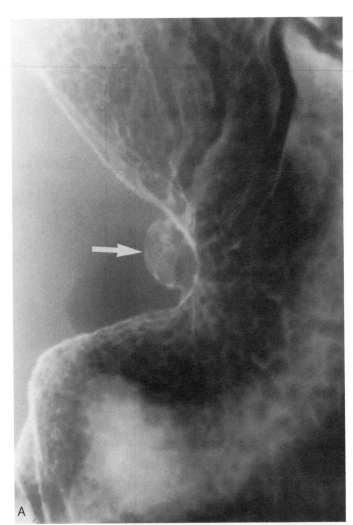

FIGURE 7–51

LESSER CURVATURE ULCERS. *A,* Smooth, round ulcer *(arrow)* projecting beyond lesser curvature. Note radiating folds and enlarged areae gastricae in adjacent mucosa due to associated inflammation and edema. (From Levine, M.S., et al.: Benign gastric ulcers: Diagnosis and follow-up with double contrast radiography. Radiology 164:9–13, 1987, with permission.)

B, Ulcer *(arrow)* straddling lesser curvature. Note smooth, symmetric folds radiating to edge of crater. Both of these cases demonstrate classic features of benign gastric ulcers.

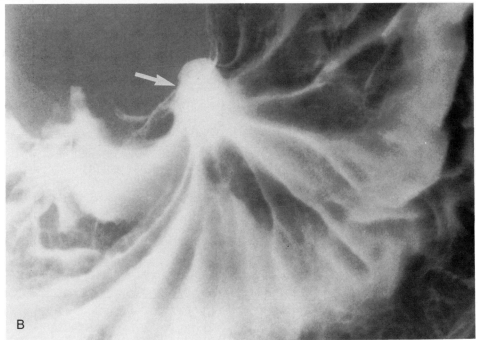

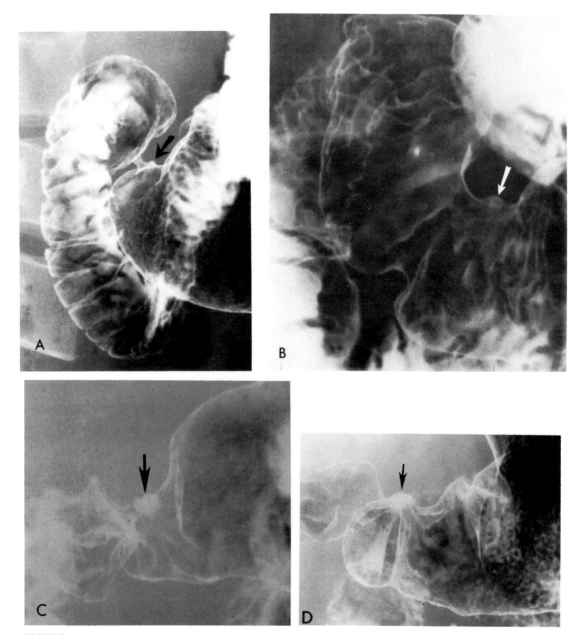

FIGURE 7–52

Four examples (A through D) of antral ulcers (arrows) in young patients.

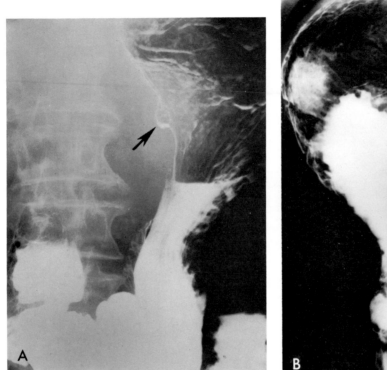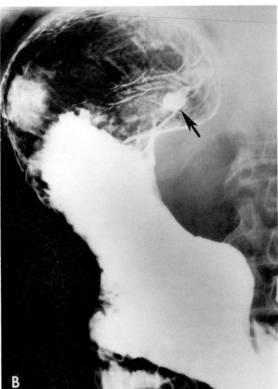

FIGURE 7–53

Elderly patient with high lesser curvature ulcer *(arrows)*, a so-called "geriatric ulcer," seen in profile *(A)* and en face *(B)* in prone position.

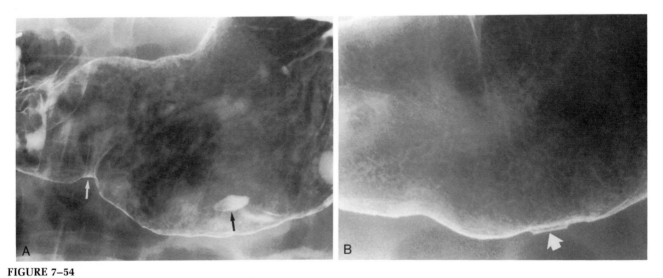

FIGURE 7–54

GREATER CURVATURE ULCERS DUE TO ASPIRIN AND INDOMETHACIN. *A,* Small ulcer *(black arrow)* in body of stomach adjacent to greater curvature. Note area of scarring more distally *(white arrow)* due to healed greater curvature ulcer in antrum.

B, Extremely shallow ulcer *(arrow)* on greater curvature due to indomethacin. Note absence of radiating folds or of other signs of inflammatory disease. This ulcer could easily be missed without optimal radiographic technique.

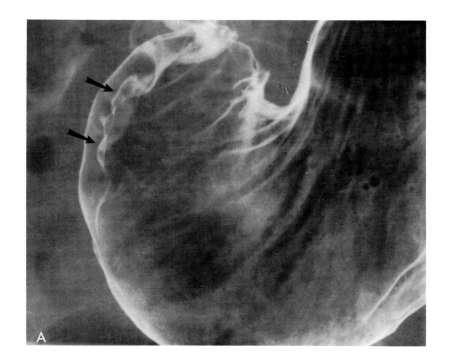

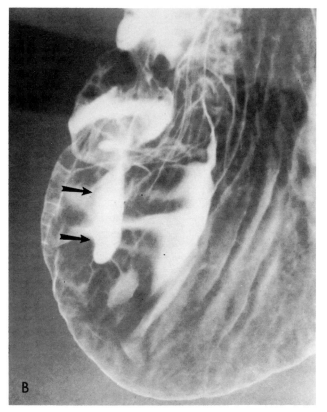

FIGURE 7–55

GREATER CURVATURE ULCER DUE TO ASPIRIN. *A,* Double contrast view of ulcer *(arrows)* on greater curvature of distal antrum. Note how ulcer crater appears to lie within contour of stomach.

B, The ulcer crater *(arrows)* has filled with barium.

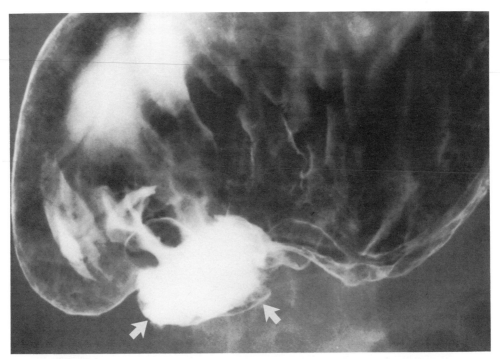

FIGURE 7–56

Giant greater curvature ulcer *(arrows)* due to aspirin. Note apparent intraluminal location of ulcer with thickened, irregular folds and considerable mass effect due to an adjacent mound of edema. These morphologic features should arouse suspicion of a malignant ulcer. However, endoscopic biopsies revealed no evidence of tumor, and following medical therapy, repeat barium study showed complete healing of ulcer.

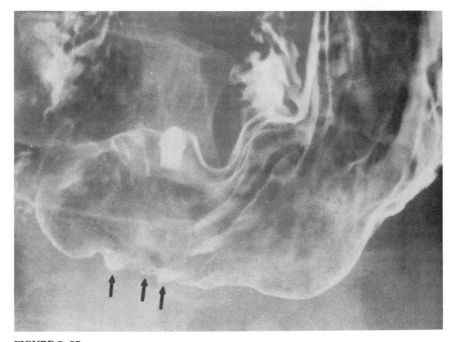

FIGURE 7–57

Multiple greater curvature ulcers *(arrows)* due to aspirin.

in considerable deformity of the adjacent gastric wall, producing one or more outpouchings that can be mistaken for active ulcers (Fig. 7–58A). Careful evaluation of the mucosa en face, however, may reveal that this appearance has resulted from radiating folds and scarring (Fig. 7–58B).

Greater curvature ulcers also have a tendency to penetrate inferiorly into the gastrocolic ligament, eventually leading to the development of a gastrocolic fistula (Fig. 7–59).[43, 45] These patients may present clinically with diarrhea, feculent vomiting, and foul-smelling eructations. With the increasing use of as-

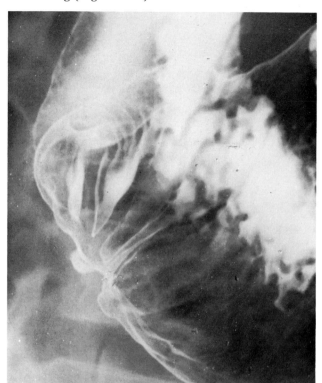

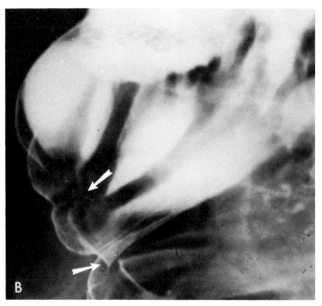

FIGURE 7–58

MULTIPLE ULCER SCARS ON GREATER CURVATURE. *A*, Several outpouchings are seen on greater curvature with radiating folds. These outpouchings could be mistaken for active ulcers.

B, In steep oblique projection, however, it is apparent that these outpouchings are two separate ulcer scars *(arrows)* associated with radiating folds.

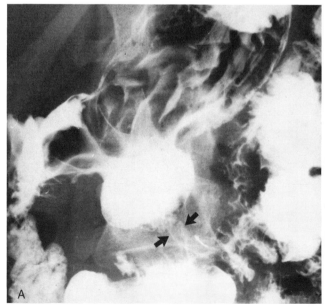

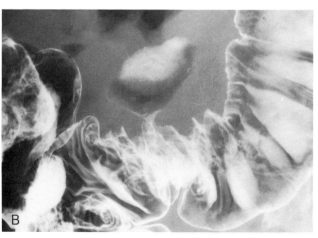

FIGURE 7–59

GASTROCOLIC FISTULA DUE TO ASPIRIN-INDUCED GREATER CURVATURE ULCER. *A*, Double contrast upper gastrointestinal study shows giant ulcer on greater curvature of stomach, with barium entering fistula *(arrows)* that communicates with transverse colon.

B, Double contrast barium enema better delineates fistula between transverse colon and greater curvature ulcer. Note inflammatory changes in transverse colon, with spiculated, tethered mucosal folds adjacent to fistula. (From Laufer, I., et al.: Gastrocolic fistula as a complication of benign gastric ulcer. Radiology *119*:7–11, 1976, with permission.)

pirin in our pill-oriented society, benign gastric ulcer is probably a more common cause of gastrocolic fistula than is carcinoma of the stomach or colon.

Benign gastric ulcers are much less common in the fundus than in the antrum or body of the stomach and are rarely found on the proximal half of the greater curvature.[36, 37, 39] Thus, any ulcer in this location should be considered malignant until proved otherwise (Fig. 7–60). Except for these ulcers high on the greater curvature, the location of the ulcer has no relationship to the presence of carcinoma.

Gastric ulcers occasionally may be found in hiatal hernias.[46] They tend to occur on the lesser curvature aspect of the hernia, where the hernial sac is compressed by the esophageal hiatus of the diaphragm.[46] Because the hernia is inaccessible to palpation, double contrast technique is particularly helpful for demonstrating these lesions (Fig. 7–61).

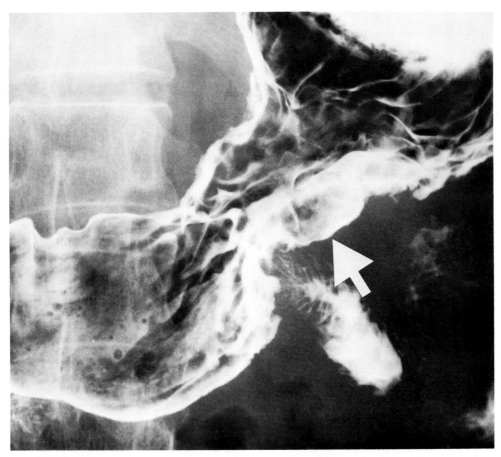

FIGURE 7–60

Malignant ulcer (arrow) on greater curvature of upper body of stomach. Note intraluminal location of ulcer with considerable mass effect and infiltration of adjacent gastric wall. Greater curvature ulcers in proximal half of stomach are almost always found to be malignant.

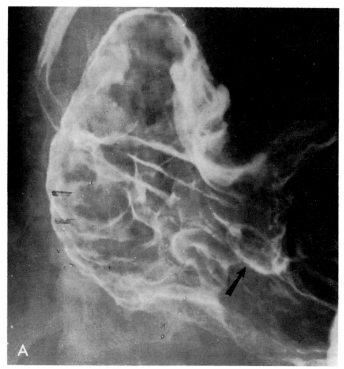 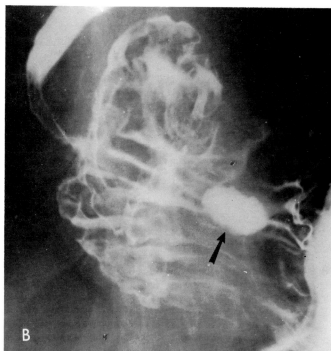

FIGURE 7–61

GASTRIC ULCER IN HIATAL HERNIA. *A*, Ring shadow *(arrow)* due to unfilled ulcer in hiatal hernia.
  B, Moments later, ulcer crater *(arrow)* has filled with barium.

Multiplicity

The frequency of multiple ulcers on conventional single contrast barium studies has ranged from 2% to 8%.[47, 48] However, data based on autopsy, surgical, or endoscopic findings indicate a much higher incidence of multiple ulcers, ranging from 20% to 30%.[49-51] Thus, it seems clear that the conventional barium study has led to underestimation of the frequency of multiple gastric ulcers. Furthermore, it has been shown that multiplicity of ulcers is not necessarily a sign of benignity. In one series of 29 patients with multiple ulcers, 20% had malignant lesions.[52] Each ulcer must therefore be evaluated separately for signs of malignancy. With double contrast technique, multiple ulcers have been detected in nearly 25% of

patients with ulcers or ulcer scars.[53] This finding more closely approximates the findings at autopsy, surgery, or endoscopy, indicating that double contrast studies are more sensitive than single contrast studies in detecting gastric ulcers.

When multiple gastric ulcers are present, they tend to be found in the antrum or body (Figs. 7–62 and 7–63). There is often a marked discrepancy between the size of the ulcers, so that one may see a small satellite ulcer adjacent to a large ulcer (Fig. 7–62). Multiple gastric ulcers or ulcer scars occur more frequently in patients who are taking aspirin or other nonsteroidal anti-inflammatory drugs (see Figs. 7–54A, 7–57, and 7–58). In one study, more than 80% of patients with multiple ulcers had a history of aspirin ingestion.[51]

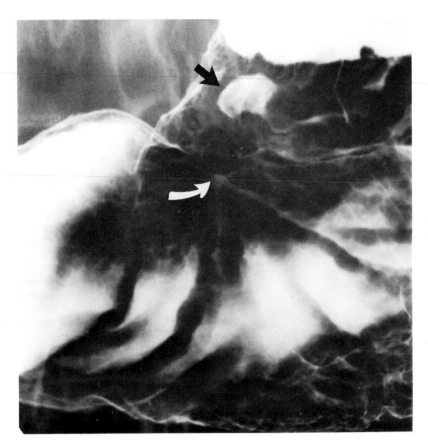

FIGURE 7–62

MULTIPLE GASTRIC ULCERS. Note small satellite ulcer *(white arrow)* adjacent to large ulcer *(black arrow)* in antrum.

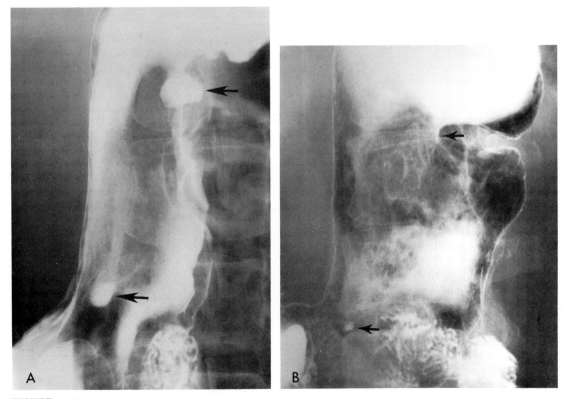

FIGURE 7–63

MULTIPLE GASTRIC ULCERS. *A*, Ulcers *(arrows)* shown in acute phase.
B, Ulcers *(arrows)* shown in healing phase.

Healing of Gastric Ulcers

The radiologic assessment of ulcer healing is important not only for evaluating the success or failure of medical therapy but also for confirming the presence of benign ulcer disease (see the next section, "Benign Versus Malignant Ulcers"). Ulcer healing may be manifested radiographically not only by a decrease in the size of the ulcer crater but also by a change in its shape. Previously round or oval ulcers often have a linear appearance on follow-up studies, so that linear ulcers presumably represent a stage of ulcer healing (Fig. 7–64).[36] Other ulcers may undergo splitting, so that the original crater is replaced by two separate ulcer niches at the periphery of the healing ulcer (Fig. 7–65).[36] This phenomenon probably occurs because the rate of healing and re-epithelialization is more rapid in the central portion of the ulcer than in the periphery.

Benign gastric ulcers usually respond dramatically to conservative medical treatment with histamine (H$_2$)-receptor antagonists. The average interval between the initial barium study showing the ulcer and the follow-up study showing complete healing is approximately 8 weeks.[36] Follow-up barium studies to document ulcer healing therefore should be performed after 6 to 8 weeks of medical treatment, because those studies performed sooner are unlikely to show complete healing.

In general, complete radiologic healing of a gastric ulcer has been considered a reliable sign that the ulcer is benign. Rarely, complete healing of malignant ulcers may occur with medical therapy.[54, 55] However, nodularity of the ulcer scar or irregularity, clubbing, or amputation of radiating folds should suggest the possibility of an underlying malignancy. The surrounding gastric mucosa therefore must be evaluated carefully after ulcer healing has occurred. If suspicious findings are present, endoscopy and biopsy are still required to rule out a malignant lesion.

Ulcer healing may be associated with the development of an ulcer scar. Although ulcer scars are not often detected on single contrast barium studies, 90% of healed gastric ulcers produce a visible ulcer scar on double contrast studies.[36] Double contrast technique is particularly well suited for demonstrating ulcer scars, as gaseous distention of the stomach permits recognition of relatively subtle areas of wall

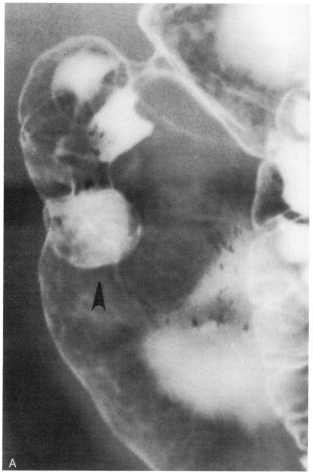

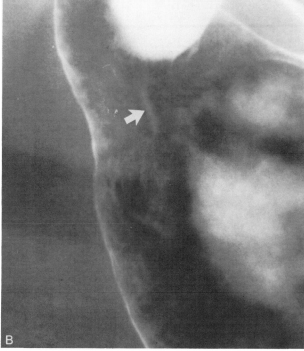

FIGURE 7–64

DEVELOPMENT OF LINEAR ULCER DURING HEALING. *A,* Large, round ulcer *(arrowhead)* on posterior wall of antrum.

B, Follow-up study 8 weeks later shows linear configuration of ulcer *(arrow)* with healing. (From Levine, M.S., et al.: Benign gastric ulcers: Diagnosis and follow-up with double-contrast radiography. Radiology *164:*9–13, 1987, with permission.)

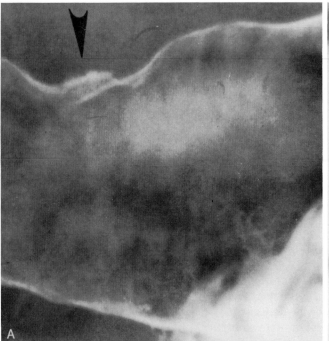
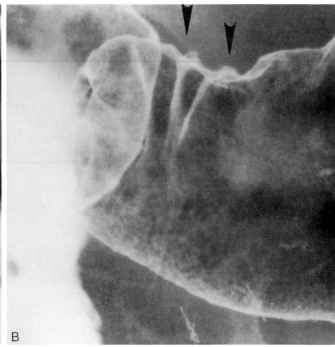
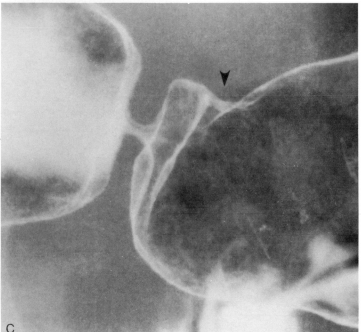

FIGURE 7–65

SPLITTING OF ULCER DURING HEALING. *A,*
Relatively flat ulcer *(arrowhead)* on lesser curvature of
antrum.

B, Follow-up study 3 weeks later shows splitting of
ulcer crater with two discrete niches *(arrowheads)* at
periphery of original crater.

C, Additional follow-up study 4 months later shows
complete ulcer healing with small ulcer scar *(arrowhead)*
manifested by retraction of adjacent gastric wall. (From
Levine, M.S., et al.: Benign gastric ulcers: Diagnosis and
follow-up with double-contrast radiography. Radiology
164:9–13, 1987, with permission.)

flattening or deformity or of abnormal folds associated
with scars. The discovery of an ulcer scar is important, because it indicates that the patient has suffered
from peptic ulcer disease in the past.

Ulcer scars may be manifested radiographically by
a central pit or depression, radiating folds, and/or
retraction of the adjacent gastric wall.[36, 56, 57] The
location of the ulcer is a major determinant of the
morphologic features of the scar. Healing of ulcers on
the lesser curvature may lead to the development of

relatively innocuous scars manifested by slight flattening or retraction of the adjacent gastric wall with
or without radiating folds (Fig. 7–66; see Figs. 7–48
and 7–65).[36, 56] In contrast, healing of ulcers on the
greater curvature or posterior wall often leads to the
development of spectacular radiating folds (Fig. 7–
67; see Fig. 7–58).[36, 56] Occasionally, healing of greater
curvature ulcers may result in some unusual or pic-
turesque scars (Fig. 7–68).

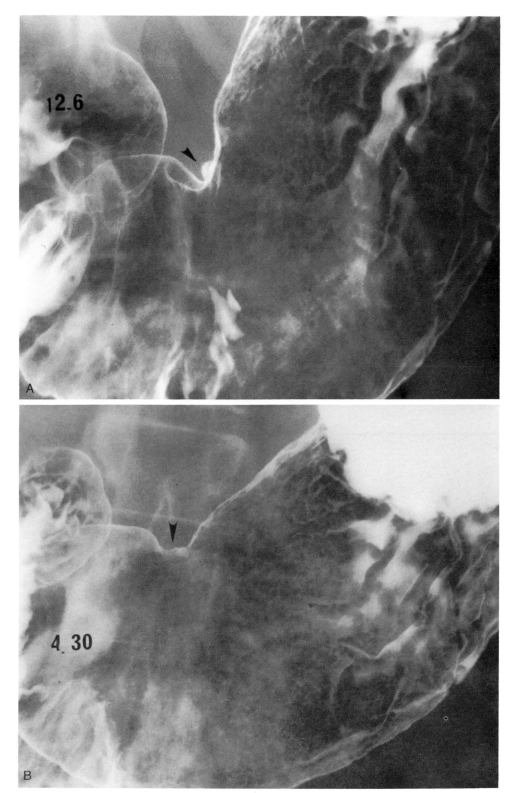

FIGURE 7–66

HEALING OF LESSER CURVATURE ULCER WITH SCARRING. *A,* Small, benign-appearing ulcer *(arrowhead)* on lesser curvature.

B, Follow-up study 5 months later shows complete healing of ulcer with slight flattening and retraction of adjacent gastric wall *(arrowhead).*

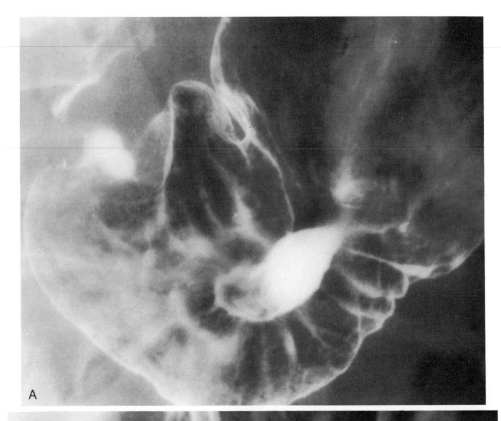

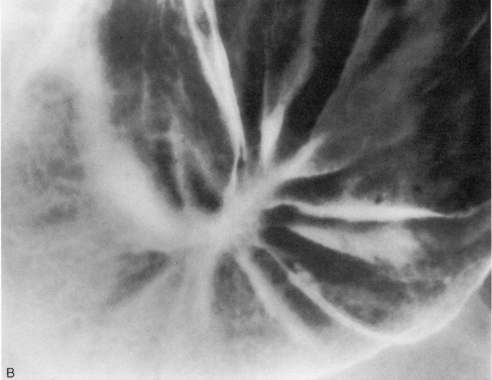

FIGURE 7–67

HEALING OF POSTERIOR WALL ULCER WITH SCARRING. *A,* Large posterior wall ulcer with multiple folds seen radiating to edge of crater.

B, Follow-up study 8 weeks later shows complete healing of ulcer with spectacular folds radiating to site of previous crater.

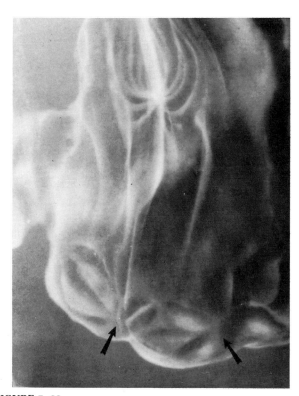

FIGURE 7-68

Multiple ulcer scars (*arrows*) on greater curvature with radiating folds and retraction.

When radiating folds are present, they may converge to a central point or to a circular or linear pit or depression. This central depression can be mistaken radiographically for a shallow, residual ulcer crater (Fig. 7–69). In other cases, this depression may have a bald, featureless appearance, so that it is

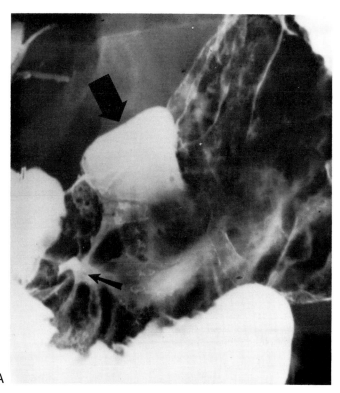

A

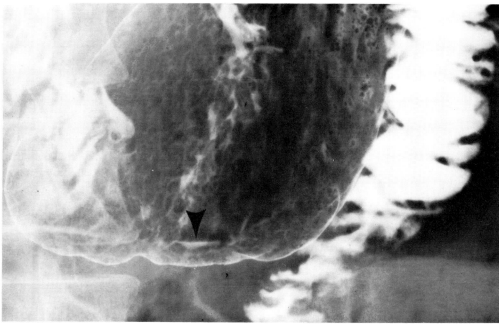

B

FIGURE 7-69

ULCER SCARS MIMICKING ACTIVE ULCERS. *A,* Ulcer scar (*small arrow*) with radiating folds and central, epithelialized depression that resembles active ulcer crater. (*Large arrow* indicates site of cystogastrostomy for decompression of pancreatic pseudocyst.)

B, Linear ulcer scar in another patient. Note linear barium collection (*arrowhead*) adjacent to greater curvature with slight retraction of gastric wall proximally and distally. Although a linear ulcer could produce identical findings, endoscopy revealed a re-epithelialized ulcer scar.

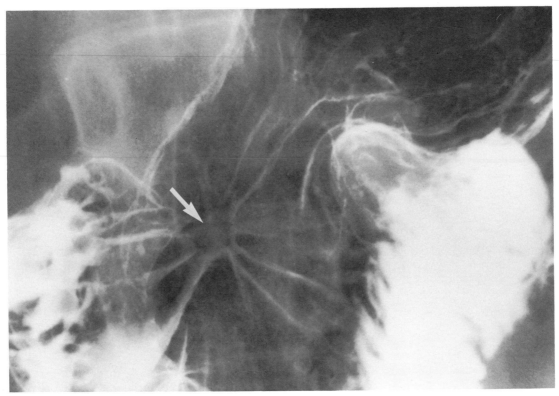

FIGURE 7–70

Ulcer scar with folds seen radiating toward a bald, featureless central area *(arrow)* that could be mistaken for a shallow, residual ulcer crater. (From Levine, M.S., et al.: Benign gastric ulcers: Diagnosis and follow-up with double-contrast radiography. Radiology *164:*9–13, 1987, with permission.)

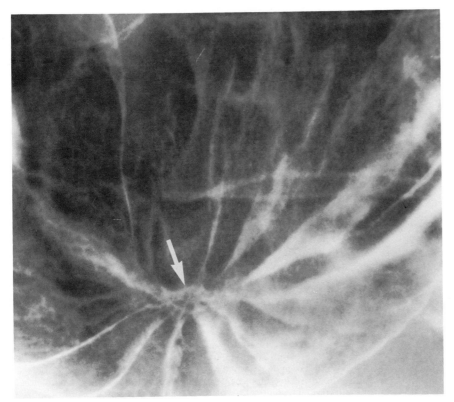

FIGURE 7–71

RE-EPITHELIALIZED ULCER SCAR WITH CENTRALLY RADIATING FOLDS. This scar can be differentiated from an active ulcer by the presence of normal areae gastricae within central portion of scar *(arrow).* (From Levine, M.S., et al.: Benign gastric ulcers: Diagnosis and follow-up with double-contrast radiography. Radiology *164:*9–13, 1987, with permission.)

unclear whether complete ulcer healing has occurred (Fig. 7–70). However, the central depression of an ulcer scar tends to have more gradually sloping margins than an ulcer crater and should remain unchanged on sequential follow-up studies. A re-epithelialized ulcer scar can also be differentiated radiographically from an active ulcer by the presence of normal areae gastricae within the central portion of the scar (Fig. 7–71).[36] The latter finding indicates complete ulcer healing, so that further radiologic or endoscopic evaluation is unnecessary.

In some patients, ulcer healing may lead to the development of severe scar formation, manifested by antral narrowing and deformity (Fig. 7–72A), or, less frequently, focal narrowing of the gastric body, producing an "hourglass" stomach (Fig. 7–72B). Although 90% of healed gastric ulcers produce a radiographically visible ulcer scar, the remaining 10% undergo healing without producing a scar (Fig. 7–73).[36] Thus, the absence of an ulcer scar in no way excludes the possibility that the patient has had ulcer disease in the past.

FIGURE 7–72

SEVERE GASTRIC SCARRING DUE TO ULCER DISEASE. *A,* Marked antral narrowing and deformity *(arrow)* due to previous antral ulcer. When scarring is this severe, gastric outlet obstruction may ensue.

B, Hourglass deformity of stomach due to scarring associated with healing ulcer *(arrowhead)* in body.

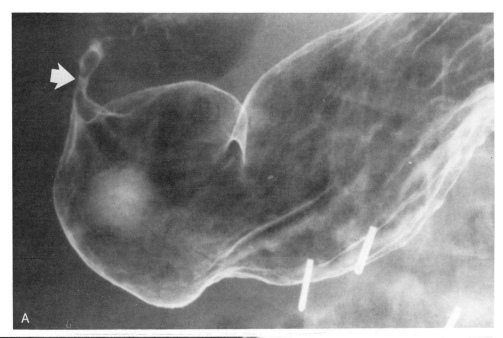

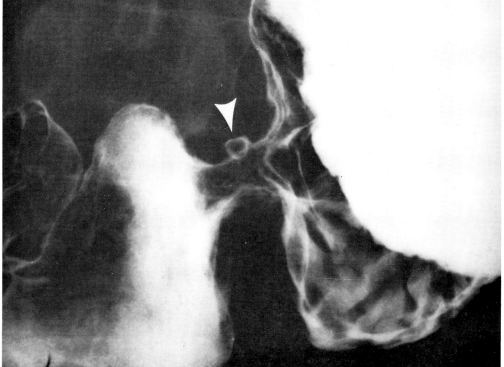

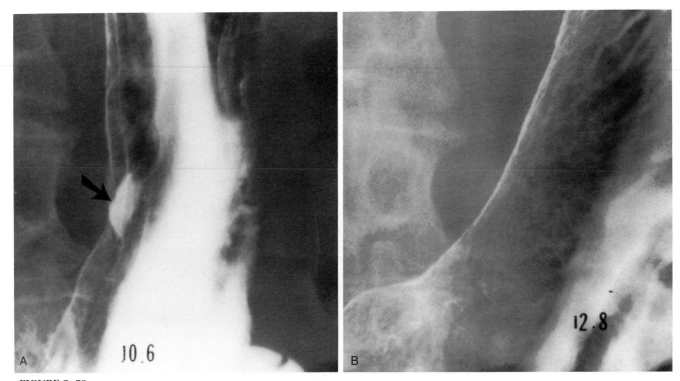

FIGURE 7–73

HEALING OF GASTRIC ULCER WITHOUT SCARRING. *A,* Relatively shallow lesser curvature ulcer *(arrow)* in body of stomach. *B,* Follow-up study 2 months later shows complete healing of ulcer without evidence of scar. (From Levine, M.S., et al.: Benign gastric ulcers: Diagnosis and follow-up with double-contrast radiography. Radiology 164:9–13, 1987, with permission.)

Benign Versus Malignant Ulcers

More than 95% of gastric ulcers diagnosed in the United States are benign.[58, 59] The typical distinguishing features of a benign ulcer demonstrated by conventional single contrast barium studies include projection of the ulcer beyond the contour of the stomach, radiating folds to the edge of the ulcer crater, Hampton's line, and intact surrounding mucosa.[58, 60] However, single contrast studies are thought to be unreliable in differentiating benign ulcers from ulcerated carcinomas. Previous reports indicate that 6% to 16% of gastric ulcers that appear benign on single contrast upper gastrointestinal examinations are malignant.[61–64] Although these studies were performed between 1955 and 1975, many gastroenterologists have used this data as justification for performing endoscopy and biopsy on all radiographically diagnosed gastric ulcers to rule out cancer in these patients.

With double contrast techniques, however, it is possible to obtain a much more detailed study of the mucosa surrounding the ulcer to detect signs of malignancy, such as irregular mass effect, nodularity, rigidity, or mucosal destruction. Several recent studies have shown that virtually all gastric ulcers with an unequivocally benign appearance on double contrast studies are in fact benign lesions.[36, 65] In those studies, about two thirds of all benign ulcers had a benign radiographic appearance, so that unnecessary endoscopy could be avoided in most patients with gastric ulcers diagnosed on double contrast examinations. This finding has enormous implications for the evaluation of gastric ulcers in general, because barium studies are safer and less expensive than endoscopy.

On double contrast studies, unequivocally benign gastric ulcers are characterized en face by a discrete ulcer crater surrounded by a smooth mound of edema or regular, symmetric mucosal folds that radiate to the edge of the crater (see Figs. 7–35, 7–64, and 7–67).[36, 65] The areae gastricae adjacent to the ulcer may be enlarged as a result of inflammation and edema of the surrounding mucosa (see Figs. 7–47 and 7–51A). However, the areae gastricae can often be seen to extend to the edge of the ulcer crater without evidence of nodularity, mass effect, or tumor infiltration. When viewed in profile, benign gastric ulcers project outside the gastric lumen and are often associated with a

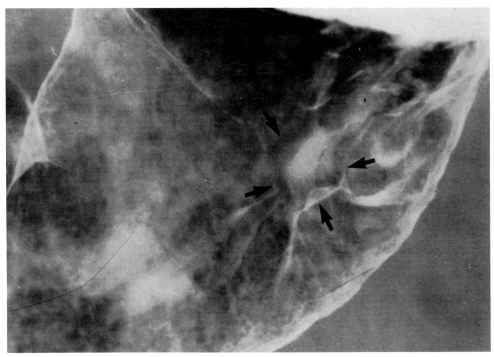

FIGURE 7–74

Malignant gastric ulcer (arrows) with tumor nodule in its wall. Note how radiating folds are nodular and irregular. (Courtesy of Frederick M. Kelvin, M.D., Indianapolis, Indiana. From Laufer, I: Double contrast radiology in the diagnosis of gastrointestinal cancer. In Glass, G.B.J. (ed.): Progress in Gastroenterology, vol. 3. New York, Grune & Stratton, 1977, p. 643, with permission.)

smooth, symmetric ulcer mound or collar or with smooth, straight mucosal folds that radiate to the edge of the ulcer crater (see Figs. 7–51 and 7–66).

In contrast, malignant ulcers are characterized en face by an irregular ulcer crater eccentrically located in an irregular mass with distortion or obliteration of the normal areae gastricae surrounding the ulcer.[36] Although radiating folds may be present, they tend to be nodular and irregular and may stop well short of the ulcer crater (Fig. 7–74). In addition, the tips of the folds may be fused, clubbed, or amputated.[66] When viewed in profile, malignant ulcers do not project beyond the expected gastric contour, and there is often a discrete tumor mass that forms acute angles with the gastric wall rather than the obtuse, gently sloping angles expected for a benign mound of edema. There may also be nodularity of the adjacent mucosa or thickened, lobulated folds radiating to the ulcer because of infiltration by tumor (Figs. 7–75 and 7–76).

Equivocal ulcers are those that have mixed features of benign and malignant disease, so that a confident diagnosis cannot be made on radiologic criteria. For example, edema and inflammation surrounding an acute ulcer may result in enlarged, distorted areae gastricae, mass effect, or thickened, irregular folds, producing an indeterminate radiographic appearance

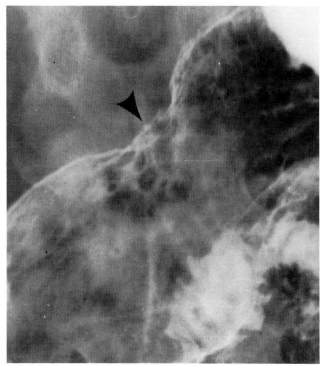

FIGURE 7–75

Early gastric cancer with lesser curvature ulcer (arrowhead). There is considerable nodularity of adjacent mucosa due to infiltration by tumor.

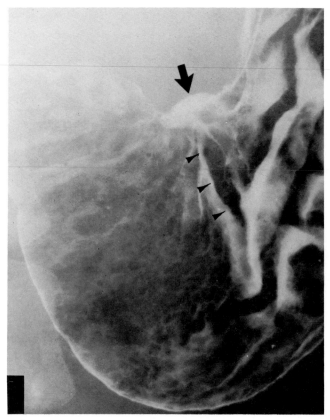

FIGURE 7-76

Early gastric cancer with lesser curvature ulcer *(large arrow)*. Note how surrounding mucosal folds *(small arrowheads)* are disorganized and lobulated and taper as they approach ulcer. (From Laufer, I: Double contrast radiology in the diagnosis of gastrointestinal cancer. *In* Glass, G.B.J. (ed.): Progress in Gastroenterology, vol. 3. New York, Grune & Stratton, 1977, p. 643, with permission.)

(Figs. 7–77 and 7–78). Similarly, greater curvature ulcers that have an apparent intraluminal location or considerable associated mass effect and shouldered edges may result in equivocal radiographic findings (see Fig. 7–56). Most ulcers that have an equivocal appearance are ultimately found to be benign.[36, 65] However, it seems prudent to err on the side of caution by suggesting the possibility of malignancy in some benign lesions to avoid missing an early carcinoma.

Gastric ulcers that have an unequivocally benign appearance on double contrast studies can be followed radiographically until complete healing without the need for endoscopic intervention.[36] However, ulcers that have an equivocal or suspicious appearance should undergo endoscopy and biopsy. Although endoscopy is a relatively accurate technique for detecting gastric carcinoma,[67] false-negative endoscopic biopsies and brushings have been reported in some patients with malignant lesions.[68] If the radiographic findings are suspicious for malignancy, negative endoscopic or cytologic findings therefore should not be taken as definitive evidence of a benign ulcer. Instead, follow-up barium studies should be performed at regular intervals until complete healing is documented. If the ulcer fails to heal with adequate medical treatment or if it continues to have a suspicious appearance, repeat endoscopy may be necessary. Even if endoscopic biopsies and brushings remain negative, surgical resection should be considered in some patients who have highly suspicious radiographic findings.

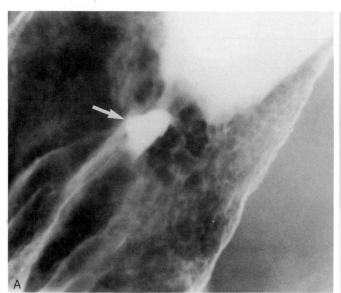
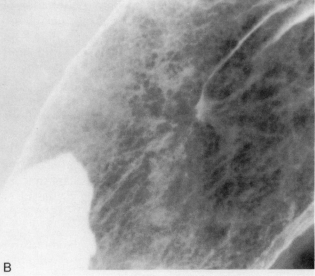

FIGURE 7-77

BENIGN ULCER WITH SUSPICIOUS RADIOGRAPHIC APPEARANCE. *A,* Posterior wall ulcer *(arrow)* in upper body of stomach. Enlarged, nodular areae gastricae adjacent to ulcer raise possibility of mucosal spread of tumor. However, endoscopic biopsies revealed no evidence of malignancy.

B, Follow-up study 3 months later shows return of normal areae gastricae in this region with ulcer healing. (From Levine, M.S., et al.: Benign gastric ulcers: Diagnosis and follow-up with double-contrast radiography. Radiology 164:9–13, 1987, with permission.)

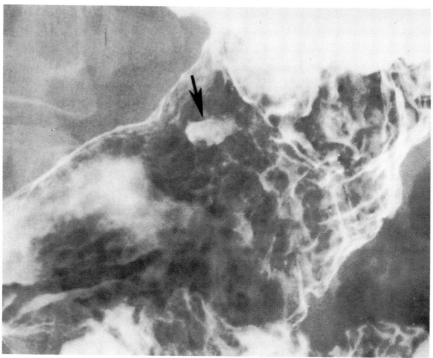

FIGURE 7–78

BENIGN ULCER WITH MALIGNANT APPEARANCE. There is a 1-cm ulcer (*arrow*) near lesser curvature with considerable mass effect surrounding ulcer. Note how adjacent mucosa has nodular appearance, suggestive of malignancy. However, endoscopic biopsies revealed no evidence of tumor, and repeat endoscopy 1 month later showed complete healing of ulcer.

REFERENCES

1. Mackintosh, C.E., and Kreel, L.: Anatomy and radiology of the areae gastricae. Gut 18:855, 1977.
2. Rubesin, S.E., and Herlinger, H.: The effect of barium suspension viscosity on the delineation of areae gastricae. AJR 146:35, 1986.
3. Rose, C., and Stevenson, G.W.: Correlation between visualization and size of the areae gastricae and duodenal ulcer. Radiology 139:371, 1981.
4. Watanabe, H., Magota, S., Shiiba, S., et al.: Coarse areae gastricae in the proximal body and fundus: A sign of gastric hypersecretion. Radiology 146:303, 1983.
5. Koga, M., Nakata, H., and Kuyonari, H.: Minute mucosal patterns in gastric carcinoma: Magnification radiography on resected gastric specimens. Radiology 120:199, 1976.
6. Levine, M.S., Palman, C.L., Rubesin, S.E., et al.: Atrophic gastritis in pernicious anemia: Diagnosis by double-contrast radiography. Gastrointest. Radiol. 14:215, 1989.
7. Keto, P., Suoranta, H., Myllarniemi, H., et al.: Areae gastricae in gastritis: Lack of correlation between size and histology. AJR 141:693, 1983.
8. Seymour, E.Q., and Meredith, H.C.: Antral and esophageal rimple: A normal variation. Gastrointest. Radiol. 3:147, 1978.
9. Cho, K.C., Gold, B.M., and Printz, D.A.: Multiple transverse folds in the gastric antrum. Radiology 164:339, 1987.
10. Freeny, P.C.: Double-contrast gastrography of the fundus and cardia: Normal landmarks and their pathologic changes. AJR 133:481, 1979.
11. Herlinger, H., Grossman, R., Laufer, I., et al.: The gastric cardia in double-contrast study: Its dynamic image. AJR 135:21, 1980.
12. Cimmino, C.V.: Sign of the burnous in the stomach. Radiology 75:722, 1960.
13. Lewis, T.D., Laufer, I., and Goodacre, R.L.: Arteriovenous malformation of the stomach: Radiologic and endoscopic features. Am. J. Dig. Dis. 23:467, 1978.
14. Gohel, V.K., Kressel, H.Y., and Laufer, I.: Double-contrast artifacts. Gastrointest. Radiol. 3:139, 1978.
15. Laufer, I., Hamilton, J., and Mullens, J.E.: Demonstration of superficial gastric erosions by double contrast radiography. Gastroenterology 68:387, 1975.
16. Lanza, F., Royer, G., and Nelson, R.: An endoscopic evaluation of the effects of non-steroidal anti-inflammatory drugs on the gastric mucosa. Gastrointest. Endosc. 21:103, 1975.
17. Laufer, I., Trueman, T., and de Sa, D.: Multiple superficial gastric erosions due to Crohn's disease of the stomach: Radiologic and endoscopic diagnosis. Br. J. Radiol. 49:726, 1976.
18. Ariyama, J., Wehlin, L., Lindstrom, C.G., et al.: Gastroduodenal erosions in Crohn's disease. Gastrointest. Radiol. 5:121, 1980.
19. Cronan, J., Burrell, M., and Trepeta, R.: Aphthoid ulcerations in gastric candidiasis. Radiology 134:607, 1980.
20. McLean, A.M., Paul, R.E., Philipps, E., et al.: Chronic erosive gastritis—clinical and radiological features. J. Can. Assoc. Radiol. 33:158, 1982.
21. Poplack, W., Paul, R.E., Goldsmith, M., et al.: Demonstration of erosive gastritis by the double-contrast technique. Radiology 117:519, 1975.
22. Laufer, I.: An assessment of the accuracy of double contrast gastroduodenal radiology. Gastroenterology 71:874, 1976.
23. Op den Orth, J.O., and Dekker, W.: Gastric erosions: Radiological and endoscopic aspects. Radiologica Clinica (Belg.) 45:88, 1976.
24. Op den Orth, J.O., and Dekker, W.: Gastric polyps or erosions. AJR 129:357, 1977.
25. Tragardh, B., Wehlin, L., and Ohashi, K.: Radiologic appearance of complete gastric erosions. Acta Radiol. [Diagn.] (Stockh.) 19:634, 1978.

26. Catalano, D., and Pagliaru, U.: Gastroduodenal erosions: Radiological findings. Gastrointest. Radiol. 7:235, 1982.

27. Kikuchi, Y., Levine, M.S., Laufer, I., et al.: Value of flow technique for double-contrast examination of the stomach. AJR 147:1183, 1986.

28. Elta, G.H., Fawaz, K.A., Dayal, Y., et al.: Chronic erosive gastritis: A recently recognized disorder. Dig. Dis. Sci. 28:7, 1983.

29. McAdam, W.A.F., Morgan, A.G., Jackson, A., et al.: Multiple persisting idiopathic gastric erosions. Gut 16:410, 1975.

30. Levine, M.S., Verstandig, A., and Laufer, I.: Serpiginous gastric erosions caused by aspirin and other nonsteroidal antiinflammatory drugs. AJR 146:31, 1986.

31. Balthazar, E.J., Megibow, A.J., and Hulnick, D.H.: Cytomegalovirus esophagitis and gastritis in AIDS. AJR 144:1201, 1985.

32. Rumerman, J., Rubesin, S.E., Levine, M.S., et al.: Gastric ulceration caused by heater probe coagulation. Gastrointest. Radiol. 13:200, 1988.

33. Lubert, M., and Krause, G.R.: The "ring" shadow in the diagnosis of ulcer. AJR 90:767, 1963.

34. Poplack, W., Paul, R.E., Goldsmith, M., et al.: Linear and rod-shaped peptic ulcers. Radiology 122:317, 1977.

35. Braver, J.M., Paul, R.E., Philipps, E., et al.: Roentgen diagnosis of linear ulcers. Radiology 132:29, 1979.

36. Levine, M.S., Creteur, V., Kressel, H.Y., et al.: Benign gastric ulcers: Diagnosis and follow-up with double-contrast radiography. Radiology 164:9, 1987.

37. Sun, D.C.H., and Stempien, S.J.: The Veterans' Administration Cooperative Study on Gastric Ulcer. Site and size of the ulcer as determinants of outcome. Gastroenterology 61:576, 1971.

38. Thompson, G., Stevenson, G.W., and Somers, S.: Distribution of gastric ulcers by double-contrast barium meal with endoscopic correlation. J. Can. Assoc. Radiol. 34:296, 1983.

39. Gelfand, D.W., Dale, W.J., and Ott, D.J.: The location and size of gastric ulcers: Radiologic and endoscopic evaluation. AJR 143:755, 1984.

40. Amberg, J.R., and Zboralske, F.F.: Gastric ulcers after seventy. AJR 96:393, 1966.

41. Sheppard, M.C., Holmes, G.K.T., and Cockel, R.: Clinical picture of peptic ulceration diagnosed endoscopically. Gut 18:524, 1977.

42. Findley, J.W.: Ulcers on the greater curvature of the stomach. Gastroenterology 40:183, 1961.

43. Kottler, R.E., and Tuft, R.J.: Benign greater curve gastric ulcer: The "sump-ulcer." Br. J. Radiol. 54:651, 1981.

44. Zboralske, F.F., Stargardter, F.L., and Harell, G.S.: Profile roentgenographic features of benign greater curvature ulcers. Radiology 127:63, 1978.

45. Laufer, I., Thornley, G.D., and Stolberg, H.: Gastrocolic fistula as a complication of benign gastric ulcer. Radiology 119:7, 1976.

46. Hocking, B.V., and Alp, M.H.: Gastric ulceration within hiatus hernia. Med. J. Aust. 2:207, 1976.

47. Welch, C.E., and Allen, A.W.: Gastric ulcer: Study of Massachusetts General Hospital cases during the 10-year period 1938–1947. N. Engl. J. Med. 240:277, 1949.

48. Smith, F.H., Boles, R.S., and Jordon, S.M.: Problem of gastric ulcers reviewed. JAMA 153:1505, 1953.

49. Portis, S.A., and Jaffee, R.H.: Study of peptic ulcer based on necropsy records. JAMA 106:6, 1938.

50. Dolphin, J.A., Smith, L.A., and Waugh, J.M.: Multiple gastric ulcers: Their occurrence in benign and malignant lesions. Gastroenterology 25:202, 1953.

51. Dagradi, A.E., Falkner, R.E., and Lee, E.R.: Multiple benign gastric ulcers. Am. J. Gastroenterol. 62:36, 1974.

52. Taxin, R.N., Livingston, P.A., and Seaman, W.B.: Multiple gastric ulcers: A radiographic sign of benignity? Radiology 114:23, 1975.

53. Bloom, S.M., Paul, R.E., Matsue, H., et al.: Improved radiologic detection of multiple gastric ulcers. AJR 128:949, 1977.

54. Sakita, T., Ogura, Y., and Takasu, S.: Observations on the healing of ulcerations in early gastric cancer. Gastroenterology 60:835, 1971.

55. Kagan, A.R., and Steckel, R.J.: Gastric ulcer in a young man with apparent healing. AJR 128:831, 1977.

56. Keller, R.J., Wolf, B.S., and Khilnani, M.T.: Roentgen features of healing and healed benign gastric ulcers. Radiology 97:353, 1970.

57. Gelfand, D.W., and Ott, D.J.: Gastric ulcer scars. Radiology 140:37, 1981.

58. Nelson, S.W.: The discovery of gastric ulcers and the differential diagnosis between benignancy and malignancy. Radiol. Clin. North Am. 7:5, 1969.

59. Wenger, J., Brandborg, L.L., and Spellman, F.A.: Cancer: Part I. Clinical aspects. Gastroenterology 61:598, 1971.

60. Wolf, B.S.: Observations on roentgen features of benign and malignant ulcers. Semin. Roentgenol. 6:140, 1971.

61. Hayes, M.A.: The gastric ulcer problem. Gastroenterology 29:609, 1955.

62. Kirsh, I.E.: Benign and malignant gastric ulcers: Roentgen differentiation. Radiology 64:357, 1955.

63. Elliott, G.V., Wald, S.M., and Benz, R.I.: A roentgenologic study of ulcerating lesions of the stomach. AJR 77:612, 1957.

64. Schulman, A., and Simpkins, K.C.: The accuracy of radiological diagnosis of benign, primarily and secondarily malignant gastric ulcers and their correlation with three simplified radiological types. Clin. Radiol. 26:317, 1975.

65. Thompson, G., Somers, S., and Stevenson, G.W.: Benign gastric ulcer: A reliable radiologic diagnosis? AJR 141:331, 1983.

66. Ichikawa, H.: Differential diagnosis between benign and malignant ulcers of the stomach. Clin. Gastroenterol. 2:329, 1973.

67. Qizilbash, A.H., Castelli, M., Kowalski, M.A., and Churly, A.: Endoscopic brush cytology and biopsy in the diagnosis of cancer of the upper gastrointestinal tract. Acta Cytol. (Baltimore) 24:313, 1980.

68. Segal, A.W., Healy, M.J.R., Cox A.G., et al.: Diagnosis of gastric cancer. Br. Med. J. 2:669, 1975.

TUMORS OF THE STOMACH

Marc S. Levine, M.D.
Igor Laufer, M.D.

8

BENIGN TUMORS

Mucosal Polyps

Gastric polyps are generally considered to be uncommon lesions. However, the routine use of double contrast technique has dramatically improved our ability to detect gastric polyps, which are found in 1% to 2% of double contrast studies.[1, 2] Since gastric polyps are usually small lesions, it is likely that most are being missed on conventional single contrast examinations.

On double contrast studies, a gastric polyp on the dependent or posterior wall typically appears as a smooth, round filling defect in the thin barium pool (Fig. 8–1). Conversely, a polyp on the nondependent or anterior wall of the stomach is etched in white due to barium coating the edge of the polyp (Fig. 8–2). As a result, anterior wall polyps may be manifested by one or more ring shadows in the stomach (Fig. 8–3). If the polyp is pedunculated, its stalk may be seen en face overlying the head of the polyp, producing the "Mexican hat" sign (Fig. 8–2). Not infrequently, a droplet of barium or "stalactite" may be seen hanging down from an anterior wall polyp.[3] When this

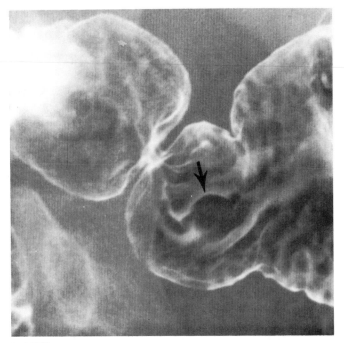

FIGURE 8–1

Polyp on posterior wall of antrum seen as radiolucent filling defect *(arrow)* in thin barium pool.

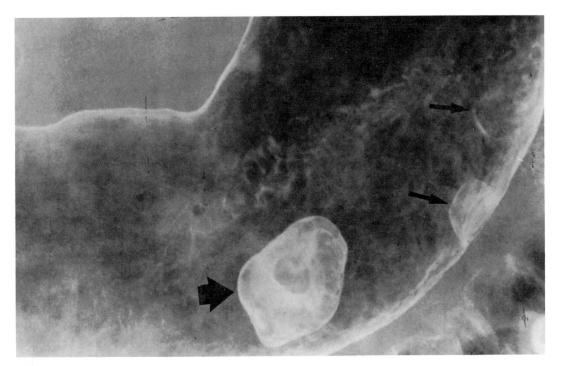

FIGURE 8–2

Anterior wall polyps are etched in white *(small arrows)* due to barium coating edge of polyp. Note that largest polyp exhibits Mexican hat sign *(large arrow)*, with central lucency representing stalk of polyp.

hanging droplet is viewed en face, it can be mistaken for a central area of ulceration (Fig. 8–3). However, it occurs as a transient finding, since the droplet of barium invariably falls off the polyp during fluoroscopic observation. Occasionally, a stalactite may be the only clue to the presence of a protruded lesion on the anterior wall (see Chapter 2).[4] When ring shadows or stalactites are observed in the stomach,

careful examination of the area with prone compression views should demonstrate the underlying polyps responsible for these findings.

The vast majority of polypoid lesions in the stomach are hyperplastic polyps.[5] They are almost always less than 1 cm in size and tend to occur as multiple lesions, most frequently in the fundus or body (Fig. 8–4).[1] Occasionally, the stomach may contain innu-

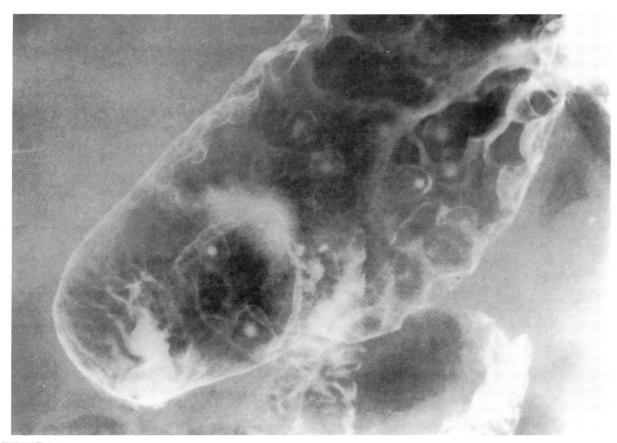

FIGURE 8–3

Multiple anterior wall polyps appearing as ring shadows in stomach. Note hanging droplets of barium or stalactites that could be mistaken for central areas of ulceration.

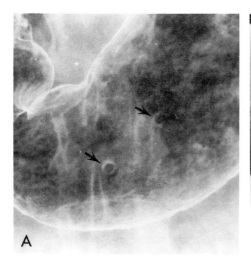

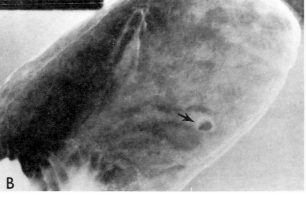

FIGURE 8–4

Multiple small hyperplastic polyps (arrows) in body (A) and fundus (B) of stomach.

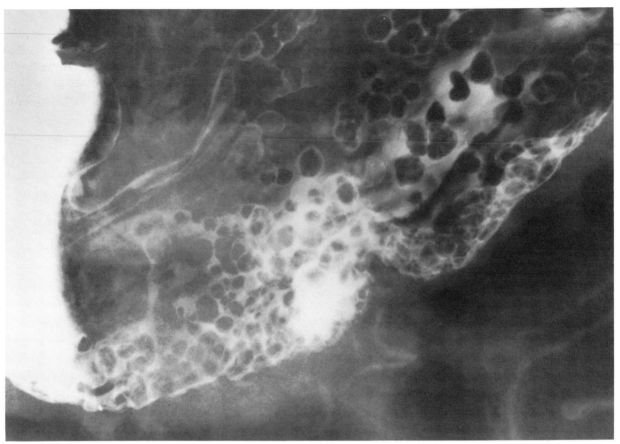

FIGURE 8–5

Innumerable hyperplastic polyps in stomach.

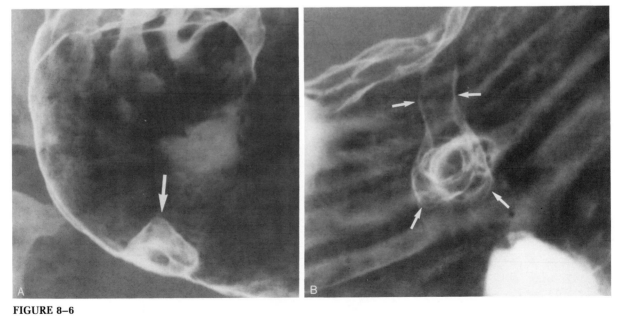

FIGURE 8–6

Two examples of solitary adenomatous polyps (*arrows*) in antrum. Note that polyp is sessile in *A* and pedunculated in *B*.

merable hyperplastic polyps (Fig. 8–5). Because these polyps are not premalignant, small (less than 1 cm), asymptomatic gastric polyps detected on double contrast studies should be considered innocuous lesions not requiring endoscopic biopsy or removal.

Although adenomatous polyps make up less than 10% of all gastric polyps,[1, 2, 5] they are dysplastic lesions that are capable of undergoing malignant degeneration via an adenoma-carcinoma sequence similar to that found in the colon. The risk of cancer is related to polyp size and becomes significant when the polyp reaches a diameter of 2 cm.[6] Nevertheless, adenocarcinoma is about 30 times more common than adenomatous polyps in the stomach, so that most gastric cancers are thought to originate de novo and not from pre-existing polyps.[7] Adenomatous polyps are almost always greater than 1 cm in size.[7, 8] The majority occur as solitary lesions, most frequently in the antrum (Fig. 8–6), but multiple lesions are occasionally found (Fig. 8–7).[8] Adenomatous polyps may

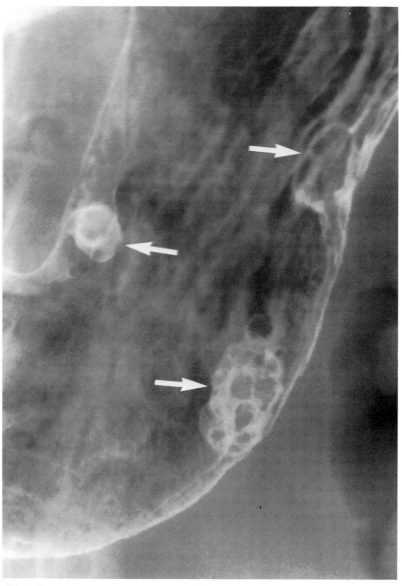

FIGURE 8–7

Multiple adenomatous polyps (*arrows*) in stomach. Note that lesions are larger and more lobulated than hyperplastic polyps.

When viewed in profile, submucosal tumors also have be sessile or pedunculated and tend to be more lobulated than hyperplastic polyps (Figs. 8–6 and 8–7). Thus, polyps that are pedunculated or lobulated or those that are greater than 1 cm in size should be evaluated by endoscopy. If biopsies confirm the presence of an adenomatous polyp, it should be resected because of the risk of malignant degeneration (Fig. 8–8). Adenomatous polyps are also important because they are associated with a high incidence of separate, coexisting gastric carcinomas.[5, 7]

Gastric involvement in the polyposis syndromes is discussed in Chapter 15.

Submucosal Tumors

Leiomyomas are by far the most common submucosal tumors in the stomach.[9] Other less common submucosal lesions include leiomyoblastomas, lipomas, hemangiomas, neurofibromas, and granular cell tumors. Even in patients with generalized neurofibromatosis, the most common submucosal tumor is a leiomyoma or lipoma rather than a neurofibroma (Fig. 8–9).[10] Although most of these lesions are discovered as incidental findings, ulcerated submucosal masses may cause abdominal pain or upper gastrointestinal bleeding. Submucosal tumors of smooth muscle origin are also important because of an associated risk of malignancy.

Submucosal tumors are often difficult to visualize at endoscopy because the overlying mucosa appears normal. However, these lesions are readily detected on double contrast studies. When viewed en face, submucosal tumors have very abrupt, well-defined borders, with adjacent mucosal folds that fade out at the periphery of the lesion (Fig. 8–10A). Because the mucosa is usually intact, a normal areae gastricae pattern can often be seen overlying these lesions. When viewed in profile, submucosal tumors also have

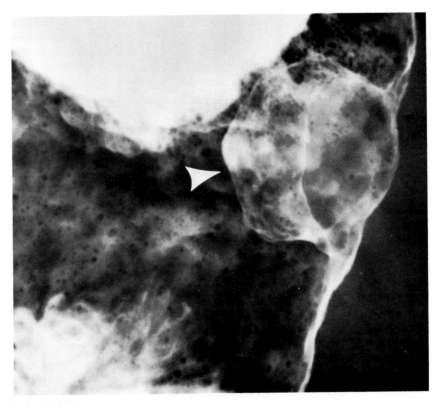

FIGURE 8–8

Giant adenomatous polyp (*arrowhead*) found to contain a central focus of adenocarcinoma.

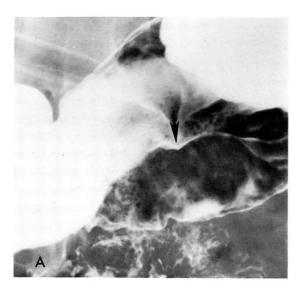

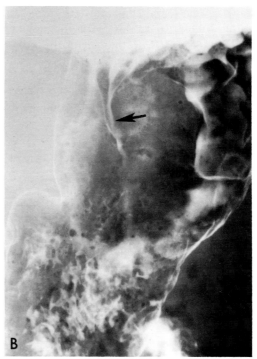

FIGURE 8–9

Gastric lipoma in patient with neurofibromatosis. The tumor, seen in profile (A) and en face (B), has a central furrow (arrows).

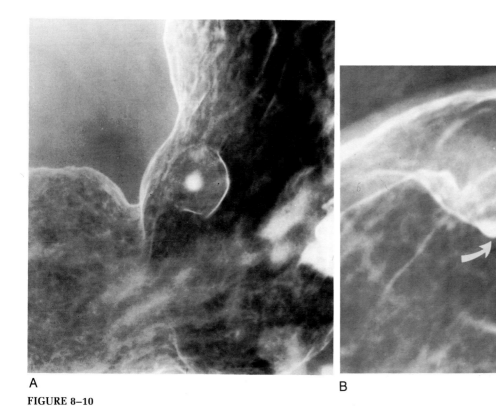

A

B

FIGURE 8–10

TWO EXAMPLES OF GASTRIC LEIOMYOMAS. A, Small leiomyoma seen en face in gastric body. This lesion has typical features of submucosal mass with smooth, well-defined borders. Also note hanging droplet of barium or stalactite on surface of this anterior wall lesion. B, Another leiomyoma seen in profile in gastric fundus. Note that borders of lesion form slightly obtuse angles with adjacent gastric wall. This view was taken with patient upright, and barium stalactite (arrow) is seen hanging down from inferior surface of lesion.

a very smooth surface, and their borders form right angles or slightly obtuse angles with the adjacent gastric wall (Fig. 8–10B). Although it is difficult to distinguish the various submucosal tumors on radiographic criteria, a lipoma may be suspected if the lesion changes in size or shape at fluoroscopy (Fig. 8–11A and B).[11] The fatty density of a lipoma can be confirmed by computed tomography (CT; Fig. 8–11C).[12, 13]

Submucosal tumors may vary in size from tiny lesions of several millimeters to enormous masses that encroach significantly upon the gastric lumen (Fig. 8–12). Some exogastric lesions may grow outward from the stomach into the peritoneal cavity.

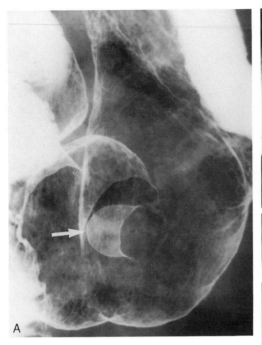

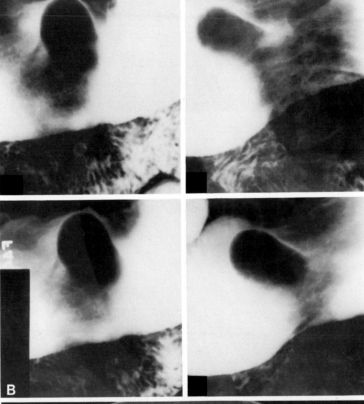

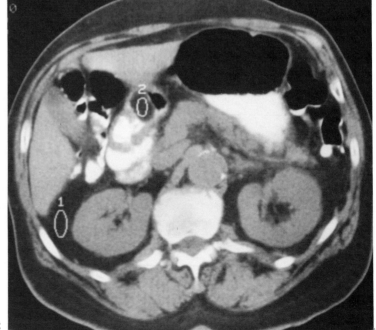

FIGURE 8–11

GASTRIC LIPOMA. *A,* Double contrast view shows smooth submucosal mass (*arrow*) in antrum.

B, Prone single contrast views show how lesion changes in size and shape with varying degrees of compression. This changing appearance should be highly suggestive of a lipoma.

C, CT scan shows how lesion in antrum (*cursor 2*) has same density as perirenal fat (*cursor 1*), confirming presence of lipoma.

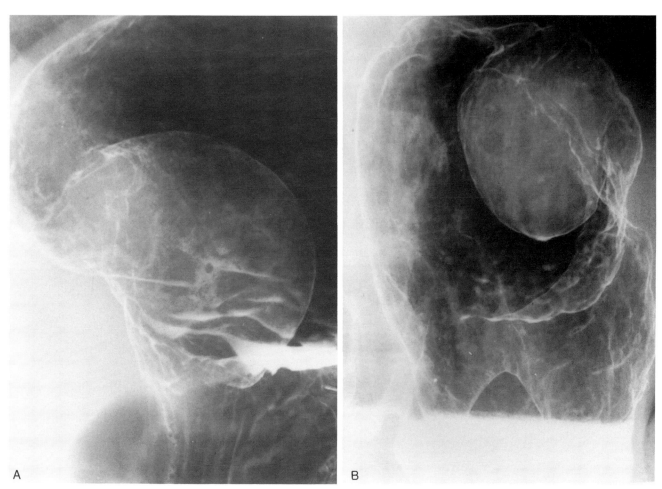

FIGURE 8–12

A and *B,* Two examples of giant leiomyomas in gastric fundus.

Tumors greater than 2 cm in size frequently contain areas of ulceration, manifested by a central barium-filled crater within the mass (Fig. 8–13A). Ulceration is generally considered an indication for surgery because of the risk of upper gastrointestinal bleeding. However, complete healing of ulceration in a gastric leiomyoma has been documented on follow-up studies (Fig. 8–13B),[14] so that conservative medical treatment may lead to cessation of bleeding when surgery is contraindicated. Occasionally, a hanging droplet of barium or stalactite on an anterior wall leiomyoma can mimic the appearance of ulceration (Fig. 8–10A). However, the stalactite can be recognized as a transient finding at fluoroscopy. Although leiomyomas and leiomyosarcomas cannot be reliably differentiated on radiologic criteria, the possibility of malignancy should be suspected when the lesion is larger than 2 to 3 cm in size or lobulated or contains extensive areas of ulceration (Fig. 8–14).[9]

Other types of lesions can mimic submucosal tumors. An ectopic pancreatic rest may be manifested radiographically by a submucosal mass, most frequently on the greater curvature of the distal antrum (Fig. 8–15).[15, 16] Approximately 50% of these lesions have a central umbilication, representing the orifice of a primitive ductal system.[15] As a result, the radiographic appearance may suggest an ulcerated submucosal tumor. An acute antral ulcer with a large

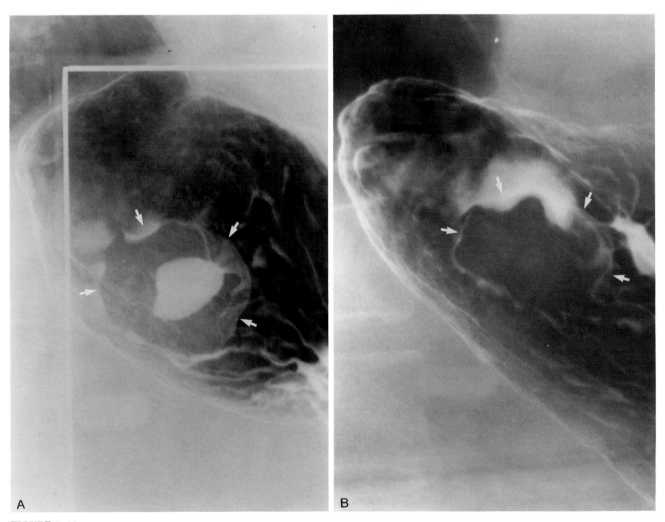

A

B

FIGURE 8–13

ULCERATED LEIOMYOMA WITH HEALING OF ULCER. *A,* Initial study shows leiomyoma *(arrows)* in fundus with central area of ulceration.

B, Follow-up study 3½ years later shows complete healing of ulcer in leiomyoma *(arrows).* (From O'Riordan, D., et al.: Complete healing of ulceration within a gastric leiomyoma. Gastrointest. Radiol. *10:*47, 1985, with permission.)

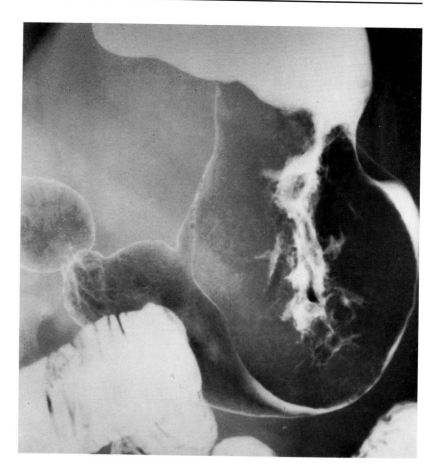

FIGURE 8–14

Large leiomyosarcoma on posterior wall of
stomach with irregular areas of ulceration.
(Courtesy of Hans Herlinger, M.D., Philadelphia,
Pennsylvania.)

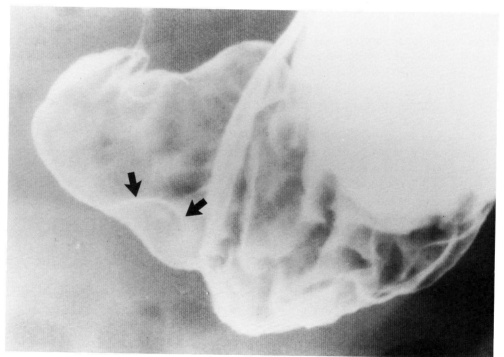

FIGURE 8–15

Ectopic pancreatic rest appearing as submucosal mass (arrows) on greater curvature of antrum.

mound of edema may also simulate an intramural lesion. With ulcers, however, there tends to be a more gradual transition between the edematous mound and the adjacent gastric mucosa. Finally, extrinsic compression of the stomach by a normal or enlarged liver, spleen, pancreas, or kidney may be indistinguishable from an exophytic submucosal tumor (Fig. 8–16). However, the presence of a central dimple or spicule at the apex of the mass should suggest an exogastric lesion such as a leiomyoma or leiomyosarcoma.[17] In such patients, CT or sonography is often helpful for establishing the correct diagnosis.

MALIGNANT TUMORS

Carcinoma

Early Tumors

Early gastric cancer is defined histologically as carcinoma in which malignant invasion is limited to the mucosa or submucosa.[18] During the past several decades, detection of early gastric cancer has increased dramatically in Japan as the result of mass screening of asymptomatic patients who undergo periodic double contrast upper gastrointestinal studies and endoscopy. This aggressive approach to gastric cancer by the Japanese has also resulted in a dramatic increase in patient survival, with 5-year survival rates as high as 95% for patients with early gastric cancer.[19] The Japanese have devised an elaborate system for classifying these tumors on the basis of the predominant morphologic (elevated, flat, or depressed) features of the lesions (see Chapter 14).[18]

Radiologists in Western countries should be aware of the various appearances of early gastric cancer, because occasional cases may be encountered (Fig. 8–17). However, the widespread use of double contrast radiographic techniques and fiberoptic endoscopy has not improved our ability to diagnose early gastric cancer in the West.[20] This discrepancy from the Japanese experience can be attributed primarily to the fact that mass screening programs are not employed in Western countries because of the lower incidence of gastric carcinoma. Thus, radiologists should recognize that they are unlikely to experience a significant increase in the detection of early gastric cancer as long as these examinations are performed predominantly on symptomatic patients.

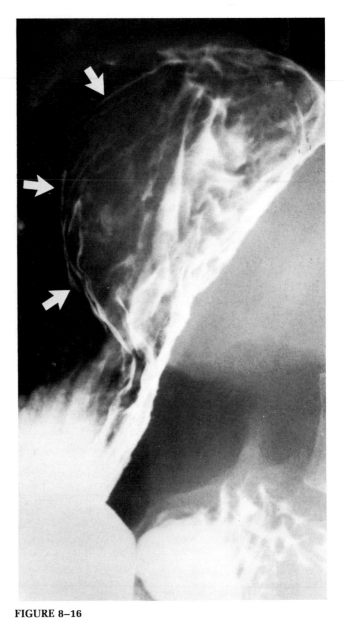

FIGURE 8–16

Pancreatic pseudocyst with extrinsic compression of posterior wall of fundus (*arrows*), simulating appearance of giant submucosal mass.

Advanced Tumors

Most symptomatic patients with gastric carcinoma present with advanced tumors. These lesions may be polypoid (Fig. 8–18), plaque-like (Fig. 8–19), ulcerated (Fig. 8–20), or infiltrating (Fig. 8–21); or, less frequently, they may be manifested by thickened, irregular folds (Fig. 8–22). Despite the advanced stage of these tumors, approximately 10% of gastric carci-

Text continued on page 264

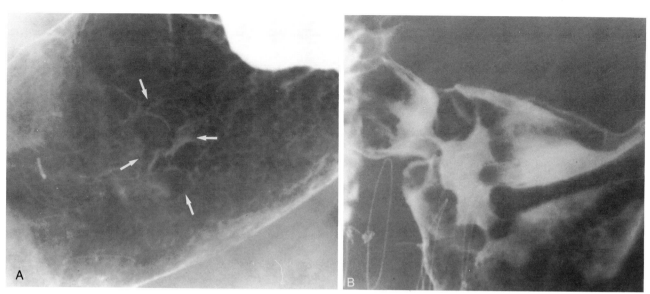

FIGURE 8–17

TWO EXAMPLES OF EARLY GASTRIC CANCER. *A*, Small, superficial cancer in gastric body manifested by nodular, irregular elevations *(arrows)*.

B, Malignant ulcer on posterior wall of antrum, with scalloped borders and nodular, clubbed folds surrounding ulcer. (*B*, From Levine, M.S., et al.: Benign gastric ulcers: Diagnosis and follow-up with double contrast radiography. Radiology *164*:9–13, 1987, with permission.)

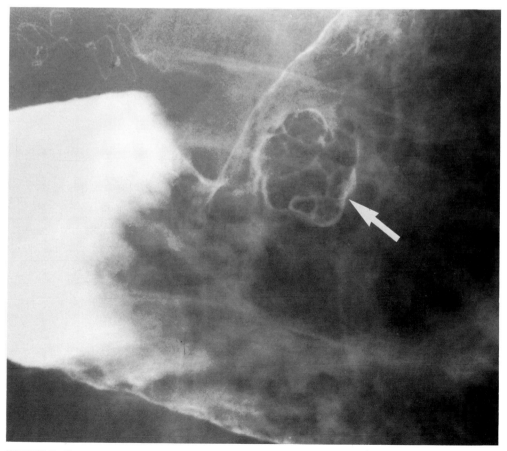

FIGURE 8–18

Small polypoid carcinoma *(arrow)* in gastric body.

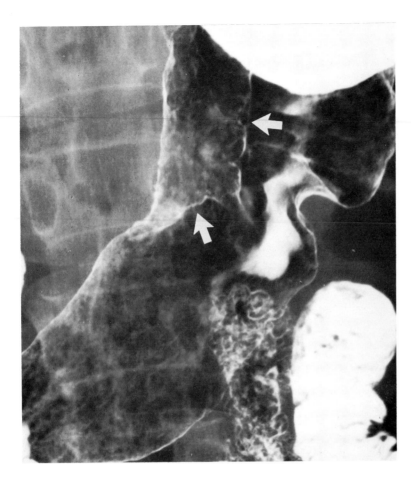

FIGURE 8–19

Plaque-like carcinoma (*arrows*) high on lesser curvature of stomach.

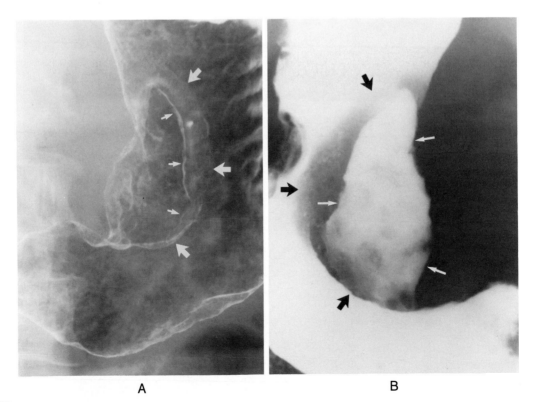

A

B

FIGURE 8–20

ULCERATED GASTRIC CARCINOMA. *A,* Double contrast view of stomach shows relatively large mass on anterior wall that is etched in white (*large arrows*). Also note second curvilinear density (*small arrows*) due to barium coating rim of unfilled central ulcer.

B, Prone compression view shows mass as radiolucent filling defect (*black arrows*) on anterior wall of stomach. Note how central ulcer fills with barium (*white arrows*) when patient is in prone position.

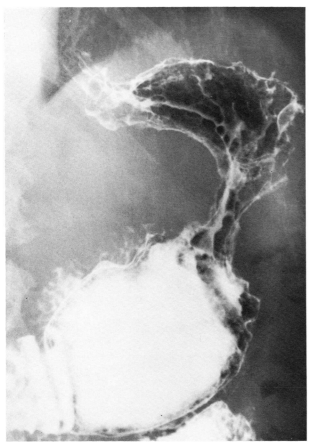

FIGURE 8–21

Advanced, infiltrating carcinoma with irregular narrowing of proximal portion of stomach.

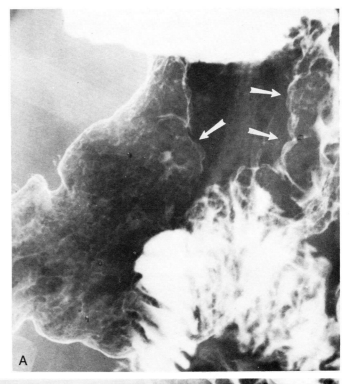

FIGURE 8–22

GASTRIC CARCINOMA WITH THICKENED FOLDS. *A,* Note large, lobulated folds (*arrows*) in gastric body.

B, Close-up view shows disorganization of folds due to infiltration by tumor.

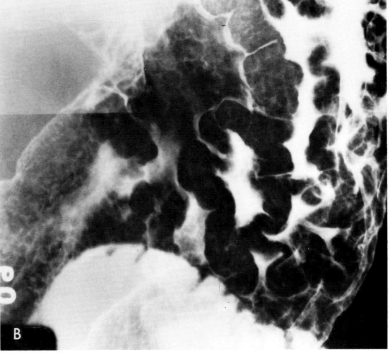

nomas are missed on conventional single contrast barium studies and an additional 15% are misdiagnosed as benign lesions.[21] Infiltrating tumors and tumors involving the proximal portion of the stomach are more likely to be missed on single contrast studies.[22] Yet these are precisely the lesions that require accurate radiologic diagnosis, since endoscopic biopsies and brushings are often negative for tumor in these patients.[23] Fortunately, double contrast studies are particularly well suited for demonstrating infiltrating lesions or lesions involving the proximal portion of the stomach (Fig. 8–23).

Localized areas of rigidity or decreased distensibil-

ity due to infiltrating tumors are accentuated by gastric distention on the double contrast examination (see Fig. 8–23). In general, the greater the degree of distention, the easier it is to detect infiltrating lesions that limit distensibility. However, it should be recognized that overdistention may obscure some of the morphologic features of the lesion that are better seen when the stomach is less distended. Conversely, inadequate gaseous distention can accentuate the appearance of the rugal folds, erroneously suggesting an infiltrating tumor (Fig. 8–24A). With adequate distention, however, normal folds usually can be effaced, ruling out the possibility of malignancy (Fig. 8–24B).

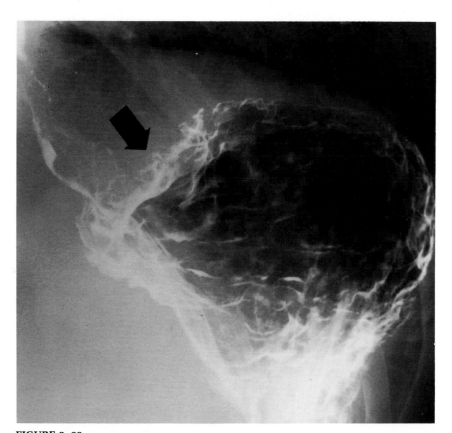

FIGURE 8–23

Gastric carcinoma with localized infiltration of medial aspect of fundus (arrow). Optimal distention of fundus is needed to demonstrate this lesion.

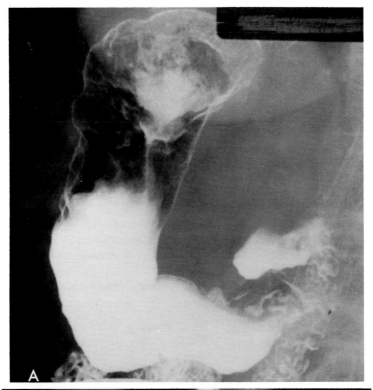

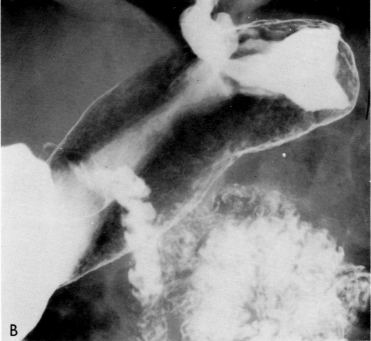

FIGURE 8–24

DANGER OF INADEQUATE GASEOUS DISTENTION. *A,* Thickened folds are seen in proximal portion of stomach, raising the possibility of tumor. However, the fundus is inadequately distended on this view.

B, With greater gaseous distention, the folds are effaced in the fundus, eliminating the possibility of tumor.

Scirrhous Tumors

Scirrhous carcinoma of the stomach is an infiltrating type of gastric cancer in which the tumor spreads predominantly in the submucosa, inciting a marked desmoplastic response in the gastric wall. Less frequently, the stomach can be infiltrated by metastatic breast cancer. Whether primary or metastatic, these scirrhous tumors are classically manifested radiographically by irregular narrowing and rigidity of the stomach, producing a "linitis plastica" or "leather bottle" appearance (Fig. 8–25). Occasionally, however, scirrhous tumors of the stomach may cause only mild loss of distensibility. Instead, these lesions may be recognized on double contrast studies primarily by distortion of the normal surface pattern of the stomach with mucosal nodularity, spiculation, ulceration, or thickened, irregular folds (Fig. 8–26).[24] Thus, some lesions are likely to be missed if the radiologist relies too heavily on gastric narrowing as the major criterion for diagnosing these tumors.

Scirrhous gastric carcinomas are classically thought to involve the distal half of the stomach, arising near the pylorus and gradually extending upward from the antrum into the body and fundus. Although some localized lesions may be confined to the prepyloric region of the antrum (Fig. 8–27),[25] it is difficult to find cases in the literature of lesions involving the proximal stomach that spare the antrum. With double contrast technique, however, nearly 40% of patients with these scirrhous tumors have localized lesions in the gastric fundus or body with antral sparing (Figs. 8–28 and 8–29).[24] Detection of these lesions is presumably related to gaseous distention of the proximal stomach on double contrast studies. In any case, radiologists should be aware that a significant percentage of patients with scirrhous

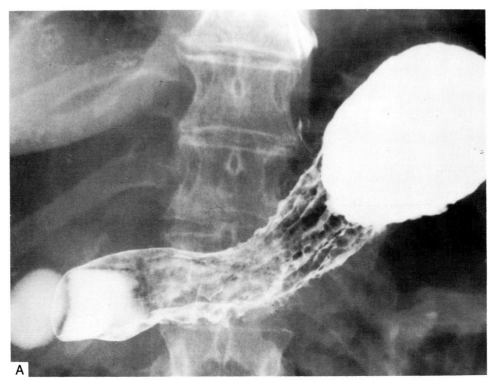

FIGURE 8–25

SCIRRHOUS TUMORS OF THE STOMACH. A, Linitis plastica with irregular narrowing of antrum and body due to metastatic breast cancer involving stomach. Note absent left breast shadow.

tumors have localized lesions involving the gastric fundus or body rather than the classic form of linitis plastica involving the distal stomach.

The limitations of endoscopy in diagnosing scirrhous carcinoma of the stomach should also be recognized. False-negative endoscopic brushings and biopsies are frequently obtained not only because these tumors are located predominantly in the submucosa but because the tumor cells are often separated by large areas of fibrosis (Fig. 8–29).[23-26] Thus, excessive reliance on negative endoscopic findings can lead to a significant delay in the diagnosis and treatment of these tumors.

The radiologic diagnosis of recurrent gastric carcinoma and primary gastric stump carcinoma following partial gastrectomy is considered in Chapter 9.

Text continued on page 273

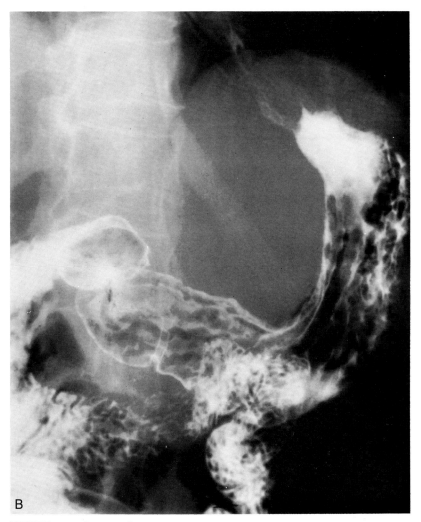

B

FIGURE 8–25 *Continued*

B, Diffuse gastric narrowing due to primary scirrhous carcinoma of stomach. There was also involvement of distal esophagus, producing an achalasia-like picture. This patient presented with dysphagia.

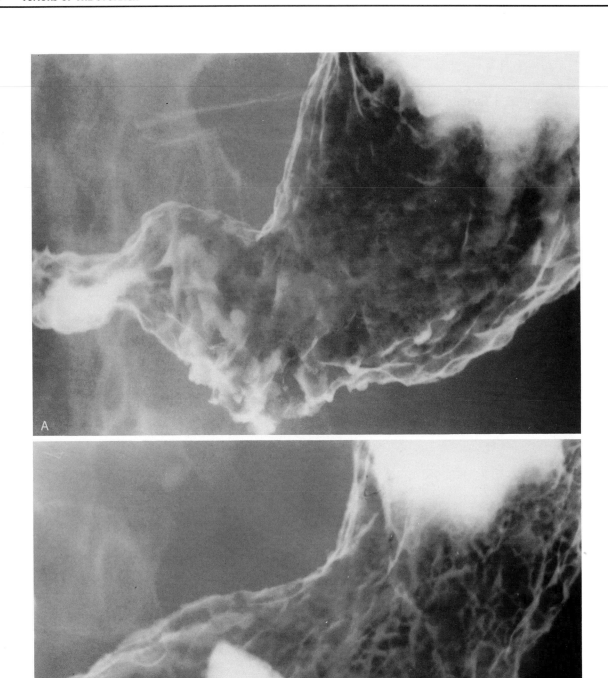

FIGURE 8–26

A and *B*, Two examples of metastatic breast cancer involving stomach with only mild loss of distensibility. However, there is distortion of normal surface pattern with nodular, irregular mucosa in both cases. (From Levine, M.S., et al.: Scirrhous carcinoma of the stomach: Radiologic and endoscopic diagnosis. Radiology *175*:151–154, 1990, with permission.)

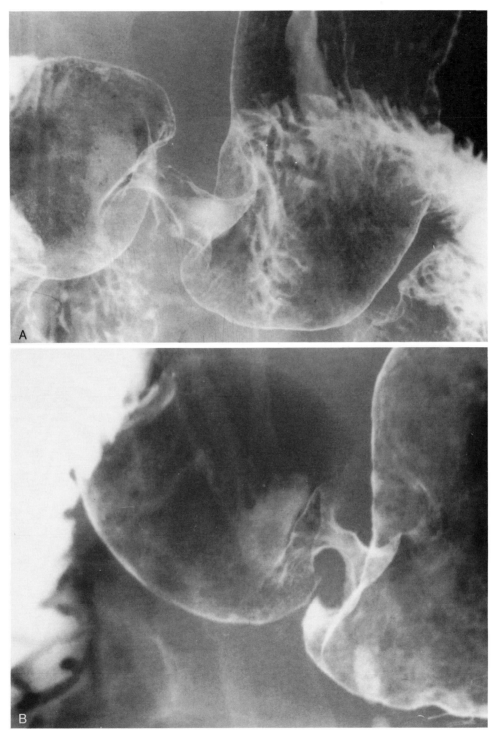

FIGURE 8–27

A and *B*, Two examples of localized scirrhous carcinoma of distal antrum. In both cases, there is a short, annular lesion in prepyloric region of antrum. Note abrupt, shelf-like borders of lesions. (*A*, From Levine, M.S., et al.: Scirrhous carcinoma of the stomach: Radiologic and endoscopic diagnosis. Radiology *175*:151–154, 1990, with permission.)

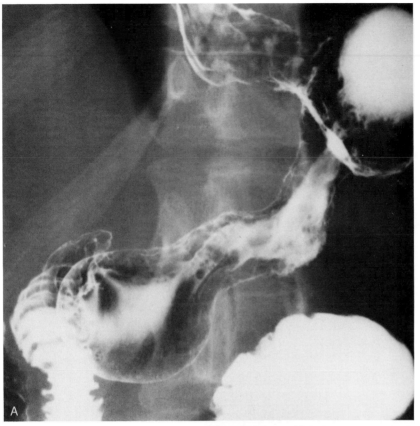

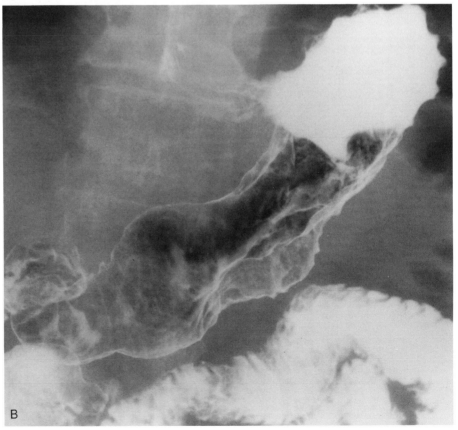

FIGURE 8–28

TWO EXAMPLES OF LOCALIZED SCIRRHOUS CARCINOMA OF PROXIMAL STOMACH. *A,* Marked narrowing of gastric body with normal distensibility of antrum and fundus.

B, Irregular narrowing of fundus and body with antral sparing. (*A,* From Levine, M.S., et al.: Scirrhous carcinoma of the stomach: Radiologic and endoscopic diagnosis. Radiology *175:*151–154, 1990, with permission.)

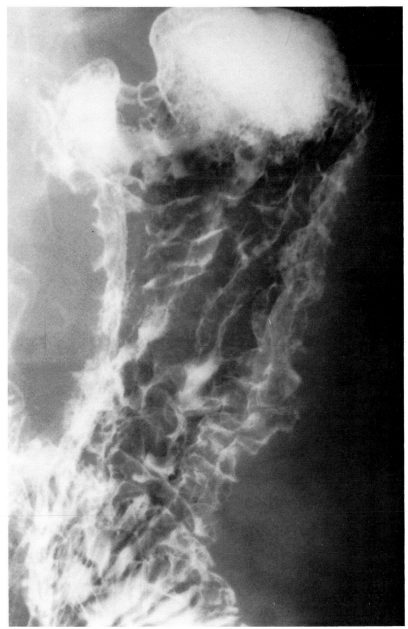

FIGURE 8–29

Metastatic breast cancer causing linitis plastica in proximal half of stomach with antral sparing. Note how gastric fundus and body have irregular contour with thickened, spiculated folds. Despite the dramatic radiographic findings, biopsies and brushings from initial endoscopic examination failed to confirm presence of tumor. (From Levine, M.S., et al.: Scirrhous carcinoma of the stomach: Radiologic and endoscopic diagnosis. Radiology *175*:151–154, 1990, with permission.)

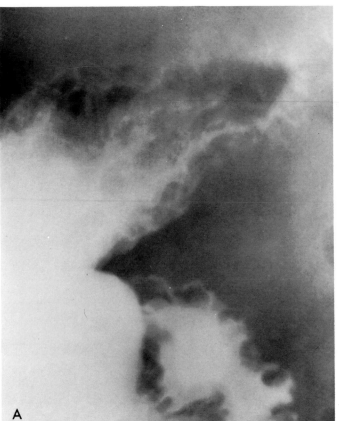
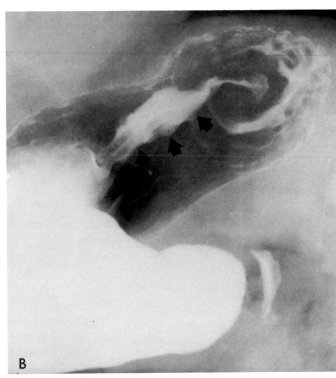

FIGURE 8–30

LIMITATION OF SINGLE CONTRAST BARIUM STUDY IN DIAGNOSIS OF CARCINOMA OF THE CARDIA. *A*, No tumor is seen in fundus on conventional single contrast study.

B, With greater gaseous distention of fundus, ulcerated lesion *(arrows)* is clearly seen adjacent to cardia on double contrast view. (From Glass, G.B.J. (ed.): Progress in Gastroenterology, vol. 3. New York, Grune & Stratton, 1977, with permission.)

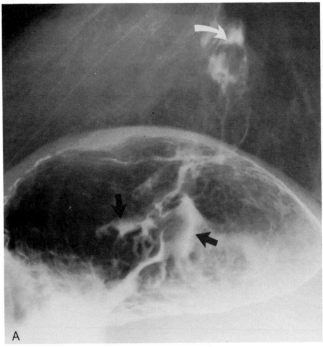
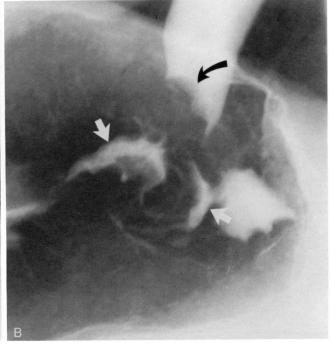

FIGURE 8–31

A and *B*, Two examples of cardiac carcinoma in which normal anatomic landmarks at cardia have been obliterated and replaced by irregular areas of ulceration *(straight arrows)*. In both cases, note polypoid extension of tumor into distal esophagus *(curved arrows)*. (*A*, From Levine, M.S., et al.: Carcinoma of the gastric cardia in young people. AJR *140*:69–72, 1983, with permission, © by American Roentgen Ray Society.)

272

Carcinoma of the Cardia

Tumors involving the gastric cardia or fundus are notoriously difficult to detect on conventional single contrast barium studies. Because the overlying rib cage precludes manual palpation or compression of the fundus, even large lesions at the cardia may be obscured by crowded folds or relatively opaque barium that prevents adequate visualization of this region (Fig. 8–30A). With gaseous distention of the fundus, however, it is possible to evaluate the normal anatomic landmarks at the cardia and the surrounding gastric mucosa for evidence of malignancy (Fig. 8–30B).

When viewed en face, the normal cardia often appears on double contrast studies as a circular elevation containing four or five stellate folds that radiate to a central button at the gastroesophageal junction (the cardiac "rosette"; see Chapter 7).[27, 28] Some lesions at the cardia may be recognized only by relatively subtle nodularity, mass effect, or ulceration in this region with distortion, effacement, or obliteration of these landmarks (Fig. 8–31).[27–31] Enlargement or lobulation of the surrounding elevation should also suggest a neoplastic lesion (Fig. 8–32). If the radiographic findings are equivocal, the patient should be instructed to swallow an additional bolus of barium.

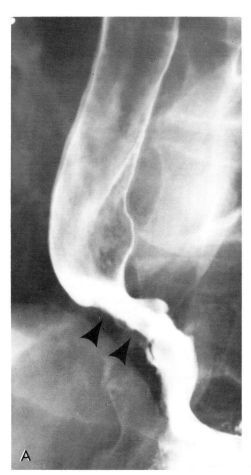

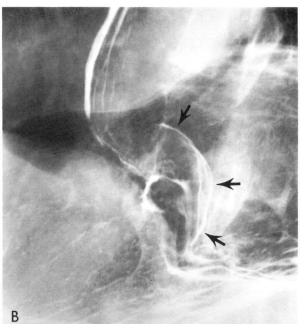

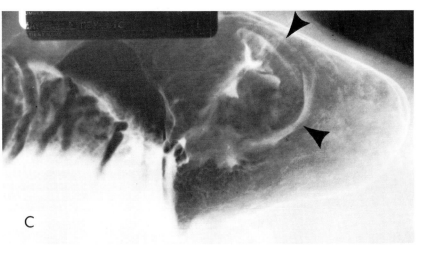

FIGURE 8–32

CARCINOMA OF THE CARDIA, CAUSING DYSPHAGIA. *A,* Upright view of esophagus shows minimal irregularity along one wall of distal esophagus *(arrowheads).*

B, Right posterior oblique view of fundus shows relatively flat polypoid lesion *(arrows)* surrounding cardia.

C, Right lateral view of fundus also shows polypoid lesion *(arrowheads)* at cardia. Note small areas of ulceration in tumor.

The protrusion surrounding a normal cardia should disappear when barium is swallowed, because this landmark is obliterated by relaxation of the lower esophageal sphincter. A lesion therefore should be suspected if this protrusion or other abnormalities persist during passage of the barium bolus at fluoroscopy. Conversely, an apparent abnormality at the cardia must be an artifact if it vanishes as the cardia opens.

Advanced carcinomas of the gastric cardia or fundus are usually exophytic or infiltrating lesions, often containing irregular areas of ulceration (Fig. 8–33B).[30, 32] Secondary esophageal involvement by advanced lesions may be manifested radiographically by a polypoid or fungating mass that extends from the fundus into the distal esophagus or by thickened folds or irregular narrowing of the distal esophagus without a discrete lesion.[30, 32] Submucosal spread of tumor may also result in "secondary achalasia" with tapered, beak-like narrowing of the distal esophagus at or just above the gastroesophageal junction (Fig. 8–

33A).[32, 33] However, careful examination of the gastric cardia and fundus almost always demonstrates the underlying gastric lesion (Fig. 8–33B). Because of the frequency of esophageal involvement, patients with carcinoma of the cardia often present clinically with dysphagia. Some of these patients may have a sensation of blockage that is referred to the upper esophagus or pharynx. The cardia therefore should be carefully evaluated in all patients with unexplained dysphagia to rule out a carcinoma of the cardia masquerading as a pharyngeal or esophageal disorder.

When a suspicious lesion is detected at the cardia, endoscopy should be performed for a definitive diagnosis. Nevertheless, radiographically diagnosed lesions at the cardia occasionally can be missed on endoscopic examination.[34] The barium study therefore should be repeated, despite a negative endoscopy, if the initial examination suggests a malignant lesion. Rarely, some patients with continuing radiologic evidence of malignancy may require surgery without preoperative histologic confirmation.

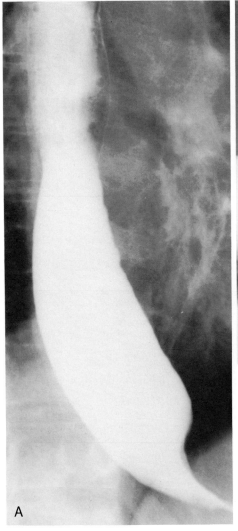

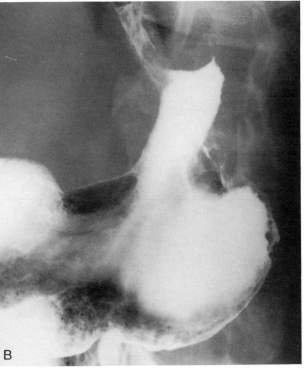

FIGURE 8–33

SECONDARY ACHALASIA CAUSED BY GASTRIC CARCINOMA. *A,* Smooth, tapered narrowing of distal esophagus, producing classic "bird-beak" appearance of achalasia.

B, However, radiograph of stomach shows advanced, infiltrating carcinoma of gastric cardia and fundus invading distal esophagus. (From Levine, M.S.: Radiology of the Esophagus, Philadelphia, W.B. Saunders, 1989, p. 179, with permission.)

Lymphoma

Gastric lymphoma accounts for about 50% of all gastrointestinal lymphomas.[35] The majority of patients have primary gastric lymphoma with disease confined to the stomach and regional lymph nodes, whereas the remainder have generalized lymphoma with associated gastric involvement. Histologically, 90% to 95% of patients have non-Hodgkin's lymphoma, and the remaining 5% to 10% have Hodgkin's disease involving the stomach.[35] Depending on their gross morphology, gastric lymphomas may appear radiographically as infiltrating, polypoid, nodular, or ulcerated lesions (Figs. 8–34 to 8–36), or they may be manifested by thickened folds (Fig. 8–37).[36–39] Occasionally, one or more submucosal masses that are centrally ulcerated may have a characteristic "bull's-eye" or "target" appearance (Fig. 8–38). How-

ever, many lesions have mixed morphologic features, so that there is considerable overlap in the radiologic classification of these tumors. The radiologist may not suggest the diagnosis of lymphoma because it is often indistinguishable from adenocarcinoma, a much more common malignant neoplasm in the stomach. However, the presence of grossly enlarged rugal folds in a stomach that retains its normal distensibility should suggest the possibility of lymphoma.[36, 37, 39]

Gastric lymphoma has a much better prognosis than gastric carcinoma, with 5-year survival rates approaching 60%.[40, 41] As a result, the failure to obtain biopsies from an advanced lesion that is assumed to be inoperable gastric cancer may deprive the patient of the opportunity for cure or long-term palliation. When the radiographic findings suggest a malignant

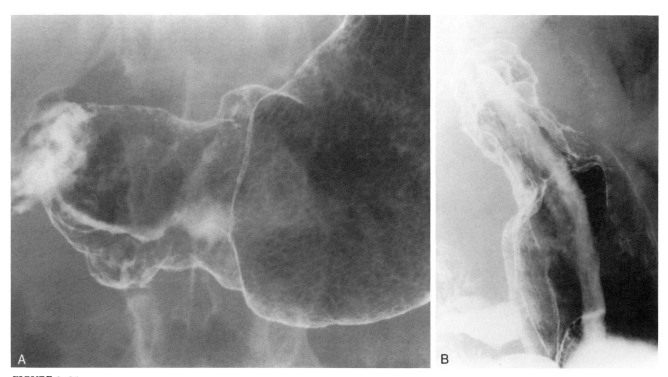

FIGURE 8–34

Two examples of infiltrating gastric lymphomas involving antrum (A) and fundus (B) of stomach.

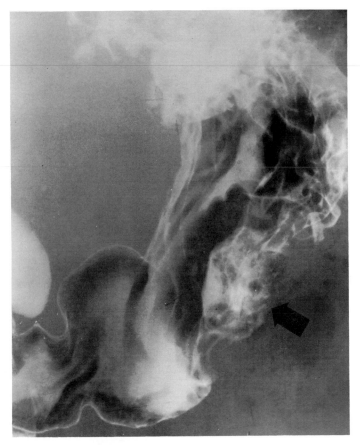

FIGURE 8–35

Gastric lymphoma manifested by polypoid mass on greater
curvature with central area of ulceration *(arrow)*.

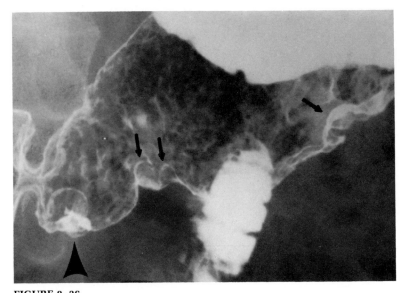

FIGURE 8–36

Gastric lymphoma with multiple small submucosal masses *(arrows)*. The
most distal mass is ulcerated *(arrowhead)*.

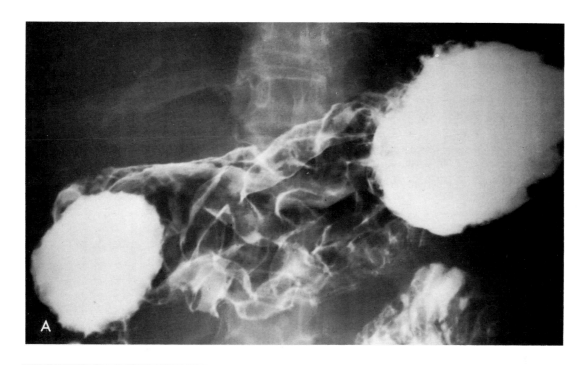

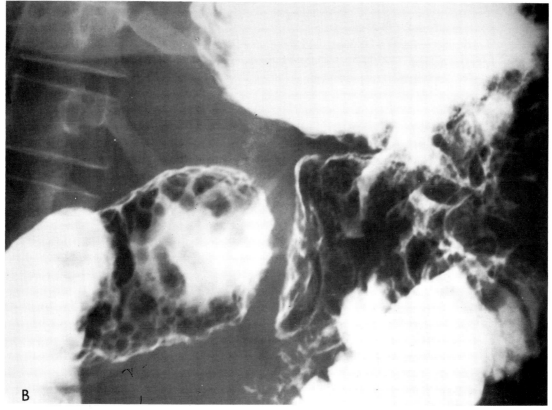

FIGURE 8–37

A and *B*, Gastric lymphoma with diffuse enlargement of rugal folds. Also note duodenal involvement in *B*. (Courtesy of Alec Megibow, M.D., and Patricia Redmond, M.D., New York, New York.)

tumor in the stomach, a histologic diagnosis therefore should be obtained because of the possibility of lymphoma. However, deep endoscopic biopsies are usually required for a definite pathologic diagnosis, because the lymphomatous tissue tends to infiltrate the gastric wall beneath an intact mucosa. With adequate cytologic and histologic specimens, the endoscopic sensitivity in diagnosing gastric lymphoma may be as high as 90%.[42, 43]

Proper staging of gastric lymphoma by CT or other diagnostic tests is important, so that a rational treatment decision can be made about the need for surgery, radiation, or chemotherapy. With the increasing use of systemic chemotherapy for advanced disease, follow-up double contrast studies may also be helpful for documenting the response to treatment and for evaluating abdominal pain or gastrointestinal bleeding after the initiation of systemic chemotherapy. In some patients, chemotherapy may lead to dramatic regression of ulcerated plaques or mass lesions with the development of a benign-appearing ulcer or ulcer scar at the site of the previous lesion (Figs. 8–39A and C).[44] However, chemotherapy may also lead to ulceration or perforation of these lymphomatous lesions with the development of massive upper gastrointestinal bleeding or peritonitis (Fig. 8–39B). These complications may necessitate discontinuation of chemotherapy, resulting in treatment failure.[45]

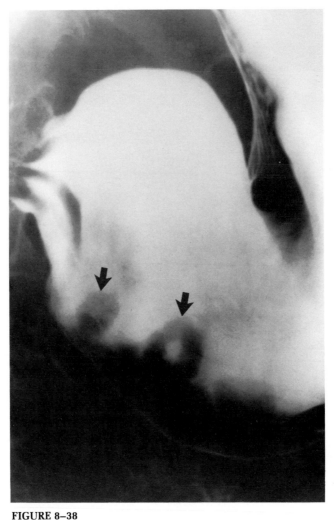

FIGURE 8–38

Gastric lymphoma with centrally ulcerated submucosal masses or bull's-eye lesions (arrows) in antrum.

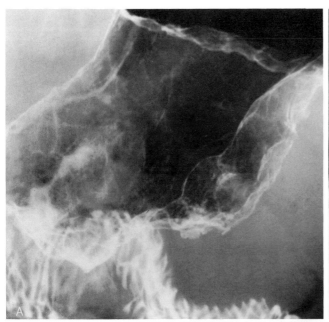

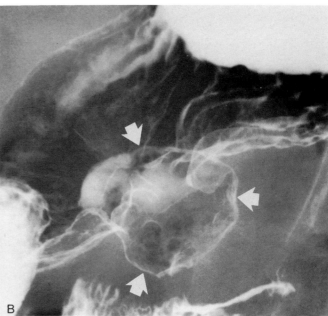

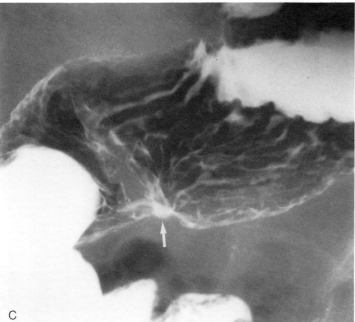

FIGURE 8–39

RESPONSE OF GASTRIC LYMPHOMA TO CHEMOTHERAPY.
A, Initial study shows thickened, irregular folds in gastric body due to lymphoma.

B, After treatment with chemotherapy, follow-up study 6 months later shows regression of lymphoma with large area of cavitation *(arrows)* adjacent to posterior wall of stomach.

C, Another follow-up study 1 year later shows further regression of lymphoma with radiating folds and tiny, benign-appearing residual ulcer *(arrow)* at site of previous excavation.

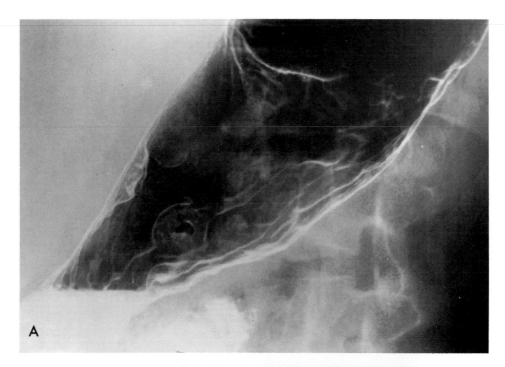

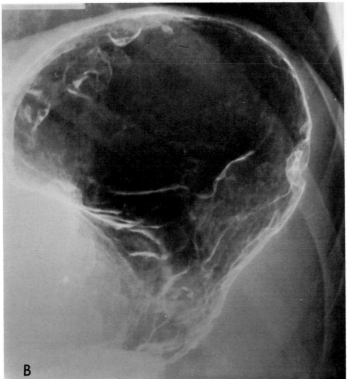

FIGURE 8–40

A and B, Multiple submucosal nodules in stomach due to metastatic melanoma. (Courtesy of Herbert Y. Kressel, M.D., Philadelphia, Pennsylvania.)

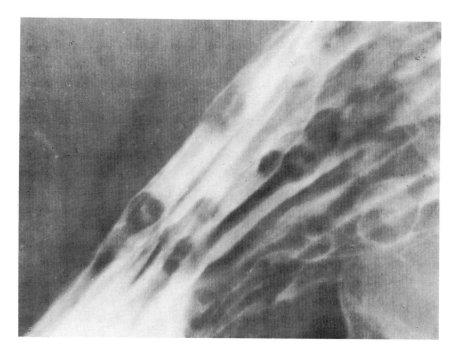

FIGURE 8–41

Multiple ulcerated metastases or bull's-eye lesions in stomach due to adenocarcinoma of unknown origin.

Metastatic Disease

Hematogenous or blood-borne metastases to the stomach may be manifested radiographically by one or more discrete submucosal masses (Fig. 8–40). As they outgrow their blood supply, these submucosal masses often undergo central necrosis and ulceration, producing characteristic "bull's-eye" or "target" lesions (Fig. 8–41).[46, 47] Bull's-eye lesions are frequently seen in patients with metastatic melanoma, but the differential diagnosis includes other metastatic lesions, lymphoma, and, most recently, Kaposi's sarcoma in patients with AIDS.[48–50] Less frequently, hematogenous metastases to the stomach may undergo excavation, producing giant, cavitated lesions (Fig. 8–42).[47] Gastric lymphoma, leiomyosarcoma, and, rarely, adenocarcinoma may produce similar findings. Metastatic breast cancer involving the stomach may also produce a linitis plastica appearance indistinguishable from that of a primary scirrhous carcinoma (see Figs. 8–25A, 8–26, and 8–29; see earlier section, "Scirrhous Tumors").[24, 46, 51]

The stomach may be directly invaded by malignant tumors arising in neighboring structures such as the esophagus and pancreas. Adenocarcinomas arising in Barrett's esophagus have a particular tendency to invade the gastric cardia and fundus.[52] These lesions may be indistinguishable radiographically from primary carcinomas of the cardia or fundus invading the esophagus (see Chapter 6). Depending on their location, carcinomas arising in the head, body, or tail of

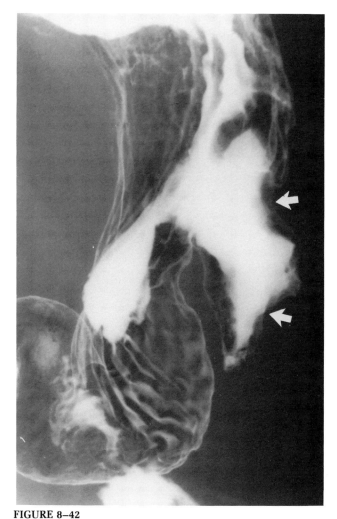

FIGURE 8–42

Metastatic breast cancer with giant, cavitated lesion *(arrows)* in stomach.

the pancreas may also invade the stomach, causing mass effect, nodularity, or spiculation of the greater curvature of the antrum or posterior wall of the body and fundus (Fig. 8–43).

The stomach may also be involved by direct extension of colonic or pancreatic carcinoma along mesenteric reflections such as the gastrocolic ligament or transverse mesocolon or by contiguous spread of tumor along the greater omentum (Fig. 8–44). Bulky omental metastases or "omental cakes" are a relatively common finding in patients with disseminated ovarian cancer or other gynecologic or gastrointestinal malignancies. These omental metastases may spread superiorly via the proximal portion of the greater omentum or gastrocolic ligament to the greater curvature of the stomach, producing mass effect, nodularity, flattening, or spiculated, tethered mucosal folds on the greater curvature of the gastric antrum or body (Figs. 8–45 and 8–46A).[53] Carcinoma of the transverse colon invading the stomach via the gastrocolic ligament may produce identical radiographic findings.[46, 54] However, patients with omental metastases involving the stomach almost always have associated colonic involvement, manifested by mass effect, nodularity, or spiculated folds on the superior border of

the transverse colon or, in advanced cases, circumferential narrowing of the bowel (Fig. 8–46B).[53, 55] Thus, a barium enema examination should differentiate omental metastases to the stomach from gastric invasion by carcinoma of the transverse colon. When gastric involvement by omental metastases is suspected on barium studies, computed tomography should be performed to better delineate the nature and extent of metastatic tumor (Fig. 8–47).[56]

Squamous cell carcinoma of the pharynx or esophagus may also spread to the stomach via submucosal esophageal lymphatics that extend subdiaphragmatically to paracardiac, lesser curvature, or celiac nodes. These squamous cell metastases to the stomach usually appear radiographically as discrete submucosal masses in the gastric fundus at a considerable distance from the primary tumor.[57, 58] The lesions may be quite large and often contain central areas of ulceration, so that they can be mistaken for ulcerated leiomyomas or leiomyosarcomas (Fig. 8–48). Because the treatment for esophageal cancer depends on the stage of the tumor at the time of diagnosis, the gastric cardia and fundus should be carefully evaluated radiographically in all patients with esophageal cancer to rule out unsuspected metastases to the stomach.

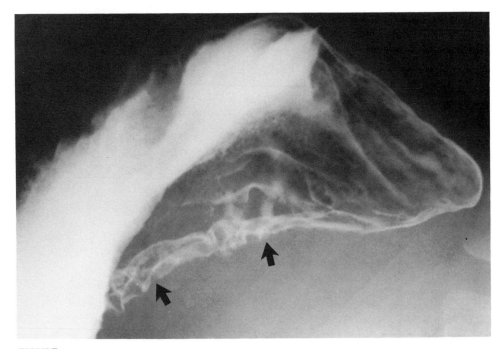

FIGURE 8–43

Carcinoma of tail of pancreas invading stomach with mass effect and spiculation of posterior wall of fundus (*arrows*).

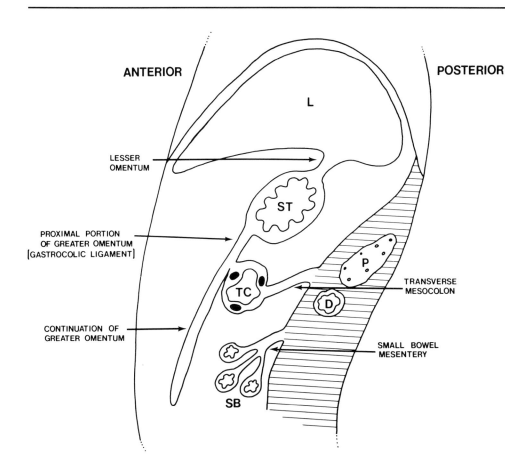

FIGURE 8–44

Sagittal diagram showing mesenteric attachments of stomach, small bowel, and colon. Because proximal portion of greater omentum or gastrocolic ligament inserts along greater curvature of stomach, contiguous spread of tumor from transverse colon or greater omentum primarily affects this region. (From Rubesin, S.E., and Levine, M.S.: Omental cakes: Colonic involvement by omental metastases. Radiology 154:593–596, 1985, with permission.)

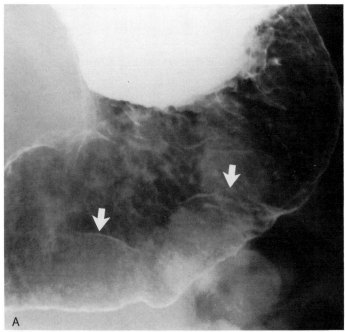

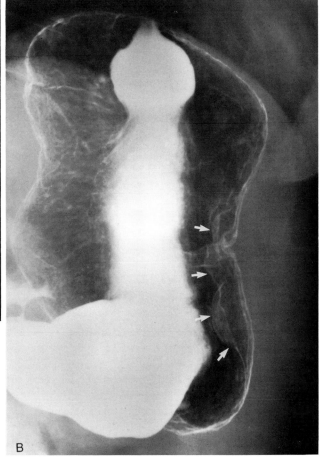

FIGURE 8–45

GASTRIC INVOLVEMENT BY OMENTAL METASTASES FROM OVARIAN CARCINOMA. *A,* Oblique view of stomach shows slight flattening and irregularity of greater curvature due to contiguous spread of tumor from greater omentum. Also note curvilinear defects *(arrows)* caused by extension of tumor anteriorly.

B, Steep oblique view better delineates metastases to anterior gastric wall *(arrows).* (From Rubesin, S.E., et al.: Gastric involvement by omental cakes: Radiographic findings. Gastrointest. Radiol. *11*:223, 1986, with permission.)

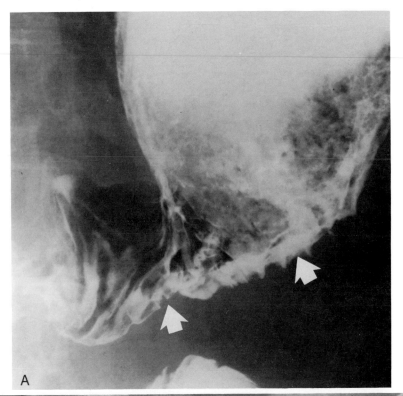

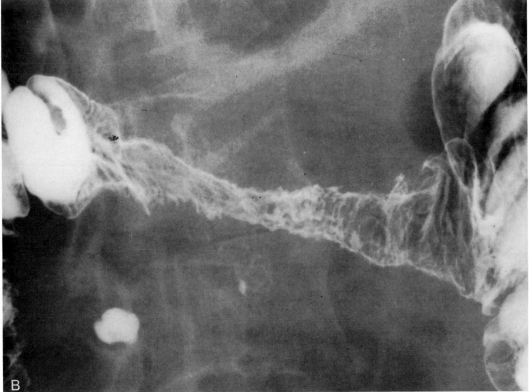

FIGURE 8–46

GASTRIC AND COLONIC INVOLVEMENT BY OMENTAL METASTASES FROM BREAST CARCINOMA. A, Double contrast view of stomach shows tethered, spiculated mucosal folds on greater curvature *(arrows)* due to direct extension of omental tumor.

B, Close-up view from double contrast barium enema shows circumferential narrowing and fixation of transverse colon with severely distorted mucosal folds due to simultaneous colonic involvement by omental tumor. (From Rubesin, S.E., et al.: Gastric involvement by omental cakes: Radiographic findings. Gastrointest. Radiol. *11*:223, 1986, with permission.)

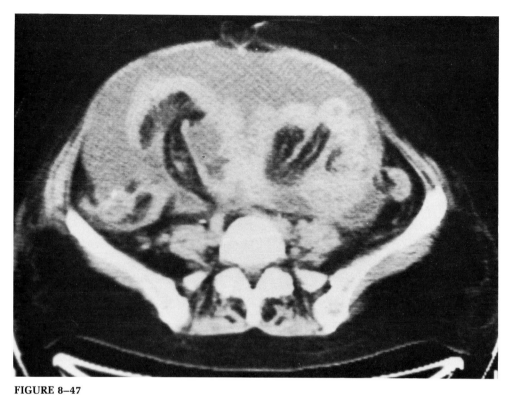

FIGURE 8–47

CT scan showing characteristic appearance of bulky omental metastases or "omental cake" in anterior portion of abdomen.

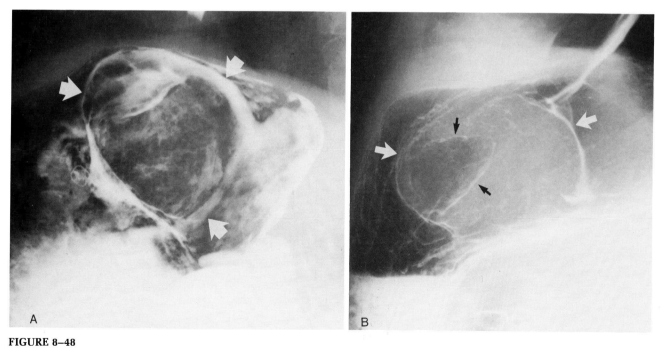

FIGURE 8–48

A and B, Two examples of squamous cell metastases to gastric cardia manifested by giant submucosal masses *(white arrows)* that could be mistaken for leiomyomas or leiomyosarcomas. Note triangular area of ulceration *(black arrows)* in B. (A, From Glick, S.N., et al.: Squamous cell metastases to the gastric cardia. Gastrointest. Radiol. *10*:339, 1985, with permission.)

REFERENCES

1. Gordon, R., Laufer, I., and Kressel, H.Y.: Gastric polyps found on routine double-contrast examination of the stomach. Radiology 134:27, 1980.
2. Feczko, P.J., Halpert, R.D., and Ackerman, L.V.: Gastric polyps: Radiologic evaluation and clinical significance. Radiology 155:581, 1985.
3. Op den Orth, J.O., and Ploem, S.: The stalactite phenomenon on double contrast studies of the stomach. Radiology 117:523, 1975.
4. Aronchick, J., Laufer, I., and Glick, S.N.: Barium stalactites: Observations on their nature and significance. Radiology 149:588, 1983.
5. Ming, S.C., and Goldman, H.: Gastric polyps: A histogenetic classification and its relation to carcinoma. Cancer 18:721, 1965.
6. Tomosulo, J.: Gastric polyps: Histologic types and their relationship to gastric carcinoma. Cancer 27:1346, 1971.
7. Ming, S.-C.: The adenoma-carcinoma sequence in the stomach and colon. II. Malignant potential of gastric polyps. Gastrointest. Radiol. 1:121, 1976.
8. Op den Orth, J.O., and Dekker, W.: Gastric adenomas. Radiology 141:289, 1981.
9. Delikaris, P., Golematis, B., Missitzis, G., et al.: Smooth muscle neoplasms of the stomach. South. Med. J. 76:440, 1983.
10. Hoare, A.M., and Elkington, S.G.: Gastric lesions in generalized neurofibromatosis. Br. J. Surg. 63:449, 1976.
11. Culver, G.J., and Toffolo, R.R.: Criteria for roentgen diagnosis of submucosal gastric lipoma. Radiology 82:254, 1964.
12. Heiken, J.P., Forde, K.A., and Gold, R.P.: Computed tomography as a definitive method for diagnosing gastrointestinal lipomas. Radiology 142:409, 1982.
13. Imoto, T., Nobe, T., Koga, M., et al.: Computed tomography of gastric lipomas. Gastrointest. Radiol. 8:129, 1983.
14. O'Riordan, D., Levine, M.S., and Yeager, B.A.: Complete healing of ulceration within a gastric leiomyoma. Gastrointest. Radiol. 10:47, 1985.
15. Kilman, W.J., and Berk, R.N.: The spectrum of radiographic features of aberrant pancreatic rests involving the stomach. Radiology 123:291, 1977.
16. Thoeni, R.F., and Gedgaudas, R.K.: Ectopic pancreas: Usual and unusual features. Gastrointest. Radiol. 5:37, 1980.
17. Herlinger, H.: The recognition of exogastric tumors: Report of six cases. Br. J. Radiol. 39:25, 1966.
18. Shirakabe, H., Nishizawa, M., Maruyama, M., et al.: Atlas of X-ray Diagnosis of Early Gastric Cancer, pp 1–18. New York, Igaku-Shoin Ltd, 1982.
19. Kaneko, E., Nakamura, T., Umeda, N., et al.: Outcome of gastric carcinoma detected by gastric mass survey in Japan. Gut 18:626, 1977.
20. White, R.M., Levine, M.S., Enterline, H.T., et al.: Early gastric cancer: Recent experience. Radiology 155:25, 1985.
21. Cooley, R.N.: The diagnostic accuracy of upper gastrointestinal radiologic studies. Am. J. Med. Sci. 242:628, 1961.
22. Fierst, S.M.: Carcinoma of the cardia and fundus of the stomach. Am. J. Gastroenterol. 57:403, 1972.
23. Winawer, S.J., Posner, G., Lightdale, C.J., et al.: Endoscopic diagnosis of advanced gastric cancer: Factors influencing yield. Gastroenterology 69:1183, 1975.
24. Levine, M.S., Kong, V., Rubesin, S.E., et al.: Scirrhous carcinoma of the stomach: Radiologic and endoscopic diagnosis. Radiology 175:151, 1990.
25. Balthazar, E.J., Rosenberg, H., and Davidian, M.M.: Scirrhous carcinoma of the pyloric channel and distal antrum. AJR 134:669, 1980.
26. Evans, E., Harris, O., Dickey, D., et al.: Difficulties in the endoscopic diagnosis of gastric and oesophageal cancer. Aust. NZ J. Surg. 55:541, 1985.
27. Freeny, P.C.: Double-contrast gastrography of the fundus and cardia: Normal landmarks and their pathologic changes. AJR 133:481, 1979.
28. Herlinger, H., Grossman, R., Laufer, I., et al.: The gastric cardia in double-contrast study: Its dynamic image. AJR 135:21, 1980.

29. Kobayashi, S., Yamada, A., Kawai, B., et al.: Study on early cancer of the cardiac region: X-ray findings of the surrounding area of the oesophago-gastric junction. Australas. Radiol. 16:258, 1972.
30. Freeny, P.C., and Marks, W.M.: Adenocarcinoma of the gastroesophageal junction: Barium and CT examination. AJR 138:1077, 1982.
31. Levine, M.S., Laufer, I., and Thompson, J.J.: Carcinoma of the gastric cardia in young people. AJR 140:69, 1983.
32. Balthazar, E.J., Goldfine, S., and Davidian, N.M.: Carcinoma of the esophagogastric junction. Am. J. Gastroenterol. 74:237, 1980.
33. Lawson, T.L., and Dodds, W.J.: Infiltrating carcinoma simulating achalasia. Gastrointest. Radiol. 1:245, 1976.
34. Milnes, J.P., Hine, K.R., Holmes, G.K.T., et al.: Limitations of endoscopy in the diagnosis of carcinoma of the cardia of the stomach. Br. J. Radiol. 55:593, 1982.
35. Brady, L.W.: Malignant lymphoma of the gastrointestinal tract. Radiology 137:291, 1980.
36. Menuck, L.S.: Gastric lymphoma: A radiologic diagnosis. Gastrointest. Radiol. 1:157, 1976.
37. Privette, J.T.J., Davies, E.R., and Roylance J: The radiologic features of gastric lymphoma. Clin. Radiol. 28:457, 1977.
38. Zornoza, J., and Dodd, G.D.: Lymphoma of the gastrointestinal tract. Semin. Roentgenol. 15:272, 1980.
39. Fork, F.T., Ekberg, O., and Haglund, U.: Radiology in primary gastric lymphoma. Acta Radiol. Diagn. 25:481, 1984.
40. Lim, F.E., Hartman, A.S., Tan, E.G.C., et al.: Factors in the prognosis of gastric lymphoma. Cancer 39:1715, 1977.
41. Mittal, B., Wasserman, T.H., and Griffith, R.C.: Non-Hodgkin's lymphoma of the stomach. Am. J. Gastroenterol. 78:780, 1983.
42. Cabre-Fiol, V., and Vilardell, F.: Progress in the cytological diagnosis of gastric lymphoma. Cancer 41:1456, 1978.
43. Spinelli, P., Gullo, C.L., and Pizzetti, P.: Endoscopic diagnosis of gastric lymphomas. Endoscopy 12:211, 1980.
44. Fox, E.R., Laufer, I., and Levine, M.S.: Response of gastric lymphoma to chemotherapy: Radiologic appearance. AJR 142:711, 1984.
45. Rosenfelt, F., and Rosenberg, S.A.: Diffuse histiocytic lymphoma presenting with gastrointestinal tract lesions. Cancer 45:2188, 1980.
46. Meyers, M.A., and McSweeney, J.: Secondary neoplasms of the bowel. Radiology 105:1, 1972.
47. Libshitz, H.I., Lindell, M.M., and Dodd, G.D.: Metastases to the hollow viscera. Radiol. Clin. North Am. 20:487, 1982.
48. Goldstein, H.M., Beydoun, M.T., and Dodd, G.D.: Radiologic spectrum of melanoma metastatic to the gastrointestinal tract. AJR 129:605, 1977.
49. Dunnick, R., Harell, G.S., and Parker, B.R.: Multiple bull's eye lesions in gastric lymphoma. AJR 126:965, 1976.
50. Rose, H.S., Balthazar, E.J., Megibow, A.J., et al.: Alimentary tract involvement in Kaposi sarcoma: Radiographic and endoscopic findings in 25 homosexual men. AJR 139:661, 1982.
51. Joffe, N.: Metastatic involvement of the stomach secondary to breast carcinoma. AJR 123:512, 1975.
52. Levine, M.S., Caroline, D., Thompson, J.J., et al.: Adenocarcinoma of the esophagus: Relationship to Barrett mucosa. Radiology 150:305, 1984.
53. Rubesin, S.E., Levine, M.S., and Glick, S.N.: Gastric involvement by omental cakes: Radiographic findings. Gastrointest. Radiol. 11:223, 1986.
54. Bachman, A.L.: Roentgen appearance of gastric invasion from carcinoma of the colon. Radiology 63:814, 1954.
55. Rubesin, S.E., and Levine, M.S.: Omental cakes: Colonic involvement by omental metastases. Radiology 154:593, 1985.
56. Levitt, R.G., Koehler, R.E., Sagel, S.S., et al.: Metastatic disease of the mesentery and omentum. Radiol. Clin. North Am. 20:501, 1982.
57. Glick, S.N., Teplick, S.K., and Levine, M.S.: Squamous cell metastases to the gastric cardia. Gastrointest. Radiol. 10:339, 1985.
58. Glick, S.N., Teplick, S.K., and Levine, M.S.: Gastric cardia metastasis in esophageal carcinoma. Radiology 160:627, 1986.

THE POSTOPERATIVE STOMACH

9

J. Odo Op den Orth, M.D.

INTRODUCTION

A radiologist examining a patient who has had previous gastric surgery should be familiar with the common gastric operations. In order to choose an appropriate examination technique he must know whether a surgical anastomosis has been performed. If there has been no anastomosis, the examination technique is essentially the same as that for the intact stomach. However, if an anastomosis has been made, the technique must be modified to prevent premature loss of contrast material through the anastomosis. It is therefore of utmost importance that the radiologist collect all available information regarding the surgical procedure. He should also review any preceding radiologic studies if these are available. It these data are not obtainable, the examination must be undertaken on the assumption that an anastomosis has been performed.

OPERATIONS WITHOUT ANASTOMOSIS

Examination Technique

The examination technique in patients without amostomosis is essentially the same as the examination in patients with an intact stomach. This has been described in detail.[1, 2] Currently we prefer a barium suspension of medium-high density, approximately 100% w/v, to provide good mucosal coating for double contrast studies and transparency for good compression studies. In cases of suspected leakage, low-osmolality contrast media such as Hexabrix (May and Baker) are indicated for the initial study; they have no adverse effects in clinical practice.[3] If such an initial study demonstrates no evidence of leakage, the examination should in most instances, be continued with a barium suspension that not only provides much better mucosal coating but may also reveal small perforations that are missed with water-soluble contrast media.[4]

Simple Closure

Simple closure of a perforated ulcer may result in a localized filling defect.[5, 6] These filling defects disappear with the passage of time.[6, 7] It has been our experience, as well as that of others,[8] that it is often impossible to differentiate the original ulcer from a simple closure, and even from a recurrent ulcer in the duodenal bulb.

Vagotomy and Pyloroplasty

The common Heineke-Mikulicz pyloroplasty has been performed as a drainage procedure in association with vagotomy. The pyloroplasty consists of a longitudinal incision extending from the antrum across the pylorus. The incision is then closed vertically. This results in a typical deformity, sometimes referred to as the beagle-ear sign (Fig. 9–1).[9, 10]

After vagotomy, peristalsis in the stomach is sluggish, and the appearance of the duodenum is similar to that seen during drug-induced hypotonic duodenography. After highly selective vagotomy, peristalsis in the stomach is virtually normal.[8]

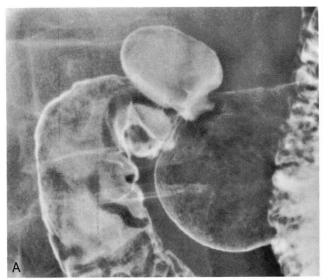
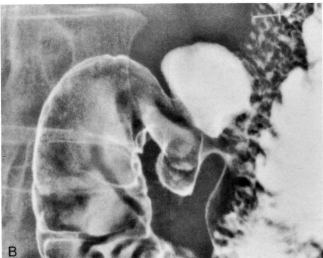

FIGURE 9–1

BEAGLE-EAR SIGN. *A* and *B*, Typical pseudodiverticulum in a patient after a Heineke-Mikulicz pyloroplasty.

Gastropexy and Localized Resections

In an anterior gastropexy, the anterior wall of the stomach is sutured to the anterior abdominal wall. Such an operation produces a characteristic deformity (Fig. 9–2).

Localized resections (wedge resections and segmental resections) result in permanent and often bizarre deformities of the stomach (Fig. 9–3). Post-surgical changes may also be seen in the stomach following cystogastrostomy for drainage of a pancreatic pseudocyst. These appearances may be mistaken for an active peptic ulcer or scarring.[11]

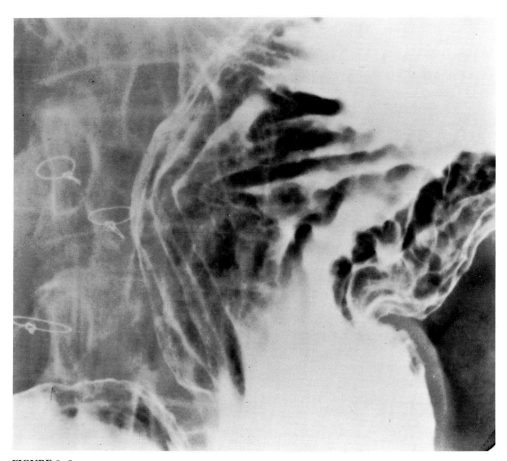

FIGURE 9–2

Angulation of gastric folds after an anterior gastropexy performed to keep a Foley catheter in place after a decompression procedure.

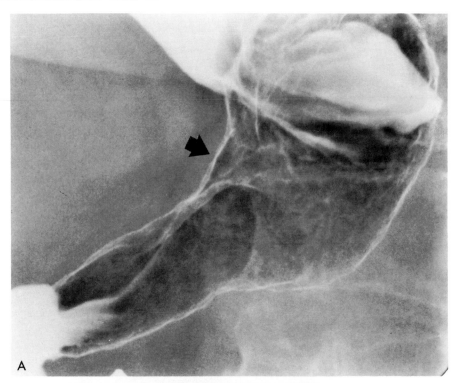

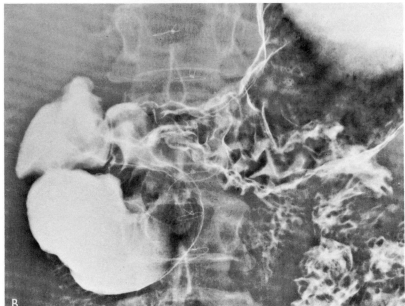

FIGURE 9–3

DEFORMITY DUE TO LOCAL EXCISION. *A,* Deformity of the lesser curvature 2 months after a wedge excision for a small polypoid carcinoma.

B, Bizarre deformity of the stomach 4 years after wedge resection of the lesser curvature for a benign gastric ulcer.

Surgery for Hiatal Hernia and Gastroesophageal Reflux

Numerous surgical techniques have been developed for the treatment of hiatal hernia and gastroesophageal reflux; an extensive review of these techniques and their radiologic aspects has been provided by Hüpscher in his recent monograph.[12]

A Nissen fundoplication[13] is often performed to prevent gastroesophageal reflux and to repair a hiatal hernia. A sleeve of the gastric fundus is wrapped around the distal esophagus and fixed there with plication sutures. On postoperative contrast studies, this produces a typical pseudotumor with variable narrowing of the abdominal esophagus (Fig. 9–4).[14–17] The pseudotumor may diminish or disappear with the passage of time. When neither the pseudotumor nor the narrowing is visualized, one may suspect that the operation has not been successful or that there has been a recurrence.[18] If the fundoplication is too tight a "gas bloat syndrome" may develop, with an inability of the patient to belch or to vomit.

In the Belsey Mark IV fundoplication the hernia is reduced, and the esophagus is sutured to the stomach and the diaphragm. This can result in a small pseudotumor. In addition, two sharp angles in the intraabdominal esophagus can be identified.[15, 19]

In the Angelchik antireflux procedure, a ring-shaped radiopaque prosthesis is placed around the esophagus after reduction of the hernia, usually below the diaphragm.[20] Complications include slipping down of the prosthesis over the stomach and erosion of the prosthesis into the esophagus or the stomach (Fig. 9–5).[20–22]

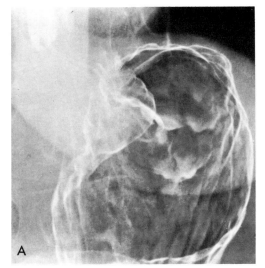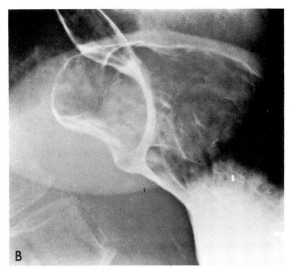

FIGURE 9–4

A and B, Typical pseudotumor and narrowing of the lower esophagus 2 months after a Nissen fundoplication.

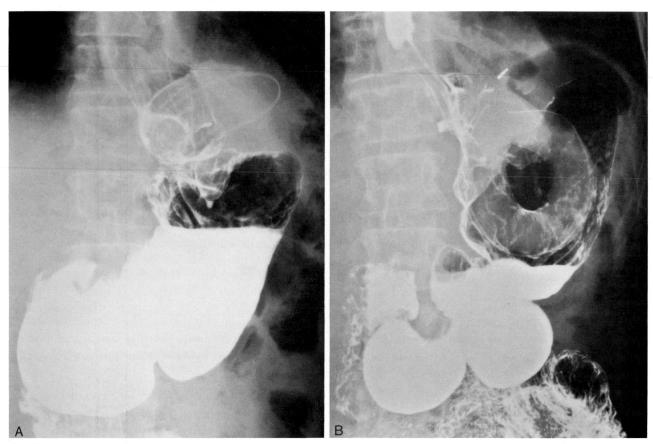

FIGURE 9–5

COMPLICATION OF ANGELCHIK ANTIREFLUX DEVICE. A, Under the left hemidiaphragm an Angelchik prosthesis perpendicular to the course of the esophagus in its normal position.
 B, Six months later the orientation has changed; endoscopy demonstrated partial erosion into the lumen.

Gastroplasty for Morbid Obesity

The radiologic aspects of current surgical procedures for the treatment of morbid obesity have recently been reviewed by Goodman and Halpert.[23]

In gastroplasty a small proximal gastric pouch is created, which communicates only by a narrow channel with the rest of the stomach. Patients who have had gastroplasty are often extremely difficult to examine, and double contrast examination is of limited use. Most authors use a single contrast technique either with a water-soluble contrast medium or a barium suspension.[23–26]

OPERATIONS WITH ANASTOMOSIS

Examination Technique: General Remarks

Drug-induced hypotonia that improves coating and distention of stomach and small bowel is essential to obtain optimal results.[27–30] In our experience an intravenous injection of 0.3 to 0.5 mg of glucagon is most effective. Tilting the table 20 to 30 degrees anti-Trendelenburg (head-up) helps to prevent loss of gas through the anastomosis.

After gastric surgery the fundus is not accessible to compression, just as in patients with an intact stomach. However, the same holds true for the greatest portion of the gastric remnant after distal partial gastrectomy, and for the small bowel segment at the esophagojejunal anastomosis following total gastrectomy. Therefore, double contrast technique is essential for the examination of these segments of the gastrointestinal tract. If an anastomotic leak is suspected, low-osmolality contrast media such as Hexabrix are indicated for the initial study.[3] If such an initial study demonstrates no evidence of leakage, the examination should be continued with a barium suspension.

Gastroenterostomy

Currently, gastroenterostomy is performed only to provide drainage in cases of distal gastric or duodenal obstruction when no other operation is possible. In most cases the obstruction is caused by a malignant lesion, and a side-to-side anastomosis is fashioned between the stomach and a loop of jejunum (Fig. 9–6). The examination technique is basically the same as that described in the following text for partial resection with anastomosis. In addition, mucosal relief films are made with the patient in the prone position.

In elderly patients one often encounters a long-standing gastroenterostomy performed for benign disease. In these patients, marked contraction of the antrum, probably due to antral and pyloric hypertrophy, is sometimes seen (Fig. 9–7).[31, 32] Differentiation of such a benign contraction of the antrum from scirrhous carcinoma is often impossible on a purely radiologic basis, so that gastroscopy and biopsy are frequently necessary. It may also be necessary to differentiate this antral contraction from a small partial distal gastrectomy with side-to-side gastrojejunostomy (Fig. 9–8).

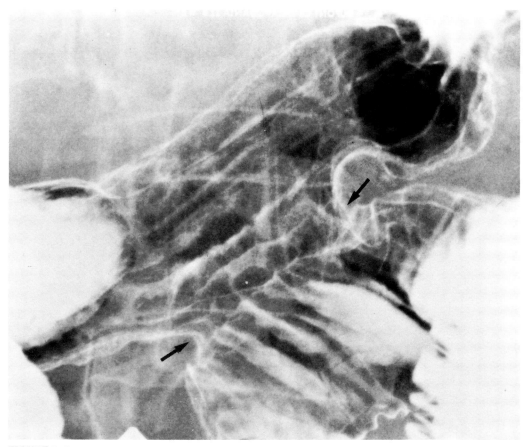

FIGURE 9–6

Typical gastroenterostomy.

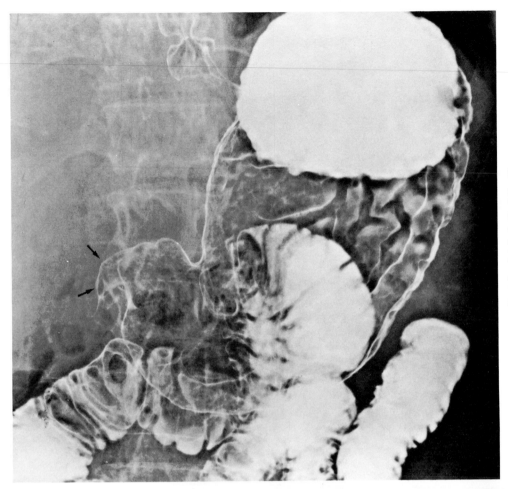

FIGURE 9–7

GASTROENTEROSTOMY WITH ANTRAL CONTRACTION. Double contrast examination in the supine position 42 years after a posterior gastroenterostomy. There is contraction of the antrum (arrows). The autopsy performed shortly after the x-ray examination demonstrated a hypertrophic pylorus.

FIGURE 9–8

BILLROTH II. Small distal partial gastrectomy with a side-to-side gastroenterostomy (patient supine). The configuration of the folds of the distal part of the stomach confirms that a blind pouch (arrows) has been formed. This makes it possible to differentiate between this kind of operation and the condition shown in Figure 9–7. This gastrojejunostomy with side-to-side anastomosis represents the original Billroth II operation.

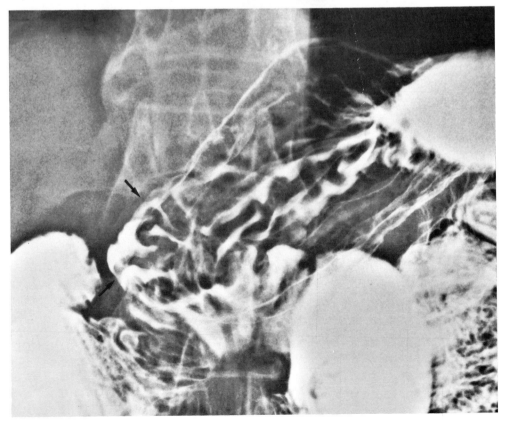

Gastric Bypass for Morbid Obesity

In gastric bypass a small proximal gastric pouch is created, which does not communicate with the rest of the stomach. The proximal pouch is anastomosed with the jejunum. As in gastroplasty, double contrast examination is only of limited use. Often only a single contrast examination either with a water-soluble contrast medium or barium is performed.[23–25, 33]

Partial Resection with Anastomosis

In common usage the eponym "Billroth I" is used to refer to any partial gastrectomy with gastroduodenos-tomy, and the eponym "Billroth II" refers to all varieties of partial gastrectomy with gastrojejunos-tomy.[34]

In a gastroduodenostomy an end-to-end anasto-mosis is generally used. The cut end of the stomach is usually partially oversewn to adapt the size of the gastric opening to the size of the duodenum. The area that is oversewn often produces a persistent deformity or plication defect along the lesser curvature in the preanastomotic area (Fig. 9–9).

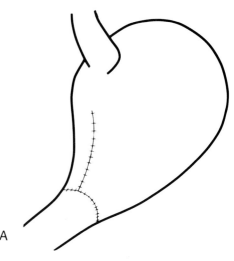

FIGURE 9–9

BILLROTH I. A and B, Typical distal partial gastrectomy and gastroduodenostomy and end-to-end anastomosis (patient supine). Despite complete distension there remains a concave defect on the lesser curvature side of the preanastomotic area (arrow), probably resulting from the surgical procedure to adapt the size of the distal cut end of the stomach to the duodenum. The surgery had been performed 38 years previously.

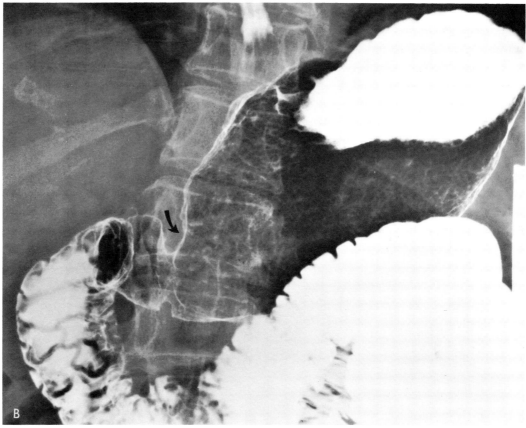

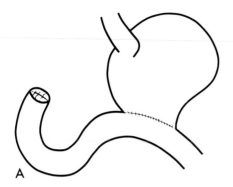

In a gastrojejunostomy the end-to-side anastomosis can be made using the entire cut end of the stomach (Fig. 9–10), or the size of the stomach can be reduced by oversewing part of the cut end (Fig. 9–11). The oversewn area produces a plication defect with this type of anastomosis as well. In the Whipple procedure the head of the pancreas and the duodenum are resected; the rest of the pancreas and the common

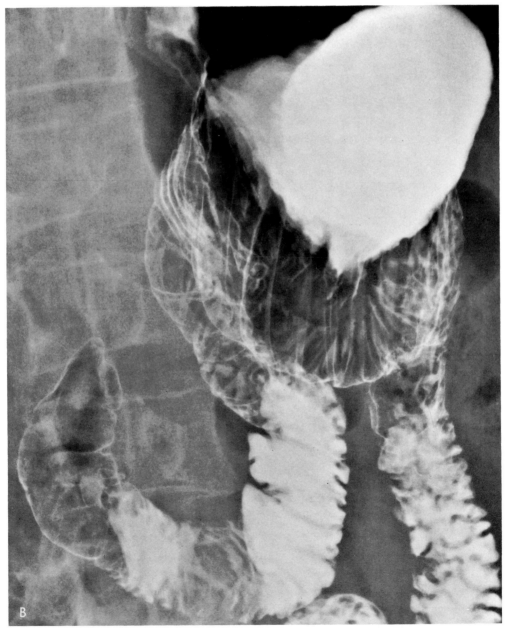

FIGURE 9–10

A and B, Typical distal partial gastrectomy and gastrojejunostomy with an end-to-side anastomosis (patient supine, right side up). The entire cut end of the stomach has been used for the anastomosis.

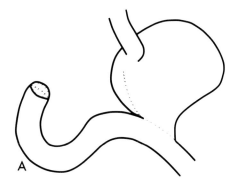

bile duct are connected by end-to-side anastomoses to the jejunum. After a partial distal gastrectomy, an end-to-side gastrojejunostomy is fashioned. During the radiologic examination of a patient after a Whipple procedure, the condition may be mistaken for a simple gastrojejunostomy; examination of the afferent loop, however, usually discloses the end-to-side choledochojejunostomy.

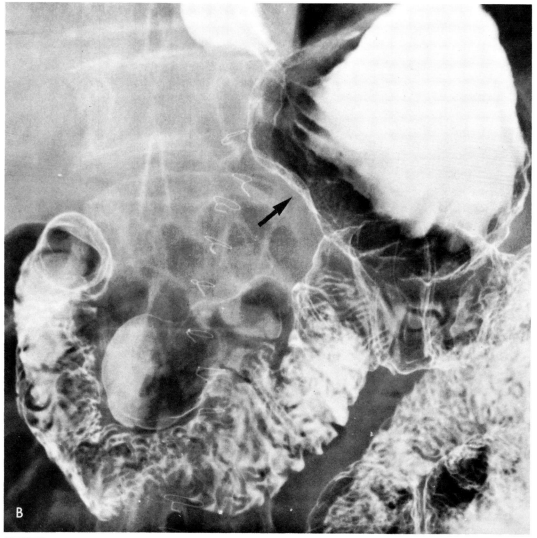

FIGURE 9–11

A and *B*, Typical distal partial gastrectomy and gastrojejunostomy with an end-to-side anastomosis with a restricted stoma formed 18 years before (patient supine). The concave contour of the gastric remnant just above the anastomosis on the lesser curvature side *(arrow)* results from the operative procedure (plication defect). There is a large diverticulum of the duodenum.

Technique

Immediately before the start of the examination, an intravenous injection of 0.3 to 0.5 mg of glucagon is given. This renders the gastric remnant and small bowel hypotonic and prevents rapid spilling of contrast material into the distal small bowel.

Adequate gaseous distention of the gastric remnant and anastomotic loops of small bowel is clearly an important component of this examination. Although satisfactory results can be obtained with the use of effervescent pellets, granules, or powders, we prefer the "bubbly barium" method. This consists of a carbonated barium suspension cocktail that is mixed in a 2-liter soda siphon. It is prepared by slowly adding 2 cartridges of carbon dioxide to 2 liters of refrigerated barium suspension. The "bubbly barium" thus prepared dissociates in 90 seconds to produce 1 part of

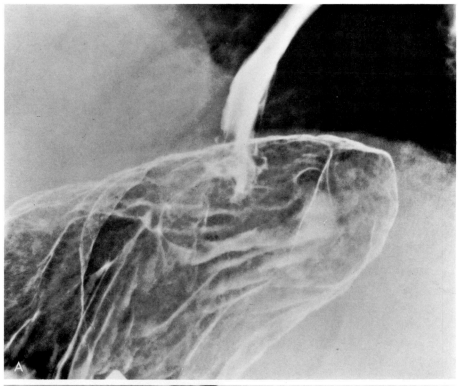

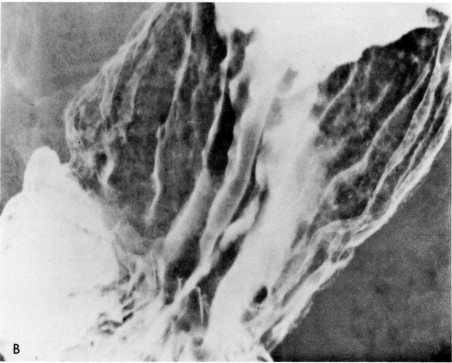

FIGURE 9–12

DOUBLE CONTRAST VIEWS OF THE GASTRIC REMNANT. A, Patient supine, left side up. Table 20 to 30 degrees anti-Trendelenburg.

B, Patient supine. Table 20 degrees anti-Trendelenburg.

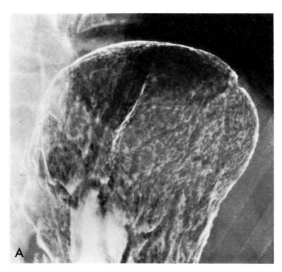
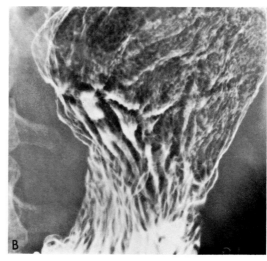

FIGURE 9–13

DOUBLE CONTRAST STUDIES OF THE GASTRIC REMNANT IN ANOTHER PATIENT. Note the surface pattern or areae gastricae. At endoscopy the appearance of the fundal mucosa was considered to be normal. *A*, Patient supine, left side up. Table 20 to 30 degrees anti-Trendelenburg.

B, Patient supine. Table 20 degrees anti-Trendelenburg.

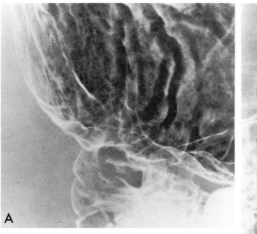
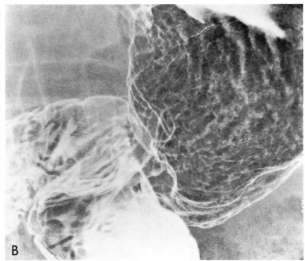

FIGURE 9–14

A and *B*, Detailed double contrast studies of the preanastomotic area in two different patients with a gastrojejunostomy (patient supine, table only slightly anti-Trendelenburg). Note the areae gastricae.

barium suspension and 2 parts of carbon dioxide.[1, 2, 35, 36]

A barium suspension of moderately high density is preferred to allow for good double contrast films (80 to 90 kV with rare earth intensifying screens) as well as for transparency on single contrast compression studies (120 to 150 kV).[1] With such a barium suspension (approximately 100% w/v), compression studies of the stomal area and the anastomotic loops of small bowel are made. The patient is placed first in the supine and semi-erect positions, and a Holzknecht spoon is used for compression. The patient is then put in the prone position, and an inflatable paddle is inserted between the patient's body and the table for compression. The patient then swallows additional barium and an effervescent agent and is placed supine, with the head of the table elevated 20 to 30 degrees. If the initial coating is inadequate we currently use a high-density (250% w/v) barium suspension (E-Z-HD, E-Z-Em Co, Westbury, NY) after the compression studies have been made.

To achieve good mucosal coating the patient rolls to and fro between the right and left decubitus positions, and double contrast films of the gastric pouch and preanastomotic area are made (Figs. 9–12 to 9–14). To obtain double contrast views of the stomal area following a Billroth II resection, it is necessary to lower the table to a nearly horizontal position (Fig. 9–15). Careful fluoroscopic control is needed to prevent loss of gas through the anastomosis. The stomal area in a Billroth I resection is easily visualized in a nearly horizontal position with the patient supine and the right side elevated. Double contrast views of the pseudobulb are similar to those of the unoperated duodenal bulb (Fig. 9–16).

The head of the table is again elevated 20 to 30 degrees. The patient lies on the right side and drinks additional barium, and, if necessary, additional effervescent agent. Frequently the barium flows spontaneously into the afferent loop to the top of the duodenum. If this does not happen, the Valsalva maneuver or coughing may be of great help. As soon as barium is seen to enter the duodenum the patient is quickly turned to the supine position with the right side up to allow gas to enter the duodenum. To provide good mucosal coating in the duodenum, the patient is rotated approximately 135 degrees between the supine LPO position to the prone position (Fig. 9–17).[35] When good coating has been obtained, films of the duodenum are made with the patient in the supine position, right side elevated and prone (Fig. 9–18). Thereafter, large-size survey films are made with the patient in the supine and erect (frontal and lateral) positions (Fig. 9–19).

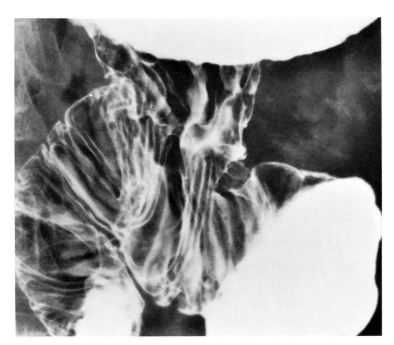

FIGURE 9–15

Detailed double contrast study of an end-to-side gastrojejunostomy (patient supine, table horizontal).

FIGURE 9–16

Detailed double contrast study of an end-to-end gastroduodenostomy (patient supine, right side slightly elevated). A pseudobulb has been formed; the transversely orientated Kerckring folds facilitate differentiation from a normal duodenal bulb.

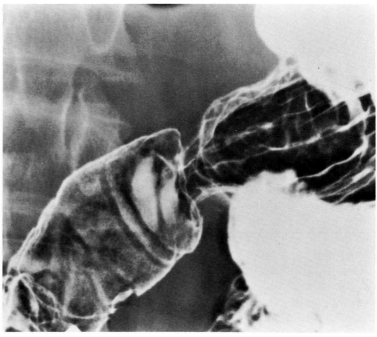

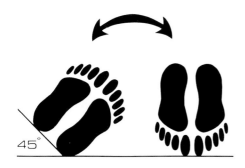

FIGURE 9–17

This schema indicates the movement that must be performed to obtain good mucosal coating of the duodenum. Owing to the dorsal position of the duodenum, there is no risk of losing gas when the movements of the patient remain between the indicated limits.

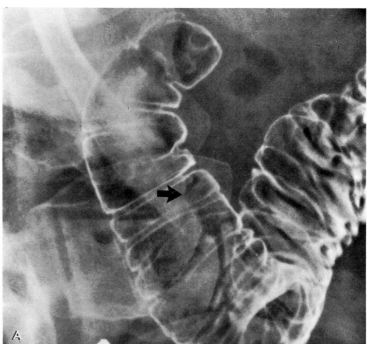

FIGURE 9–18

THE AFFERENT LOOP. Note the inverted stump at the top of the duodenum. The major papilla is well visualized in A (arrow) (patient supine, right side up). The major papilla can also be identified in the prone position in B (large arrow). The minor papilla (small arrow) can generally be visualized only in the prone position because it is a shallow protrusion which usually has gently sloping edges and is situated on the anterior wall of the descending duodenum.[81] The minor papilla lies cephaloventral of the major papilla, the mean distance 18 to 20 mm.[82, 83]

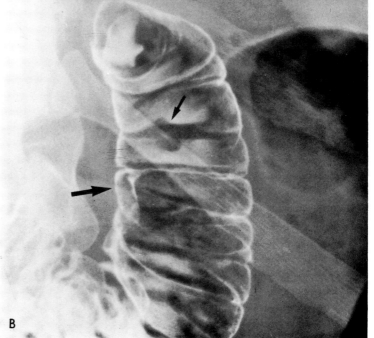

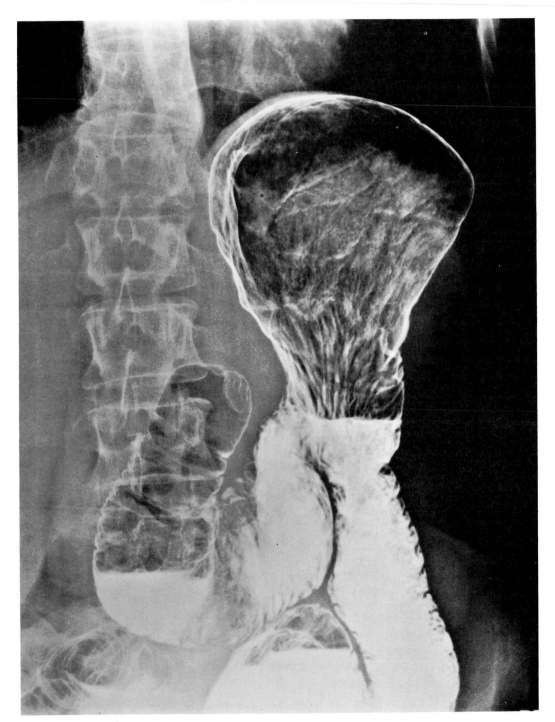

FIGURE 9–19

Survey film after a distal partial gastrectomy and a right-to-left, end-to-side gastrojejunostomy (patient erect). Note the inverted stump at the top of the duodenum.

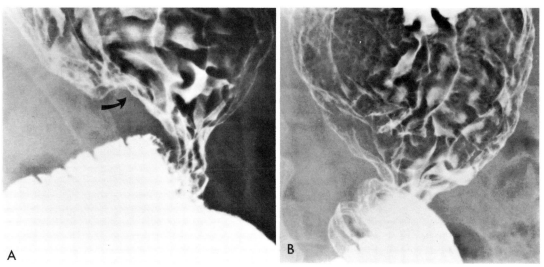

FIGURE 9–20

A, Profile view of the lesser curvature 11 years after a distal partial gastrectomy with an end-to-side gastrojejunostomy: filling defect on the lesser curvature side of the preanastomotic area *(arrow).*

   B, Same patient, face-on view. Gastroscopy and biopsy proved that this was a plication defect.

Plication Defects and Other Pseudolesions

In both the Billroth I and the Billroth II resections, a portion of the cut end of the stomach may be oversewn and inverted to restrict the size of the stoma. These produce typical deformities or plication defects (Figs. 9–9, 9–11, 9–20).[37–39] In the differential diagnosis of such defects, foreign body granuloma must also be considered (Fig. 9–28).[40, 41] Typical defects due to an inverted stump with or without a foreign body granuloma also occur in the stump of the duodenum after a Billroth II operation (Figs. 9–18, 9–19, 9–21).

At any place where sutures have been placed, distortion of the mucosal relief may occur, causing crater-like patterns (pseudoulcers) that cannot be distinguished from true ulcers on a radiologic basis (Fig. 9–27). Mass-like lesions may be encountered following removal of a surgical gastrostomy tube.[42]

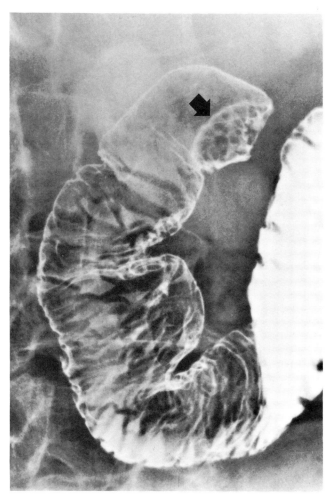

FIGURE 9–21

Afferent loop 6 years after a distal partial gastrectomy with gastrojejunostomy (patient supine, right side up). Large filling defect at the top of the duodenum *(arrow)* caused by a plication defect or a foreign body granuloma.

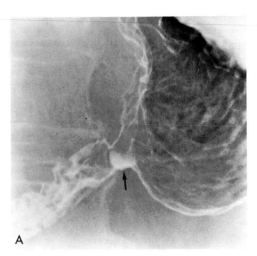
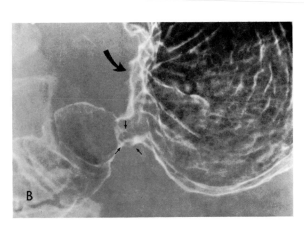

FIGURE 9–22

STOMAL ULCER. *A,* Ulcer niche at the stoma *(arrow),* endoscopically confirmed 12 years after distal partial gastrectomy with end-to-end duodenostomy.

B, The niche is visible only as a ring shadow *(small arrows)* after the barium flows out of the niche. Note the large plication defect on the lesser curvature side of the preanastomotic area *(curved arrow).*

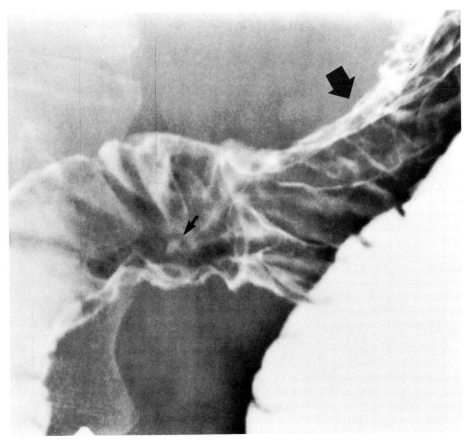

FIGURE 9–23

DUODENAL ULCER. Niche in the pseudobulb *(small arrow)* 29 years after a distal partial gastrectomy with end-to-end gastroduodenostomy. Note the large plication defect on the lesser curvature side of the preanastomotic area *(large arrow).* Several weeks after the radiologic examination endoscopy showed inflammation and the remnant of an ulcer niche.

Postoperative Ulcer

Postoperative ulcers occur more frequently after an operation for duodenal ulcer than for gastric ulcer. In the case of gastrojejunostomy the small bowel just distal to the anastomosis is the site of predilection. The efferent loop is affected more frequently than the afferent loop. Ulceration may also occur in the anastomotic ring. In a gastroduodenostomy the anastomotic ring is affected most commonly, but localiza-tion in the pre- and postanastomotic area also occurs. A recurrent ulcer in the rest of the gastric remnant is rare in gastrojejunostomy and in gastroduodenostomy.[43, 44]

Just as in the nonoperated stomach, the radiologic diagnosis of such ulcers depends upon the demonstration of an ulcer niche (Figs. 9–22 and 9–23). Both the double contrast and the positive contrast compression studies should be used (Figs. 9–24 and 9–25). An ulcer crater in a gastric remnant discovered many years after an operation for a benign condition

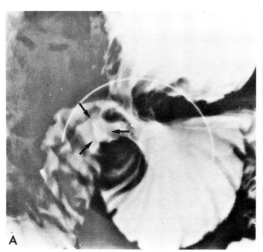
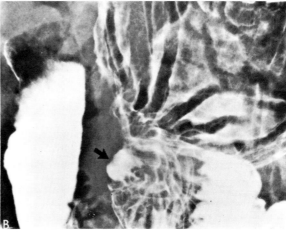

FIGURE 9–24

A and *B*, Jejunal ulcer. Endoscopically confirmed jejunal ulcer 9 years after distal partial gastrectomy with end-to-side gastrojejunostomy. The ulcer is demonstrated by both the complete filling/compression technique (*A, arrows*) and the double contrast technique (*B, arrow*).

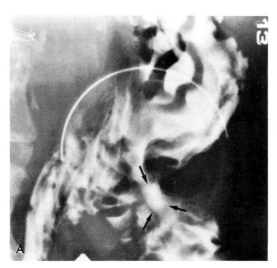
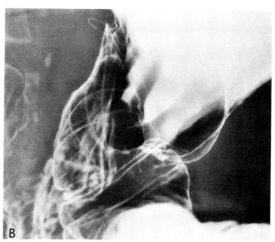

FIGURE 9–25

JEJUNAL ULCER SHOWN ONLY BY COMPRESSION. *A,* Jejunal ulcer (*arrows*) in the efferent loop 3 years after a distal partial gastrectomy with end-to-side gastrojejunostomy.

B, The double contrast technique failed to demonstrate the ulcer.

may be benign but should be considered potentially malignant (Fig. 9–26).

In the preanastomotic area, pseudolesions resembling an ulcer may be caused by barium trapped between distorted gastric folds. Only the endoscopist can decide whether there is intact mucosa at the base of such a crater-like lesion (Fig. 9–27).

A review of the literature regarding the accuracy of radiologic diagnosis of marginal ulcer shows percentages of correct positive diagnosis ranging from 28% to 40%.[45–49] In our experience, for demonstrating a *small* marginal ulcer situated in the jejunum, fiberendoscopy is superior to radiology.[50]

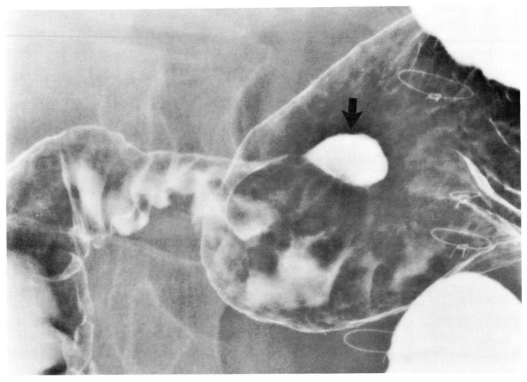

FIGURE 9–26

GASTRIC ULCER. Large ulcer crater (*arrow*) on the posterior wall (patient supine) of a gastric remnant 28 years after a small distal partial gastrectomy with end-to-end gastroduodenostomy for hypertrophic pyloric stenosis. Because the swollen folds end fairly far from the crater and because of the long postoperative interval, this ulcer was considered to be malignant. However, acid production was demonstrated, and at endoscopy the ulcer looked benign. This was confirmed by multiple biopsies.

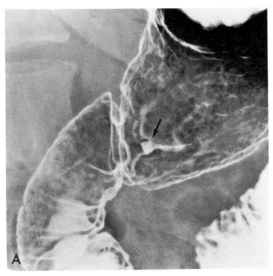 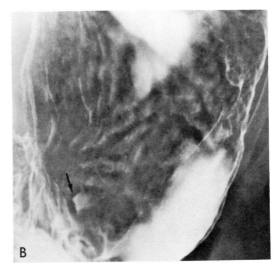

FIGURE 9–27

PSEUDOULCERS. *A*, A collection of barium in the preanastomotic area of a gastric remnant (*arrow*) 4 years after a distal partial gastrectomy with end-to-end gastroduodenostomy. Gastroscopy showed an intact epithelium. The crater-like pattern is caused by barium trapped between gastric folds.

B, A crater-like collection (*arrows*) 16 years after a distal partial gastrectomy with end-to-side gastrojejunostomy. Endoscopy demonstrated a configuration of folds which accounted for the radiologic finding. The epithelium at the base of the crater-like lesion was intact.

Carcinoma

The radiologic diagnosis of carcinoma involving the gastric remnant encompasses two distinct conditions. Secondary postgastrectomy carcinoma or recurrent carcinoma refers to those patients who have had surgery for a primary gastric carcinoma. Primary postgastrectomy or gastric stump carcinoma refers to a carcinoma arising in the gastric remnant of a patient in whom the original surgery was for a lesion other than carcinoma. In both cases the detection of carcinoma is difficult, because of the surgical deformity and because the absence of the pylorus makes it difficult to retain contrast in the gastric remnant.

The diagnosis of secondary postgastrectomy carcinoma (recurrent cancer) can be extremely difficult,[51] especially shortly after the operative procedure (Fig. 9–28). An early postoperative baseline study is of great help for comparison with later studies.

Primary postgastrectomy carcinoma or gastric stump carcinoma is often defined as a primary cancer of the gastric remnant arising at least 5 years after a partial gastrectomy in which there was no evidence of malignant disease in the resected portion of the stomach.[52] The incidence seems to be much higher in Europe than in the United States.[52, 53] Stalsberg and Taksdal[54] in Norway studied the frequency of gastric cancer at necropsy after previous gastric surgery (Billroth II resection and gastroenterostomy). Patients who had had their operation less than 15 years prior to death had a lower incidence of gastric carcinoma than matched unoperated controls. However, patients with operations 25 years or more prior to death had a sixfold increase in gastric carcinoma. There was no evidence of a difference in this respect between patients operated on for gastric ulcer and patients operated on for duodenal ulcer, or between partial gastrectomy with gastrojejunostomy and gastrojejunostomy alone. A Swiss study by Clémençon and associates[55] reports 21 cases of primary gastric stump carcinoma among 326 patients with a Billroth II resection for benign lesions. The incidence of stump carcinoma after 10 years was 15.1% and after 20 years was 21.43%. These authors advise that gastric resection for benign disease should be avoided whenever

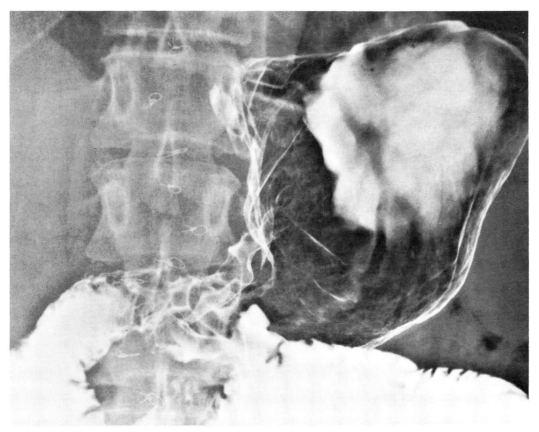

FIGURE 9–28

INFLAMMATION SIMULATING CARCINOMA. Distorted lesser curvature 1 year after distal partial gastrectomy with end-to-end gastroduodenostomy for carcinoma (early gastric cancer). It is often impossible to exclude secondary postgastrectomy carcinoma (recurrent cancer) on radiologic grounds. The patient refused endoscopy. Shortly after the radiologic examination the patient died. Autopsy showed a large plication defect, swollen folds, gastritis and perigastritis, and persistent sutures with no recurrent carcinoma.

possible. An annual endoscopic examination is recommended starting 10 years after the resection. Terjesen and Erichsen[56] in Norway advise that gastric resection be avoided in young patients. They recommend a regular follow-up, thorough x-ray examinations, and gastroscopy starting after a postoperative interval of 15 years.

Opinions on the accuracy of the radiologic examination vary greatly,[52, 56–60] although good results were reported by Saegesser and Jämes.[58] In our experience a hypotonic double contrast examination is a very reliable screening method for the detection of potentially malignant lesions of the operated stomach to determine which patients should be subjected to biopsy (Figs. 9–29 to 9–31). Positive contrast studies of the gastric stump beneath the thoracic cage are of limited value because compression is impossible. However, compression studies of the anastomotic region may offer essential information and should be obtained whenever possible (Fig. 9–32).

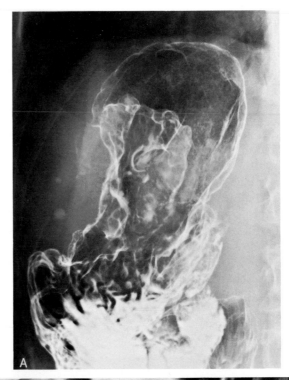

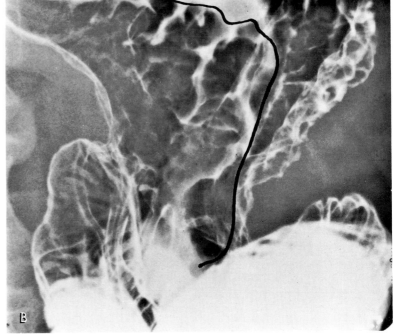

FIGURE 9–29

PRIMARY GASTRIC CARCINOMA FOLLOWING BILLROTH II RESECTION. *A,* Irregular filling defect on the lesser curvature side (prone film) 52 years after a distal partial gastrectomy with end-to-side anastomosis. Gastric biopsy showed adenocarcinoma.

B, Another patient, 30 years after a distal partial gastrectomy with end-to-side gastrojejunostomy. Distortion of folds and nodularity in the preanastomotic area raised the radiologic suspicion of primary postgastrectomy carcinoma which was confirmed by gastrobiopsy.

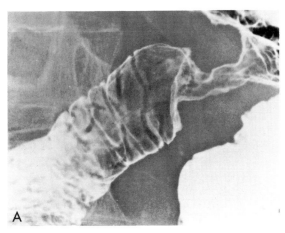
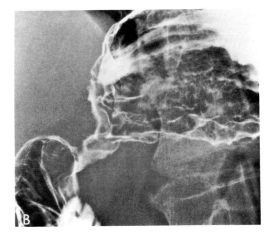

FIGURE 9–30

A and *B*, Gastric stump carcinoma following Billroth I resection. Irregular stricture of the anastomotic area 30 years after a distal partial gastrectomy with end-to-end gastroduodenostomy. The radiologic diagnosis of primary postgastrectomy carcinoma was confirmed by gastroscopy and biopsy.

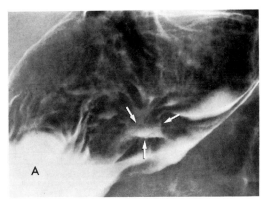
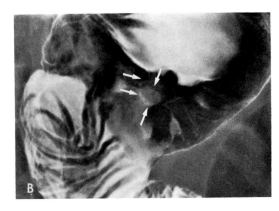

FIGURE 9–31

ULCERATED STUMP CARCINOMA. *A* and *B*, Crater *(arrows)* with converging thickened folds on the posterior wall (patient supine) of the gastric remnant 30 years after a distal partial gastrectomy with end-to-side gastrojejunostomy. Gastroscopy and biopsy showed an adenocarcinoma.

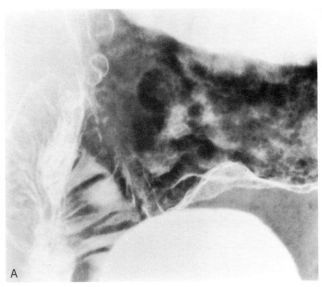
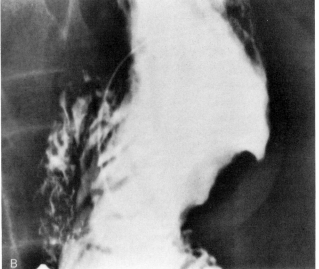

FIGURE 9–32

PRIMARY GASTRIC CARCINOMA FOLLOWING BILLROTH II RESECTION. *A*, On the lesser curvature side just above the anastomosis, there are small polyps. On the greater curvature side just above the anastomosis there is a smoothly demarcated filling defect.

   B, The positive contrast graded compression study of the same patient facilitates the diagnosis of a malignant tumor. At earlier postoperative examinations of this patient, who had been operated on more than 10 years before for a benign condition, no abnormalities had been demonstrated. Gastric biopsy showed adenocarcinoma.

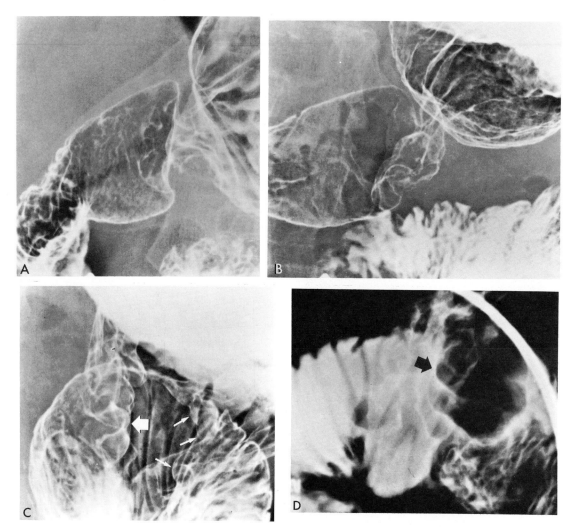

FIGURE 9–33

PROLAPSE OF GASTRIC MUCOSA INTO THE DUODENUM. *A,* Fifteen years after a distal partial gastrectomy with end-to-end gastroduodenostomy. The patient complained of intermittent obstruction. On several occasions gastric retention was found. During the radiologic examination the passage of contrast material through the gastroduodenostomy was unusually slow for such an operation. Gastroduodenal prolapse is obvious.

B, Eighteen years after a distal partial gastrectomy with end-to-end gastroduodenostomy. There is a mass on the greater curvature side of the anastomosis and in the pseudobulb. Gastroscopy and biopsy showed that the mass was caused by prolapsed gastric mucosa.

C, Gastrojejunal prolapse 30 years after a distal partial gastrectomy with an end-to-side gastrojejunostomy. Double contrast study, patient supine. There is a mass on the lesser curvature side *(large arrow)* and several smaller masses on the greater curvature side of the anastomosis *(small arrows).*

D, Positive contrast compression study, patient prone. Note the transparency due to the medium high density barium suspension. Gastroscopy and biopsy showed prolapse of gastric mucosa into the jejunum.

Mucosal Prolapse and Intussusception

Gastrojejunal or gastroduodenal mucosal prolapse is a relatively rare condition.[61-64] Its incidence seems to be greater after a restricted stoma has been fashioned. In a series of 24 cases described by Seaman[64] the median time between the initial surgery and the detection of the prolapse was 6 years. It is not an acute condition; bleeding is the most common clinical manifestation, and partial obstruction may occur. In some cases, awareness of this condition is sufficient for the radiologic diagnosis (Fig. 9-33A and B). When there is an extensive mass, gastric biopsy may be needed to exclude a malignant lesion (Fig. 9-33C and D).

True gastrojejunal intussusceptions are seldom found.[65] Jejunogastric intussusceptions occur more frequently (Fig. 9-34).[66-71] The acute form is a potentially lethal condition because of the risk of incarceration. The radiologic diagnosis depends upon the identification of a striated filling defect, representing a part of the small bowel in the gastric remnant.

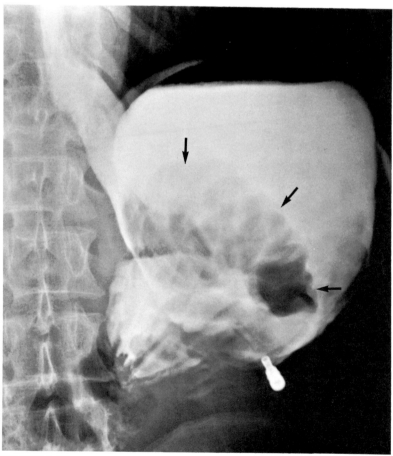

FIGURE 9-34

RETROGRADE JEJUNOGASTRIC INTUSSUSCEPTION. Three years following the Billroth II resection, there was sudden onset of abdominal cramps and vomiting. The x-ray study shows obstruction of the gastric remnant owing to retrograde jejunogastric intussusception (arrows). The diagnosis was confirmed at laparotomy. (Courtesy of Professor E. Ponette, University Hospital, Leuven, Belgium.)

Afferent Loop

With hypotonic technique the afferent loop can be examined much more easily than ever before.[35] Apart from the pathology that is found in hypotonic duodenography (Figs. 9–35 and 9–36), the relationship between the gastric remnant and the anastomosed loop can be studied very easily. According to Burhenne,[72] an iatrogenic afferent loop syndrome can occur if the afferent loop has been attached to the greater curvature instead of to the lesser curvature. Such a left-to-right anastomosis can, particularly when an oblique plane of anastomosis exists, result in preferential filling of the afferent loop, which might cause symptoms (Fig. 9–37). There is, however, sometimes a striking discrepancy between the radiologic findings and the absence of complaints (Fig. 9–38).

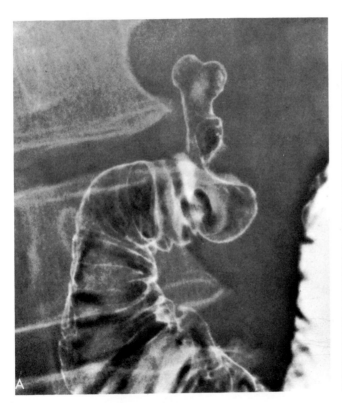

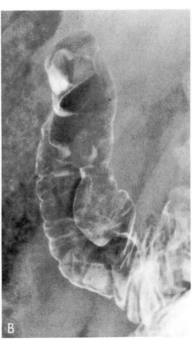

FIGURE 9–35

SCARRED DUODENAL BULB. A, Hypotonic duodenogram of the afferent loop after a distal partial gastrectomy with gastrojejunostomy (patient supine, right side up) showing an irregular configuration of the proximal part of the duodenum. Probably the remnants of the deformed duodenal bulb; confirmation by duodenoscopy.

B, Extramucosal mass. Hypotonic duodenogram of the afferent loop, 35 years after a distal partial gastrectomy with gastrojejunostomy (patient supine, right side up). Smooth-surfaced indentation along the inner aspect of the descending duodenum. Duodenoscopy showed an extramucosal indentation.

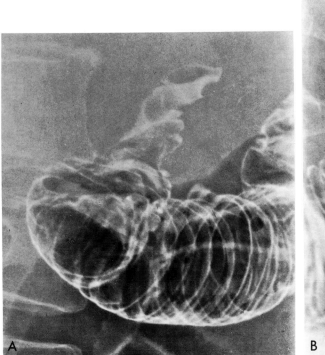
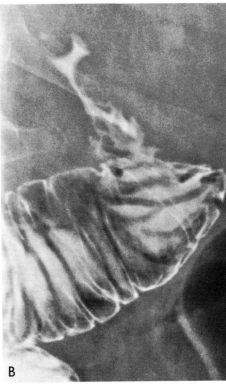

FIGURE 9–36

DUODENAL INVOLVEMENT BY CHOLECYSTITIS. Hypotonic duodenogram in a patient with a distal partial gastrectomy and gastrojejunostomy with clinical features of cholecystitis. A, Supine, right side up.
   B, Prone position. Compression of the duodenum by pericholecystitis caused by a perforation of the gallbladder.

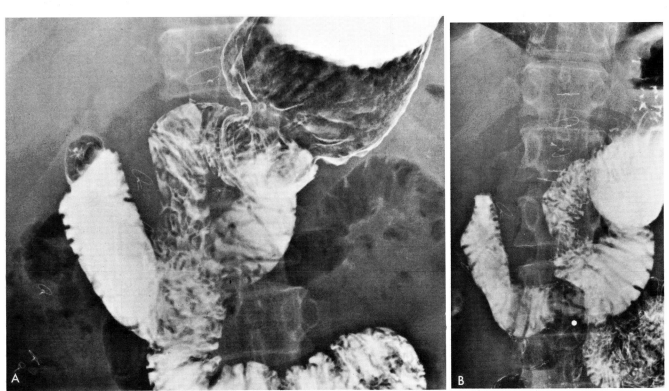

FIGURE 9–37

AFFERENT LOOP SYNDROME. A, Distal partial gastrectomy with end-to-side gastrojejunostomy. There is a left-to-right anastomosis resulting in preferential filling of the afferent loop. Following the operation the patient complained of nausea and vomiting after meals.
   B, Follow-up film after 90 minutes showed hyperperistalsis of the afferent loop, which was still filled with barium. An example of an iatrogenic afferent loop syndrome.

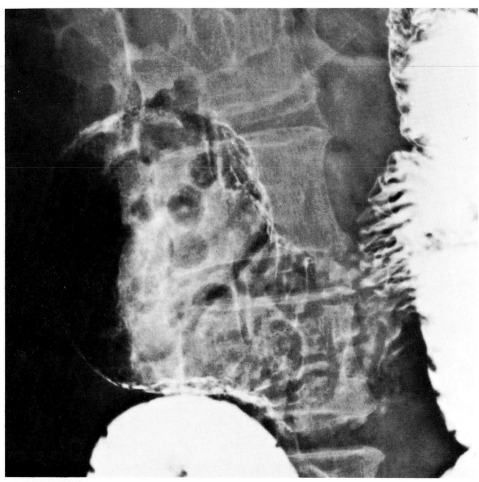

FIGURE 9–38

Afferent loop obstruction 19 years after a distal partial gastrectomy with gastrojejunostomy. Patient supine, right side up. There is huge dilatation of the afferent loop with dilution of the barium suspension and residual food (green peas). The patient denied any complaints.

Retained Antrum

In the top of the afferent duodenal loop after a Billroth II resection, typical defects are observed. They are caused by the inverted stump with or without postoperative edema or foreign body granuloma (see Figs. 9–18, 9–19, 9–21). Although these defects are usually of no clinical importance, they are useful for the radiologist to demonstrate that he has really filled a closed duodenal stump, which is mandatory if a retained antrum has to be excluded. In this condition there is surgical retention of the gastric antrum with a high incidence of recurrent ulcers.[73–75] The diagnosis is suspected when a complete duodenal bulb is seen without a filling defect caused by an inverted stump. Then the examination should be continued and every effort should be made to see whether there is reflux from the duodenum by way of the pylorus into the gastric antrum (Fig. 9–39).

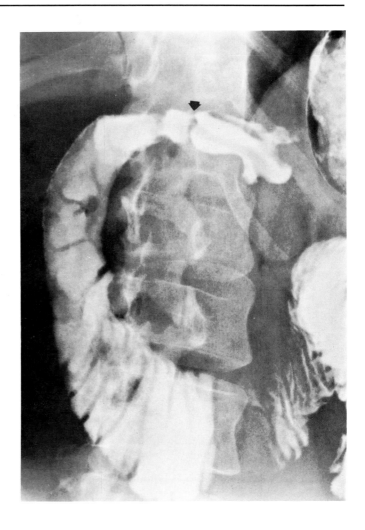

FIGURE 9–39

RETAINED GASTRIC ANTRUM. During examination of the afferent loop of a patient with recurrent marginal ulceration after a Billroth II resection, there is reflux of contrast material through the pylorus (arrow) into a retained gastric antrum. Note the gastric folds characteristic of a retained antrum.

FIGURE 9–40

Forty years after a distal partial gastrectomy with end-to-side gastrojejunostomy. Small polypoid lesions (arrows) on the greater curvature side of the preanastomotic area. Gastroscopy and biopsy showed that they were benign.

Limitations of Radiologic Examination

Because of the many surgical procedures and their variations, it is not possible to describe the normal stomach after partial distal gastrectomy. Examples of plication defects and other pseudolesions have been given in this chapter (see Figs. 9–20, 9–21, and 9–27). Furthermore, acute and chronic inflammatory changes of the mucosa of the gastric remnant due to bile reflux frequently complicate the picture.[76, 77] Benign polypoid lesions, the significance of which is uncertain, are often found in the stomal area after gastrojejunostomy (Fig. 9–40).[78, 79] Glick and colleagues have reported the development of large hyperplastic polyps in the gastric remnant following Billroth II gastrectomy.[80] These lesions can be distinguished from carcinoma only by endoscopic biopsy. Figures 9–41 to 9–43 illustrate the limitations of the radiologic examination, the need for baseline studies, and in many instances the need for endoscopy with multiple biopsies.

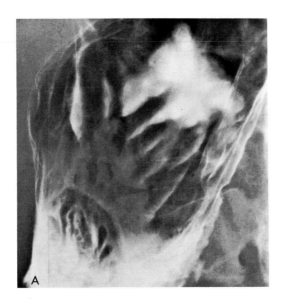

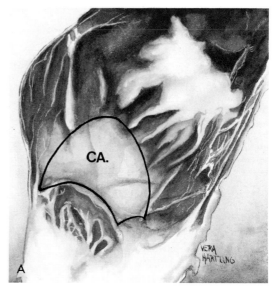

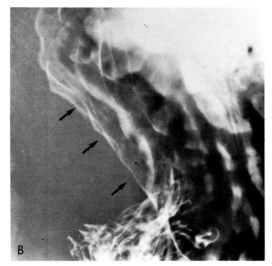

FIGURE 9–41

EARLY CANCER OF THE GASTRIC REMNANT. *A,* Radiograph and artist's representation of a face-on view of the lesser curvature of the gastric remnant 9 years after a distal partial gastrectomy with gastrojejunostomy. The mucosal folds are interrupted by an area of flattened mucosa.

B, Same patient, profile view. Unusual appearance on the lesser curvature side of the preanastomotic area *(arrows)*. Radiologic diagnosis indeterminate; no baseline studies. Gastroscopy and biopsy: adenocarcinoma. Resected specimen: carcinoma restricted to the mucosa (i.e., early cancer of the gastric remnant).

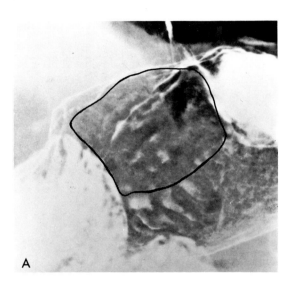
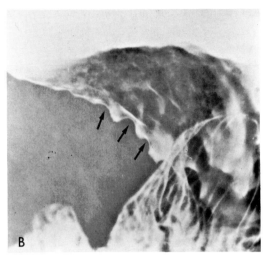

FIGURE 9–42

GASTRITIS. *A*, Face-on view of the lesser curvature of a gastric remnant 25 years after a distal partial gastrectomy with gastrojejunostomy.

B, Same patient, profile view. Swollen irregular folds on the lesser curvature side. No radiologic diagnosis. Gastroscopy: swollen folds. Gastroscopy and biopsy: inflammatory changes.

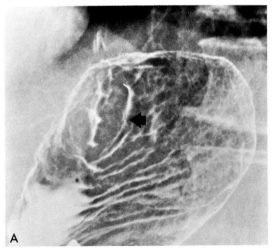
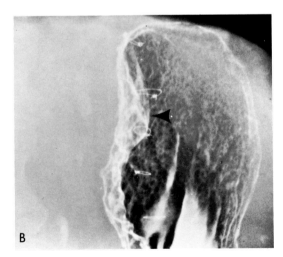

FIGURE 9–43

PLICATION DEFECT SIMULATING CARCINOMA. *A*, Face-on view of the gastric remnant 17 years after a distal partial gastrectomy.

B, Same patient, profile view. Large filling defect on the lesser curvature side, suggestive of carcinoma. In this case, however, postoperative baseline and follow-up studies were available and demonstrated that the lesion had not changed over many years. A malignant lesion was therefore excluded.

Total Gastrectomy

A detailed description of the large number of operative techniques used to restore continuity in the digestive tract after total gastrectomy is beyond the scope of this chapter. We feel, however, that the hypotonic double contrast technique is of help in the visualization of the postoperative result, as shown in Figure 9–44.

CONCLUSION

An optimal hypotonic double contrast study, complemented with a positive contrast compression study of those parts of the gastric stump and small bowel that allow effective compression, prove or exclude most instances of ulceration and neoplasm. As in nonoperated patients, an initial radiologic examina-

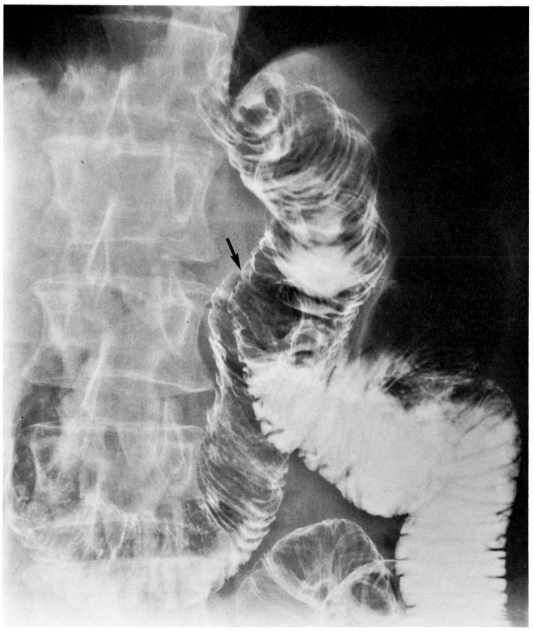

FIGURE 9–44

Esophagojejunostomy 12 days after a total gastrectomy. The hypotonic examination clearly demonstrates the end-to-side jejunojejunal (Roux-en-y) anastomosis (arrow).

tion may therefore serve as a screening method to determine whether endoscopy is necessary. However, in operated patients endoscopy is indicated in a higher percentage than in nonoperated patients. After surgery, artifacts may occur which in some cases cannot be differentiated from malignant tumors or ulcer craters on a purely radiologic basis, although postoperative baseline studies may be helpful. Furthermore in our experience endoscopy has proved to be superior to radiology for detecting small jejunal ulcers, following a Billroth II resection.

The possibility of *recurrent* carcinoma must be considered even after a short interval following surgery for gastric carcinoma. However, if the surgery was undertaken for a benign lesion, a higher rate of malignancy (primary gastric stump carcinoma) is not to be expected before a postoperative interval of at least 5 years.

The hypotonic technique allows for excellent visualization of the afferent loop, the normal anatomic landmarks, the sequelae, and the complications of surgery as well as unrelated diseases affecting the duodenum.

REFERENCES

1. Op den Orth, J.O., and Ploem, S.: The standard biphasic-contrast gastric series. Radiology *122*:530, 1977.
2. Op den Orth, J.O.: The Standard Biphasic-Contrast Examination of the Stomach and Duodenum: Method, Results and Radiological Atlas. Boston, Martinus Nijhoff, 1979.
3. Ginai, A.Z.: Clinical use of Hexabrix for radiological evaluation of leakage from the upper gastrointestinal tract based on experimental study. Br. J. Radiol. *60*:343, 1987.
4. Foley, M.J., Ghahremani, G.C., and Rogers, L.F.: Reappraisal of contrast media used to detect upper gastrointestinal perforations. Radiology *144*:231, 1982.
5. Burhenne, H.J.: Postoperative defects of the stomach. Semin. Roentgenol. *6*:182, 1971.
6. Prévôt, R.: Die Röntgendiagnostik des operierten Magens. Dtsch. Med. Wochenschr. *88*:942, 1963.
7. Norberg, P.B.: Results of the surgical treatment of perforated peptic ulcer: A clinical and roentgenological study. Acta Chir. Scand. *249*(Suppl):24, 1959.
8. Nahum, H., and Fékété, F.: Radiologie de l'appareil digestif opéré. pp. 54–58. Paris. Masson et Cie., 1976.
9. Gleeson, J., and Ellis, H.: Vagotomy and pyloroplasty, a cineradiographic study. Am. J. Dig. Dis. *14*:84, 1969.
10. Toye, D.K.M., Hutton, J.F.K., and Williams, J.A.: Radiological anatomy after pyloroplasty. Gut *11*:358, 1970.
11. Balthazar, E.J.: Radiographic examination of the stomach following surgery for pancreatic pseudocyst: A source of diagnostic error. Gastrointest. Radiol. *4*:23, 1979.
12. Hüpscher, D.N.: Radiology of the Esophagus, pp. 95–100. Stuttgart, New York, Georg Thieme-Verlag, 1988.
13. Nissen, R., and Rossetti, M.: Surgery of hiatal and other diaphragmatic hernias. J. Int. Coll. Surg. *43*:663, 1965.
14. Cohen, W.N.: The fundoplication repair of sliding esophageal hiatus hernia: Its roentgenographic appearance. AJR *104*:625, 1968.
15. Feigin, D.S., James, A.E., Stitik, F.P., et al.: The radiological appearance of hiatal hernia repairs. Radiology, *110*:71, 1974.
16. Kuyk, P.J., van: Diagnostic radiology in fundoplication according to Nissen. Radiol. Clin. *45*:115, 1976.
17. Thoeni, R.F., and Moss, A.A.: The radiographic appearance of complications following Nissen fundoplication. Radiology *131*:17, 1979.
18. Kuyk, P.J., van: Fundoplication according to Nissen. Personal communication, 1978.
19. Skucas, J., Mangla, J.C., Adams, J.T., et al.: An evaluation of the Nissen fundoplication. Radiology, *118*:539, 1976.
20. Lewis, R.A., Angelchik, J.P., and Cohen, R.: A new surgical prosthesis for hiatal hernia repair. Radiology *135*:630, 1980.
21. G. Curtis, D.J., Benjamin, S.B., Kerr, R., et al.: Angelchik anti-reflux device: Radiographic appearance of complications. Radiology *151*:311, 1984.
22. H. Martens, F., van Rooy, W.J., Tytgat, G.N.J., et al.: Radiographic follow-up of erosion of an Angelchik anti-reflux prosthesis into the esophagus and subsequent endoscopic removal: a case report. J. Med. Imaging *1*:218, 1987.
23. Goodman, P., and Halpert, R.D.: Radiological evaluation of gastric stapling procedures for morbid obesity. Crit. Rev. Diagn. Imaging *32*:37, 1991.
24. Agha, F.P., Eckhauser, F.E., Strodel, W.E., et al.: Mason's vertical banded gastroplasty for morbid obesity. Radiology *150*:825, 1984.
25. Smith, C., Gardiner, R., Kubicka, R.A., et al.: Gastric restrictive surgery for obesity: Early radiologic evaluation. Radiology *153*:321, 1984.
26. Smith, C., Gardiner, R., Kubicka, R.A., et al.: Radiology of gastric restrictive surgery. RadioGraphics *5*(2):193, 1985.
27. Régent, D., Bigard, M.A., Hodez, Cl., et al.: Exploration radiologique en double contraste de l'estomac opéré. J. Radiol. Electrol. *57*:683, 1976.
28. Gold, R.P., and Seaman, W.B.: The primary double-contrast examination of the postoperative stomach. Radiology, *124*:297, 1977.
29. Op den Orth, J.O.: Experiences with a standard biphasic-contrast examination after partial gastrectomy. RSNA Educational Materials Center: Audiovisual program RS 88, 1977.
30. Gohel, V.K., and Laufer, I.: Double contrast examination of the postoperative stomach. Radiology *129*:601, 1978.
31. Carter, T.L., and Martel, W.: Contraction of the gastric antrum following a long-term gastroenterostomy. Radiology *91*:514, 1968.
32. Hajdu, N., Hyde, D.M.R.I., and Riddell, V.: Antro-pyloric hypertrophy in patients with longstanding gastroenterostomies: A study of thirteen cases. Br. J. Radiol. *41*:49, 1968.
33. Koehler, R.E., and Halverson, J.D.: Radiographic abnormalities after gastric bypass. AJR *138*:267, 1982.
34. Burhenne, H.J.: Roentgen anatomy and terminology of gastric surgery. AJR *91*:731, 1964.
35. Op den Orth, J.O.: Tubeless hypotonic examination of the afferent loop of the Billroth II stomach. Gastrointest. Radiol. *2*:1, 1977.
36. Pochaczevsky, R.: "Bubbly barium," a carbonated cocktail for double-contrast examination of the stomach. Radiology, *107*:465, 1973.
37. Kim, S.Y., and Evans, J.A.: The roentgen appearance of the stomach and duodenum following the Billroth I gastric resection. AJR *81*:576, 1959.
38. Fisher, M.S.: The Hofmeister defect: A normal change in the postoperative stomach. AJR *84*:1082, 1960.
39. Sasson, L.: Tumor-simulating deformities after subtotal gastrectomy. JAMA *174*:142, (280–283), 1960.
40. Eklöf, O., and Ohlsson, S.: Postoperative plication deformity with foreign-body granuloma simulating tumour of the stomach: Report of three cases. Acta Chir. Scand. *123*:125, 1962.
41. Gueller, R., Shapiro, H.A., Nelson, J.A., et al.: Suture granulomas simulating tumors. Am. J. Dig. Dis. *21*:223, 1976.
42. Hammerman, A.M., Shady, K., Fry, R., and Cohen, E.: Postgastrostomy tube deformity on upper GI series. Gastrointest. Radiol. *16*:13, 1991.
43. Frik, W.: Digestive Tract. *In:* Schinz, H.R., Baensch, W.E., Frommhold, W., et al. (eds): Lehrbuch der Röntgendiagnosik. Band V., p. 223. Stuttgart, Georg Thieme-Verlag, 1965.
44. Wychulis, A.R., Priestley, J.T., and Foulk, W.T.: A study of 360 patients with gastrojejunal ulceration. Surg. Gynecol. Obstet. *122*:89, 1966.

45. Schulman, A.: Anastomotic gastrojejunal ulcer: Accuracy of radiological diagnosis in surgically proven cases. Br. J. Radiol. 44:422, 1971.

46. Demling, L., Ottenjann, R., and Elster, K.: Endoskopie und Biopsie der Speiseröhre und des Magens, p. 121. Stuttgart, F.K., Schattauer Verlag, 1972.

47. Burhenne, H.J.: The postoperative stomach. In: Margulis, A.R., and Burhenne, H.J. (eds.): Alimentary Tract Roentgenology, vol 1, p. 766. St. Louis, C.V. Mosby, 1973.

48. Moulinier, B., Lambert, R., Russo, A., et al.: Diagnostic endoscopique de l'ulcère anastomotique après chirurgie gastrique: À propos de 150 cas. Ann. Gastroentérol. Hépatol. 11:209, 1975.

49. Ott, D.J., Munitz, H.A., Gelfand, D.W., et al.: The sensitivity of radiography of the postoperative stomach. Radiology 144:741, 1982.

50. Dekker, W., and Op den Orth, J.O.: Correlations and discorrelations between endoscopy and radiology of the upper GI tract. Scientific exhibit shown at the Scientific Assembly and Annual Meeting of the Radiological Society of North America, Chicago, 1977.

51. Bachman, A.L., and Parmer, E.P.: Radiographic diagnosis of recurrence following resection for gastric cancer. Radiology, 84:913, 1965.

52. Feldman, F., and Seaman, W.B.: Primary gastric stump cancer. AJR 115:257, 1972.

53. Dahm, K., and Werner, B.: Das Karzinom im operierten Magen. Dtsch. Med. Wochenschr. 100:1073, 1975.

54. Stalsberg, H., and Taksdal, S.: Stomach cancer following gastric surgery for benign conditions. Lancet 2:1175, 1971.

55. Clémençon, G., Baumgartner, R., Leuthold, E., et al.: Das Karzinom des operierten Magens. Dtsch. Med. Wochenschr. 101:1015, 1976.

56. Terjesen, T., and Erichsen, H.G.: Carcinoma of the gastric stump after operation for benign gastroduodenal ulcer. Acta Chir. Scand., 142:256, 1976.

57. Pygott, F., and Shah, V.L.: Gastric cancer associated with gastroenterostomy and partial gastrectomy. Gut, 9:117, 1968.

58. Saegesser, F., and Jämes, D.: Cancer of the gastric stump after partial gastrectomy (Billroth II principle) for ulcer. Cancer 29:1150, 1972.

59. Kriedeman, E., Rotte, K.-H., Mateev, B., et al.: Probleme der Diagnostik des magenstumpfkarzinoms und des Tumorrezidivs: ein Vergleich zwischen Röntgen diagnostik und Endoskopie. Arch. Geschwulstforsch., 45:552, 1975.

60. Dobroschke, J., Feustel, H., and Filler, D.: Das Karzinom am resezierten Magen: Secondary carcinoma after gastric resection. Akt. Gastrologie, 5:369, 1976.

61. LeVine, M., Boley, S.J., Mellins, H.Z., et al.: Gastrojejunal mucosal prolapse. Radiology, 80:30, 1963.

62. Grimoud, M., Moreau, G., and Lemozy, J.: Le prolapse postopératoire transanastomotique de la muqueuse gastrique. Arch. Mal. Appar. Diag. 53:649, 1964.

63. Shane, M.D., Amberg, J.R., and Szemes, G.: Gastrojejunal mucosal prolapse after subtotal gastrectomy. Calif. Med. 111:177, 1969.

64. Seaman, W.B.: Prolapsed gastric mucosa through a gastrojejunostomy. AJR, 110:403, 1970.

65. Poppel, M.H.: Gastric intussusceptions. Radiology 78:602, 1962.

66. Aleman, S.: Jejuno-gastric intussusception—a rare complication of the operated stomach. Acta Radiol. 29:384, 1948.

67. Bradford, B., and Boggs, J.A.: Jejunogastric intussusception—an unusual complication of gastric surgery. Arch. Surg. 77:201, 1958.

68. Bret, P., Amiel, M., and Lescos, L.: Les images lacunaires des moignons de gastrectomie. Ann. Radiol. 7:519, 1964.

69. Reyelt, W.P., Jr., and Anderson, A.A.: Retrograde jejunogastric intussusception. Surg. Gynec. Obstet. 119:1305, 1964.

70. Devor, D., and Passaro, E.: Jejunogastric intussusception: Review of 4 cases—diagnosis and management. Ann. Surg. 173:93, 1966.

71. Waits, J.O., Beat, R.W., and Charboneau, J.W.: Jejunogastric intussuception. Arch. Surg. 115:1449, 1980.

72. Burhenne, H.J.: The iatrogenic afferent loop syndrome. Radiology, 91:942, 1968.

73. Burhenne, H.J.: The retained gastric antrum—a preoperative roentgenologic diagnosis of an iatrogenic syndrome. AJR 101:459, 1967.

74. Beneventano T.C., Glotzer, P., and Messenger, N.H.: Retained gastric antrum. Am. J. Gastroenterol. 59:361, 1973.

75. Dunlap, J.A., McLane, R.C., and Roper, T.J.: The retained gastric antrum. Radiology 117:371, 1975.

76. Bushkin, F.L., Wickbom, G., DeFord, J.W., et al.: Postoperative alkaline reflux gastritis. Surg. Gynecol. Obstet. 138:933, 1974.

77. Drapanas, T., and Bethea, M.: Reflux gastritis following gastric surgery. Ann. Surg. 179:618, 1974.

78. Kobayashi, S., Prolla, J.C., and Kirsner, J.B.: Late gastric carcinoma developing after surgery for benign conditions: Endoscopic and histologic studies of the anastomosis and diagnostic problems. Am. J. Dig. Dis. 15:905, 1970.

79. Domellöf, I., Eriksson, S., and Janunger, K-G.: Carcinoma and possible precancerous changes of the gastric stump after Billroth II resection. Gastroenterology 73:462, 1977.

80. Glick, S.N., Teplick, S.K., and Amenta, P.S.: Giant hyperplastic polyps of the gastric remnant simulating carcinoma. Gastrointest. Radiol. 15:151, 1990.

81. Op den Orth, J.O.: Radiologic visualization of the normal duodenal minor papilla. Fortschr. Roentgenstr. 128:572, 1978.

82. Baldwin, M.: The pancreatic duct in man, together with a study of the microscopical structure of the minor duodenal papilla. Anat. Rec. 5:197, 1911.

83. Poppel, M.H., Jacobson, H.R., and Smith, R.W.: The Roentgen Aspects of the Papilla and Ampulla of Vater, pp. 4–8, 12–20, 110. Springfield, Charles C Thomas, 1953.

DUODENUM

10

Marc S. Levine, M.D.
Igor Laufer, M.D.
Giles Stevenson, M.D.

INTRODUCTION

Fiberoptic endoscopy has exposed the limitations of conventional single contrast radiography in evaluating the duodenum, as 20% to 35% of lesions may be missed with single contrast technique.[1, 2] However, the double contrast study has increased our radiologic sensitivity in this area to more than 90%.[3-5] Most false negatives occur with examinations that the radiologist can recognize and report as less than ideal. The first part of this chapter therefore is devoted to some aspects of technique and anatomy that may help radiologists to indicate with confidence that the duodenum is normal. The finding of a normal duodenum depends upon the clear demonstration of normal anatomic landmarks in this region. The second part of the chapter deals with some of the common abnormalities found in and around the duodenum.

TECHNIQUE

In the past, double contrast duodenography was performed as a selective technique, utilizing a duodenal tube and hypotonia for evaluation of suspected pancreaticoduodenal disorders.[6, 7] However, it is possible to perform "tubeless" hypotonic duodenography by using an effervescent agent to introduce gas into the stomach and duodenum.[8, 9] With appropriate positioning of the patient, double contrast views of the duodenum can be readily obtained. The modified technique of double contrast hypotonic duodenography described in this chapter is included in our routine upper gastrointestinal examination.

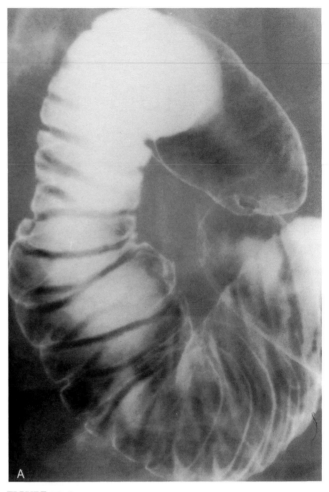

FIGURE 10–1

NORMAL DUODENUM. *A*, Ideal visualization of duodenum in LPO projection. Note smooth, featureless appearance of bulb.

Routine Study

In ideal circumstances, radiologic examination of the duodenum would include meticulous fluoroscopic observation, single contrast films with low-density barium, compression spot films, mucosal relief films, and double contrast films with high-density barium. However, it is not feasible to use all of these techniques in a single examination. We therefore rely primarily on double contrast technique for examining the duodenum. At the same time, it is important to recognize that overreliance on double contrast technique may result in errors, particularly if mucosal coating is inadequate or if lesions are suspected on the anterior wall of the duodenum. Instead, the study should be performed as a biphasic examination that includes double contrast views of the duodenum with high-density barium and single contrast prone or upright compression views of the duodenum with low-density barium.

The materials and techniques for performing a

double contrast examination of the upper gastrointestinal tract are described in detail in Chapter 3. Hypotonic agents are particularly important for optimal delineation of the normal anatomic landmarks in the duodenum. A standard dose of 0.1 mg of glucagon or 20 mg of Buscopan (hyoscine N-butyl bromide) is routinely administered at the beginning of the study to produce adequate hypotonia of the stomach and duodenum.[10] By the time that double contrast views of the stomach have been obtained, barium usually has emptied into the duodenum. The patient is then turned to the left posterior oblique (LPO) position for 4-on-1 spot films of the duodenal bulb and vertically split 2-on-1 spot films of the descending duodenum (Fig. 10–1A). In some patients, gaseous distention of the stomach creates difficulties by rotating the duodenum more posteriorly. This problem can be overcome by turning the patient to the right posterior oblique (RPO) position (Fig. 10–1B) or to a steep LPO

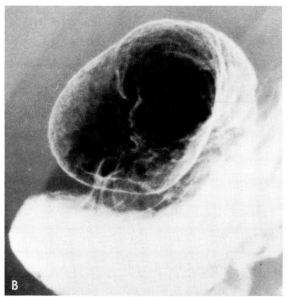

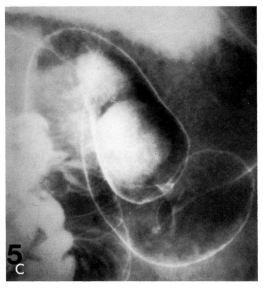

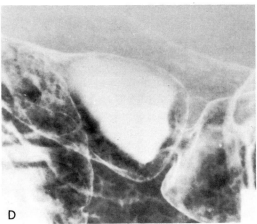

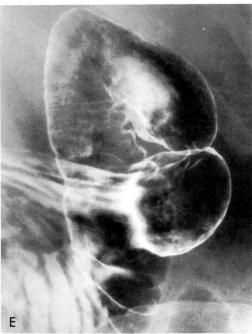

FIGURE 10–1 *Continued*

B, Duodenal bulb in RPO projection.

C, Steep LPO view, projecting duodenum between stomach and jejunum.

D, Left lateral view, projecting duodenum through gas-filled stomach.

E, Semi-prone LAO view with pad between patient's abdomen and table to show bulb clear of stomach.

F, Upright RPO view of bulb.

(Fig. 10–1C), left lateral (Fig. 10–1D), or even semi-prone left anterior oblique (LAO) position (Fig. 10–1E), so that the duodenal bulb and descending duodenum are seen through the gas-filled stomach. If, despite these maneuvers, the bulb is inadequately distended with gas or obscured by barium, it may be necessary to elevate the table to a semi-upright or fully upright position. This causes barium to pool in the antrum or descending duodenum and gas to rise into the duodenal bulb, which tends to assume a vertical configuration, so that adequate double contrast views of the bulb can be obtained (Fig. 10–1F). However, mucosal coating may deteriorate rapidly in the upright position, so that superficial lesions can sometimes be missed on these views.

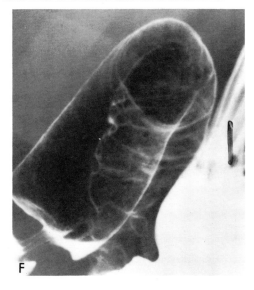

When the double contrast portion of the examination is completed, the patient drinks a low-density barium suspension, and additional 4-on-1 prone or right anterior oblique (RAO) spot films of the duodenum are obtained with varying degrees of compression using an inflatable balloon or other prone compression device that is positioned beneath the patient's abdomen. These views are particularly helpful for showing depressed or protruded lesions on the anterior wall of the duodenum. In other patients, it may also be helpful to obtain upright 4-on-1 spot films of the duodenum with varying degrees of compression. The single contrast examination is particularly important when the double contrast portion of the study is unsuccessful.

Selective Hypotonic Duodenography

The technique just described is suitable for evaluating the duodenum during routine double contrast upper gastrointestinal examinations. If there is a high clinical suspicion of disease in the duodenum or if the routine examination is equivocal, however, a modified technique for hyptonic duodenography can be used to obtain a more detailed examination of the duodenum. For this technique, the patient is given the effervescent agent and then asked to drink the high-density barium suspension while lying on the right side. In this position, barium should empty rapidly into the duodenum. As soon as the duodenum is seen to fill with barium, a larger dose of hypotonic agent (usually 1.0 mg of glucagon) is given intravenously to relax the duodenum. The patient is then turned to the left to allow gas to enter the duodenum and achieve adequate duodenal distention. If this technique is unsuccessful, hypotonic duodenography may be performed with a duodenal tube as a last resort.[6, 7]

NORMAL APPEARANCES

Duodenal Bulb

With intravenous administration of glucagon or Buscopan, the pylorus is frequently seen as a circular ring with a diameter varying from a few millimeters to more than 1 cm (Fig. 10–2A). It normally has a central location at the base of the duodenal bulb. An eccentric location of the pylorus in relation to the stomach and duodenum may indicate scarring from peptic ulcer disease (Fig. 10–2B).

The duodenal bulb usually has a smooth, featureless appearance on double contrast studies (see Fig. 10–1). In about 5% to 10% of patients, however, a lacy, reticular mucosal pattern may be observed in the duodenum as a normal variation (Fig. 10–3).[11] This appearance results from tiny, interlacing circles of barium surrounding 1 to 2 mm lucencies that represent normal villous structures on the duodenal mucosa (Fig. 10–4).[11, 12] Occasionally, these surface

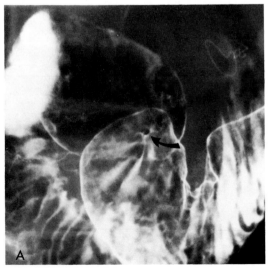
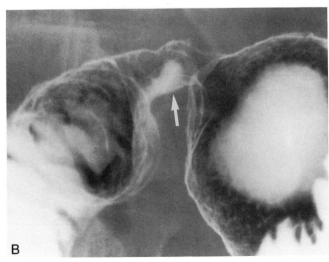

FIGURE 10–2

THE PYLORUS. *A,* Normal pylorus seen as circular lucency *(arrow)* with folds radiating to this site.
B, Widened, eccentric pylorus *(arrow)* due to scarring from peptic ulcer disease.

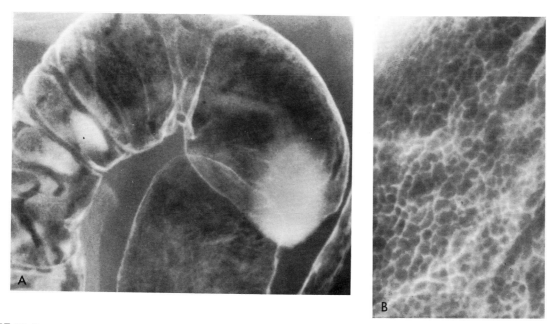

FIGURE 10–3

NORMAL MUCOSAL SURFACE PATTERN OF DUODENUM. *A*, Fine villous pattern seen in duodenal bulb as normal variation. *B*, In contrast, much coarser surface pattern (i.e., the areae gastricae) is seen in stomach.

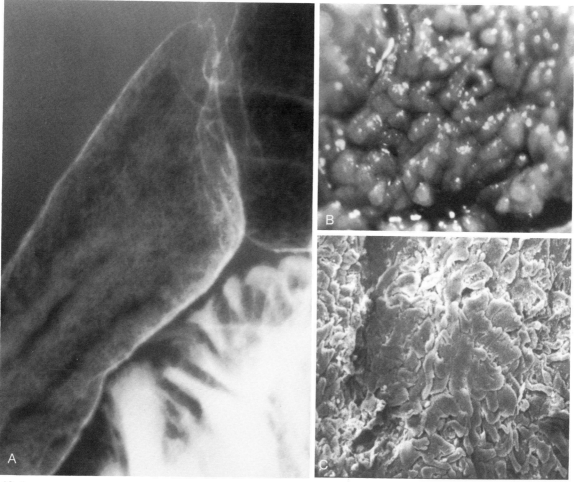

FIGURE 10–4

NORMAL MUCOSAL SURFACE PATTERN OF DUODENUM. *A*, Lacy reticular pattern is present in duodenal bulb.

B, In another patient, photograph of mucosal surface of bulb with dissecting microscope (× 10) shows tiny villous structures with sulci in between.

C, Scanning electron microscopy at low power (× 20) shows numerous villi surrounded by tiny sulci. Trapping of barium in these sulci or grooves presumably accounts for the fine reticular pattern seen on double contrast studies. (*B* and *C*, From Bova, J.G., et al.: The normal mucosal surface pattern of the duodenal bulb: Radiologic-histologic correlation. AJR 145:735–738, 1985, with permission, © by American Roentgen Ray Society.)

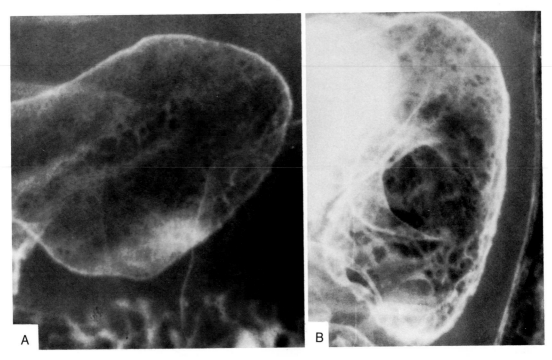

FIGURE 10–5

A and *B,* Two examples of larger, more irregular surface elevations in bulb. In both cases, endoscopic biopsies revealed normal duodenal mucosa.

elevations may be larger and more irregular (Fig. 10–5). In patients with a coarsely nodular mucosa, the findings can be confused with pathologic conditions such as duodenitis, Brunner's gland hyperplasia, and benign lymphoid hyperplasia (see later sections, "Duodenitis" and "Duodenal Tumors"). In other patients, punctate collections of barium may be observed in the duodenum both en face and in profile due to trapping of barium in normal mucosal pits (Fig. 10–6).[11, 12] This finding should not be mistaken for erosive duodenitis (see later section, "Duodenitis").

Heaped-up areas of redundant mucosa are sometimes identified as a normal finding on the inner aspect of the superior duodenal flexure between the duodenal bulb and the proximal descending duodenum.[13, 14] In some projections, this finding can mimic a polypoid mass or ulcer in the duodenum (Fig. 10–7). However, these "flexural pseudolesions" can be differentiated from true pathologic lesions by their characteristic location and changeable appearance at fluoroscopy.[13, 14]

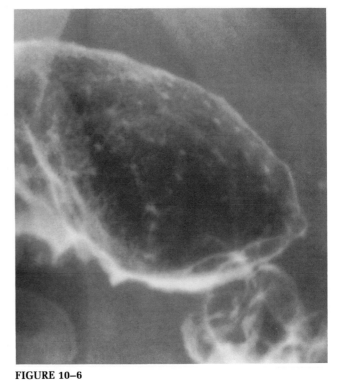

FIGURE 10–6

NORMAL MUCOSAL PITS IN DUODENUM. Punctate collections of barium trapped in these pits can be mistaken for duodenal erosions. (From Bova, J.G., et al.: The normal mucosal surface pattern of the duodenal bulb: Radiologic-histologic correlation. *AJR 145:*735–738, 1985, with permission, © by American Roentgen Ray Society.)

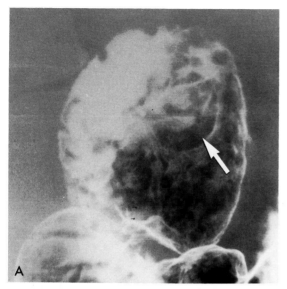

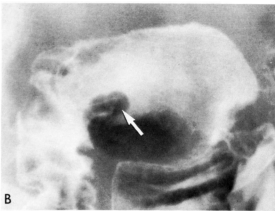

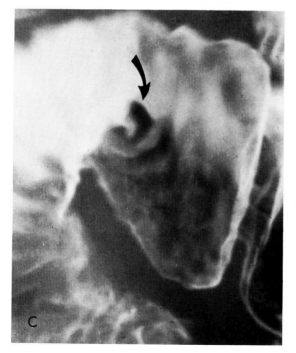

FIGURE 10–7

A to *C,* Three examples of duodenal pseudolesions *(arrows)* due to redundant mucosa at superior duodenal flexure. This redundant mucosa sometimes can simulate polyps or ulcers.

Duodenal Loop

The major landmarks of the duodenal sweep are the circular valvulae conniventes and the papillae.[15] The ampulla of Vater usually lies on the medial aspect of the second portion of the duodenum and is approximately 5 mm in diameter (Fig. 10–8). Its position may vary from the midpoint of the second portion of the duodenum to as far distally as the third portion. Endoscopic analysis of the ampulla has revealed three common types: hemispheric, flat, and papillary (Fig. 10–9). The ampulla is often recognized radiographically by its associated mucosal folds (Fig. 10–10). A distal longitudinal fold and hooding fold are present in approximately 90% of patients. A proximal longitudinal fold and oblique folds are identified less frequently.

The minor or accessory papilla is located adjacent to the orifice of the minor pancreatic duct or Santorini's duct and usually is not patent. It seldom has a distal longitudinal fold, and even the hooding fold is rarely prominent. The minor papilla lies approximately 1 cm proximal to the major papilla and 30 to 45 degrees anterior to it. Thus, in the supine oblique position, the major papilla can often be seen lying posteriorly in the second portion of the duodenum, whereas the minor papilla, when identifiable, is seen tangentially on the medial wall of the duodenum (see Fig. 10–8A). Conversely, in the prone position, the major papilla can often be identified lying on the medial aspect of the second portion of the duodenum, whereas the minor papilla is seen anteriorly a short distance proximal to the major papilla (see Fig. 10–8B). This relationship between the major and minor

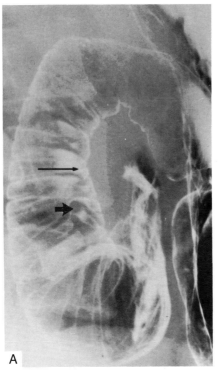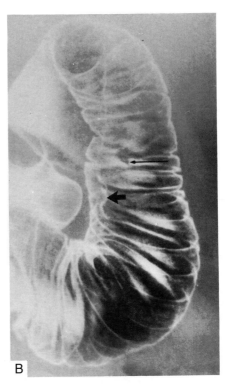

A   B

FIGURE 10–8

DUODENAL LOOP WITH MAJOR AND MINOR PAPILLAE. *A,* Supine LPO view shows major papilla *(short arrow)* on posterior wall of descending duodenum with minor papilla *(long arrow)* seen tangentially on medial wall 1 to 2 cm proximal to major papilla.

B, Prone view shows major papilla *(short arrow)* on medial wall of descending duodenum with minor papilla *(long arrow)* seen anteriorly above this level.

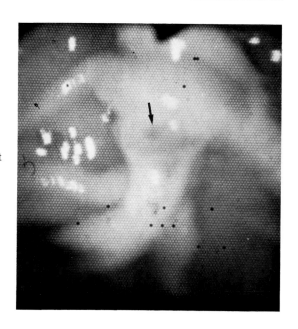

FIGURE 10–9

ENDOSCOPIC APPEARANCE OF NORMAL PAPILLA. Note flat
papilla with dark central area *(arrow)* representing the orifice.
Hooding fold, distal longitudinal fold, and oblique folds are all
clearly visible (see text).

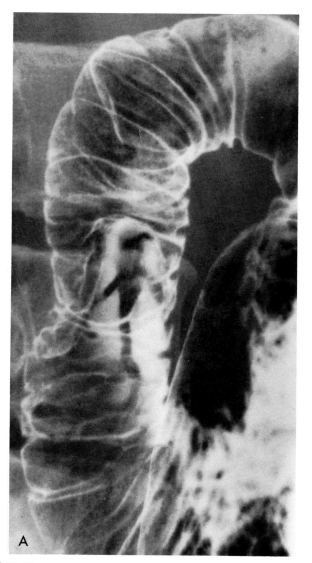

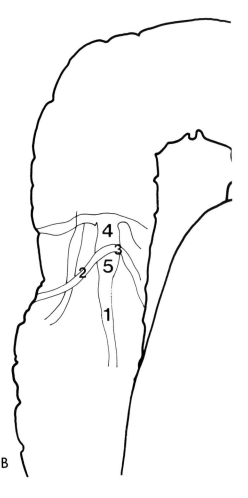

FIGURE 10–10

A and *B*, The ampulla of Vater and its associated folds. 1, Distal longitudinal fold, present in majority of patients. 2, Oblique folds—
variable. 3, Hooding fold, also present in majority of patients. 4, Proximal longitudinal fold—variable. 5, Ampulla of Vater.

papillae is amazingly constant. However, the minor papilla varies greatly in size and is sometimes as large as the major papilla (Fig. 10–11A). The minor papilla may be patent and draining a significant portion of the pancreas, particularly in patients with pancreas divisum (Fig. 10–11B).

Demonstration of the major or minor papilla or the normal villous surface pattern of the duodenal bulb is seldom important. However, clear delineation of these anatomic landmarks indicates that the examination has been technically satisfactory and therefore increases the reliability of the radiologic diagnosis of a normal duodenum.

Extrinsic Impressions

Neighboring structures may produce a variety of extrinsic impressions on the gas-filled duodenum, particularly in thin patients. A smooth indentation may be observed on the superolateral border of the duodenal bulb from the gallbladder or on the posterolateral border of the descending duodenum from the right kidney (Fig. 10–12A). An enlarged kidney or polycystic kidney occasionally may produce a more prominent or lobulated area of mass effect posteriorly or laterally on the duodenum (Fig. 10–12B). Although the pancreas normally may cause some flattening of

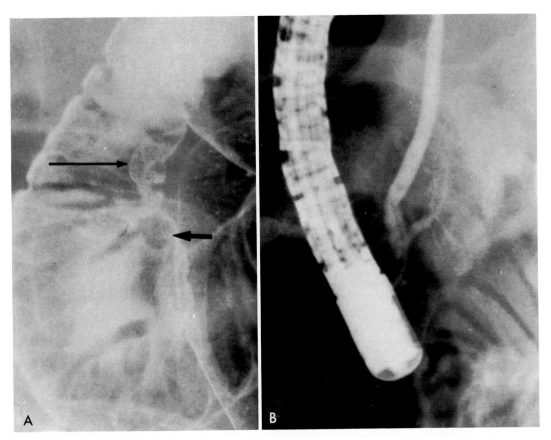

FIGURE 10–11

UNUSUALLY LARGE MINOR PAPILLA IN PATIENT WITH PANCREAS DIVISUM. A, Major papilla *(short arrow)* and unusually large minor papilla *(long arrow)* are seen in descending duodenum.

B, Injection of major papilla at endoscopic retrograde cholangiopancreatography (ERCP) shows filling of common bile duct and small dorsal pancreatic duct system in head of pancreas. No communication is seen with major portion of pancreatic duct, which must be draining through the enlarged minor papilla in this patient with pancreas divisum.

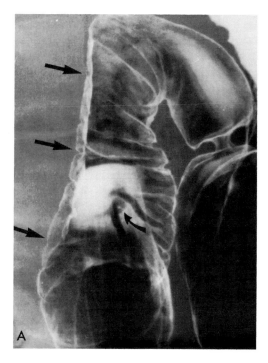 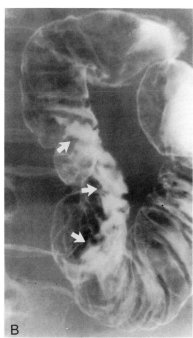

FIGURE 10–12

EXTRINSIC IMPRESSIONS ON DESCENDING DUODENUM. *A,* Normal impression *(arrows)* along lateral aspect of descending duodenum from right kidney.

B, More lobulated area of extrinsic mass effect *(arrows)* on duodenum from renal cell carcinoma.

the medial border of the descending duodenum, significant compression or effacement of the duodenum in this region should suggest pancreatic disease (see later section, "Pancreatic Diseases").

DUODENAL ULCERS

Duodenal ulcers, unlike gastric ulcers, are virtually always benign. When these lesions are detected radiographically, treatment with H_2-receptor antagonists therefore can be initiated without need for endoscopy. However, a significant percentage of duodenal ulcers are located on the anterior wall of the duodenal bulb,

so that a definitive diagnosis is best made on the compression phase of the examination. Furthermore, duodenal ulcers may be obscured by edema, spasm, or scarring of the bulb. Radiologists therefore should be aware of the limitations of double contrast technique in the search for duodenal ulcers and of the need for performing a biphasic examination in these patients.

Technical Considerations

Adequate mucosal coating is essential for the detection of duodenal ulcers, because an ulcer crater can easily be missed in a poorly coated bulb (Fig. 10–13).

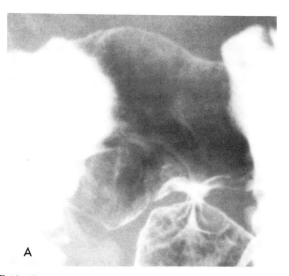 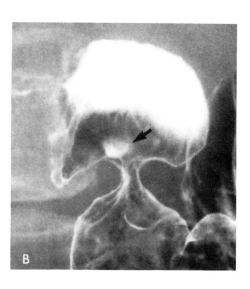

FIGURE 10–13

IMPORTANCE OF MUCOSAL COATING FOR DEMONSTRATING DUODENAL ULCERS. *A,* Well-distended but poorly coated duodenal bulb. No ulcer is seen.

B, With better mucosal coating, ulcer crater *(arrow)* is now clearly visible at base of bulb.

Duodenal spasm and deformity can also mask an ulcer crater, so that hypotonic agents such as glucagon are used to facilitate detection of ulcers by relaxing the duodenum (Fig. 10–14). Finally, the radiologic examination should include prone or upright compression views of the duodenum with low-density barium to detect ulcers on the anterior wall of the bulb (see following section).[16] Thus, double contrast technique complements but in no way replaces conventional techniques for the diagnosis of duodenal ulcers.

Features of Duodenal Ulcers

Location

About 95% of duodenal ulcers are located in the duodenal bulb and the remaining 5% in the postbulbar duodenum.[17] Bulbar ulcers may involve the apex, central portion, or base of the bulb (Fig. 10–15). Unlike gastric ulcers, which rarely occur on the anterior wall, as many as 50% of duodenal ulcers are located on the anterior wall of the bulb.[2, 18] When they occur, postbulbar ulcers are usually located in the proximal descending duodenum above the papilla of Vater (see later section, "Postbulbar Ulcers").

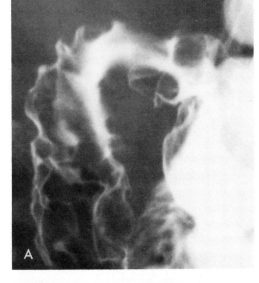

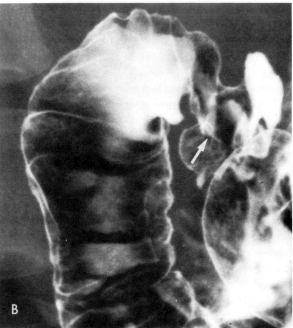

FIGURE 10–14

VALUE OF HYPOTONIA FOR DEMONSTRATING DUODENAL ULCERS. *A*, Initial view of duodenum shows poorly distended bulb without definite ulcer.

B, Following intravenous glucagon, there is much better distention of duodenum. As a result, the deformed bulb and ulcer crater *(arrow)* can now be recognized.

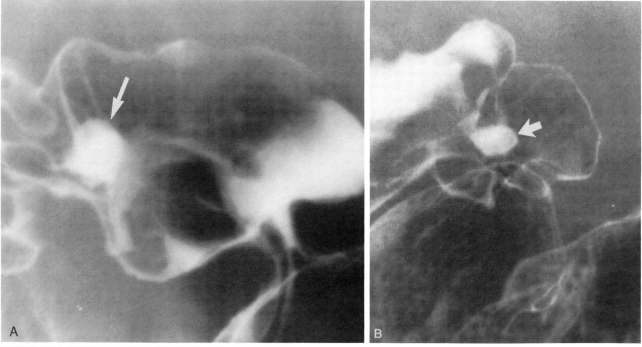

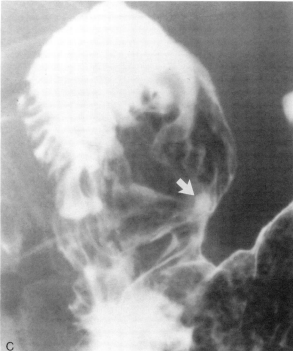

FIGURE 10–15

Duodenal ulcers (*arrows*) in various locations, including apex (*A*), central portion (*B*), and base (*C*) of bulb. In all cases, note folds radiating toward ulcer crater.

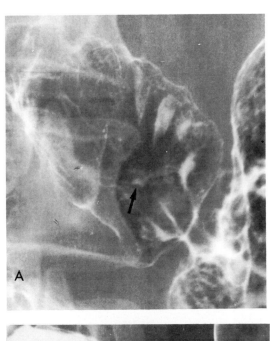

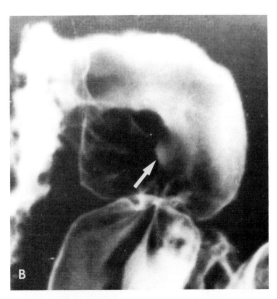

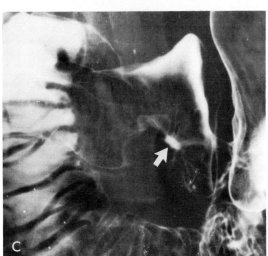

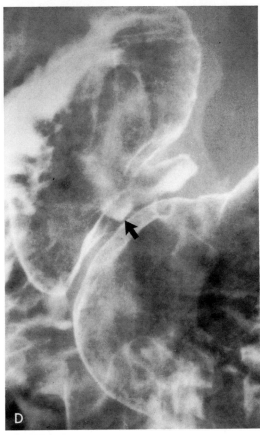

FIGURE 10–16

VARIETY OF SMALL DUODENAL ULCERS (ARROWS).
A and B, With little or no deformity of bulb.
C and D, With bulbar deformity.

Size

The vast majority of duodenal ulcers diagnosed on double contrast studies are less than 1 cm in size. A major advantage of double contrast technique is its ability to demonstrate small duodenal ulcers, frequently no more than several millimeters in diameter (Fig. 10–16). Conversely, giant ulcers (ulcers greater than 2 cm) are occasionally detected in the duodenum.[19] These ulcers can be so large that they replace virtually the entire duodenal bulb (Fig. 10–17). Paradoxically, giant ulcers can be mistaken for a normal or scarred bulb. However, their constant size and shape at fluoroscopy should help to differentiate these lesions from the changing appearance of the bulb.[19]

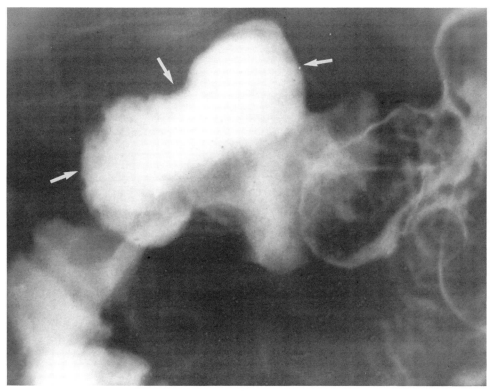

FIGURE 10–17

Giant duodenal ulcer (*arrows*) replacing duodenal bulb. Note radiolucent band of edema at base of bulb. Although this collection could be mistaken for a deformed duodenal bulb, its constant size and shape at fluoroscopy should help differentiate a giant ulcer from a scarred bulb.

Shape

Most duodenal ulcers appear radiographically as round or ovoid barium collections. However, about 5% of duodenal ulcers have a linear configuration (Fig. 10–18).[20, 21] These linear ulcers tend to be located near the base of the duodenal bulb, and they frequently have a transverse orientation in relation to the bulb (Fig. 10–18A).[21] As in the stomach, linear ulcers are thought to represent a stage of ulcer healing.[21, 22] In fact, they may be indistinguishable from linear ulcer scars.

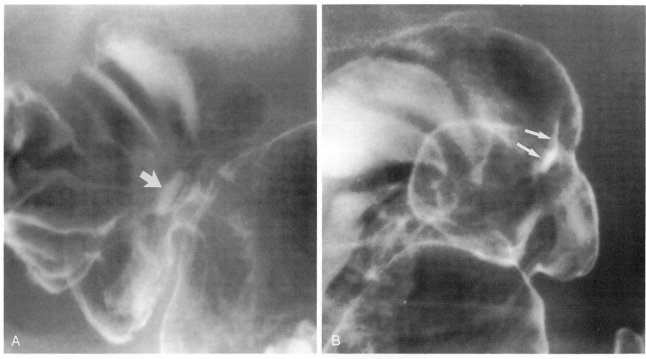

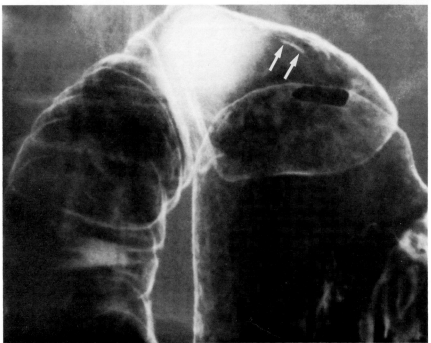

C

FIGURE 10–18

LINEAR DUODENAL ULCERS. *A,* Linear ulcer *(arrow)* at base of bulb with transverse orientation in relation to bulb. Also note folds radiating toward ulcer crater.

B and *C,* Two patients with linear ulcers *(arrows)* near apex of bulb.

Morphology

Ulcers in the duodenal bulb usually appear as discrete niches that can be seen en face or in profile on double contrast radiographs (Figs. 10–13 to 10–18). The ulcer crater is often surrounded by a smooth, radiolucent mound of edematous mucosa. Bulbar ulcers also tend to be associated with radiating folds that converge centrally at the edge of the crater (Figs. 10–15 and 10–16). In patients with shallow ulcers or small, healing ulcers, the ulcer crater may be visible only with optimal radiographic technique. Thus, the presence of radiating folds should prompt a careful search for an active ulcer at the site of fold convergence before attributing these folds to an ulcer scar.

As in the stomach, ulcers on the anterior wall of the duodenal bulb may be difficult to detect on routine double contrast views (Fig. 10–19A). Other anterior wall (nondependent) ulcers may be manifested by a ring shadow due to barium coating the rim of the unfilled ulcer crater (Fig. 10–20A).[23] These anterior wall ulcers can be demonstrated by turning the patient into the prone position or by compressing the bulb in either the prone or upright positions to fill the crater with barium (Figs. 10–19B and 10–20B).

Duodenal ulcers are often associated with significant deformity of the bulb due to edema and spasm accompanying the ulcer or scarring from a previous ulcer (Figs. 10–16C, 10–16D, and 10–21).[16] This deformity sometimes can obscure small ulcers in the bulb. Conversely, barium trapped in the crevices of a deformed bulb occasionally can be mistaken for an active ulcer crater. Thus, it is important to recognize the limitations of the radiologic diagnosis of duodenal ulcers in the presence of a deformed bulb. Although a confident diagnosis of "peptic ulcer disease" can be made in patients with bulbar deformity, it is often unclear whether an active ulcer is present. Nevertheless, symptomatic patients with a deformed bulb on barium studies probably should be treated for an active duodenal ulcer because of the high risk of ulcer disease, whether or not an ulcer is demonstrated with certainty.

Multiplicity

About 15% of patients with duodenal ulcers have multiple ulcers.[24] Most of these ulcers are located in the duodenal bulb.

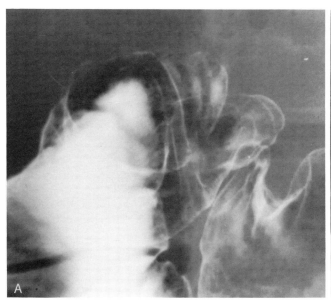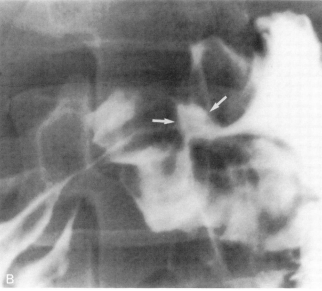

FIGURE 10–19

VALUE OF PRONE COMPRESSION FOR DEMONSTRATING ANTERIOR WALL DUODENAL ULCERS. A, Double contrast view of duodenum shows deformity of bulb and radiating folds without definite ulcer.

B, Prone compression view shows filling of anterior wall ulcer (arrows).

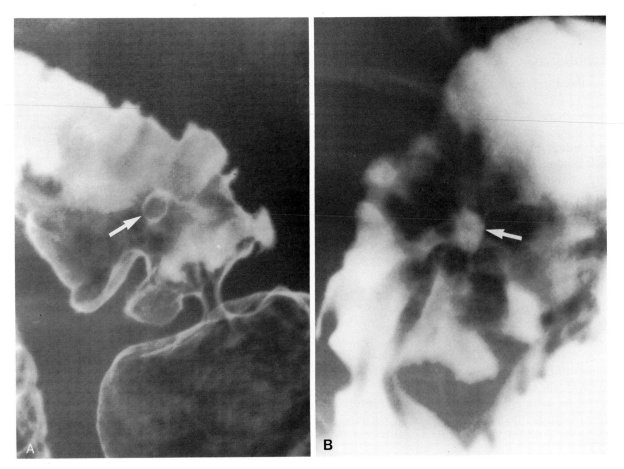

FIGURE 10–20

RING SHADOW IN DUODENUM DUE TO ANTERIOR WALL ULCER. *A,* Double contrast view of duodenum shows ring shadow (*arrow*) in bulb due to barium coating rim of unfilled ulcer on nondependent surface.

 B, Prone compression view shows filling of anterior wall ulcer (*arrow*).

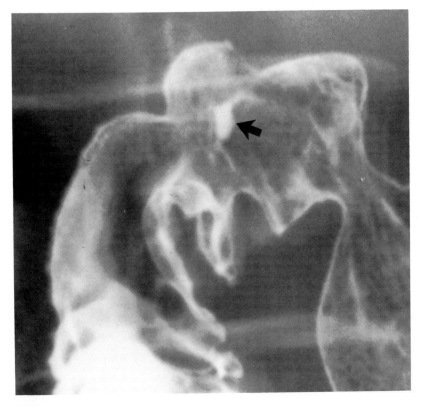

FIGURE 10–21

Duodenal ulcer (*arrow*) associated with marked deformity of bulb.

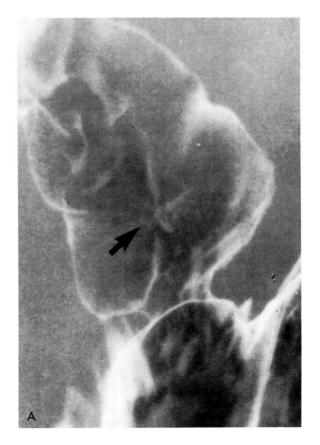

Ulcer Healing

Duodenal ulcers usually heal rapidly during treatment with H_2-receptor antagonists. Ulcer healing is often associated with the development of an ulcer scar, manifested by radiating folds or bulbar deformity. When radiating folds are present, they almost always converge at the site of the previous ulcer (Fig. 10–22). In some patients, a residual depression in the central portion of the scar may simulate an active ulcer crater.

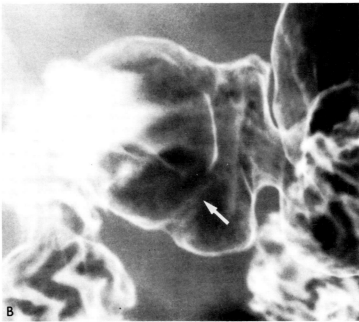

FIGURE 10–22

A and *B,* Two examples of ulcer scars *(arrows)* in duodenum with folds radiating to site of previous ulcer.

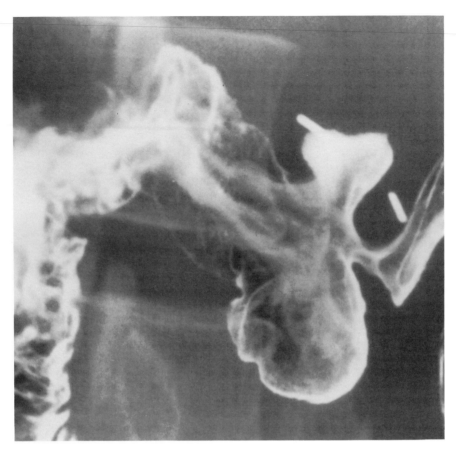

FIGURE 10–23

Scarred duodenal bulb with multiple pseudodiverticula, producing "clover leaf" appearance.

Bulbar deformity results from asymmetric scarring of the bulb. Uninvolved segments of the bulb may balloon out between areas of fibrosis, producing one or more pseudodiverticula. These pseudodiverticula usually can be differentiated from ulcers by their tendency to change in size and shape at fluoroscopy. When multiple pseudodiverticula are present, the duodenal bulb may have a classic "clover leaf" appearance (Fig. 10–23).

Postbulbar Ulcers

Postbulbar ulcers are usually located on the medial wall of the proximal descending duodenum above the papilla of Vater (Fig. 10–24A).[17, 25] These ulcers are notoriously difficult to demonstrate on barium studies, presumably because of severe edema and spasm accompanying the ulcer that prevent visualization of the ulcer crater. This edema and spasm often results in a smooth, rounded indentation on the lateral wall of the proximal descending duodenum opposite the crater (Fig. 10–24A).[25] Other patients may develop a "ring-stricture" with eccentric narrowing of the postbulbar duodenum due to scarring and fibrosis from previous ulcers in this region (Fig. 10–24B).[26] Hypotonic duodenography may be performed to better delineate postbulbar ulcers when these lesions are suspected on routine studies (see earlier section, "Technique").

Because most postbulbar ulcers are located above the papilla of Vater, the presence of one or more ulcers distal to the papilla should suggest the possibility of Zollinger-Ellison syndrome (Fig. 10–25).[27]

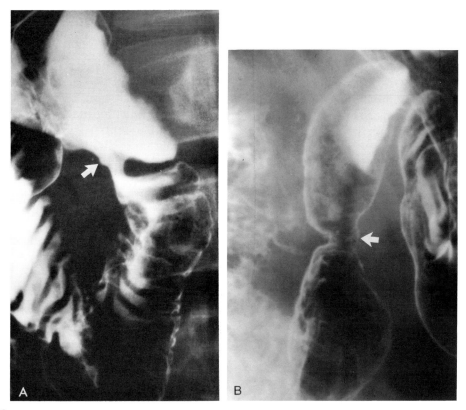

FIGURE 10–24

POSTBULBAR ULCERS. *A*, Postbulbar ulcer *(arrow)* on medial wall of proximal descending duodenum with smooth, rounded indentation of opposite wall.

B, Different patient with postbulbar "ring stricture" *(arrow)* but no definite ulcer.

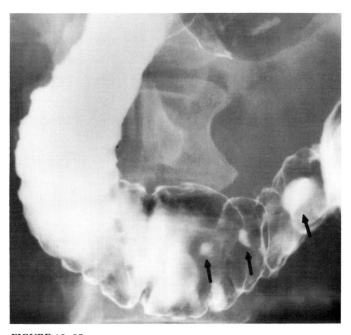

FIGURE 10–25

Multiple postbulbar duodenal ulcers *(arrows)* in patient with Zollinger-Ellison syndrome. Note how ulcers are located distal to papilla. (Courtesy of Wylie J. Dodds, M.D., Milwaukee, Wisconsin.)

DUODENITIS

It is unclear whether duodenitis represents part of the spectrum of peptic ulcer disease or a separate pathologic entity. The clinical significance of duodenitis has also been a subject of controversy. However, many investigators believe that it is a major cause of dyspepsia in the adult population.[28, 29] Less frequently, erosive duodenitis may be associated with upper gastrointestinal bleeding. In some patients, hemorrhagic duodenitis may occur as a complication of myocardial infarction or congestive heart failure.[30] Occasionally, the site of bleeding in the duodenum can be documented by angiography.[31, 32]

The diagnosis of duodenitis may be suggested radiographically in patients who have a spastic, irritable duodenal bulb or thickened, nodular folds in the proximal duodenum (Fig. 10–26A).[33] For reasons that are unclear, patients with chronic renal failure who are on dialysis often have enlarged duodenal folds to a degree rarely encountered in other patients with duodenitis (Fig. 10–26B).[34, 35] In most cases, however, thickened folds and spasm are nonspecific findings, so that the upper gastrointestinal examination generally has not been considered to be an accurate technique for diagnosing duodenitis.

With double contrast technique, it is possible to demonstrate more subtle signs of inflammatory disease in the duodenum.[11, 36–38] This inflammation may be manifested by mucosal nodules or nodular folds (Fig. 10–27) or by diffuse coarsening of the mucosal surface pattern of the bulb with lucent areas surrounded by barium-filled grooves that resemble the areae gastricae (Fig. 10–28).[11, 37, 38] With double contrast technique, it is also possible to diagnose erosive

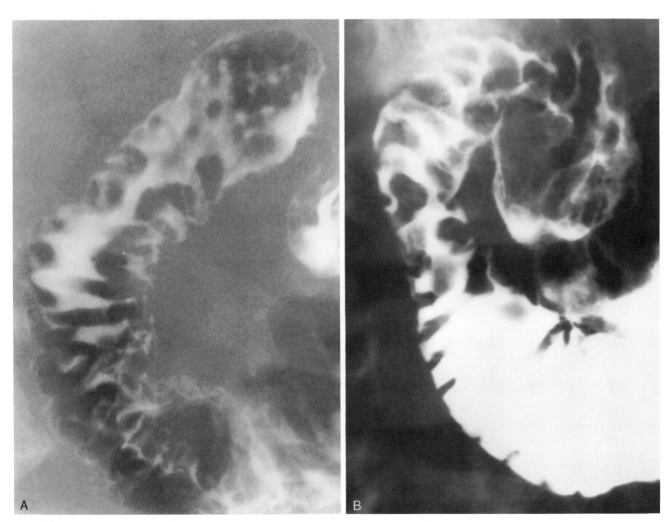

FIGURE 10–26

DUODENITIS WITH THICKENED FOLDS. A, Thickened, nodular folds are seen in descending duodenum. Also note erosions in bulb.
   B, Another patient with grossly thickened, polypoid folds associated with chronic renal failure.

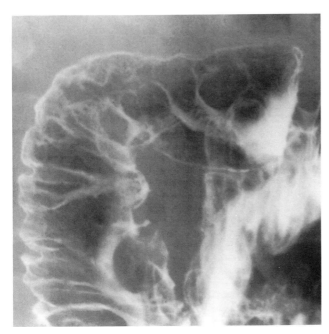

FIGURE 10–27

Duodenitis with nodular mucosa in proximal duodenum.

FIGURE 10–28

Duodenitis with coarse reticular pattern in bulb. This patient had Crohn's disease.

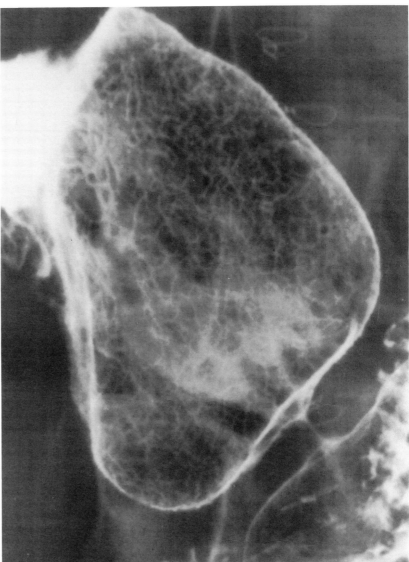

duodenitis, a condition previously thought to be solely in the domain of the endoscopist.[36–38] These erosions may be found in the duodenal bulb or, less frequently, in the descending duodenum. As in the stomach, incomplete erosions in the duodenum appear as tiny flecks of barium (Fig. 10–29A), whereas complete or varioliform erosions appear as central barium collections surrounded by radiolucent halos of edematous mucosa (Fig. 10–29B).[36] False-positive radiologic diagnoses occasionally may result from normal mucosal pits in the duodenum that are mistaken for incomplete erosions on double contrast studies (Fig. 10–30).[12, 38] Barium precipitates may also resemble incomplete erosions. Thus, a confident diagnosis of erosive duodenitis can be only made when true varioliform erosions are demonstrated.

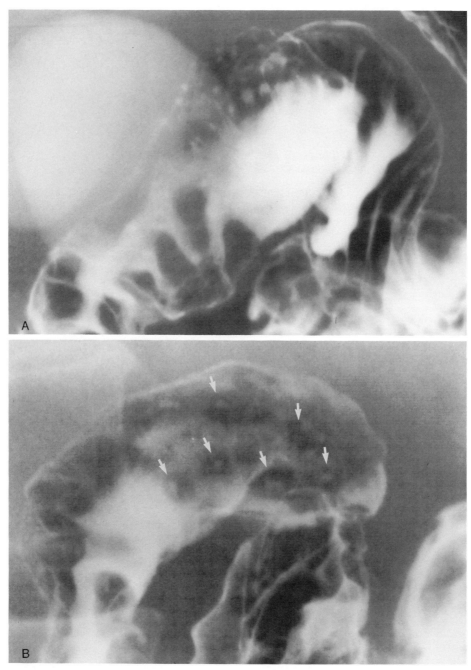

FIGURE 10–29

EROSIVE DUODENITIS. *A,* Incomplete erosions in bulb manifested by tiny flecks of barium seen both en face and in profile. (Note contrast in gallbladder adjacent to duodenum.)

B, Complete erosions (*arrows*) appearing as central barium collections with surrounding mounds of edema. (*B,* From Levine, M.S., et al.: Double-contrast upper gastrointestinal examination: Technique and interpretation. Radiology *168:*593–602, 1988, with permission.)

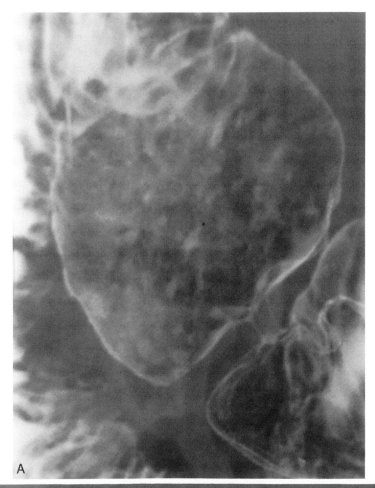

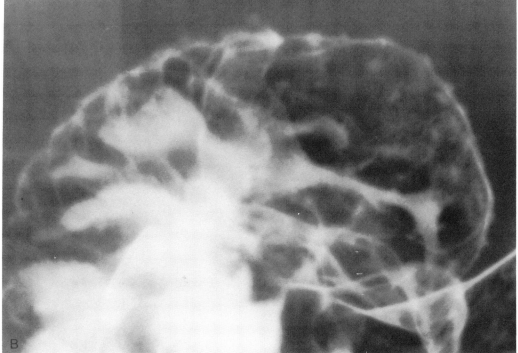

FIGURE 10–30

A and *B*, Two examples of normal mucosal pits in duodenal bulb simulating erosions. In both cases, endoscopic biopsies revealed normal duodenal mucosa. (*B*, From Levine, M.S., et al.: Double-contrast upper gastrointestinal examination: Technique and interpretation. Radiology *168*:593–602, 1988, with permission.)

CROHN'S DISEASE

Only 1% to 3% of patients with Crohn's disease have evidence of upper gastrointestinal involvement on conventional single contrast barium studies.[39, 40] These patients usually have advanced disease in the stomach and duodenum, manifested by thickened folds, ulcers, narrowing, and scarring.[39–41] In our experience, however, early signs of gastroduodenal Crohn's disease may be detected on double contrast studies in more than 20% of patients with granulomatous ileocolitis. Occasionally, the onset of upper gastrointestinal involvement may coincide with or even precede the onset of ileal or colonic involvement, so that these patients do not necessarily have known Crohn's disease when they seek medical attention. Endoscopic biopsies from the duodenum may fail to reveal granulomas due to the superficial nature of the biopsies and the patchy distribution of the disease.[42] Thus, the absence of definitive histologic findings should not discourage a diagnosis of duodenal Crohn's disease if the clinical and radiographic findings suggest this condition.

The earliest lesions of duodenal Crohn's disease are "aphthous ulcers" similar to those found else-where in the gastrointestinal tract in this disease.[43–45] Although these lesions may be indistinguishable from duodenal erosions associated with peptic duodenitis (see previous section, "Duodenitis"), the latter condition typically involves the duodenal bulb, whereas the aphthous ulcers of Crohn's disease may be located anywhere in the duodenum from the bulb to the ligament of Treitz (Fig. 10–31). Most patients with duodenal Crohn's disease have concomitant involvement of the small bowel or colon, so that a small bowel follow-through or barium enema should be performed when duodenal involvement is suspected.

More advanced duodenal Crohn's disease may be manifested radiographically by thickened folds (Fig. 10–32A), "cobblestoning" of the mucosa (Fig. 10–32B), ulceration (Fig. 10–32C), or strictures (Fig. 10–32D).[40] At this stage of disease, most patients have continuous involvement of the gastric antrum, pylorus, and duodenum. Duodenal strictures often appear as smooth, tapered areas of narrowing involving the apical portion of the duodenal bulb and adjacent segment of the postbulbar duodenum (Fig. 10–32D).[40] Severe duodenal disease is almost always associated with severe Crohn's disease involving the small bowel or colon.

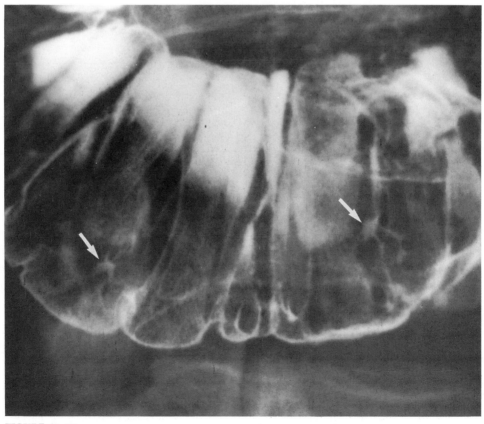

FIGURE 10–31

Duodenal Crohn's disease with discrete aphthous ulcers (*arrows*) in distal duodenum near ligament of Treitz. (Courtesy of Louis Engelholm, M.D., Brussels, Belgium. From Levine, M.S.: Crohn's disease of the upper gastrointestinal tract. Radiol Clin North Am 25:79, 1987, with permission.)

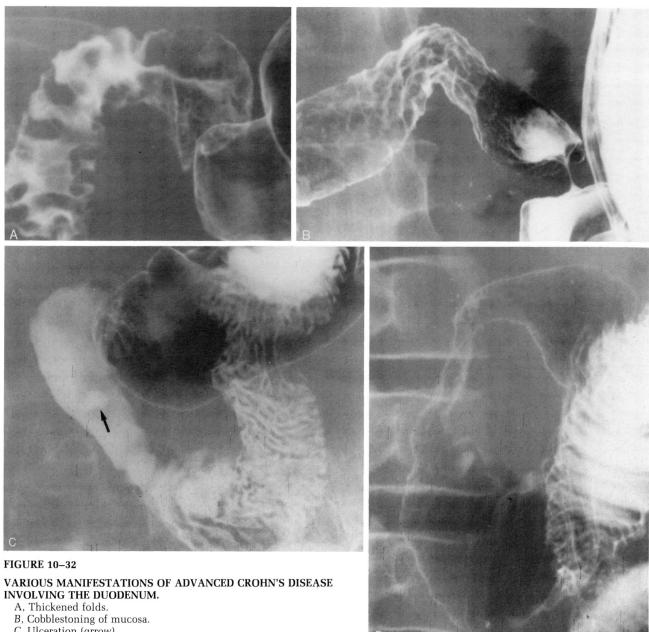

FIGURE 10–32

VARIOUS MANIFESTATIONS OF ADVANCED CROHN'S DISEASE INVOLVING THE DUODENUM.

A, Thickened folds.
B, Cobblestoning of mucosa.
C, Ulceration (*arrow*).
D, Postbulbar stricture.

CELIAC DISEASE

Celiac disease (nontropical sprue) typically involves the jejunum and ileum (see Chapter 11). However, it may also produce striking abnormalities in the duodenum. Some patients may have small (1 to 4 mm), hexagonal filling defects in the duodenal bulb, producing a distinctive mosaic pattern or "bubbly" bulb (Fig. 10–33).[46] Unlike heterotopic gastric mucosa, which predominantly affects the juxtapyloric region of the bulb (see later section, "Mass-like Lesions"), these nodules tend to be located more diffusely throughout the bulb. They may reflect the underlying changes of celiac disease in the duodenum or Brunner's gland hyperplasia due to associated peptic duodenitis.[46] Other patients with celiac disease may have thickened folds or nodular mucosa in the descending duodenum (Fig. 10–34).[47] Thus, the presence of a bubbly bulb or thickened duodenal folds in patients with malabsorption should suggest the possibility of celiac disease. A small bowel enema or small bowel biopsy may be required for a more definitive diagnosis (see Chapter 11).

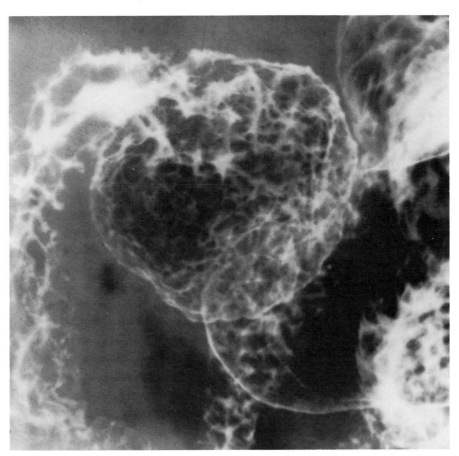

FIGURE 10–33

CELIAC DISEASE WITH "BUBBLY" BULB. Note multiple hexagonal filling defects in bulb and thickened folds in descending duodenum. (From Jones, B., et al.: "Bubbly" duodenal bulb in celiac disease: radiologic-pathologic correlation. AJR 142:119–122, 1984, with permission, © by American Roentgen Ray Society.)

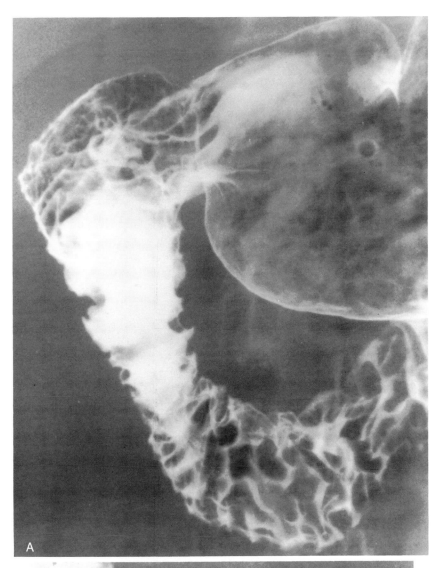

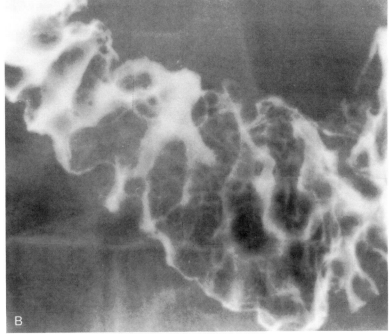

FIGURE 10–34

CELIAC DISEASE WITH DUODENITIS. *A,* Thickened, nodular folds are seen in distal descending duodenum.

B, Close-up view of this region shows polypoid folds and coarse nodularity of mucosa.

DUODENAL TUMORS

Polyps are much less common in the duodenum than in the stomach. They tend to be adenomatous or hyperplastic lesions. The vast majority are asymptomatic, so that duodenal polyps are almost always detected as incidental findings on radiologic or endoscopic examinations. They usually appear as smooth, sessile filling defects or ring shadows in the first or second portions of the duodenum (Fig. 10–35). Most duodenal polyps occur as solitary lesions, but multiple adenomatous, hyperplastic, or inflammatory polyps may be found in the duodenum as part of a diffuse polyposis syndrome (see Chapter 15).

Brunner's gland hyperplasia is another condition that may be manifested by multiple rounded nodules in the duodenal bulb and proximal duodenum, producing a characteristic "Swiss cheese" appearance (Fig. 10–36).[48] Benign lymphoid hyperplasia may also produce multiple nodular elevations in the duodenum, but the lesions tend to be smaller (1 to 2 mm) and more uniform in size (Fig. 10–37).[49] These patients often have generalized lymphoid hyperplasia of the small bowel or colon due to an underlying immunologic disorder. Both conditions should be differentiated from heterotopic gastric mucosa in the duodenal bulb (see next section, "Mass-like Lesions").

Although villous tumors are typically found in the colon, they also have a predilection for the duodenum, most frequently near the papilla of Vater.

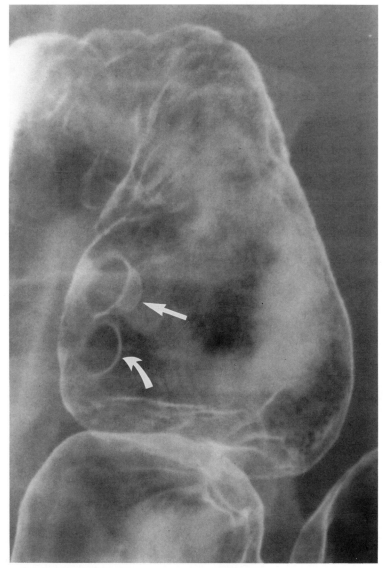

FIGURE 10–35

DUODENAL POLYPS. Note that lower polyp appears as ring shadow (*curved arrow*), whereas higher polyp can be recognized as bowler hat (*straight arrow*).

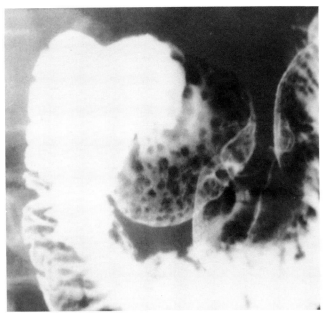

FIGURE 10–36

Brunner's gland hyperplasia with multiple round nodules in duodenal bulb, producing "Swiss cheese" appearance.

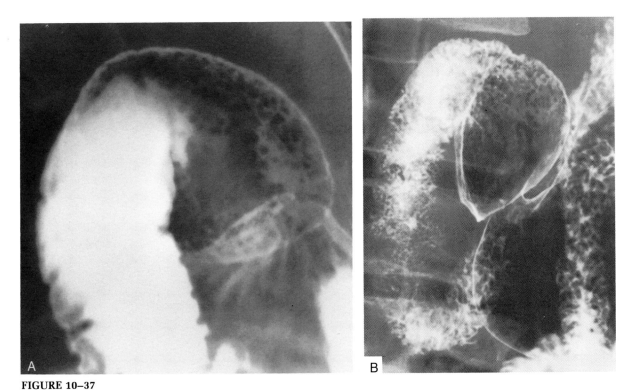

FIGURE 10–37

A and B, Two examples of benign lymphoid hyperplasia with innumerable tiny nodules in duodenum. In B, the patient had hypogammaglobulinemia.

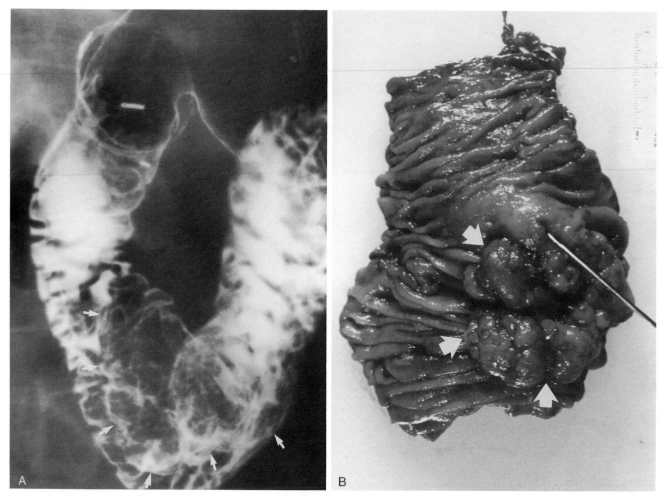

FIGURE 10–38

VILLOUS ADENOMA IN DUODENUM. *A,* Large polypoid lesion *(arrows)* is seen in descending duodenum below level of papilla. Note reticular appearance due to trapping of barium between frond-like projections of tumor.

B, Photograph of gross specimen shows large villous adenoma adjacent to papilla. (Note placement of probe with tip in orifice of papilla.)

These villous tumors may have a reticular or "soap bubble" appearance due to barium trapped in multiple clefts between the frond-like projections of the tumor (Fig. 10–38).[50, 51] Because these lesions may be obscured by superimposed mucosal folds, optimal distention of the duodenum is often required for their detection. As in the colon, villous tumors in the duodenum should be resected because of the high risk of malignant degeneration as these lesions enlarge.[52]

Primary malignant tumors of the duodenum are rare lesions. When they occur, they tend to be located at or below the ampulla of Vater.[53–55] Duodenal carcinoma or lymphoma may be manifested by a polypoid, ulcerated, or annular lesion (Figs. 10–39 and 10–40). Both carcinoma and lymphoma of the duodenum or small bowel may occur as complications of long-standing celiac disease.[56] Unfortunately, treatment with a gluten-free diet has not been effective in preventing the development of these tumors. Thus,

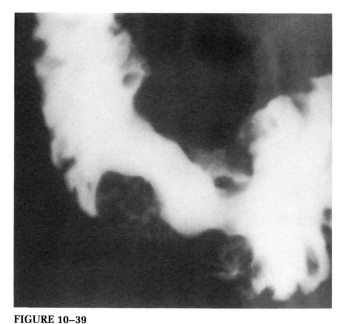

FIGURE 10–39

ANNULAR CARCINOMA OF DISTAL DUODENUM. Note abrupt, shelf-like borders of lesion.

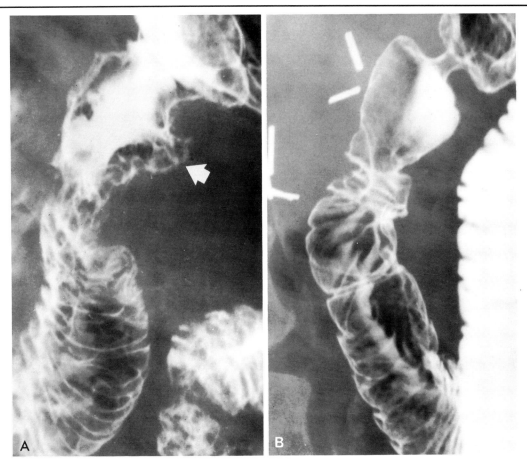

FIGURE 10–40

DUODENAL LYMPHOMA. *A,* Polypoid mass lesion is seen on medial wall of proximal descending duodenum. Note large area of ulceration *(arrow)* in lesion. At surgery, this was found to be duodenal lymphoma.

B, Follow-up study after radiation therapy shows regression of lesion with postbulbar scarring in region of previous ulcer. Note prominent longitudinal and oblique folds associated with duodenal papilla.

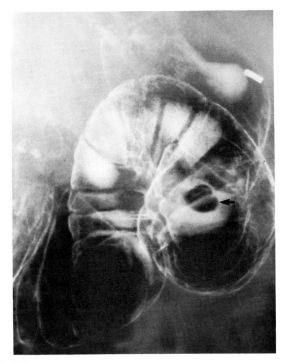

FIGURE 10–41

Small polypoid ampullary carcinoma *(arrow)* found in elderly man who presented with obstructive jaundice.

radiologic surveillance of the small bowel has been advocated in patients with celiac disease to detect these lesions at the earliest possible stage.

Carcinoma of the ampulla of Vater may also involve the duodenum.[54] These tumors may appear as polypoid masses in the region of the papilla. Because of the location of these lesions, affected patients usually present with obstructive jaundice. However, some ampullary carcinomas may be quite small at the time of clinical presentation (Fig. 10–41). Even when the

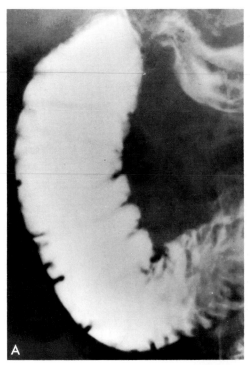
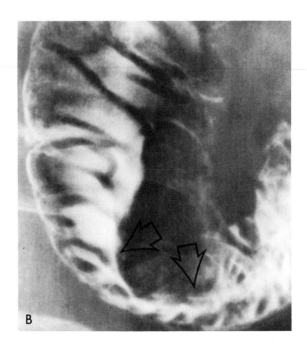

FIGURE 10–42

AMPULLARY CARCINOMA WITH DILATED COMMON BILE DUCT. *A,* Barium-filled view of duodenum shows no abnormality.

B, Hypotonic duodenography shows broad impression *(arrows)* on medial aspect of distal descending duodenum due to dilated common bile duct in patient with small ampullary carcinoma that was obstructing the duct. (From Laufer, I.: Double contrast radiology in the diagnosis of gastrointestinal cancer. *In* Glass, G.B.J. (ed.): Progress in Gastroenterology, vol. 3. New York, Grune & Stratton, 1977, p. 643, with permission.)

tumor itself is not visible, dilatation of the common bile duct may cause a broad impression on the medial aspect of the descending duodenum (Fig. 10–42).

MASS-LIKE LESIONS

Duodenal tumors may be simulated by a variety of innocuous findings such as see-through artifacts (Fig. 10–43), surgical defects (Fig. 10–44), prolapsed gastric mucosa (Fig. 10–45), prolapsed gastric tumors (Fig. 10–46), and heterotopic gastric mucosa in the duodenum (Fig. 10–47). Occasionally, gastric mucosa that has prolapsed into the duodenum can be mistaken for a polypoid lesion (Fig. 10–45A). However, prolapsed gastric mucosa is usually characterized by a mushroom-shaped defect at the base of the bulb that is observed as a transient finding at fluoroscopy (Fig. 10–45B).[57] Apparent polypoid lesions in the duodenum may also represent gastric tumors that

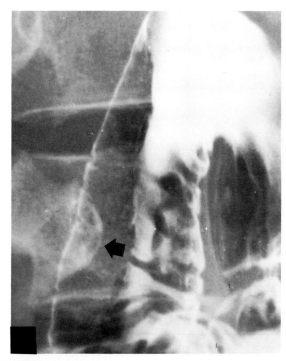

FIGURE 10–43

SEE-THROUGH ARTIFACT. Note vertebral pedicle *(arrow)* simulating polypoid lesion in descending duodenum.

have prolapsed through the pylorus into the duodenal bulb (Fig. 10–46). Heterotopic gastric mucosa in the duodenum is another benign condition manifested by polygonal or angulated 1- to 5-mm nodules or plaques that tend to be clustered near the base of the duodenal bulb (Fig. 10–47).[58, 59] Prolapsed gastric mucosa and heterotopic gastric mucosa in the duodenum both have such characteristic findings on barium studies that endoscopy usually is unnecessary in these patients.

In patients with an impacted common duct stone or pancreatitis, the ampulla of Vater occasionally becomes large and edematous, simulating a duodenal tumor. A prominent longitudinal fold seen tangentially may also suggest an intrinsic or extrinsic mass lesion involving the medial aspect of the descending duodenum (Fig. 10–48A). By manipulating the barium pool in the proper projection, however, the true nature of this longitudinal fold can be recognized (Fig. 10–48B).

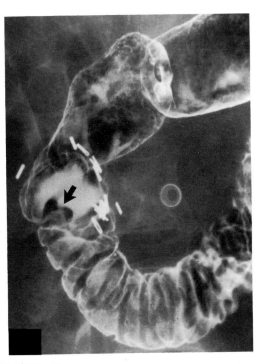

FIGURE 10–44

Surgical defect (*arrow*) appearing as small polypoid lesion in descending duodenum.

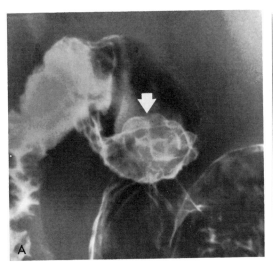 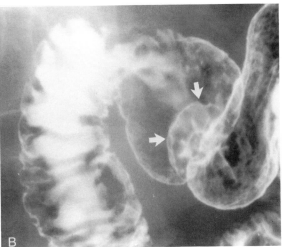

FIGURE 10–45

PROLAPSED GASTRIC MUCOSA. *A*, Prolapsed antral mucosa appearing as polypoid mass lesion (*arrow*) at base of bulb. *B*, More typical appearance of prolapsed gastric mucosa with mushroom-shaped defect (*arrows*) at base of bulb.

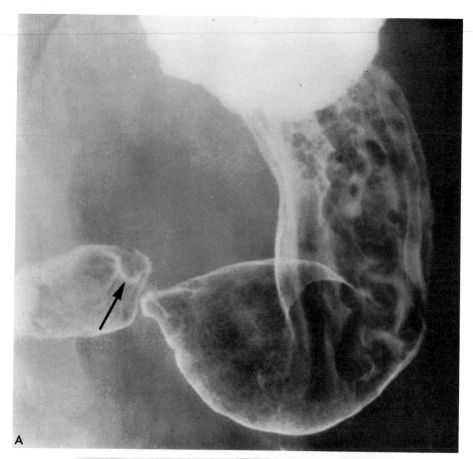

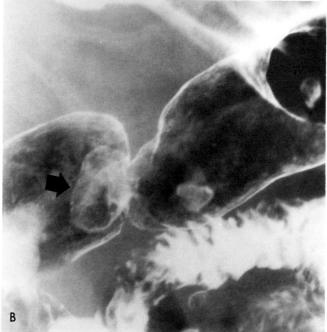

FIGURE 10–46

PROLAPSED GASTRIC TUMORS. *A*, Small gastric polyp *(arrow)* prolapsed into duodenal bulb.

B, Mass lesion *(arrow)* in bulb due to polypoid gastric carcinoma that has prolapsed into duodenum.

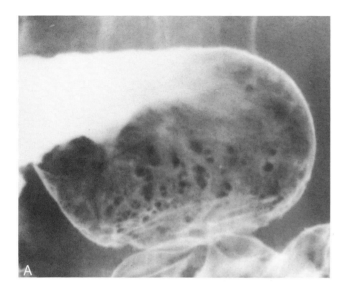

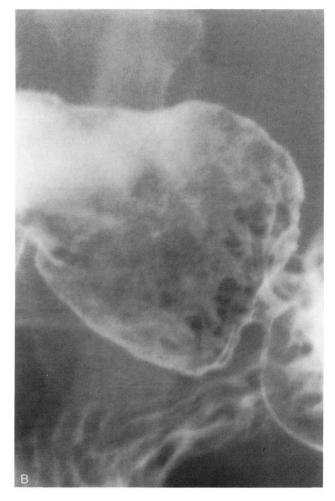

FIGURE 10–47

A and B, Two examples of heterotopic gastric mucosa manifested by discrete, angulated filling defects near base of bulb. This appearance is so characteristic that a confident diagnosis can be made on double contrast studies without need for endoscopy. (B, From Levine, M.S., et al.: Double-contrast upper gastrointestinal examination: Technique and interpretation. Radiology 168:593–602, 1988, with permission.)

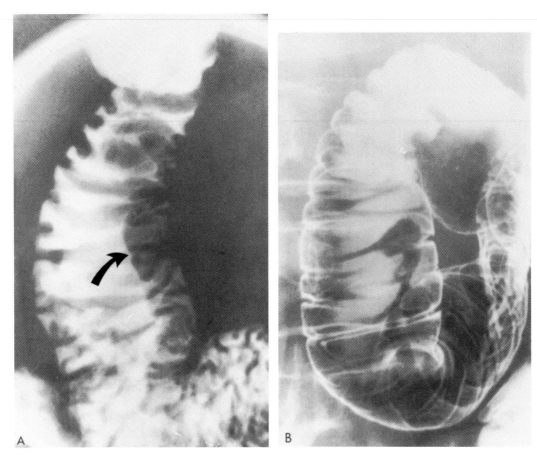

FIGURE 10–48

PROMINENT LONGITUDINAL FOLD MIMICKING MASS LESION IN DUODENUM. *A*, Initial view shows possible mass lesion *(arrow)* in medial wall of duodenum or head of pancreas.

   B, Hypotonic double contrast duodenography shows prominent longitudinal fold adjacent to major papilla without evidence of mass lesion. (Courtesy of Harvey M. Goldstein, M.D., San Antonio, Texas.)

PANCREATIC DISEASES

Inflammatory or neoplastic diseases of the pancreas are best evaluated by cross-sectional imaging techniques such as computed tomography and ultrasound. However, duodenal manifestations of pancreatic disease are sometimes seen on double contrast studies. In patients with acute or chronic pancreatitis, an enlarged head of the pancreas may cause widening of the duodenal sweep, compression of the medial aspect of the duodenum, or thickened, spiculated duodenal folds (Figs. 10–49 and 10–50). In other patients, pancreatitis may cause circumferential narrowing of the descending duodenum with varying degrees of obstruction. Pancreatic carcinoma may also result in compression and nodularity of the medial wall of the duodenum (Fig. 10–51A). As the tumor erodes into the bowel, ulceration eventually may occur (Fig. 10–51B). The "reverse 3" sign is a classic sign of advanced pancreatic carcinoma involving the duodenum. However, this sign occasionally may be simulated by underfilling of the duodenum, particularly in the presence of a duodenal diverticulum (Fig. 10–52). Finally, annular pancreas is a congenital abnormality that occasionally may be manifested in adults by focal narrowing or obstruction of the descending duodenum.

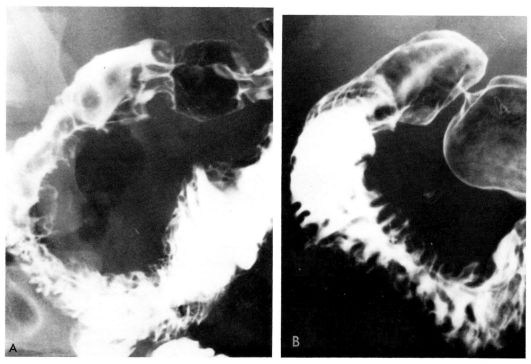

FIGURE 10–49

TWO EXAMPLES OF ACUTE PANCREATITIS INVOLVING DUODENUM. *A*, Widening of duodenal loop with compression of medial aspect of duodenum and thickened folds.
B, Different patient with thickened, spiculated folds in descending duodenum.

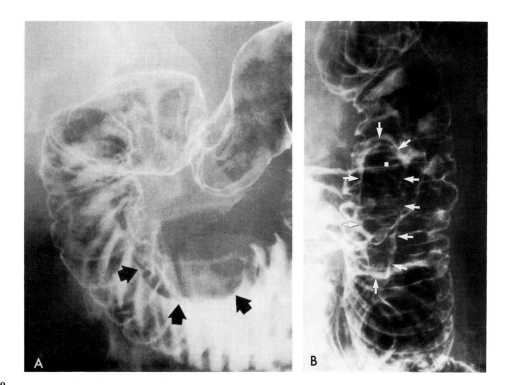

FIGURE 10–50

CHRONIC PANCREATITIS INVOLVING DUODENUM. *A*, Hypotonic duodenography shows area of mass effect *(arrows)* on medial aspect of descending duodenum.
B, Prone oblique view shows outline of periampullary mass en face *(arrows)*. Mucosal biopsies were normal. Although the ampulla was not identifiable at endoscopy, orifice of major papilla was found in mass, as indicated by dot. ERCP revealed chronic pancreatitis, which was confirmed by the patient's subsequent clinical course.

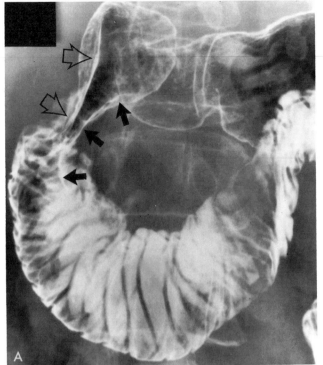

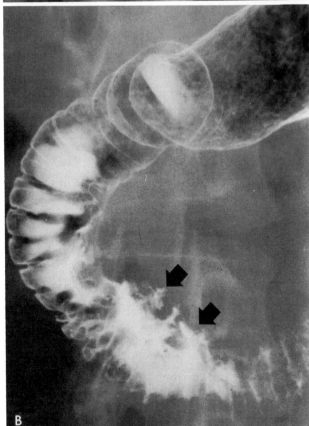

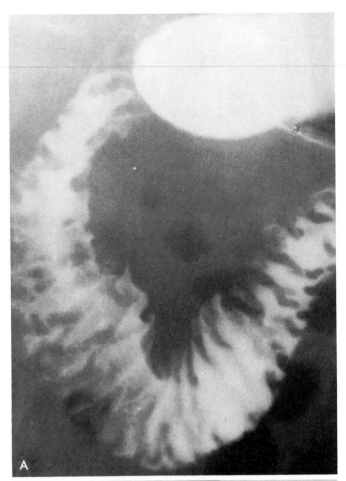

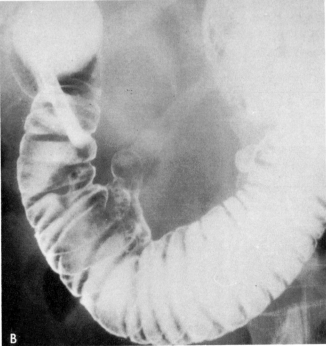

FIGURE 10–51

TWO EXAMPLES OF PANCREATIC CARCINOMA INVOLVING DUODENUM. *A,* Area of mass effect *(closed arrows)* is seen on medial aspect of proximal descending duodenum. There is also compression of lateral aspect of postbulbar duodenum by an enlarged gallbladder *(open arrows).* (Courtesy of Harvey M. Goldstein, M.D., San Antonio, Texas.)

B, Different patient with irregular ulceration *(arrows)* of descending duodenum due to invasion by pancreatic carcinoma.

FIGURE 10–52

SPURIOUS "REVERSE 3" SIGN DUE TO DUODENAL DIVERTICULUM. *A,* Initial view shows apparent compression of medial aspect of duodenum with "reverse 3" sign.

B, However, hypotonic duodenography with a tube shows a duodenal diverticulum without evidence of pancreatic or duodenal disease.

REFERENCES

1. Salmon, P.R., Brown, P., Htut, T., et al.: Endoscopic examination of the duodenal bulb: Clinical evaluation of forward- and side-viewing fibreoptic systems in 200 cases. Gut 13:170, 1972.
2. Classen, M.: Endoscopy in benign peptic ulcer. Clin. Gastroenterol. 2:315, 1973.
3. Herlinger, H., Glanville, J.N., and Kreel, L.: An evaluation of the double contrast barium meal (DCBM) against endoscopy. Clin. Radiol. 28:307, 1977.
4. Laufer, I., Mullens, J.E., and Hamilton, J.: The diagnostic accuracy of barium studies of the stomach and duodenum: Correlation with endoscopy. Radiology 115:569, 1975.
5. Laufer, I.: Assessment of the accuracy of double contrast gastroduodenal radiology. Gastroenterology 71:874, 1976.
6. Bilbao, M.K., Frische, L.H., and Dotter, C.T.: Hypotonic duodenography. Radiology 89:438, 1967.
7. Eaton, S.B., Benedict, K.T., Ferruci, J.T., et al.: Hypotonic duodenography. Radiol. Clin. North Am. 8:125, 1970.
8. Martel, W., Scholtens, P.A., and Lim, L.W.: "Tubeless" hypotonic duodenography: Technique, value, and limitations. AJR 107:119, 1969.
9. Sear, H.S., and Friedenberg, M.J.: Simplified technique for tubeless hypotonic duodenography. Radiology 103:210, 1972.
10. Miller, R.E., Chernish, S.M., Greenman, G.F., et al.: Gastrointestinal response to minute doses of glucagon. Radiology 143:317, 1982.
11. Glick, S.N., Gohel, V.K., and Laufer, I.: Mucosal surface patterns of the duodenal bulb. Radiology 150:317, 1984.
12. Bova, J.G., Kamath, V., Tio, F.O., et al.: The normal mucosal surface pattern of the duodenal bulb: Radiologic-histologic correlation. AJR 145:735, 1985.
13. Nelson, J.A., Sheft, D.J., Minagi, H., et al.: Duodenal pseudopolyp: The flexural fallacy. AJR 123:262, 1975.
14. Burrell, M., and Toffler, R.: Flexural pseudolesions of the duodenum. Radiology 120:313, 1976.
15. Ferruci, J.T., Benedict, K.T., Page, D.L., et al.: The radiographic features of the normal hypotonic duodenogram. Radiology 96:401, 1970.
16. Stein, G.N., Martin, R.D., Roy, R.H., et al.: Evaluation of conventional roentgenologic techniques for demonstration of duodenal ulcer craters. AJR 91:801, 1964.
17. Rodriquez, H.P., Aston, J.K., and Richardson, C.T.: Ulcers in the descending duodenum: Postbulbar ulcers. AJR 119:316, 1973.
18. Sheppard, M.C., Holmes, G.K.T., and Cockel, R.: Clinical picture of peptic ulceration diagnosed endoscopically. Gut 18:524, 1977.
19. Eisenberg, R.L., Margulis, A.R., and Moss, A.A.: Giant duodenal ulcers. Gastrointest. Radiol. 2:347, 1978.
20. Braver, J.M., Paul, R.E., Philipps, E., et al.: Roentgen diagnosis of linear ulcers. Radiology 132:29, 1979.
21. de Roos, A., and Op den Orth, J.O.: Linear niches in the duodenal bulb. AJR 140:941, 1983.
22. Poplack, W., Paul, R.E., Goldsmith, M., et al.: Linear and rod-shaped peptic ulcers. Radiology 122:317, 1977.
23. Lubert, M., and Krause, G.R.: The "ring" shadow in the diagnosis of ulcer. AJR 90:767, 1963.
24. Kawai, K., Ida, K., Misaki, F., et al.: Comparative study for duodenal ulcer by radiology and endoscopy. Endoscopy 5:7, 1973.
25. Ball, R.P., Segal, A.L., and Golden, R.: Postbulbar ulcer of the duodenum. AJR 59:90, 1948.
26. Bilbao, M.K., Frische, L.H., Rosch, J., et al.: Postbulbar duodenal ulcer and ring-stricture. Radiology 100:27, 1971.
27. Nelson, S.W., and Christoforidis, A.J.: Roentgenologic features of the Zollinger-Ellison syndrome: Ulcerogenic tumor of the pancreas. Semin. Roentgenol. 3:254, 1968.
28. Thomson, W.O., Robertson, A.G., Imrie, C.W., et al.: Is duodenitis a dyspeptic myth? Lancet 1:1197, 1977.
29. Greenlaw, R., Sheehan, D.G., DeLuca, V., et al.: Gastroduodenitis: A broader concept of peptic ulcer disease. Dig. Dis. Sci. 25:660, 1980.
30. Katz, A.M.: Hemorrhagic duodenitis in myocardial infarction. Ann. Intern. Med. 51:212, 1959.
31. Baum, S., Ward, S., and Nusbaum, M.: Stress bleeding from the mid-duodenum: An often unrecognized source of gastrointestinal hemorrhage. Radiology 95:595, 1970.
32. Blakemore, W.S., Baum, S., and Nusbaum, M.: Diagnosis and management of massive hemorrhage from postoperative stress ulcers of the descending duodenum. Surg. Clin. North Am. 50:979, 1970.
33. Fraser, G.M., Pitman, R.G., Lawrie, J.H., et al.: The significance of the radiological finding of coarse mucosal folds in the duodenum. Lancet 2:979, 1964.
34. Wiener, S.N., Vertes, V., Shapiro, H.: The upper gastrointestinal tract in patients undergoing chronic dialysis. Radiology 92:110, 1969.
35. Zukerman, G.R., Mills, B.A., Koehler, R.E., et al.: Nodular duodenitis: Pathologic and clinical characteristics in patients with end-stage renal disease. Dig. Dis. Sci. 11:1018, 1983.
36. Catalano, D., and Pagliari, U.: Gastroduodenal erosions: Radiological findings. Gastrointest. Radiol. 7:235, 1982.
37. Gelfand, D.W., Dale, W.J., Ott, D.J., et al.: Duodenitis: Endoscopic-radiologic correlation in 272 patients. Radiology 157:577, 1985.
38. Levine, M.S., Turner, D., Ekberg, O., et al.: Duodenitis: A reliable radiologic diagnosis? Gastrointest. Radiol. 16:99, 1991.
39. Legge, D.A., Carlson, H.C., and Judd, E.S.: Roentgenologic features of regional enteritis of the upper gastrointestinal tract. AJR 110:355, 1970.
40. Thompson, W.M., Cockrill, H., and Rice, R.P.: Regional enteritis of the duodenum. AJR 123:252, 1975.
41. Marshak, R.H., Maklansky, D., Kurzban, J.D., et al.: Crohn's disease of the stomach and duodenum. Am. J. Gastroenterol. 77:340, 1982.
42. Danzi, J.T., Farmer, R.G., Sullivan, B.H., et al.: Endoscopic features of gastroduodenal Crohn's disease. Gastroenterology 70:9, 1976.
43. Ariyama, J., Wehlin, L., Lindstrom, C.G., et al.: Gastroduodenal erosions in Crohn's disease. Gastrointest. Radiol. 5:121, 1980.
44. Kelvin, F.M., and Gedgaudas, R.K.: Radiologic diagnosis of Crohn's disease (with emphasis on its early manifestations). CRC Crit. Rev. Diagn. Imaging 16:43, 1981.
45. Levine, M.S.: Crohn's disease of the upper gastrointestinal tract. Radiol. Clin. North Am. 25:79, 1987.
46. Jones, B., Bayless, T.M., Hamilton, S.R., et al.: "Bubbly" duodenal bulb in celiac disease: Radiologic-pathologic correlation. AJR 142:119, 1984.
47. Marn, C.S., Gore, R.M., and Ghahremani, G.G.: Duodenal manifestations of nontropical sprue. Gastrointest. Radiol. 11:30, 1986.
48. Weinberg, P.E., and Levin, B.: Hyperplasia of Brunner's glands. Radiology 84:259, 1965.
49. Govoni, A.F.: Benign lymphoid hyperplasia of the duodenal bulb. Gastrointest. Radiol. 1:267, 1976.
50. Ring, E.J., Ferruci, J.T., Eaton, S.B., et al.: Villous adenoma of the duodenum. Radiology 104:45, 1972.
51. Miller, J.H., Gisvold, J.J., Weiland, L.H., et al.: Upper gastrointestinal tract: Villous tumors. AJR 134:933, 1980.
52. Spira, I.A., and Wolff, W.I.: Villous tumors of the duodenum. Am. J. Gastroenterol. 67:63, 1977.
53. Bosse, G., and Neeley, J.A.: Roentgenologic findings in primary malignant tumors of the duodenum. AJR 170:111, 1969.
54. Blumgart, L.H., and Kennedy, A.: Carcinoma of the ampulla of vater and duodenum. Br. J. Surg. 60:33, 1973.
55. Balikian, J.P., Nassar, N.T., Shamma'a, M.H., et al.: Primary lymphomas of the small intestine including the duodenum. AJR 107:131, 1969.
56. Collins, S.M., Hamilton, J.D., Lewis, T.D., et al.: Small bowel malabsorption and gastrointestinal malignancy. Radiology 126:603, 1978.
57. Feldman, M., and Myers, P.: The roentgen diagnosis of prolapse of gastric mucosa into the duodenum. Gastroenterology 20:90, 1952.
58. Langkemper, R., Hoek, A.C., Dekker, W., et al.: Elevated lesions in the duodenal bulb caused by heterotopic gastric mucosa. Radiology 137:621, 1980.
59. Agha, F.P., Ghahremani, G.G., Tsang, T.K., et al.: Heterotopic gastric mucosa in the duodenum: Radiographic findings. AJR 150:291, 1988.

SMALL BOWEL

11

Hans Herlinger, M.D.

The small intestine, a winding tube of uncertain length and variable position within the abdomen, is an environment potentially hostile to ingested barium suspensions. A torrent of fluid that contains most substances present in plasma and about 250 g of shed epithelial cells pours into its lumen every day, most of it being continuously reabsorbed together with ingested materials.[1] Added to this are pancreatic secretions containing protein and electrolytes, gastric juices, and bile with pigments, salts, and mucus. In the fasting state this outpouring diminishes considerably, although there is still an estimated daily outflow that includes 10 to 25 ml of fat,[2] most of it reabsorbed. Little is known about the mucus that covers the whole of the mucosa.[3] In this environment even flocculation-resistant barium may occasionally flocculate in patients whose fecal fats are normal.[4]

Normal variation of bowel tone[5] and transit time[6] can affect the radiologic appearance of the mucosal surface, showing the valvulae conniventes either as circular bands surrounding a wider lumen or as a feathery pattern in the collapsed small bowel.

The variable appearance of the normal surface of the small bowel, coating difficulties due to gut contents, unpredictable transit time, and problems caused by overlap of loops have made it difficult to be confident either of normality or of the early changes in disease. Moreover, even the most carefully done small bowel studies produce a very low yield of organic disease. It is not surprising that many radiologists show little interest in the small bowel and that clinicians have been induced to accept, as sufficient radiodiagnostic effort, follow-through examinations based mostly on overview radiographs of barium-filled loops with the assurance that major pathology had not been revealed.

The purpose of this chapter is to describe an intubation method that produces a biphasic, single as well as double contrast form of lumen delineation. However, not every patient requires the intubation-based technique. An alternative method, the fluoroscopic follow-through, is briefly described and its limited indications are mentioned. Since the investigation of the duodenum forms part of the upper gastrointestinal barium routine, the term *small intestine* in the context of this chapter refers to the jejunum and ileum only. This chapter is concerned primarily with the examination of adolescents and adults. Nevertheless, the early recognition of small bowel disease is of special importance in children because it can be associated with growth retardation. A modified enteroclysis technique has been described for application in children.[7]

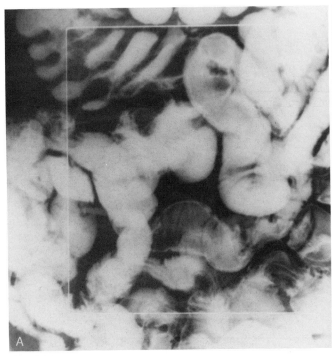
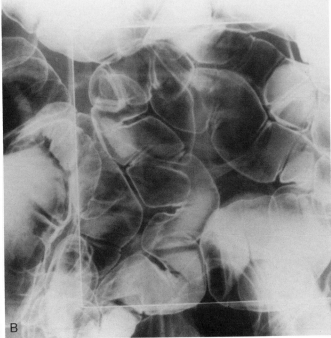

FIGURE 11–1

VALUE OF PERORAL PNEUMOCOLON. *A,* Spot film of distal ileum during a fluoroscopic follow-through examination has insufficient detail.

B, The peroral pneumocolon outlines the normal terminal ileum and distal ileum in excellent double contrast.

TECHNIQUES

Fluoroscopic Follow-Through

Since reliance on overhead films of barium-filled and overlapping loops of small bowel has been shown to result in missed lesions,[8] it is essential that repeated spot films be taken during fluoroscopy. Transit acceleration and type and quantity of barium used are important factors for success.

Metoclopramide accelerates gastric emptying and passage through the intestine and can be administered as two 10 mg tablets about 20 minutes before the barium.[9] At least 500 ml of barium at 40% w/v, such as Entrobar (E-Z-EM Co., Westbury, NY 11590) should be ingested. The upper gastrointestinal tract can be examined in single contrast, but the emphasis of this examination and of its clinical indications should be on the small bowel. Compression spot films are taken of most small bowel loops with the patient in suitable rotation. Attention should be paid to the mobility and pliability of such loops. Overhead views of the abdomen can be taken at intervals but serve mainly for orientation. Most examinations can be completed in 60 minutes.

Distal segments of ileum are often suboptimally shown by this method. The peroral pneumocolon can then usefully supplement the examination.

Limitations

Acceleration of small bowel transit is associated with a reduction of the lumen diameter. This method cannot, therefore, test the distensibility of the bowel. In the absence of lumen distention and the associated straightening of mucosal folds, this method does not allow for a confident diagnosis of morphologic normality.

Indications

The fact that intubation is not required constitutes the major advantage of the fluoroscopic follow-through over the small bowel enema (SBE). The fluoroscopic study may be used in the routine follow-up of known Crohn's disease; in the demonstration of the degree and level of an obstruction; and in the assessment of diseases that extend over longer segments of intestine, such as radiation enteritis.

Peroral Pneumocolon

Peroral pneumocolon (PNC) technique[10–12] can significantly improve detail and information quality in the distal ileum, cecum, and right colon. It follows the peroral barium examination of the small bowel and

is used after the ileum and cecum have become well opacified. An intravenous injection of 1 mg of glucagon is given. A small rectal catheter is then inserted, an insufflator is attached, and air is introduced with the patient supine. The patient is then turned to the left to fill the right colon with air. To get air into the terminal ileum, it may be necessary to turn the patient prone. After good distention has been achieved, compression spot films are taken of the areas of interest. Surprisingly good views can be obtained of the right colon and distal ileum (Fig. 11–1).

Double Contrast Enema

Excellent double contrast views of the terminal ileum can be obtained during the course of the double contrast enema. Reflux of air and barium into the terminal ileum is promoted by the use of intravenous glucagon. These views are particularly valuable for the diagnosis of early changes of Crohn's disease.

SMALL BOWEL ENEMA

A catheter, passed into the distal duodenum or first loop of jejunum, makes possible the introduction of contrast materials direct into the small bowel, bypassing the delaying and limiting action of the pylorus. The rate of injection influences both speed of transit and distention. This should be a biphasic examination. The barium suspension, later propelled by an infusion of methyl cellulose (MC), forms the single contrast phase. Gradually, the MC produces the required double contrast effect against a continuing barium coating of the mucosal surface. *Enteroclysis*, a term originally used for the single contrast intubation method, has now become virtually interchangeable with the term *SBE*, because both are biphasic and tend to use MC.

Historical Review

The history of the development of intubation techniques for the examination of the small bowel has previously been described in detail.[13] Important contributions were made by Cole,[14] Einhorn,[15] Pribram and Kleiber,[16] Pesquera,[17] Gershon-Cohen and Shay,[18] Schatzki,[19] and Lura.[20]

Earlier intubation had been made by means of an Einhorn or a Rehfuss tube; more easily managed types of tube now became available. In 1960, Scott-Harden[21] described a coaxial tube system with an outer catheter to be taken to the vicinity of the pylorus and a more pliable inner tube to advance into the duodenum. The long, 1.5-mm lumen inner tube allowed the introduction of only dilute barium, given in surpris-

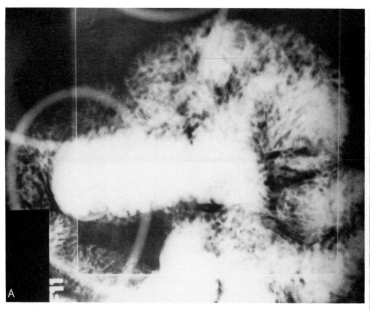

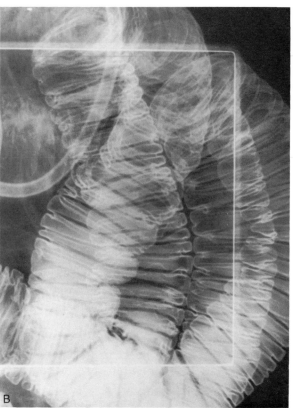

FIGURE 11–2

VALUE OF DISTENTION. *A*, Before infusion of methyl cellulose (MC), pseudonodules are produced by the intersection of superimposed folds in contracted loops.

B, Distention and double contrast demonstrate normal appearances without nodules.

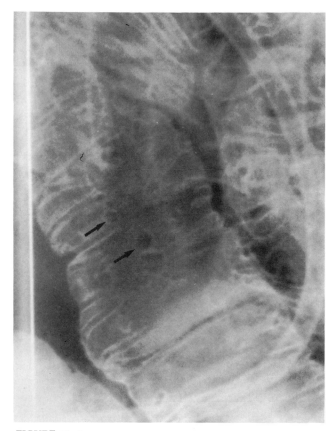

FIGURE 11–3

VALUE OF DOUBLE CONTRAST. Several small inflammatory polyps *(arrows)* are shown together with an interruption of mucosal folds. These are features of early Crohn's disease.

ingly small amounts and then flushed along with injected water.[22, 23] Intubation was further facilitated by Gianturco's[24] application of a modified Volkswagen speedometer cable to serve as a guide in a duodenal tube described by Bilbao and co-workers.[25]

The small bowel enema came of age with the publications of Sellink.[26–28] His method essentially consisted of the infusion of barium by gravity through a nasoduodenal tube. The density of the suspension was adjusted to the patient's body thickness, the whole small bowel was filled with an uninterrupted column, and the examination could be completed with the injection of water.

Most publications concerning the intubation examination of the small bowel have come from innovators and enthusiasts who have not critically questioned the clinical value of this more complex procedure. Fleckenstein and Pedersen[29] in 1975 were the first to report a series of small bowel enemas and follow-through examinations carried out in the same patients. In 52 evaluation pairs they considered the enema to be superior in the jejunum and upper ileum but found no significant difference in the terminal ileum. Sanders and Ho[30] were able to compare the conventional small bowel examination with the small bowel enema in 26 patients; the latter gave relevant additional information in 50% of their patients. In a comparison of the oral technique with the double contrast small bowel enema in 43 patients with Crohn's disease, intubation was found to demonstrate pathology more clearly and to delineate the proximal extension of disease more accurately.[31] Fistulae were shown equally well by both modalities. A more recent prospective comparison study confirmed the significantly greater accuracy of intubation-based examinations over peroral methods.[32]

Technical Considerations

Distention

Distention is an integral part of the SBE and is associated with a few disadvantages that are greatly outweighed by its benefits. Disadvantages are that dilatation is rendered less obvious as a sign of disease and that the small bowel is crowded into the peritoneal cavity. The advantages are that distention causes small bowel folds to straighten so that they can be assessed and measured. Misinterpretations can be avoided (Fig. 11–2); tiny surface alterations become visible (Fig. 11–3); and by testing distensibility, attention is drawn to even mildly narrowed or rigid segments (Fig. 11–4).

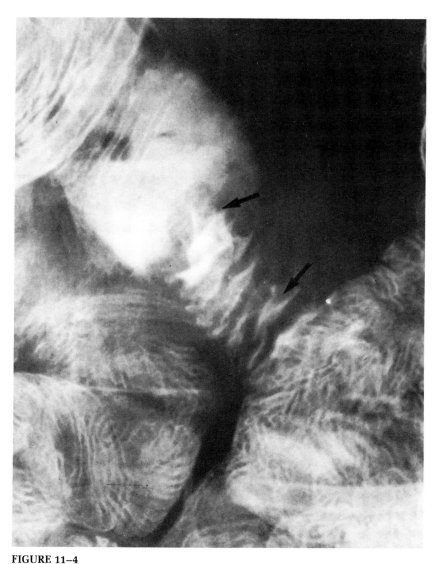

FIGURE 11–4

Short segment of early Crohn's disease in lower jejunum (*arrows*) presents a nondistensible lumen with swollen folds, readily identified against the distended bowel above. Such a lesion might not be recognized in a follow-through examination.

Transradiancy of Loops

Small bowel loops normally overlap within the abdominal cavity. This situation is aggravated when the loops are distended. When distended loops are filled with high-density barium, mucosal detail will be inadequate even when abdominal compression is applied. Transradiancy can be achieved by the use of barium of lower density together with a high kV technique. This forms the basis of single contrast enteroclysis. The double contrast method combines transradiancy, distention, and the demonstration of mucosal surface detail by barium coating even at the site of overlapping bowel loops (Fig. 11–5).

Double Contrast Agents

The double contrast effect requires that the barium mucosal coating be highlighted against a distending agent of lower density. Water and air have been the radiolucent agents most frequently used in the past.

Water

Sellink[22] often introduced 600 ml or more of water after barium had reached the distal ileum. This was found to produce distention of ileal loops at a desired level of contrast medium dilution. A true state of double contrast was confined to the jejunum, where it would persist for about 1 minute.

Recently infusion of water has again been recommended to achieve double contrast in the jejunum at the end of a single contrast enteroclysis; however, to prevent too rapid flushing of barium from the mucosal surface, the prior introduction of an additional amount of high-density barium was recommended.[33]

Air

Air should be the ideal double contrast medium because its density difference against barium is maximal and diffusion between them can never be a problem. Though well proved in the esophagus, stomach, and colon, air double contrast for the small bowel has presented problems in our hands.

1. Air does not propel barium through the small bowel. Rather, air percolates through the small bowel loops without advancing the barium, which remains in dependent pools, separated from the nondependent bowel wall.

2. As could be shown in the colon, a vertical x-ray beam may fail to demonstrate lesions submerged in a barium pool or may show them inadequately against a background of pooled barium. In the colon this can be corrected by taking opposing lateral decubitus views with a horizontal beam. This cannot be usefully applied to the small bowel, where the lateral decubitus position increases loop crowding and the alteration of loop distribution within the abdomen in response to position change would render orientation between decubitus film pairs an impossible task.

Nevertheless, the air double contrast method can produce the most subtle surface detail. This method is the best way to image the terminal ileum, whether air is introduced as part of a barium enema or as part of the peroral pneumocolon method.

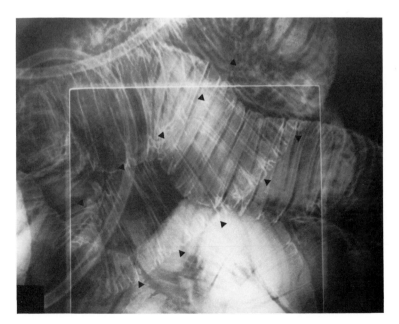

FIGURE 11–5

IMPORTANCE OF TRANSRADIANCY. Two superimposed segments of jejunum seen in double contrast (*arrowheads* outline one of the segments). Mucosal fold detail of both segments is clearly shown. Compression spot film.

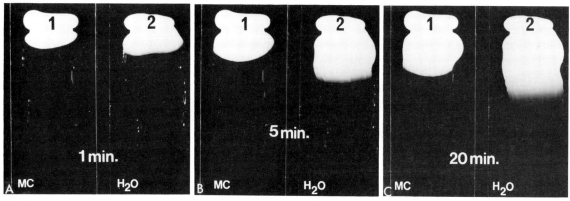

FIGURE 11-6

DIFFUSIVITY EXPERIMENT. Barium suspension that is MC-compatible has been placed at one end of slides 1 and 2. Slide 1 was then covered with 0.5% MC, and slide 2 with water in amounts sufficient to make contact with the barium. Both slides were left undisturbed and were photographed at intervals. A, At 1 minute, a sharp interface between barium and MC and barium and water is maintained, with no diffusion into the liquid.

B, At 5 minutes, there is lack of sharpness of the interface in slide 2, indicating early diffusion of barium into water.

C, At 20 minutes, there is increased diffusion on slide 2 while the interface between barium and MC in slide 1 has remained sharp.

Methyl Cellulose

Historical Review

Having found the "water flush" method[22, 23] to produce too much dilution of barium in the ileum, Trickey and co-workers[35] searched for a "flush" that would not readily mix with barium, that would be able to propel the barium toward the colon, and that would distend the lumen while rendering it radiolucent. They introduced a 0.7% solution of water containing hydroxyethylcellulose with a wetting agent, a proprietary preparation no longer available. A 1% suspension of methyl cellulose (MC) in water had been employed as a contrast agent for barium enemas,[36] with the claim that removal of barium coating from the bowel wall was minimized in this way. For their method of double contrast SBE, Gmuendner and Wirth[37] used a "flush" of 2 tsp of MC in 900 ml of water, following the injection of only 50 ml of Micropaque (Nicholas Laboratories, Slough, England).

Methyl Cellulose for the Small Bowel Enema

A 0.5% solution of MC in water is used as a double contrast agent for the SBE for the following reasons:

1. Used with compatible barium suspensions, such as Entero-H (E-Z-EM Co., Westbury, NY 11590), Micropaque liquid (Nicholas Laboratories, Slough, England) or Micropaque reconstituted powder (Picker Co., Cleveland, OH 44143), the MC solution shows a very low degree of diffusivity compared with that of water. This can be demonstrated on a slide test (Fig. 11–6) and, more important, confirmed by in vivo experience.

2. The MC solution efficiently propels an unbroken though gradually diluting barium column toward the cecum while maintaining an uninterrupted barium coating of the mucosal surface. Although the density difference from barium to MC cannot ap-

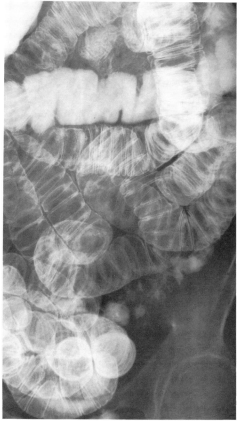

FIGURE 11-7

EFFECT OF MC ON THE SMALL BOWEL. An overhead film taken 20 minutes after the instillation of contrast shows a relaxed, coated small bowel even though barium has progressed to fill the colon.

proach that of barium to air, the MC method can produce excellent surface detail without interference by barium pools.

3. Small bowel loops distended with MC tend to remain in a state of relaxation or low activity and retain their double contrast pattern for 15 to 20 minutes (Fig. 11–7).

4. The combination of compatible barium and 0.5% MC has been shown to resist unacceptable degrees of flocculation long enough for the examination to be completed, even in severe cases of malabsorption (Fig. 11–8).

5. On entry into the colon the desiccation-resistant MC and barium mixture provoke rapid evacuation.

It is essential to use MC powder of correct viscosity, correctly prepared. We use methyl cellulose (US or BP) graded to produce a viscosity of 350 to 550 centistokes in a 2% solution at 20°C. We prepare this solution by adding 10 g of MC powder to about 400 ml of water at 85° to 90°C, stirring well until the powder is fully wetted and dispersed.[38] Cold water with ice cubes is then added, with continued stirring until a total quantity of 1.6 liters is reached and all dispersed powder is in solution. For immediate use, 400 ml of warm water should be added so that all the fluid is at room temperature. If not used immediately, it is important to keep the solution in a refrigerator because it lacks fungistatic activity. Before later use, warm water should be added as just described.

As an alternative to its preparation in the department, MC can be obtained ready made as 1% Methocel (E-Z-EM Co., Westbury, NY 11590), which needs to be diluted with an equal amount of water.

Barium Flocculation

Commercial barium preparations are held in suspension by additives that provide a protective coating to individual particles preventing particle-to-particle contact.[39] Nevertheless, even protected particles may flocculate in the presence of mucin or secretion from inflamed mucosa. In some cases, flocculation develops for no known reason. Flocculated barium does not provide a reliable image of the mucosal surface. A mild degree of flocculation appears as a granular pattern, whereas severe degrees of flocculation present patterns that reflect the physical chemical change in the barium rather than the mucosal surface ("segmentation," "moulage").

A direct relationship could be demonstrated in vitro among the degree of flocculation, the relative quantity of interacting fluids, and the duration of exposure to them.[40] In our experience the comparatively small quantities of barium intermittently leaving the stomach in a follow-through examination and passing rather slowly through the small intestine are readily overwhelmed by small bowel contents in even moderate cases of steatorrhea. In the SBE the larger quantity of barium introduced almost as a bolus and pushed along rapidly is usually able to coat the mucosa and produce images before any flocculation develops.[41]

Laws and co-workers[4] have been able to show lack of correlation between the degree of flocculation and the degree of steatorrhea or villous atrophy. In fact, patients passing as much as 20 g of fat per day did not have flocculation, whereas others with normal fat contents did. Although flocculation eventually occurs even with SBE in the presence of abnormal fluid material, the longer it is delayed, the higher the probability of adequate imaging of the small bowel. Information on morphologic normality or disease can thus be obtained (see Fig. 11–8).

Patient Preparation

We agree that a clean right colon is important.[17, 27] The presence of feces in the right colon is often associated with the presence of similar material in the terminal ileum and tends to retard the passage of barium. It increases the amount of barium required for the examination because the distal ileum has to be cleared of debris before useful double contrast can be achieved.[39]

Whenever possible, the preparation should consist of a non-residue liquid diet the day before the examination and four bisacodyl (Dulcolax) tablets in the afternoon. No further food or fluid is allowed until the examination has been completed. The reduction of normal fluid and cell outpouring into the small bowel lumen as a result of diet restriction[1] improves the quality of the examination. Drugs that decrease bowel activity should be discontinued until after the examination.

Except in cases of high-grade obstruction, we ask the patient to take 20 mg of metoclopramide (two 10-mg tablets) 20 minutes before starting the SBE.[40] Preliminary sedation with midazolam (Versed), 1 to 2 mg given intravenously, is now used for the more apprehensive patients when someone is available to accompany them home.

Intubation

Local anesthesia is given either to the throat as a 20% benzocaine spray (for peroral intubation) or to the nasal passages as 2% lidocaine viscous gel (for transnasal intubation). We now prefer to use a 13F catheter with a balloon and side holes distal to it (Maglinte/Herlinger catheter, E-Z-EM Co., Westbury, NY 11590). A Teflon-coated, rotationally rigid guide wire with a curved tip can be advanced to the closed end of the catheter. The balloon can be inflated with up to 20 ml of air and serves to control reflux from the jejunum or duodenum. Before use, the catheter system should be lubricated inside and out with a silicone spray. The integrity of the balloon should be tested before it is introduced.

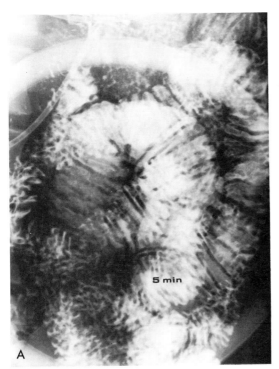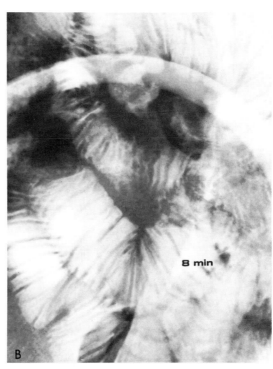

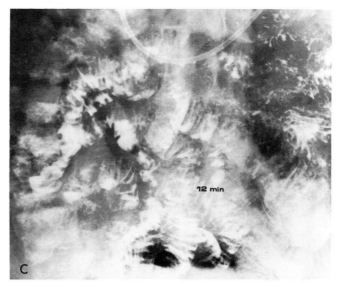

FIGURE 11–8

EFFECT OF TIME ON BARIUM FLOCCULATION IN CELIAC DISEASE.

A, At 5 minutes, adequate imaging of the jejunum is seen.

B, At 8 minutes, ileal detail is still shown to acceptable standard.

C, At 12 minutes, flocculation is pronounced; imaging is no longer possible.

With the patient sitting on the x-ray examination table, the catheter is introduced until slight resistance is felt, indicating that the fundus or body of the stomach has been reached. The patient is then turned supine and the position of the catheter is checked by fluoroscopy. A routine method of intubation and some of its variations are illustrated in Figures 11–9 through 11–12.

We aim to position the level of the balloon of the tube either in the fourth part of the duodenum or beyond the duodenojejunal junction. The balloon is then inflated and infusion of contrast materials can commence (Fig. 11–13).

Several problems may be encountered during the course of intubation.

Catheter Coiled in the Fundus. The tube is withdrawn until its tip lies at the cardia. The guide is then introduced fully and the patient is turned to the right. The outer end of the guide is bent over to make it possible to rotate it and direct the catheter into the body of the stomach (see Fig. 11–9). The catheter is then advanced over the guide wire.

Catheter Doubled Back in the Antrum. When advancing the catheter toward the pylorus, the guide is held back at the level of the angulus. The gloved hand applies craniad pressure to the greater curvature of the antrum to form a caudad concavity of the catheter to aid its passage through the pylorus and the superior duodenal flexure. At times this fails and the catheter doubles back within the stomach. The catheter is then withdrawn slowly while the guide is advanced until the tube end flicks forward again (see Fig. 11–10).

Catheter Held Up at the Pylorus. By rotating the patient well to the left, air normally present in the stomach frequently outlines the position of the duodenal bulb. Then it is usually possible, either by simply advancing the tube or by taking the wire to the tip of the tube and turning its curved end, to enter the duodenum (see Fig. 11–11). Rotation of the patient to the left helps by widening the occasionally tight superior duodenal flexure. Rarely it may be necessary to remove the guide wire and inject a bolus of air with the patient still turned well to the left. Air

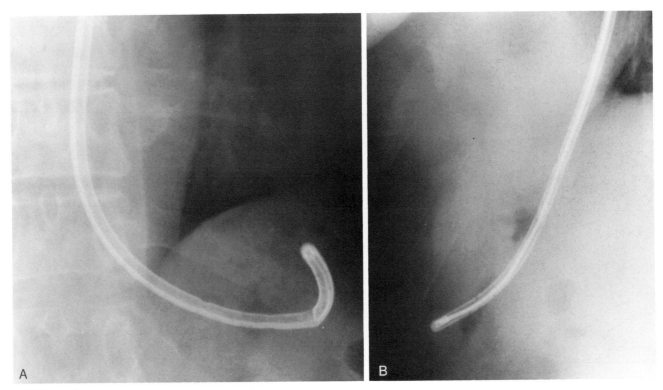

FIGURE 11–9

INTUBATION TECHNIQUE. A, Tube introduced with the patient sitting has coiled in the gastric fundus.

B, The patient is turned sharply to the right, the tube is pulled back to the cardia, and the wire is advanced and rotated toward the body of the stomach. Tube and wire can then be introduced further.

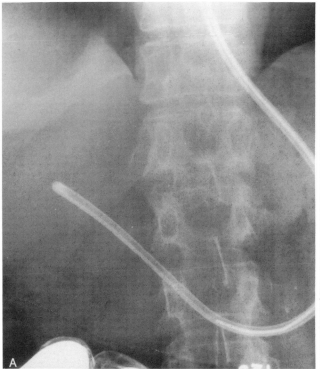

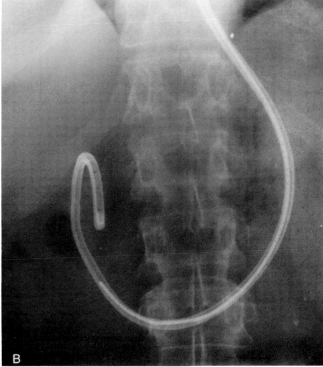

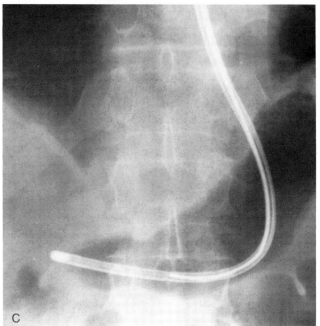

FIGURE 11–10

Intubation (continues description of technique begun in Fig. 11–9 legend). *A,* The tube now approaches the pylorus, the wire is held back, and gloved-hand pressure is applied to produce a downward concavity of the tube to help its advance through the bulb and upper flexure of the duodenum.

B, This attempt failed, and the tube folded back into the gastric antrum.

C, The catheter was withdrawn somewhat, and the wire was advanced to straighten the tube again.

Catheter Through the Duodenojejunal Junction. After the catheter has reached the expected position of the duodenojejunal junction, the patient is turned left or right laterally and then slightly farther toward a posterior oblique position. This allows the first loop of jejunum to fall forward from the retroperitoneally fixed duodenum and widens the flexure. The patient is also asked to take deep breaths and to cough while the tube is slowly advanced with the guide wire held back at the upper or lower duodenal flexure (see Fig. 11–12). The final position of the catheter is confirmed with the patient supine, and the balloon can be inflated (see Fig. 11–13). If the progress of the catheter is arrested at an unexpected level, it is important to investigate the cause by injecting a small amount of barium. In one patient a duodenal leiomyoma was discovered in this way. (For greater detail regarding intubation methods and problems, see reference 41.)

excites peristalsis and outlines the pyloric area, thus showing and promoting the way out of the stomach.

Catheter Stopped at the Inferior Duodenal Flexure. If possible, the guide is advanced beyond the superior flexure. Pressure by the gloved hand helps the end of the catheter round the retroperitoneally fixed inferior flexure.

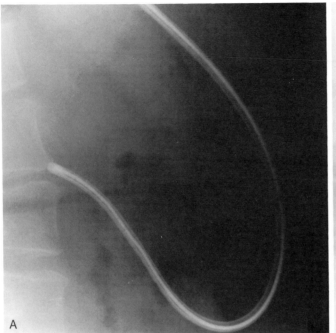

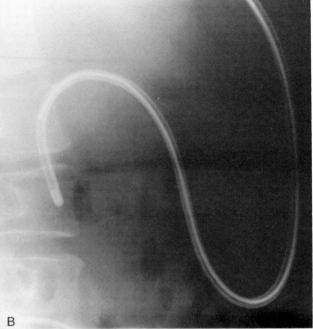

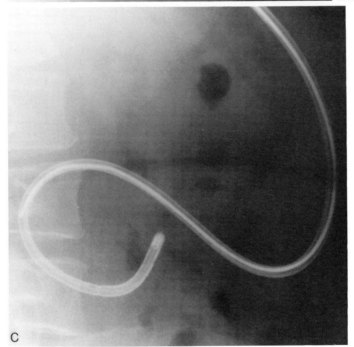

FIGURE 11–11

Intubation (continues description of technique begun in Fig. 11–9 legend). *A,* The patient is now turned to the left, the wire is taken to the end of the tube, and the tip of the tube is bent into the usually visible duodenal bulb and upper flexure.

B, The wire is held at the flexure, and the catheter is advanced over it.

C, The tube continues to move into the ascending duodenum.

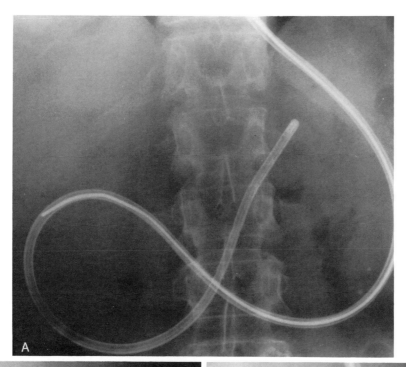

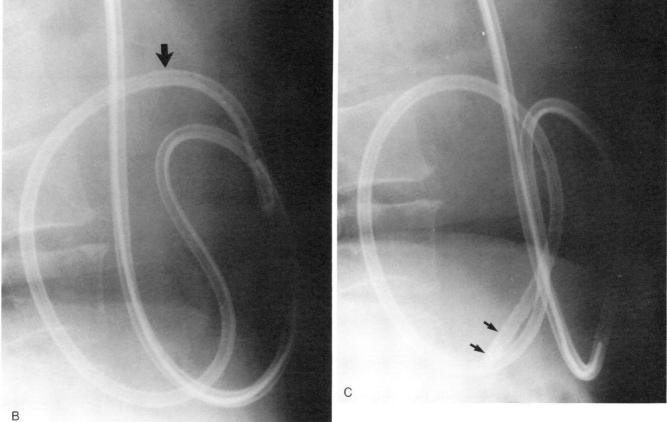

FIGURE 11–12

Intubation (continues description of technique begun in Fig. 11–9 legend). *A,* The tip of the tube approaches the duodenojejunal flexure.
　B, The patient is turned fully to the left and is asked to breathe deeply while the tube continues its advance into the jejunum (*arrow* at duodenojejunal flexure).
　C, The tube has now entered far enough into the jejunum (*arrows* mark end of tube).

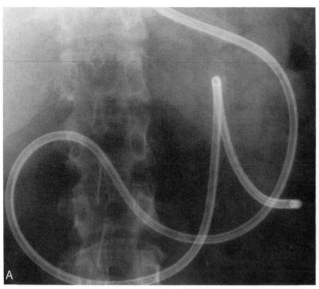
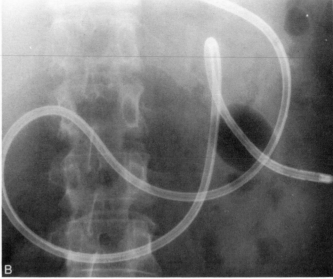

FIGURE 11–13

Intubation (continues description of technique begun in Fig. 11–9 legend). *A,* The patient is placed supine to confirm the correct position of the tube.

   B, The balloon of the catheter is now inflated with 20 ml of air. The balloon is situated beyond the ligament of Treitz.

Barium Injection

We use 60-ml syringes for the injection of the barium suspension, either Entero-H at 80% w/v or Micropaque at 85% w/v. A total of 180 to 200 ml is normally injected, somewhat less when the patient is very thin or has had a small bowel resection; more when the patient is stout or when the diagnostic problem relates to the distal ileum. Considerably more barium may have to be given (up to 400 ml) if there is small bowel dilatation with fluid excess (Fig. 11–14).

Barium should not be injected at a rate that will cause undue jejunal distention because this may delay forward flow. The aim is to achieve forward movement of an uninterrupted column of barium. We normally turn patients halfway to the left during barium injection to delay the entry into ileal loops. If the barium column stops advancing, the patient may be turned prone, because peristaltic activity usually improves in this position.

Patients with bowel atony due to neuromuscular disease or prolonged obstruction are a special problem. Overinjection and overdistention of the jejunum is to be avoided. Instead, careful turning of the patient may promote onward flow of the heavier barium even through fluid-filled loops.

Methyl Cellulose Infusion

The 0.5% solution of methyl cellulose (MC) is best infused by an electric pump, which assures a steady inflow at an accurately adjustable rate, usually be-

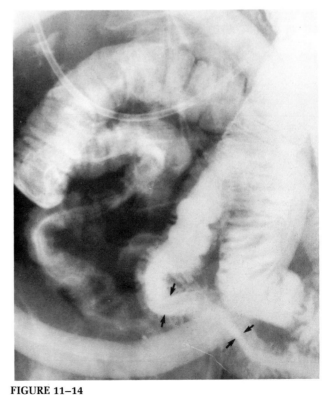

FIGURE 11–14

EVIDENCE OF EXCESS FLUID. Streaming of barium (*arrows*) and increasing barium dilution indicate excess fluid. A larger than usual amount of barium is required in such cases.

tween 70 and 110 ml/min. This is continued until sufficient transradiancy and distention have been achieved in the distal and terminal ileum. If progress is too rapid and distention is inadequate, the rate of inflow of MC should be increased to cause proximal jejunal distention with its slowing effect on the more distal bowel loops.

Normally up to 2 liters of MC are injected. If barium reaches the sigmoid and rectum before adequate transradiancy has been attained in the distal small bowel (transit in the colon is rapid), a barium enema–type catheter may be inserted into the rectum and its contents gradually siphoned into an attached empty enema bag.

The balloon of the catheter must be deflated before it is withdrawn. In certain circumstances such as occult bleeding, we withdraw the catheter into the duodenum and inject barium. It is also possible to take the catheter back into the stomach and carry out a limited double contrast study of the stomach and duodenum, although barium in the transverse colon often interferes with this examination.

Filming

Although we observe the progress and appearance of the barium column by intermittent fluoroscopy and abdominal compression—the single contrast phase— we do not usually expose films unless an abnormality is seen or suspected. More frequent films are taken in the double contrast phase, usually with compression. It is, however, important to compress and release compression gradually to avoid forcible mixing of barium and MC, which would lead to dilution of

barium and negate the double contrast result. The patient should also be instructed to turn slowly or slide gently when changing position.

The jejunum and upper ileum are usually shown with the patient turned slightly to the right (Figs. 11–15 and 11–16); the more distal ileum is shown with the patient turned to the left. The demonstration of the terminal ileum can be a problem. Because the accumulation of barium in the cecum may interfere with visualization, it may be important to film the terminal ileum during the passage of the first bolus into the cecum (Fig. 11–17). A valuable part of the examination can be the observation of peristaltic activity, best seen before distention with MC. It is also important to carefully palpate all accessible loops. We particularly evaluate the mobility of loops to identify any adhesive processes and their pliability, that is, the ability to change shape in response to compression. Mural infiltration stiffens loops and reduces or abolishes pliability.

A prone overhead view on a 14/17 film (Fig. 11–18) and often a film angled 30 degrees caudad (Fig. 11–19B) are taken at the end of the fluoroscopic examination. In cases of obstruction or in adynamic states, it may be necessary to follow up with later spot and overhead films. Such an examination may have to continue intermittently for as long as 24 hours.

A successful SBE presents the whole of the small bowel in double contrast, with the density difference between barium on the mucosa and the MC in the lumen often showing a gradual but slight decrease in the distal ileum. It gives measurable evidence of normality or of disease.

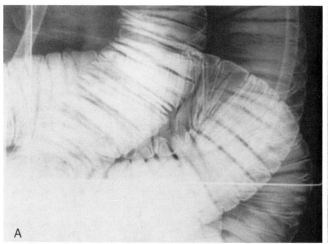 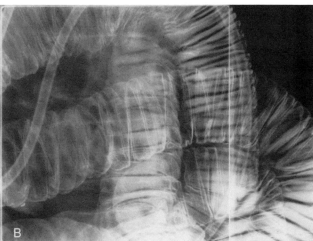

FIGURE 11–15

DEVELOPMENT OF DOUBLE CONTRAST IN PROXIMAL JEJUNUM. *A,* Proximal jejunum in single contrast.
B, Same segments in double contrast after infusion of MC.

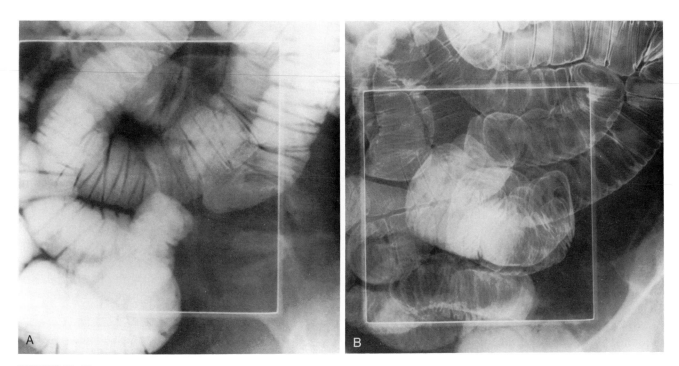

FIGURE 11–16

DOUBLE CONTRAST DEVELOPMENT IN MID–SMALL BOWEL. *A*, Mid–small bowel in single contrast.
  B, Same segments in double contrast.

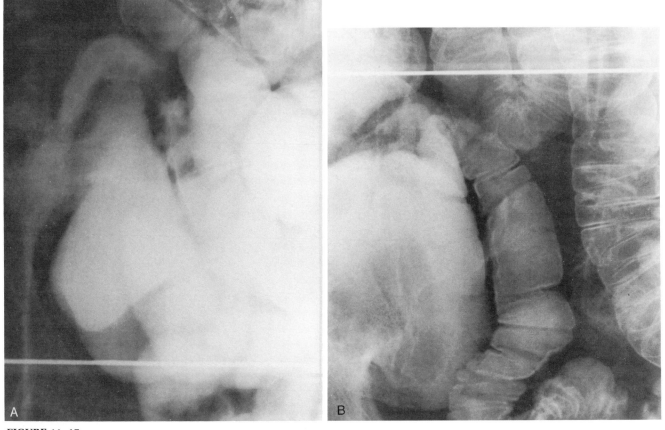

FIGURE 11–17

DEVELOPMENT OF DOUBLE CONTRAST IN TERMINAL ILEUM. *A*, Area of terminal ileum in single contrast.
  B, Same area in double contrast.

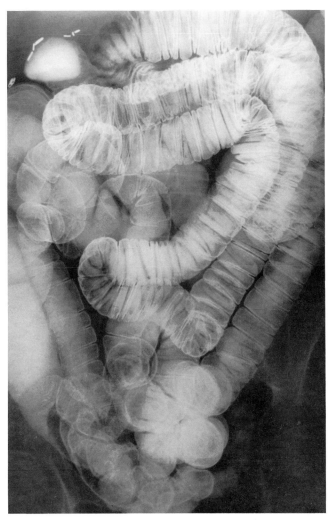

FIGURE 11–18

COMPLETION OF FLUOROSCOPIC EXAMINATION. A final prone overhead image is obtained.

Problems of Examination

Misjudged Quantities. If too little barium has been introduced, visualization of the distal ileum suffers and MC may actually overtake the barium column. It is then difficult to salvage the examination, although an attempt should be made to inject an additional quantity of barium before resuming the infusion of MC. If too much barium has been given, filling of the colon may occur before double contrast has extended into the distal ileum. Barium in the rectosigmoid may then have to be evacuated, as suggested earlier. If in doubt regarding the amount of barium to be given, it is better to give too much than too little.

Reflux Into the Stomach. Reflux of methyl cellulose was a more serious problem before balloon catheters became available. Occasionally reflux may still occur even with an inflated balloon, especially when the balloon has been inflated in the duodenum. The rate of injection of MC must then be reduced and the patient turned well to the left during injection. However, slowing the injection of MC necessarily causes less adequate distention of bowel loops and compromises the quality of the examination. Massive reflux can be dangerous to older or enfeebled patients because aspiration into the lung may follow. It is important to watch out for this complication, stop the examination, and aspirate stomach contents if it has occurred.

Ileal Loops in the Pelvis. Patients ought to be advised not to empty the bladder immediately before the examination. Not infrequently, however, especially after hysterectomy, ileal loops can be found lying deep in the pelvis, inaccessible to compression. For a successful examination it is then necessary to extend double contrast throughout these ileal loops and to take spot films of the pelvis with the patient in lateral or off-lateral positions (see Fig. 11–19A). The prone-angled view is also helpful (see Fig. 11–19B).

Small Bowel Enema Through a Long Intestinal Tube

Patients in whom a long intestinal tube, such as a Miller-Abbott (MA) tube, has been inserted in the clinical management of small bowel obstruction may require a barium study to demonstrate the level, degree, and cause of the obstructing lesion. The MA tube can be used for the introduction of contrast material provided that attention is given to the following points.

A. The tip of the tube should reach fairly close to the expected level of obstruction. At the very least it

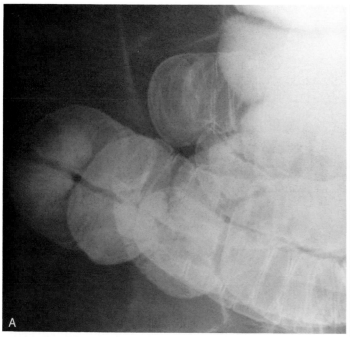

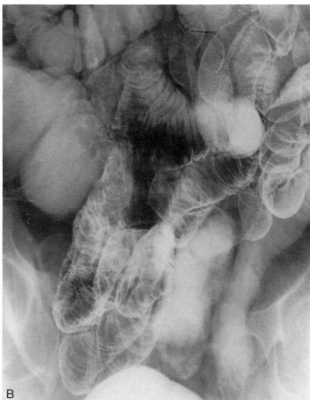

FIGURE 11–19

PROBLEM OF BOWEL LOOPS PROLAPSED DEEP INTO THE PELVIS. *A,* Good mucosal detail is obtained by taking a lateral or off-lateral view of pelvis after full double contrast development in prolapsed bowel loops.

B, A caudad angled prone film can be useful.

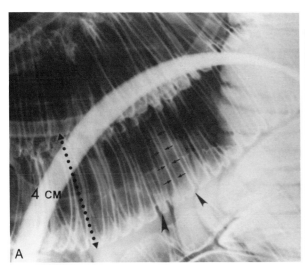 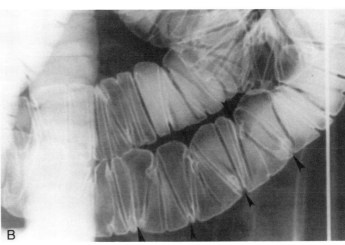

FIGURE 11–20

NORMAL APPEARANCES: FOLD PATTERNS. *A*, Straightened mucosal folds form slightly rounded corners at their junctions with the bowel wall *(arrowheads)*. Normal lumen diameter of the jejunum is indicated by *dots* and normal thickness of straight folds by *arrows*.
  B, Triangular fold patterns in a normal ileum *(arrowheads)*.

must reach 6 inches into the jejunum to insure that all its side holes are beyond the ligament of Treitz.

  B. The balloon, if inflated, must be emptied.

  C. Whenever possible, enough barium should be introduced to reach the site of obstruction. A maximum amount of 400 ml should not be exceeded.

  D. MC infusion is begun only after barium has reached the obstructing lesion or after as much as 400 ml of barium has failed to get to that level (however, see an earlier note on the careful introduction of barium in patients with bowel atony). In the absence of bowel atony, an infusion of MC can be started to try to propel the barium onward. Whenever possible, the object is to produce double contrast at the obstruction site and reach a more accurate diagnosis of the nature of the obstructing lesion. In the presence of excessive amounts of retained fluid in distended bowel loops, however, the addition of MC would serve little purpose and the examination may have to be continued as a follow-through study with delayed

filming. (For further reading on all aspects of the SBE technique, see reference 42.)

Normal Appearances

The combination of distention, double contrast, and abdominal compression makes it possible to study the shape of folds and to measure several parameters.

Fold Shape. Valvulae conniventes are found throughout the small bowel but can be less pronounced or absent in the ileum. With the bowel distended, these folds run fairly straight across the long axis, their sides parallel, joining the bowel wall in the form of "rounded corners" (Fig. 11–20*A*).[28] At times, more often in the ileum, a few of the folds crowd together on the concave side of a bend in a bowel loop. Such triangular fold patterns can be found even in straight segments of ileum, when their direction of convergence is seen to alternate (Fig. 11–20*B*).

Fold Thickness. Folds are normally slightly thicker in the nondistended bowel and become thinner with distention. In distended loops, jejunal folds are normally up to 1.8 mm thick, and ileal folds are up to 1.5 mm thick (Fig. 11–21). Fold thickness is considered pathologic when it exceeds 2.5 mm in the distended jejunum and 2.0 mm in the distended ileum.

Number of Folds. In the more distended, possibly somewhat elongated small bowel as seen in this form of SBE, the number of circular folds per inch of length was found to be less than previously reported by Sellink.[28] We have found four to seven folds per inch in the distended proximal jejunum (Fig. 11–22A) and two to five folds per inch in the more distal ileum (see Fig. 11–21B). In the occasional patient in whom small bowel tone appears to be increased, particularly in young persons, a greater number of folds was seen in what appeared to be shortened bowel.

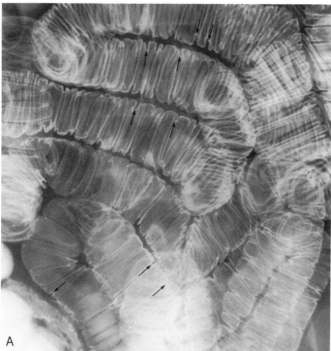

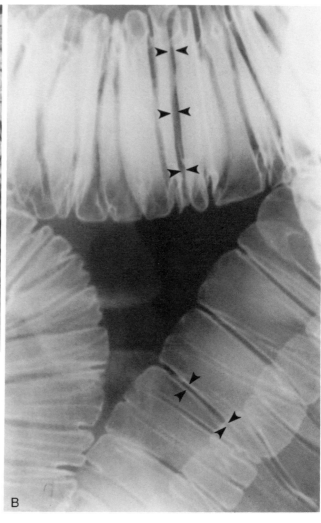

FIGURE 11–21

NORMAL FOLD THICKNESS AND HEIGHT. *A,* Overview of a small bowel study. Fold thickness, height, and luminal diameter gradually diminish from jejunum to ileum. Profile views of fold height are indicated by *arrows.*

B, A close-up view of a segment of jejunum above and proximal ileum below shows their normal fold thicknesses *(arrowheads).*

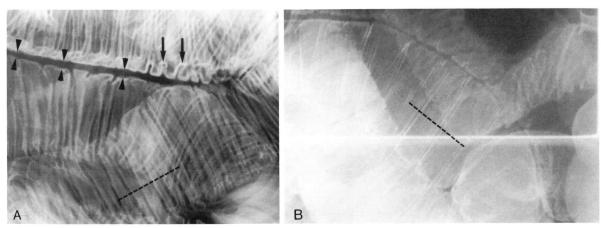

FIGURE 11–22

NORMAL APPEARANCES. *A*, A segment of jejunum illustrating normal fold height *(arrows)*. Fold density is illustrated by the 1-inch *interrupted line*, which crosses seven folds. The *arrowheads* outline an area of apposition of two segments of bowel. The distance between the two mucosal surfaces therefore represents their combined bowel wall thickness.

   B, A segment of ileum showing only three folds per inch *(interrupted line)*.

Fold Height. Jejunum and ileum also differ significantly in the height of folds, which usually varies from 3 to 7 mm in the jejunum and from 1.5 to 3.5 mm in the ileum. The decrease in height occurs gradually in a caudad direction (see Fig. 11–21). However, fold height may vary considerably within the same segment of bowel.

Lumen Diameter. Because of the lumen distention of the SBE, diameters for the upper jejunum are from 3.0 to 4.0 cm, from 2.5 to 3.5 cm in the lower jejunum, and from 2.0 to 2.8 cm in the ileum (see Figs. 11–20 and 11–21). Diameters are considered abnormal when they exceed 4.5 cm in the upper jejunum, 4.0 cm in the mid-small bowel, and 3.0 cm in the ileum. Diameters should not be measured in front of a wave of contraction.

Wall Thickness. Wall thickness can be measured if two barium-coated luminal surfaces are seen to be parallel over at least 4 cm on a film taken with abdominal compression. We then consider the loops to lie in the same plane and regard the distance between the two mucosal surfaces to represent the combined thickness of the two bowel walls. Half this measurement then gives the thickness of a single bowel loop (see Fig. 11–22A). Of normal patients, 75% showed a wall thickness of 1.0 to 1.5 mm, 12.5% showed a thickness of 1.5 to 2.0 mm, and 12.5% showed a thickness below 1 mm. This measurement was found to be the same throughout the small bowel. A wall thickness greater than 2 mm is considered abnormal.

Length of the Small Bowel. No accurate estimate can be made of this three-dimensional reality of the small bowel on the basis of two-dimensional x-ray films. There is no doubt that length of bowel varies greatly according to the individual. Muscle tone is likely to be an important factor. Withdrawing an MA tube under x-ray control has shown that approximately two thirds of it can be pulled back through an increasingly telescoping gut before the tip of the tube even begins to move.

Variations and Anomalies

Malrotation. Malrotation is the most common anomaly occurring in the second stage of re-entry into the abdominal cavity. This process can be arrested at any stage. If there is no rotation at all, the mesenteric small bowel is situated on the right side of the abdomen. Symptoms may then be produced by bands extending from the medially placed right colon to the right lateral abdominal wall.

Anomalies of Fixation. Premature fixation of the cecum occurs frequently. More commonly, there is a freely mobile cecum with its own mesentery. It may be found folded upward, in which case the terminal ileum appears to enter from below and from the right. Such a cecum may also prolapse into the pelvis, where it fills with barium and obscures the terminal ileum.

Lymph Follicles. Numerous 2- to 3-mm rounded elevations scattered over an otherwise normal mucosa can be found in the terminal ileum (Fig. 11–23); these extend more proximally in children and in some

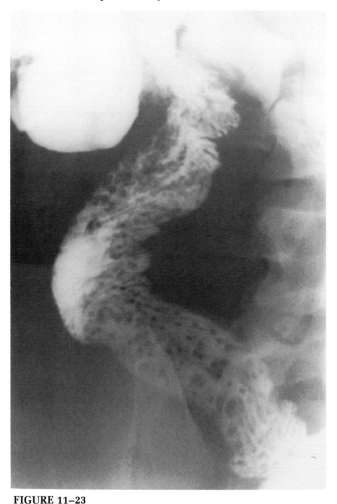

FIGURE 11–23

LYMPH FOLLICLES IN THE TERMINAL ILEUM. The elevations, each 2 to 3 mm in diameter, are distributed fairly evenly against a background of normal mucosa.

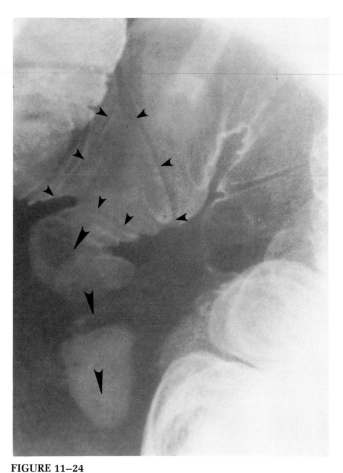

FIGURE 11–24

MECKEL'S DIVERTICULUM. A 5-cm-long diverticulum (*large arrowheads*) arises at the antimesenteric aspect of a loop of ileum. A triangular fold pattern (*small arrowheads*) outlines a mucosal plateau at the origin of the diverticulum.

adults. These follicles become particularly prominent in patients with immune deficiency.

SMALL BOWEL ENEMA IN DISEASE

Examples rather than complete descriptions of disease processes are presented here. The purpose is to show the versatility and increased accuracy of the double contrast method and its relevance to clinical management.

Meckel's Diverticulum

Meckel's diverticulum is found in 1% to 3% of autopsies. Its demonstration by follow-through barium examination has been infrequent. It is a true diverticulum arising from the antimesenteric border of the ileum within 90 cm of the ileocecal valve (Fig. 11–24). The SBE is the most reliable method for its demonstration in the adult.[43]

Malabsorption States

The term "malabsorption" refers to the failure of transport of digested or maldigested nutrients as well as of vitamins and minerals from the gut into body fluids. Most generalized small bowel diseases are accompanied by a degree of malabsorption, which may be accentuated by actual loss of nutrients in increased secretions. The disturbance of absorption is usually multifactorial, although in mild forms of even generalized small bowel disease it may be limited to selected materials. More localized disease affects only substances that are normally absorbed at those levels. In most conditions, steatorrhea, the disturbance of fat absorption, is the distinctive clinical marker of malabsorption. Secondary immunodeficiencies may accompany malabsorption states.

Pattern recognition based x-ray diagnosis is not often possible in the small bowel, and is even less likely in malabsorption states. It is therefore necessary to be aware of and to be able to evaluate a patient's clinical presentation to relate x-ray findings to this background.

Clinical Diagnosis

The amount of fat excreted is expressed as grams per day. Reported upper limits of normality vary between 5 and 12 g.[44, 45] The fact that fecal fat content varies with the amount of dietary fat ingested may explain this considerable difference. According to Losowsky and co-workers,[1] a fat excretion of 7% of intake would express the upper limit of normality more accurately. However, quantitative fecal fat analyses are now not often requested, and a qualitative fecal fat test is often used instead. More widely used in patients believed to have impairment of fat absorption is the ^{14}C-triolein breath analysis. A positive test does not, however, give information as to cause or site of the underlying abnormality. A positive D-xylose absorption test would indicate more proximal intestinal mucosal disease as a cause for steatorrhea. The same test would also be useful in patients with intestinal bacterial overgrowth when it may also be supplemented by a hydrogen breath test.

Mucosal biopsies are the most important method for positive diagnosis in many conditions presenting with malabsorption. Until recently, perorally passed tubes using a suction technique had been the standard method for obtaining biopsies. Endoscopic sampling has now largely replaced it and has the added advantage of direct visualization of the biopsy site. However, endoscopic biopsies are mostly taken in the duodenum rather than the proximal jejunum, which is the predominant site of the majority of the pathologies.

To simplify radiologic diagnosis, several authors have presented lists of x-ray findings in steatorrhea.[46–48] The list presented here is based on the increased imaging accuracy of the SBE (Table 11–1).

TABLE 11–1. Small Bowel Enema in Malabsorption States

X-ray Feature	No Fluid Increase	Fluid Increase
Folds of normal thickness	Maldigestion—pancreatic enzyme or bile salt deficiency; gastric surgery; alactasia	Adult celiac disease and dermatitis herpetiformis (fold separation in proximal jejunum); tropical sprue
Dilatation of lumen	Scleroderma (hide-bound bowel sign); dermatomyositis; amyloidosis	Celiac disease; obstruction; pseudo-obstruction; jejunal diverticulosis (fluid in diverticula)
Folds, thickened, straight	Radiation enteropathy; eosinophilic enteritis; macroglobulinemia	Edema (including celiac disease hypoalbuminemia); Zollinger-Ellison syndrome (duodenum mostly); abetalipoproteinemia; giardiasis (increased irritability)
Folds, uneven, thickened, nodular	Amyloidosis; lymphoma; extensive Crohn's disease (ulceration); Whipple's disease (1–3 mm nodules); mastocytosis (gastric antrum)	Lymphangiectasia (1–3 mm grouped nodules); giardiasis (if associated IgA deficiency); Whipple's disease (infrequently)
Other structural lesions	Stasis and bacterial overgrowth associated with strictures, blind loop, blind pouch, diverticulosis, pseudo-obstruction, short bowel syndrome	

Role of Radiology

Clinical awareness that a state of malabsorption exists should precede referral for a SBE. The purpose of radiology is to demonstrate or at least suggest a cause for malabsorption. It is important to defer the possible onset of flocculation so that mucosal surfaces can be imaged in sufficient detail. The technique of the SBE needs to be slightly modified:

1. The balloon of the catheter should be inflated in the fourth part of the duodenum to include the entire duodenojejunal flexure in the imaging process.

2. More barium is infused at a slightly higher rate of flow.

3. Compression spot films are taken early during the infusion of MC, without waiting for full development of double contrast.

It should be a rare event for radiology to suggest the presence of a clinically unsuspected malabsorption state on the basis of flocculation of barium, an unreliable sign.

Celiac Disease

Clinical Diagnosis

The clinical diagnosis of celiac disease can be difficult because not every patient presents with steatorrhea. An increasing number of patients show atypical or minimal features, such as only hematologic abnormalities in 38% of diagnosed cases.[49] Essential to definitive diagnosis is the demonstration of subtotal villous atrophy in the jejunum or, somewhat less adequately, in the duodenum. There should also be clinical and histologic return to normality after a period of gluten withdrawal.

Radiologic Findings

The SBE can play an important diagnostic function, especially in cases with atypical clinical presentation. In 75% of patients with adult celiac disease, there is a wider than normal separation of mucosal folds in the distended proximal jejunum. A finding of three or fewer folds over the length of 1 inch is highly diagnostic of celiac disease (Fig. 11–25A), whereas

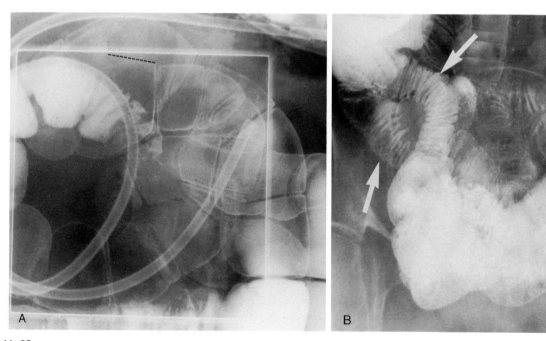

FIGURE 11–25

CELIAC DISEASE. *A*, Separation of folds. The 1-inch *interrupted line* touches only one fold. Two folds, at most, would be crossed if the line had been placed elsewhere. This finding is characteristic of celiac disease.

B, Ileal folds are crowded and slightly thicker than those normally seen in the ileum (*arrows*). This appearance has been termed "jejunization" of the ileum.[51]

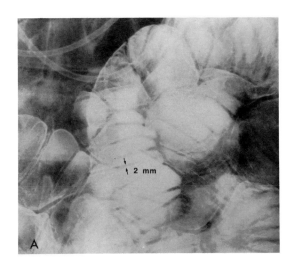

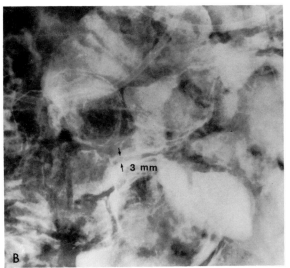

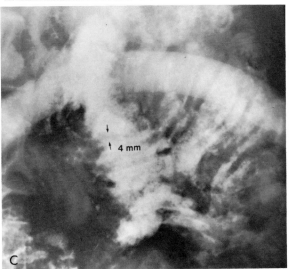

FIGURE 11–26

Misleading impression of fold thickening in active celiac disease. *A,* Initial film shows straight jejunal folds *(arrows)* that measure only 2 mm in thickness.

B, A few minutes later, the same fold *(arrows)* appears to be 3 mm thick.

C, Later still, the fold outline *(arrows)* has become unsharp and uneven, with a thickness of 4 mm. This apparent thickening has been caused by accumulation of secretions between mucosa and barium.

the presence of five or more folds per inch strongly refutes this diagnosis. The demonstration of four folds per inch of proximal jejunum would be equivocal.[50] A further SBE feature aiding the diagnosis of celiac disease is the presence of an increased number of slightly thickened folds in the ileum (jejunization, Fig. 11–25*B*), a feature of adaptation to the reduced absorptive capacity of the diseased jejunum.[51]

It is a not infrequent misconception that mucosal folds are thickened in uncomplicated celiac disease.

It is true that apparent fold thickening may develop in the course of the SBE and is due to an increased output of secretions (Fig. 11–26).[52] However, real fold thickening may occur and be due to edema caused by malabsorption-related hypoalbuminemia.[53]

Transient intussusceptions are commonly seen during fluoroscopy in patients with celiac disease.[54] They are not seen with the SBE. Dilatation can be a feature of celiac disease, but is more difficult to appreciate on the SBE.

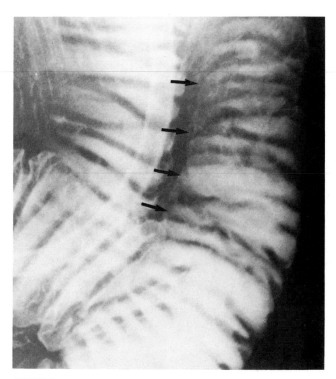

FIGURE 11–27

T-CELL LYMPHOMA COMPLICATING CELIAC DISEASE.
Jejunal folds are generally increased in thickness. One segment
(*arrows*) shows irregular nodularity of the folds.

Complications

Patients with prolonged celiac disease may occasionally present with strictures, probably a result of prior ulcerative jejunoileitis. A more acute form of ulcerative jejunoileitis has been described in patients with celiac disease. It involves a segment of variable length and causes thickening of its wall and of its folds, with ulceration. It not only resembles lymphoma but may also be its precursor. It has also been encountered in nonceliac patients.

The relationship of celiac disease to gastrointestinal malignancy has been well documented.[55, 56] A significantly increased incidence of esophageal, gastric, and rectal carcinoma and to a lesser degree of small bowel carcinoma occurs in patients with long-established celiac disease. Males are particularly at risk. Lymphoma has long been known to complicate celiac disease, and its prevalence does not seem to be affected by gluten in the diet. It has been suggested that depression of cell-mediated immunity may relate to this increased risk.[57] T-cell lymphoma seems to predominate and progress rapidly. Its radiologic features can be subtle, a mere nodular thickening of folds over a limited length of bowel (Fig. 11–27).

Other patients with celiac-related lymphoma may show the more typical findings of larger nodules and endoenteric and exoenteric masses. Splenic atrophy tends to accompany long-standing celiac disease. Hyposplenism is associated with a reduced size of the spleen, which can be adequately estimated by computed tomography (CT).

Dermatitis Herpetiformis

Dermatitis herpetiformis is associated with the small bowel abnormalities of celiac disease. Clinically, this may vary from asymptomatic villous atrophy to florid celiac disease. The radiologic appearances are indistinguishable from those of celiac disease, and the symptoms and small bowel abnormalities respond to gluten withdrawal.[1]

Tropical Sprue

Jejunal or duodenal biopsy findings resemble those in celiac disease. We have not had the opportunity to perform an SBE in such patients nor do we know whether jejunal fold separation reliably occurs in them. Improvement follows folic acid administration, not gluten withdrawal.

Diseases with Lumen Dilatation

Progressive Systemic Sclerosis (Scleroderma)

Systemic sclerosis is a progressive disorder affecting multiple systems. The esophagus is commonly affected with changes caused by replacement of the muscle layer by collagen. In over 40% of cases, the small bowel is similarly involved. Dilatation, atony, and delayed emptying are more likely to be found in the duodenum and upper jejunum. Malabsorption develops in a small number of patients and may be due to stasis with bacterial overgrowth or to the accumulation of collagen around small vessels in the submucosa.

Dilated loops may show sacculation (Fig. 11–28A). Highly characteristic for systemic sclerosis is the "hidebound" small bowel sign,[58] tightly packed folds of normal thickness within a dilated segment (Fig. 11–28B). It occurs in over 60% of cases and is most helpful in differentiating it from other conditions that present with small bowel atony.

In patients with dermatomyositis, involvement of the smooth muscle of the gastrointestinal tract resembles that seen in scleroderma, and radiologic findings are similar.

Chronic Intestinal Pseudo-obstruction

Chronic intestinal pseudo-obstruction has been defined as a condition with clinical manifestations of small bowel obstruction in the absence of mechanical obstruction. Barium passes through extremely slowly and without appreciable peristaltic activity. The examination of such patients may commence as an SBE, but this may soon have to be abandoned and replaced by follow-through filming, which may have to continue for well over 24 hours.

Chronic intestinal pseudo-obstruction may be the expression of numerous underlying pathologies. These are the collagen diseases, amyloidosis, endocrine and neurologic disorders, effects of drugs, and other conditions.[59] An idiopathic subgroup includes rare cases with neuropathy or myopathy and those without demonstrated pathology.[60]

Diseases with Thickened Folds

Amyloidosis

Gastrointestinal tract involvement is common in the primary as well as the secondary forms of amyloidosis.[61] Yet, malabsorption is unusual. The small bowel, if affected, may present a normal SBE appearance or may show a variety of changes. Uniform fold thickening is not the typical finding it was once believed to be. Nodular deposits may produce polypoid changes, the lumen may be contracted with thickening of its wall and folds, or there may be decreased motor activity presenting as pseudo-obstruction. Rectal or gingival biopsy can confirm the diagnosis.

Waldenström's Macroglobulinemia

The principal clinical features of Waldenström's macroglobulinemia are monoclonal IgM protein peaks in plasma, hepatosplenomegaly, lymphadenopathy, and anemia. Small bowel involvement is rare and associated steatorrhea is rarer still. Macroglobulin deposition in villi and secondary lymphangiectasia due to lymphatic blockage by IgM monoclonal protein can produce an SBE picture of widespread fine surface nodulation.[62] The condition is likely to progress to lymphomatous involvement of bowel and mesentery.

Abetaliproproteinemia

Abetaliproproteinemia is a rare inherited disease that combines steatorrhea with acanthocytosis, retinal abnormalities, and central nervous system damage. Betalipoproteins are absent from the plasma.[1] The SBE has shown dilatation, fluid increase, fold thickening, and a fine granular pattern. Appreciation of the clinical background is essential for inclusion of this radiologic diagnosis among several others.

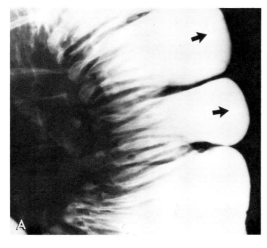
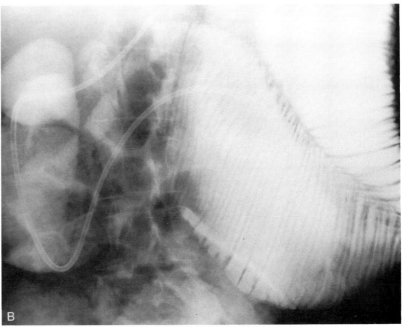

FIGURE 11–28

TWO FEATURES OF SYSTEMIC SCLEROSIS.
A, Sacculations *(arrows)* are seen on the antimesenteric border of a moderately dilated loop of jejunum. The mesenteric border shows crowding of mucosal folds.

B, The "hidebound" small bowel sign, a combination of dilatation and crowding of circular folds.

IgA Deficiency and Giardiasis

IgA deficiency is not a rare condition but may be masked by a compensatory increase of secretory IgM.[63] Nodular lymphoid hyperplasia may be the only radiologic presentation of IgA deficiency.[64] If there is associated infection with *Giardia lamblia*, inflammatory changes mostly of the duodenum and jejunum are superimposed.[65] Giardiasis can also occur in the absence of immunodeficiency.

Whipple's Disease

Whipple's disease is a rare multisystem disease mostly affecting white males, with preferential involvement of joint capsules, the small bowel and its regional nodes, heart valves, and the central nervous system.[66] With small bowel involvement, steatorrhea is usually present and characteristic Whipple's bacilli can be found in the lamina propria, usually within macrophages. Villi are distended by macrophages filled with PAS-positive material derived from the capsules of the bacilli. Mesenteric nodal masses may contain bacilli and abundant fatty material. An immunodeficiency of limited degree is usually part of the clinical picture.

A successful small bowel enema shows extensive 1- to 2-mm surface nodulation representing the distended villi. Folds tend to be irregularly thickened (Fig. 11–29A). CT may show low attenuation of fat-containing masses in the mesentery (Fig. 11–29B) whereas ultrasonography shows these masses to be highly echogenic.[67] Diagnosis should not be unduly delayed, because specific treatment with tetracycline is available for this otherwise fatal disease. Radiology can suggest the diagnosis if SBE findings are evaluated against the patient's clinical background.

Intestinal Lymphangiectasia

Intestinal lymphangiectasia is a rare but important condition, with protein loss into the gut resulting in hyoalbuminemia and hypogammaglobulinemia. It is usually due to a congenital malformation of intestinal lymphatics. A secondary immune deficiency is generally present, resulting from the loss of B and T lymphocytes into the gut lumen.

The valvulae conniventes are extensively thickened and nodular (Fig. 11–30). There is considerable fluid increase. It is important to avoid premature flocculation of barium, and the SBE needs to be

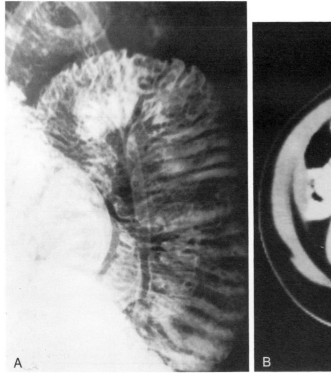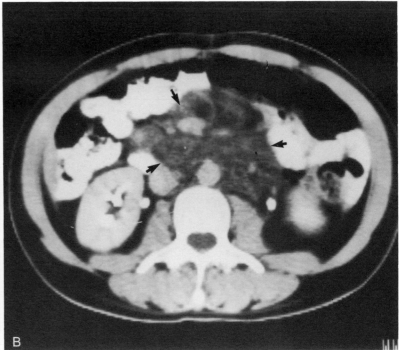

FIGURE 11–29

WHIPPLE'S DISEASE. *A*, In addition to irregular thickening of folds, there is a focally crowded pattern of nodularities measuring between 1 and 3 mm. Nodules represent distended villi. (Courtesy of E. Salomonowitz, M.D., Vienna, Austria.)

B, A mass of matted fat containing lymph nodes (*arrows*) is shown by computed tomography (CT) in another case of Whipple's disease.

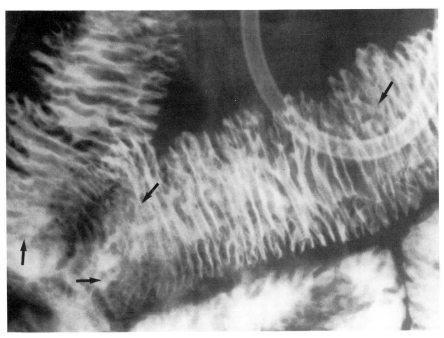

FIGURE 11–30

PRIMARY INTESTINAL LYMPHANGIECTASIA. Folds are extensively thickened. Grouped micronodules (some indicated by *arrows*) are due to distention of villi by engorged lymphatics.

modified in the way described earlier. It may then be possible to outline a patchy, 1- to 2-mm nodular pattern of the mucosa (see Fig. 11–30), representing villi distended by engorged lymphatics.[68] In cases in which lymphangiectasia is secondary to an obstructing, usually malignant process, CT may demonstrate mesenteric nodal enlargement and other masses.

Mastocytosis

Mastocytosis is a rare systemic disorder, not necessarily associated with urticaria pigmentosa. Acid peptic disease with gastric acid hypersecretion occurs in about 50% of patients. Malabsorption is common but of mild degree.[69]

Segments of the small intestine may show fold thickening with nodules. Thickening of the bowel wall may also be seen.[70] Peptic ulceration and inflammatory changes may be demonstrated in the stomach and duodenum. Endoscopic biopsy can establish the diagnosis by demonstrating an excess of mast cells in the lamina propria and submucosa. Mostly osteoblastic bone lesions are seen in almost 70% of cases.

Zollinger-Ellison Syndrome

Maximum secretion of gastric acid is stimulated by a usually malignant gastrin secreting tumor most often situated in the pancreas. The highly acidic hypersecretion is responsible for duodenitis and for inflammatory changes that may extend into the jejunum. Reflux esophagitis occurs in 60% of patients with Zollinger-Ellison syndrome.[71]

In addition to gastric hyperrugosity and fluid increase, single or multiple peptic ulcers are usually present. The widened descending duodenum may show characteristically thickened folds,[52] typically with erosions.[72] Fold thickening extends into the proximal jejunum.

Structural Lesions

Structural lesions are mostly the result either of surgery or of inflammation. The formation of a blind loop with stasis of intestinal contents allows for bacterial overgrowth and malabsorption. If the structural abnormality cannot be corrected, treatment with antibiotics provides symptomatic relief.

Jejunal Diverticulosis

Jejunal diverticula are acquired herniations of mucosa through the muscularis at the mesenteric border of the bowel. These atonic sacs can result in significant metabolic abnormalities, even when few or solitary.[73] The reported incidence of jejunal diverticulosis varies between 0.06% and 1.3% of autopsy series and between 0.02% and 0.042% of diagnosis by radiology.[74]

Erect views taken in the course of the SBE readily show characteristic fluid levels within numerous atonic sacs (Fig. 11–31). Malabsorption may be present because of stasis and bacterial overgrowth. Motility disturbance is common and may amount to acute or repeated pseudo-obstruction in 10% to 25% of patients.[74] Bleeding and diverticulitis with perforation are among the possible but rare complications.

INFLAMMATORY DISEASES

Crohn's Disease

A chronic nonspecific granulomatous process, Crohn's disease, when fully developed, involves and thickens the entire wall of a small bowel segment together with its mesentery and lymph nodes. Segments with established disease can be readily identified by the fluoroscopic follow-through, because they stand away from one another and from noninvolved, closely folded loops of bowel. However, the SBE has distinctly useful applications in Crohn's disease:

A. It is more accurate in showing the proximal limit of the disease process (Fig. 11–32). This is particularly relevant in patients in whom surgery is contemplated.

B. In addition to the obvious disease, at least 1 in 10 patients have additional, proximal skip lesions with the disease usually at an earlier stage (see Fig. 11–4). The SBE can show these more subtle lesions, thus providing valuable information for planning of surgery.

C. Features of early Crohn's disease are best demonstrated by the SBE (see text that follows). In patients with an uncertain history of Crohn's disease, the SBE is capable of either ruling out or confirming this diagnosis.

D. At least one third of patients with Crohn's disease have some degree of steatorrhea and malabsorption.[1] Its causation is multifactorial: loss of ab-

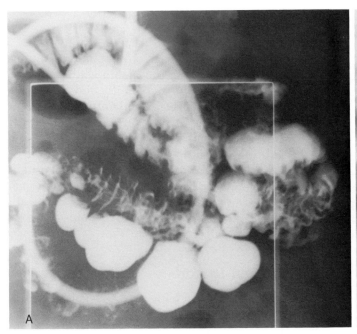 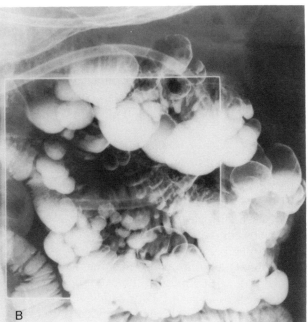

FIGURE 11–31

JEJUNAL DIVERTICULOSIS. *A,* Supine film in the single contrast phase of the small bowel enema (SBE). Diverticula begin to opacify.
    B, Erect view in the fully distended double contrast phase. A large number of diverticula are now visible, showing fluid levels between barium and methyl cellulose.

sorptive surface by disease; resection or bypass; stagnation in loops with abnormal bacterial flora; and increased gastrointestinal loss of nutrients.[75] As explained earlier, SBE is the method of choice for barium imaging in malabsorption.

E. Postresection problems seem to be shown more accurately by SBE.

F. Testing the distensibility of strictures by the lumen-distending SBE can be relevant to surgical management.

G. Crohn's disease of proximal distribution occurs in 2% to 3% of cases. The SBE may demonstrate such diseased segments in the face of a normal distal small bowel.

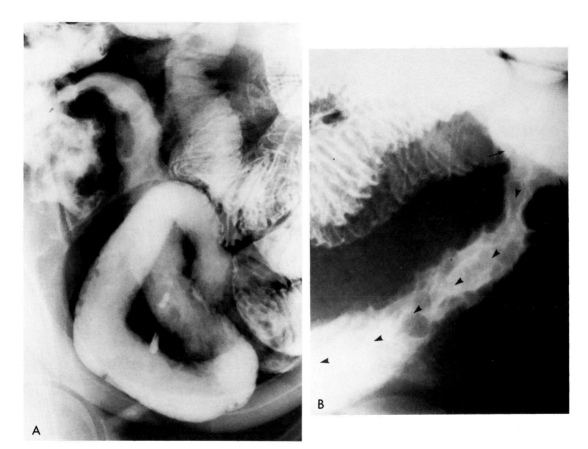

FIGURE 11–32

CROHN'S DISEASE OF THE TERMINAL ILEUM. *A,* Involvement of the terminal ileum is clearly shown by the follow-through examination.

B, Proximal extent of disease *(arrow)* is best shown with the SBE. *Arrowheads* delineate the fissured segment of Crohn's disease.

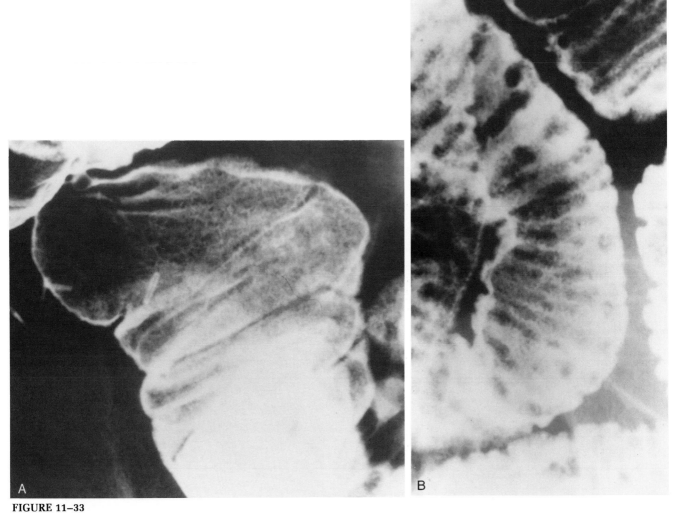

FIGURE 11–33

COARSE GRANULAR MUCOSAL PATTERN IN CROHN'S DISEASE. *A*, Coarse granularity seen in the terminal ileum.

B, Segment of ileum showing the coarse granular pattern, thickening of folds, and aphthous ulcers. (Courtesy of Dr. O. Ekberg, Malmo, Sweden.)

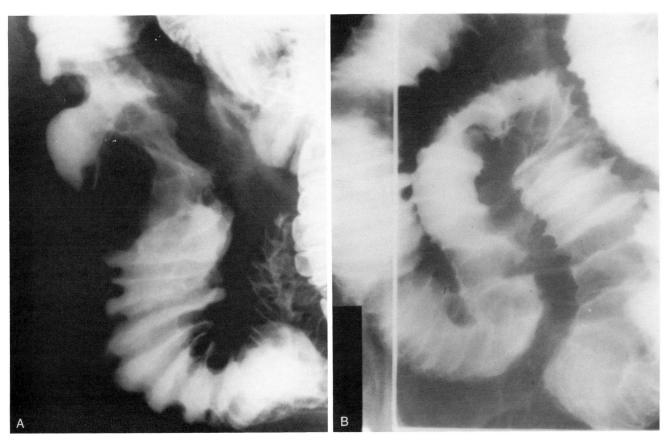

FIGURE 11–34

MUCOSAL CHANGES IN CROHN'S DISEASE. *A,* Recurrence in neoterminal ileum. Mucosal folds are thickened, and numerous aphthous ulcers are demonstrated, in the area of anastomosis.

B, Segment of ileum proximal to advanced Crohn's disease in the terminal ileum. Folds are thickened; some are fused, interrupted, or absent. Few nodules are present.

Early Changes

A coarse granular pattern due to thickened and fused villi is frequently present in Crohn's disease (Fig. 11–33).[76] However, this pattern may also occur in other inflammatory conditions and in ischemia or radiation enteropathy. Mucosal folds may be thickened, distorted, fused, interrupted, or even absent (Figs. 11–33B and 11–34). Aphthous ulcers, as described histopathologically by Morson,[77] are an early feature of Crohn's disease in the small bowel (Fig. 11–33B), as they are also in the colon. However, follow-up of some cases that presented with aphthous lesions in the terminal ileum did not show progression to established Crohn's disease.[78] Nodules, representing inflammatory polyps, are less common than in the colon. When numerous, these nodules can produce a nodular pattern that superficially resembles "cobblestones" but is still an expression of the relatively early, nonulcerated and nonstenotic disease (Fig. 11–35A).[79] Uncommon in the small bowel are postinflammatory polyps, some of them filiform and associated with distortion and interruption of mucosal folds (Fig. 11–35B).

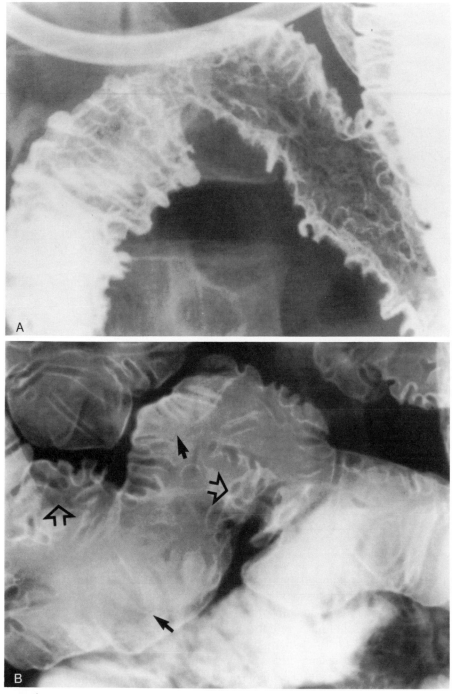

FIGURE 11–35

NODULES IN CROHN'S DISEASE. *A,* Segment of mid–small bowel showing a crowded pattern of inflammatory nodules, which are separated by barium-filled grooves.

B, Proximal ileum shows few filiform postinflammatory polyps *(open arrows);* folds are interrupted and distorted by scarring *(solid arrows).*

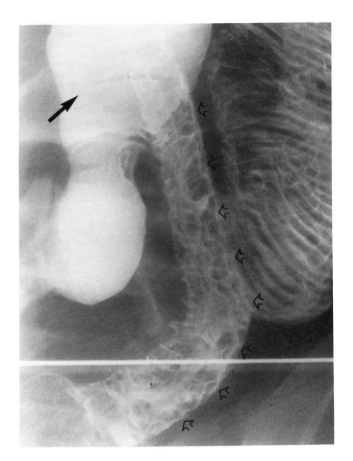

Ulcerative Changes

Linear ulcers or fissures are the hallmark of the transmural stage of Crohn's disease. The ulceronodular or "cobblestone" pattern is produced by extensive linear ulcerations that separate inflamed islands of surviving mucosa, elevated by submucosal edema (Fig. 11–36). Characteristic of small bowel Crohn's disease are linear ulcers extending along the mesenteric border, often with a margin of edema (Fig. 11–37).[80] These ulcers cause shortening and straightening of the mesenteric border and an associated redundancy of the antimesenteric side.[81] Antimesenteric sacculation continues until the disease process gradually extends transaxially to produce uniformly narrowed, ulcerated segments (Fig. 11–38).

FIGURE 11–36

"COBBLESTONE" APPEARANCE IN CROHN'S DISEASE. The cobblestone appearance is due to a pattern of linear ulcers separated by elevated islands of inflamed mucosa *(open arrows)*. Because of transmural extension of disease, the bowel segment is no longer distensible. Adjacent to the cobblestoned segment is a dilated loop of less advanced disease with interrupted and absent folds *(solid arrow)*.

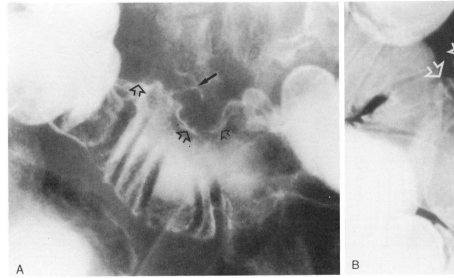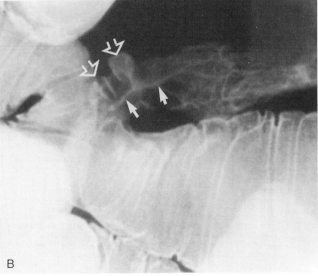

FIGURE 11–37

ULCERATION OF THE MESENTERIC BORDER IN CROHN'S DISEASE. A, Characteristic linear ulceration parallels the mesenteric border *(open arrows)* and extends even into the mesentery *(solid arrow)*. Shortening of this border causes redundancy and pleating of the antimesenteric side.

B, Skip lesion in mid–small bowel. Here, too, is a linear ulcer along the mesenteric border *(solid arrows)*, with redundancy shown at the antimesenteric border *(open arrows)*.

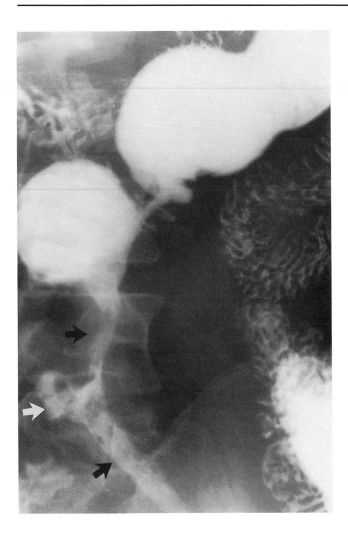

FIGURE 11–38

The shortened mesenteric border, a result of linear ulceration, is associated with antimesenteric sacculation. More distally, the Crohn's disease has become circumferential to produce ulcerated strictures *(black arrows)* and virtual elimination of a saccule *(white arrow).*

Complications

The SBE, by testing distensibility, can distinguish fibrous strictures from ulcerated, stenotic disease (Fig. 11–39). It also unmasks the "string sign" an appearance caused by spasm related to surrounding inflammation (Fig. 11–40).[82] Fistulae are well outlined, including those that lead to the sigmoid or the duodenum, in which only nonspecific focal changes are produced at the entry site of the fistula (Fig. 11–41).[83] Phlegmons or abscesses may be outlined by barium or air-containing tracts but are best demonstrated by CT.[84]

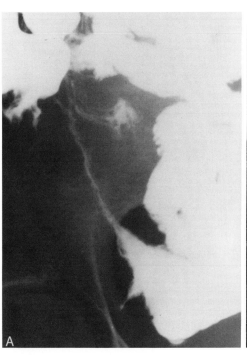
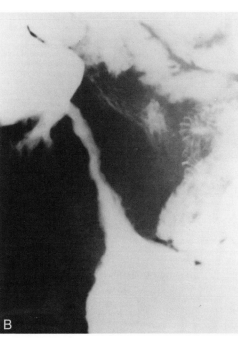

FIGURE 11–39

FIBROUS STRICTURE OF THE TERMINAL ILEUM IN CROHN'S DISEASE. A, Early stage of the single contrast phase of an SBE shows a thin, frayed 6-cm-long narrowed segment.

B, The distensibility of the stricture is tested by the infusion of methyl cellulose, but there is only minimal distention of this fibrotic stricture.

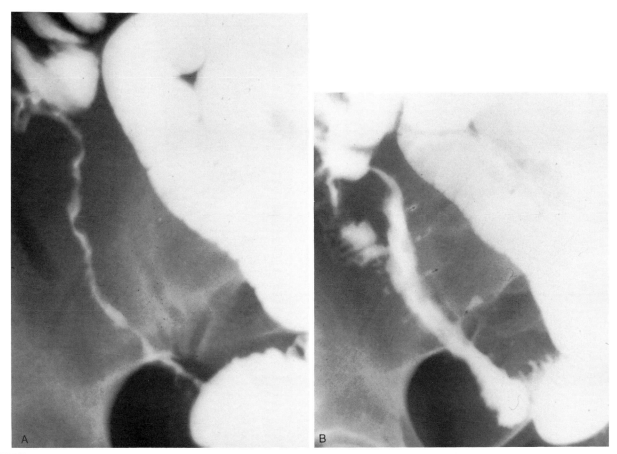

FIGURE 11–40

THE "STRING SIGN" IN CROHN'S DISEASE. *A,* In the single contrast phase, the terminal ileum has the appearance of an irregularly frayed string.

B, Following infusion of methyl cellulose, significant widening of the lumen and numerous tracks extending into an inflammatory mass are seen. The distention achieved by methyl cellulose proves that this lesion is not a fibrous stricture.

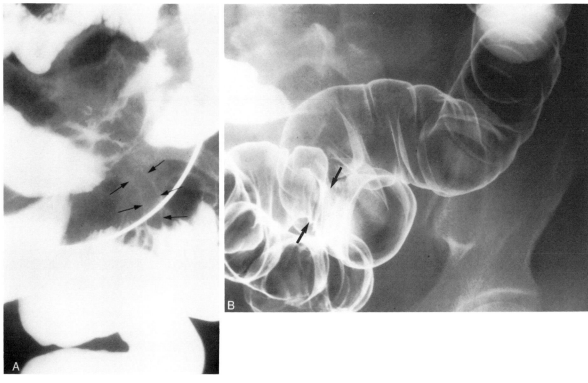

FIGURE 11–41

ILEOSIGMOID FISTULAE. *A,* From an area of ileum affected by Crohn's disease, at least two fistulae *(arrows)* lead to and penetrate the wall of the sigmoid colon, where fold thickening is observed.

B, Double contrast barium enema shows a short segment of sigmoid with limited distensibility and slight thickening of folds, marking the site of entry of Crohn's fistula *(arrows).* There is no evidence of sigmoid Crohn's disease. The sigmoid colon returned to a normal appearance after resection of the diseased ileum and of the fistula.

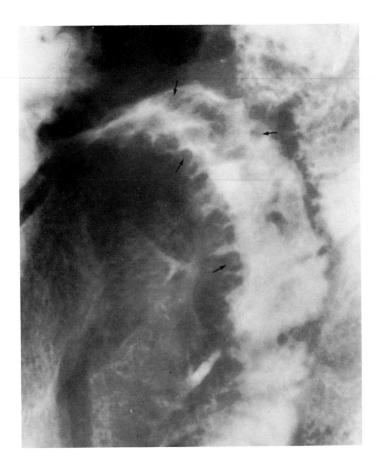

FIGURE 11–42

***YERSINIA* ILEITIS.** Numerous nodules (*arrows*) and thickened folds are seen. The appearance returned to normal after 6 weeks.

FIGURE 11–43

ILEOCECAL TUBERCULOSIS.
A, Terminal ileum is slightly dilated but normal in appearance until the thickened ileocecal valve is reached (*arrow*). The cecum is totally contracted. The extensively ulcerated ascending colon (*dots*) seems to be in direct continuation with the terminal ileum.

B, Multiple strictures (*arrows*) of the distal ileum in another patient.

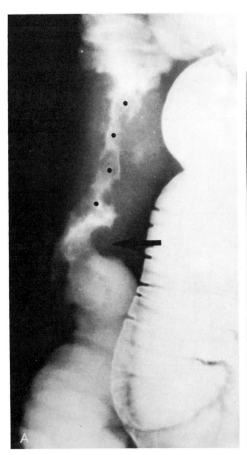

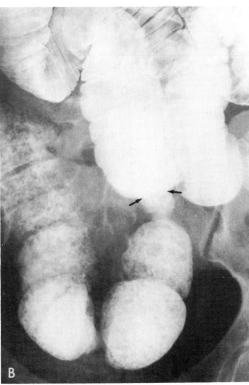

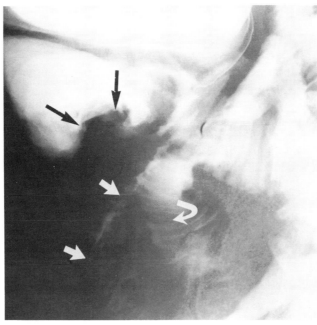

FIGURE 11–44

APPENDIX ABSCESS. *White arrows* indicate a compressed and displaced terminal ileum with thickened folds. An adjacent segment of ileum *(curved arrow)* also shows fold thickening. The medial border of the cecum is indented *(black arrows)* and the appendix has not been opacified. (From Herlinger, H., and Maglinte, D.D.T.: Miscellaneous disorders. *In* Herlinger, H., and Maglinte, D.D.T. (eds.): Clinical Radiology of the Small Intestine. Philadelphia, W.B. Saunders, 1989, p. 512, with permission.)

Yersinia Ileitis

Yersinia ileitis is a self-limited, benign disease. The diagnosis is based on positive bacteriology or serology for *Yersinia enterocolitica*. In adults the more severe disease tends to involve more of the small bowel and may also affect the colon. The radiologic features are wall and fold thickening with mucosal nodularity (Fig. 11–42); ulcers may be seen in the acute stage of the disease.[85]

Ileocecal Tuberculosis

A rare condition in developed countries, ileocecal tuberculosis is of frequent occurrence throughout much of the world, where Crohn's disease is an unusual diagnosis. Only a minority of patients with abdominal tuberculosis show features of active pulmonary infection.[86]

The diagnosis should be based on a demonstration of *Mycobacterium* tuberculosis of typical histology. In North America and Europe, the main issue is to differentiate an occasional tuberculosis from Crohn's disease. Radiologic features that suggest tuberculosis rather than Crohn's disease are the following:[87, 88]

A. Cecal involvement exceeding that of the terminal ileum; the latter may even be spared.

B. Cephalad retraction of the cecum leading to straightening of the ileocecal junction (Fig. 11–43A)

C. A fairly abrupt change from normality to disease with inflammatory exudate in the diseased portion (Fig. 11–43B).

D. Mesenteric adenopathy on CT scans may be more pronounced than in Crohn's disease; ascites of increased CT density may be present.

E. Ulcers larger than in Crohn's disease, of oval shape, and of transaxial alignment; these may result in annular strictures.

Appendix Abscess

An appendiceal abscess may affect the adjacent terminal ileum.[83] The folds of the terminal ileum may be edematous, displaced, and compressed by the adjacent inflammatory mass (Figs. 11–44 and 11–45). Graded compression ultrasonography is a valuable alternative to barium studies in patients with suspected acute appendicitis.[89] The main differential diagnosis is the distinction between appendiceal abscess and Crohn's disease. The latter would be associated more often with extensive mucosal changes including ulceration in the terminal ileum and narrowing of the terminal ileum (see Fig. 11–45).

TUMORS

Small bowel tumors are rare. They account for between 1.0% and 5.0% of all tumors of the gastrointestinal tract.

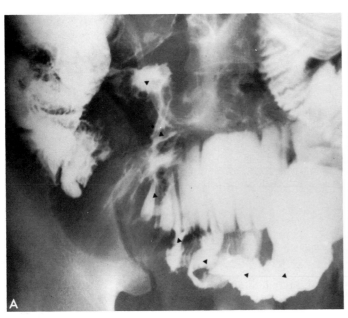

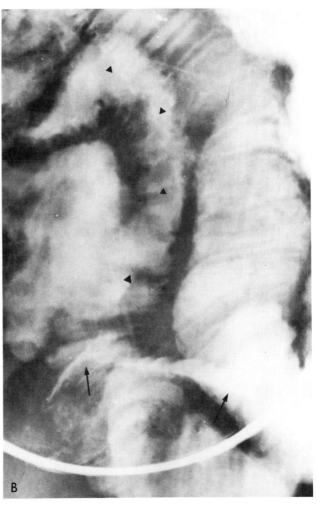

FIGURE 11–45

APPENDIX ABSCESS VERSUS CROHN'S DISEASE. *A,* The terminal ileum *(arrowheads)* was considered abnormal and Crohn's disease was suggested. Patient was given steroids and initially improved.

B, On SBE, there was no evidence of Crohn's disease *(arrowheads* indicate relatively normal ileum), but there was displacement of the more proximal part of the terminal ileum *(arrows)*, which shows an intact mucosa and swollen, compressed folds. Appendix abscess was suggested and confirmed at laparotomy.

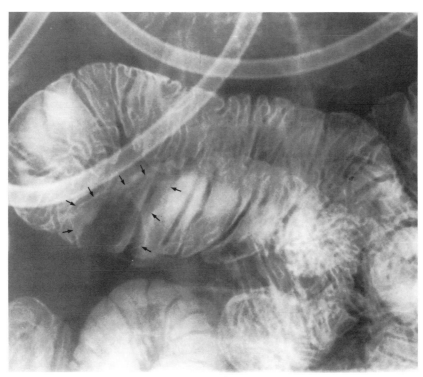

FIGURE 11–46

JEJUNAL LIPOMA. A broad-based, 3-cm-long polyp (*arrows*) was found in a patient who complained of intermittent crampy abdominal pain. The polyp could be slightly flattened by compression. It had also been demonstrated with an SBE 2 years before and had grown very little. A lipoma was later resected.

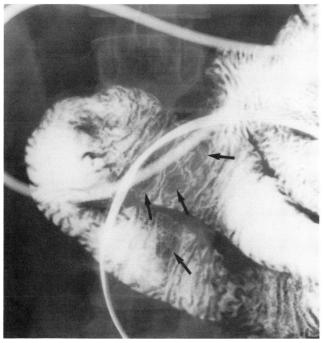

FIGURE 11–47

ADENOMATOUS POLYPS. A spot film of the jejunum shows several adenomatous polyps (*arrows*) in a patient with polyposis coli. (From Herlinger, H., and Maglinte, D.D.T.: Tumors of the small intestine. *In* Herlinger, H., and Maglinte, D.D.T. (eds.): Clinical Radiology of the Small Intestine. Philadelphia, W.B. Saunders, 1989, p. 406, with permission.)

Benign Tumors[90]

Leiomyomas, lipomas, adenomas, and hamartomas are the more common benign tumors of the small bowel. Only about 50% cause symptoms. Pain is usually due to intussusception, more often intermittent than lasting. Bleeding is the other likely presentation. The tumors are fairly evenly distributed throughout the small bowel. Lipomas protrude into the lumen, and may be shown to be soft and compressible (Fig. 11–46). CT scan can confirm their fat composition.[91] Adenomatous polyps may be found in the duodenum of patients with polyposis coli and may extend into the jejunum (Fig. 11–47).

An antegrade barium demonstration of an intussuscepting lipoma of the ileum shows the dilated lumen narrowing abruptly to a beak-like shape. Barium passing through this obstruction outlines the lumen distally, possibly demonstrating the leading tumor at the apex of the intussusceptum. The "coiled-spring" appearance of stretched folds is faintly visible only after retrograde entry of barium into the space

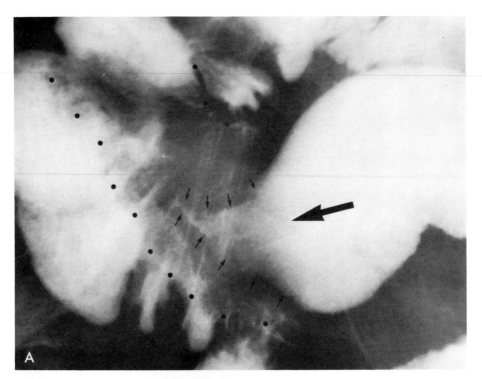

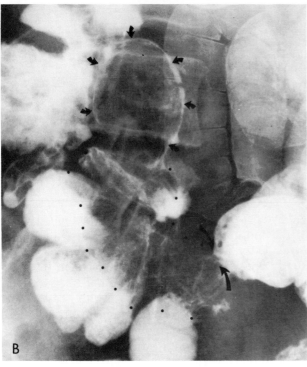

FIGURE 11–48

INTUSSUSCEPTION OF A LIPOMA OF TERMINAL ILEUM.
A, Beak-shaped narrowing at entry into the intussusception
(*arrows*). Barium flowing back from beyond the intussusception
outlines its soft tissue mass (*dots*) and faintly shows the stretched
"coiled spring" pattern of folds.
B, Lipoma outlined by barium at the apex of the intussusception
(*small arrows*).

between intussusceptum and intussuscipiens (Fig.
11–48). CT can clearly demonstrate an intussusception in longitudinal and in cross sections.[92] In institutions where ultrasonography tends to be the primary radiologic study in patients with abdominal
symptoms, the method has been reported to be able
to identify small bowel tumors with increasing accuracy.[93]

Peutz-Jeghers Syndrome

Peutz-Jeghers syndrome is an important cause of
abdominal pain and bleeding in adolescents. Multiple

lobulated hamartomatous tumors occur mostly in the
jejunum and intussuscept intermittently (Fig. 11–49).
Malignant degeneration is rare.[94]

Malignant Tumors

Carcinoid

The carcinoid is a common small bowel neoplasm
that occurs more frequently in the distal and terminal
ileum and is seen twice as often in males as in
females. These tumors are multiple in 30% of cases.

Ileal carcinoids tend to grow through the bowel wall and invade the mesentery, where they form masses that become larger than the primary tumor. Hormonal substances produced by the primary tumor and its mesenteric deposits cause an intense, focal desmoplastic process. This can be well demonstrated by SBE with regard to the primary tumor and by CT for the mesenteric metastases. A CT examination is mandatory whenever barium studies show lesions that might represent a carcinoid. Hormonally active liver metastases develop in only 10% of patients and produce the carcinoid syndrome of flushing, diarrhea, and bronchospasm.

A smoothly rounded polyp seen in the terminal ileum should always be considered a probable carcinoid. Such tumors may be asymptomatic at this early stage. At a somewhat later stage, the SBE shows desmoplastic changes affecting mucosal folds and the bowel wall. At the same time CT may demonstrate a mesenteric mass together with adjacent, thick-walled bowel loops (Fig. 11–50). CT can also identify liver metastases if the carcinoid syndrome has developed.[95]

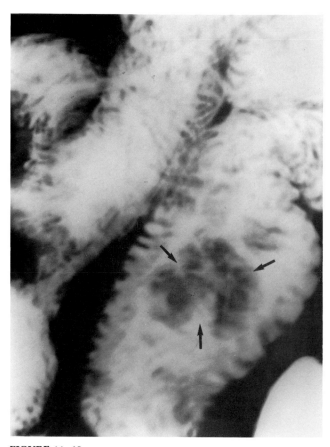

FIGURE 11–49

Peutz-Jeghers syndrome with jejunal hamartoma. (Courtesy of Dr. Grant Saunders, Winnipeg, Manitoba.)

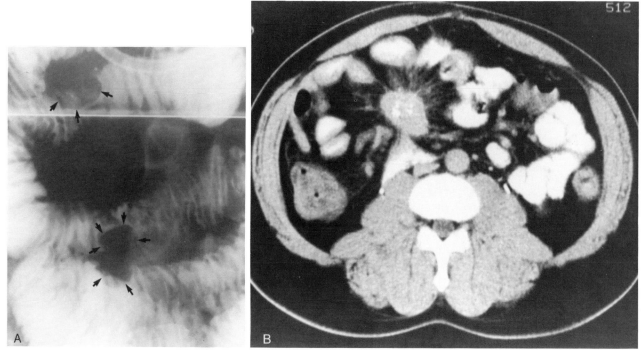

FIGURE 11–50

MULTIPLE CARCINOIDS. A, The SBE outlines three carcinoids (arrows), the largest being 2 cm wide. Separation of bowel loops can also be seen.

B, Computed tomography outlines a calcium-containing mesenteric mass surrounded by pronounced lines of retraction. Adjacent small bowel loops have thickened walls.

Adenocarcinoma

The majority of carcinomas are found in the proximal jejunum. They soon encircle the gut to produce "applecore" lesions (Fig. 11–51). Since gut contents are fluid, obstruction is usually low grade. The presenting features are pain, anemia, occult blood, and weight loss.

It is important to recognize adenocarcinomas by radiology, and SBE is the best method for this purpose. It should be possible, if clinical referral has not been unduly delayed, to make this diagnosis before mesenteric nodal metastases have developed.[95]

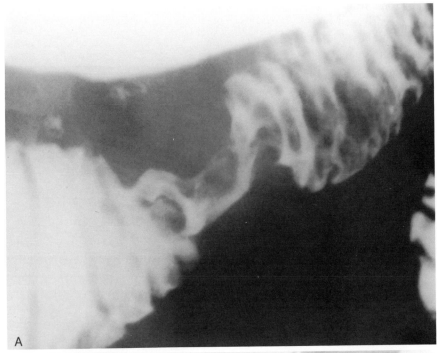

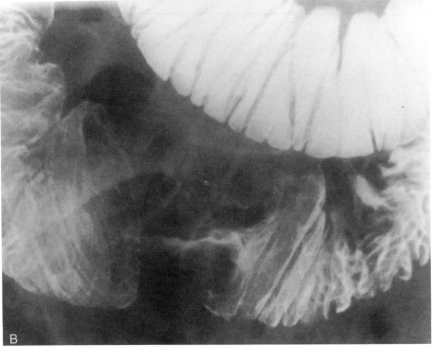

FIGURE 11–51

ADENOCARCINOMA. *A,* An annular carcinoma. Remnants of a fold pattern are still visible in the lumen of the tumor.

B, More advanced, typical "apple core" carcinoma.

Lymphoma[95–97]

Lymphomas involving the small bowel are non-Hodgkin's lymphoma (NHL). NHL affecting the small intestine can be grouped in the following way:

A. *Nodal lymphoma with secondary involvement of small bowel.* In the course of dissemination of the nodal form of NHL, the gastrointestinal tract becomes involved in 30% to 50% of cases, the most common site being the small bowel. Although a definite SBE differentiation between primary and secondary NHL of the small bowel may not always be possible, certain guidelines have emerged. Multiple nodules, usually of varying sizes, are a feature of dissemination (Fig. 11–52); less definite is the finding of segmental mural infiltration at multiple sites. A special form of secondary involvement is by an extrinsic mesenteric nodal mass of NHL, at first producing displacement and later infiltration of a small bowel segment (Fig. 11–53).

B. *Primary small bowel lymphoma.* Primary small bowel NHL of extranodal growth type has been found

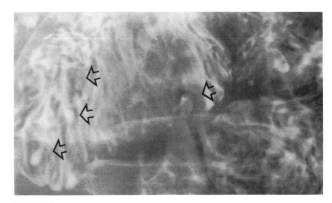

FIGURE 11–52

DISSEMINATED NON-HODGKIN'S LYMPHOMA (NHL). In addition to target lesions in the stomach, there are numerous, somewhat smaller lesions of the same type in the proximal jejunum *(arrows)*.

to present two different appearances on SBE examination. Some lesions show mural infiltration of a limited segment with obliteration of mucosal folds, outline irregularity, and, at times, dilatation; shallow

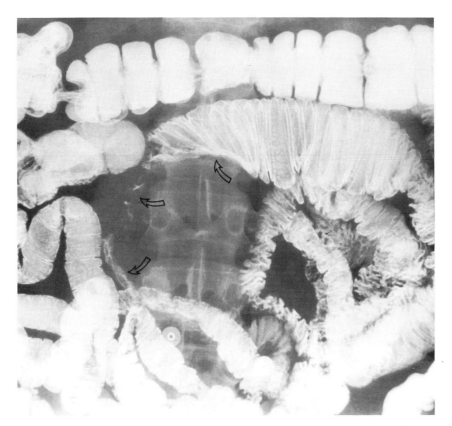

FIGURE 11–53

SECONDARY INVOLVEMENT OF JEJUNUM BY NHL. An extrinsic nodal mass compresses and infiltrates the jejunum *(arrows)*.

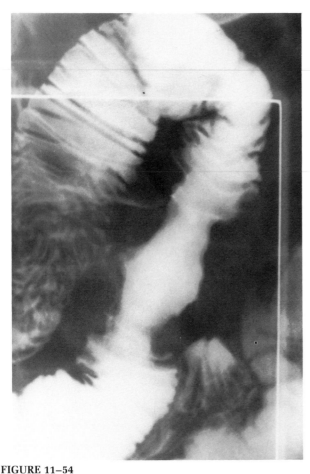

FIGURE 11-54

PRIMARY SMALL BOWEL NHL. There is an 8-cm segment of jejunum with effaced mucosal folds. The outline of the involved segment is irregular because of ulceration, and slight widening of the lumen can be seen in the center of the lesion.

ulcers are present (Fig. 11-54). Alternatively, a mural infiltrate may ulcerate and produce an exoenteric collection surrounded by lymphomatous tissue; such a lesion may extend between the leaves of the mesentery or may be found between bowel loops (Fig. 11-55).

C. *Lymphoma complicating celiac disease.* For NHL complicating adult celiac disease, see earlier in this chapter (see Fig. 11-27).

D. *Lymphoma associated with other diseases.* There is an increased incidence of NHL in patients with AIDS, lupus erythematosus, Waldenström's macroglobulinemia and in organ transplant recipients. A special type of lymphoma, Mediterranean lymphoma, is associated with alpha heavy chain disease.

Computed tomography is an essential additional radiologic method that can provide a more complete diagnosis of NHL and can aid the staging of the disease.

Seeded Carcinoma Metastases

Meyers[98] has shown that areas within the peritoneal cavity in which the ascitic fluid flow tends to slow down and stagnate become favorite sites for the deposition and implantation of cancer cells. Such areas include the ileocecal region, the ruffles of the mesentery, and the pelvic cavity. The most frequent primary sources for seeded metastases to the small bowel are the ovary and cervix in women and the colon, pancreas, and stomach in men.

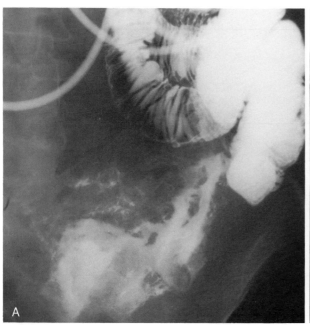
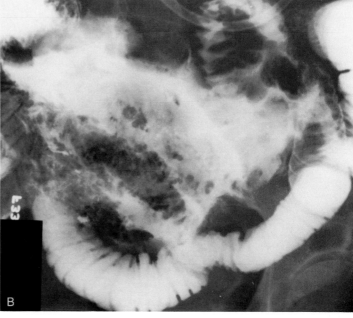

FIGURE 11-55

PRIMARY SMALL BOWEL NHL. A, Extravasation of barium from a segment of jejunum into a large space containing debris.
B, Late film shows the extent of the cavity, which contains barium, debris, and air.

Small bowel enema features of metastases deposited on serosal surfaces of the small intestine are the following:

A. Initially, a rounded protrusion toward the lumen (Fig. 11–56A).

B. Later, signs of mural infiltration with tethering of the mucosa (Fig. 11–56B);[99] when viewed en face, mucosal folds may then appear thickened or flattened or transaxially stretched or curved (Fig. 11–57); when viewed in profile, the distended lumen may show crowded fixation of folds at the side of the implant with normal separation of folds toward the opposite side (Fig. 11–56B).[95]

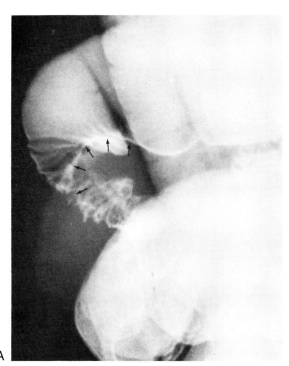
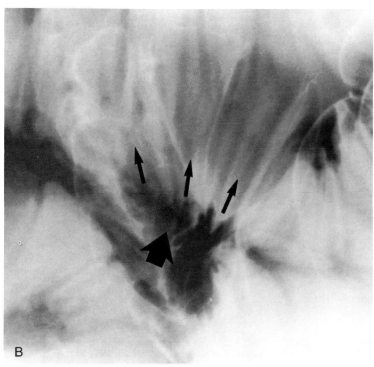

A   B

FIGURE 11–56

SEEDED METASTASES. *A,* Metastatic deposit from cervical carcinoma. Protrusion into the lumen *(arrows)* causes a partial bowel obstruction.

   B, Profile view of metastasis from endometrial carcinoma. Fixed and crowded mucosal folds at the site of infiltration *(broad arrow)* fan out toward the opposite, unaffected, and distensible side *(thin arrows).*

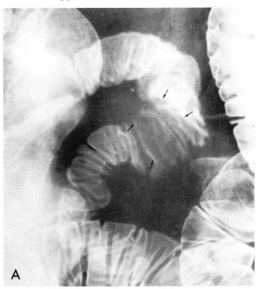
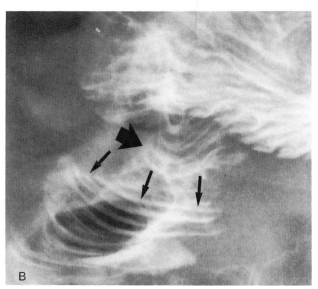

A   B

FIGURE 11–57

SEEDED METASTASES. *A,* En face view of a seeded deposit from carcinoma of the cervix. There is sharp demarcation of the lesion *(arrows),* and the folds are flattened.

   B, En face view of a metastasis from cervical carcinoma that is causing reduction of the lumen *(broad arrow)* in the center and curved, stretched folds at the edge *(thin arrows).* (*B,* From Herlinger, H., and Maglinte, D.D.T.: Tumors of the small intestine. *In* Herlinger, H., and Maglinte, D.D.T. (eds.): Clinical Radiology of the Small Intestine. Philadelphia, W.B. Saunders, 1989, p. 424, with permission.)

C. Frequently desmoplastic changes and angulation, kinking, stricture formation; high-grade small bowel obstruction may ensue (Fig. 11–58).

D. Seeded metastases, usually multiple and grouped as already described (Fig. 11–59); ascites is usually present.

E. Mesenteric carcinomatosis resulting from advanced and aggressive malignancy, often ovarian carcinoma; shortening of the mesentery then causes crowding of folds while, at the same time, the presence of interloop metastases causes separation of some of the loops.[100]

In addition to peritoneal seeding, metastatic tumor may involve the small bowel by hematogenous spread, or by direct invasion.

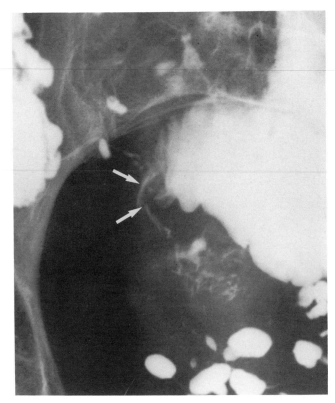

FIGURE 11–58

SMALL BOWEL OBSTRUCTION DUE TO METASTASIS FROM COLON CARCINOMA. A 24-hour film shows marked dilatation of the small bowel. The severity of obstruction is due to the combination of annular growth type and desmoplastic effect *(arrows)*.

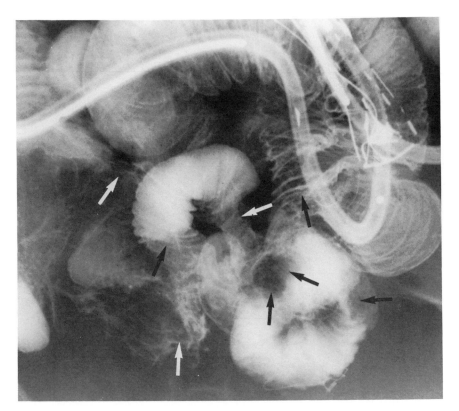

FIGURE 11–59

Small bowel obstruction due to multiple seeded metastases from carcinoma of the cervix grouped in the ileocecal area *(arrows)*. (From Herlinger, H., and Maglinte, D.D.T.: Tumors of the small intestine. *In* Herlinger, H., and Maglinte, D.D.T. (eds.): Clinical Radiology of the Small Intestine. Philadelphia, W.B. Saunders, 1989, p. 426, with permission.)

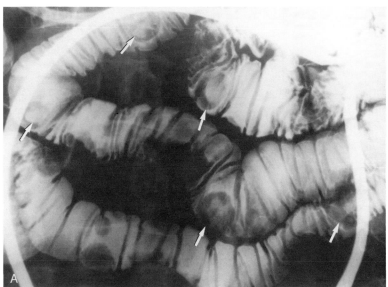
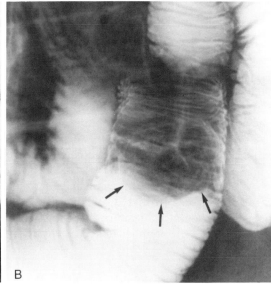

FIGURE 11–60

HEMATOGENOUS METASTASES FROM MELANOMA. *A,* There are multiple lesions on the antimesenteric border of the small bowel, many with a large central ulceration *(arrows)*. These metastases produce typical bull's-eye or target lesions characteristic of metastatic melanoma. (Courtesy of Dr. L. Costopoulos, Edmonton, Alberta.)

   B, Intussusception due to metastatic melanoma *(arrows)*. Such intussusceptions are usually transient and rarely produce small bowel obstruction.

Hematogenous Metastases

Hematogenous metastases occur less often than seeded metastases. Malignant melanoma shows a preference for small bowel localization. Carcinomas of the breast and lung show no particular predilection for small bowel involvement, but because they are so common, they account for a high proportion of cases of metastatic disease to the small bowel.

   Tumor emboli are mostly deposited at the antimesenteric aspect of small bowel loops (Fig. 11–60A). They are usually multiple and grouped in several stages of growth. Melanoma metastases tend to ulcerate and are soft and highly cellular.[101] These metastases often intussuscept but rarely obstruct (Fig. 11–60B). CT is a valuable addition to the investigation because it may show further metastases in the abdomen, such as in the liver, spleen, and mesentery.[102]

   Bronchogenic metastases may cause desmoplastic changes and occasionally a localized extravasation. Breast metastases are more likely to involve the colon and the stomach and occasionally cause strictured lesions in the small bowel.

   Direct extension of the primary carcinoma or of its involved nodes may invade and constrict a segment of small bowel, usually ileum.

VASCULAR LESIONS

Radiation Enteropathy

The small intestine is highly radiosensitive.[103] With higher radiation doses to the pelvis, the small intestine will escape injury only if free to move out of the x-ray beam. Bowel tethered by previous surgery is likely to suffer damage from a dose as low as 5000 rads.

   Chronic radiation damage makes its appearance 1 to 12 years after treatment and demonstrates recognizable changes on barium examination. The injury essentially involves endothelial cells of arterioles, leading to progressive ischemia of the mucosa and submucosa. The bowel wall becomes thickened by edema and fibrosis.

   The SBE demonstrates the associated radiologic changes. Folds are thicker than the compressed spaces between them (Figs. 11–61 and 11–62). The lumen shows limited distensibility, fixation, and poor peristaltic activity. At times, nodular defects occur and differentiation from metastases may be difficult (Figs. 11–62 and 11–63). At other times, severe damage may result in segments becoming almost devoid of folds, with shallow ulceration and a history of bleeding. Small bowel obstruction can become an important late feature, infrequently due to a radiation stricture (Fig. 11–64); more often obstruction relates to the extent of involvement and to the degree to which loops have become matted and encased by fibrosis (Fig. 11–65), lacking peristalsis and distensibility.[104] In such cases it may be necessary to abandon the SBE because further infusions of MC would not be accommodated and reflux into the stomach would occur. Follow-through over several hours may have to take its place.

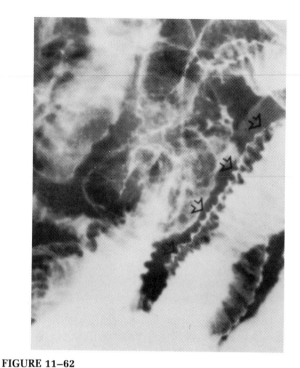

FIGURE 11–62

RADIATION ENTEROPATHY. Sharp projections of barium between evenly thickened folds represent the compressed interfold spaces (*arrows*). More proximally, there is irregular fold thickening, which is also due to radiation damage.

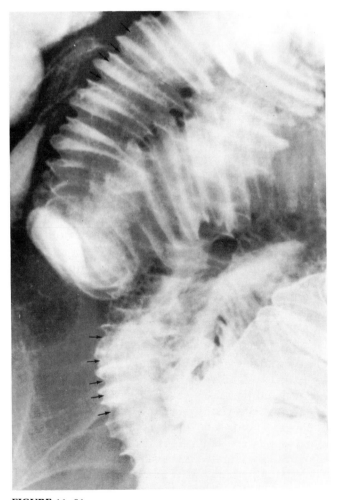

FIGURE 11–61

RADIATION ENTEROPATHY. Ileal folds are thick, straight, and parallel. Compressed interfold spaces appear as short projections of barium between the thickened folds (*arrows*).

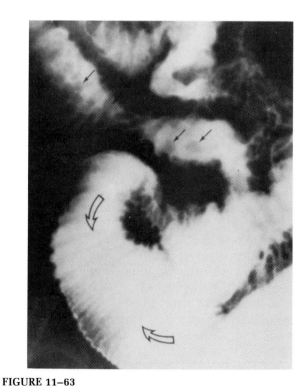

FIGURE 11–63

RADIATION ENTEROPATHY. Nodular fold thickening (*small arrows*) is seen in a narrowed segment of ileum. In a more distal segment, less thickened folds are crowded by longitudinal shortening (*curved, open arrows*).

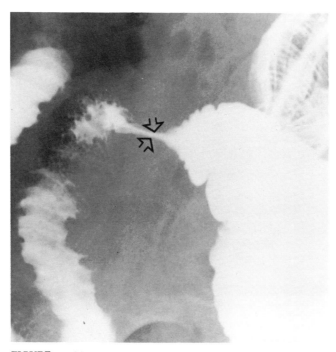

FIGURE 11–64

RADIATION STRICTURE. Short stricture *(arrows)* causes partial small bowel obstruction. Thick folds are seen in the incompletely filled segment distal to the stricture.

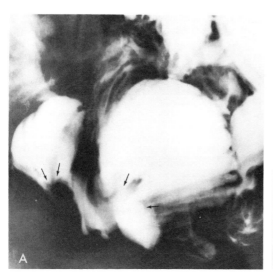
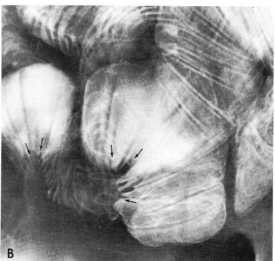

FIGURE 11–65

RADIATION DAMAGE OR MALIGNANCY? Previous surgery for carcinoma of the cervix with extensive resection was followed by radiotherapy. The patient presented with malabsorption and intermittent bleeding. *A*, Fixed loop of ileum at pelvic inlet is shown in single contrast phase. Is the lesion benign or malignant?

B, Fully developed double contrast with distention. Slightly thickened mucosal folds are demonstrated *(arrows)*, with fixation due to radiation-related adhesions and not malignant infiltration.

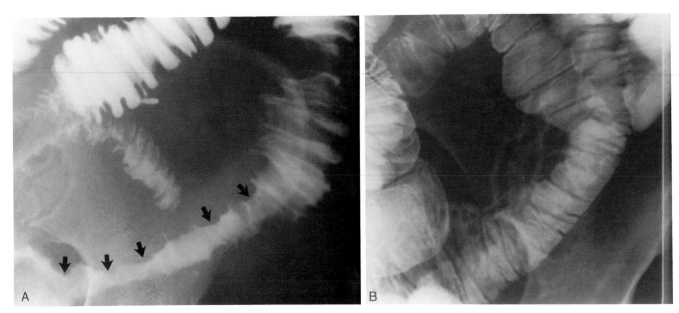

FIGURE 11-66

ISCHEMIA WITH REVERSIBLE CHANGES. *A,* Beyond thickened folds, a narrowed segment shows multiple indentations (thumbprints) of its mesenteric border *(arrows)* and barely identifiable outlines of very thick folds.

B, An SBE 4 weeks later shows the same bowel segments now with a normal appearance.

Ischemia

Acute ischemic processes due to embolic or thrombotic occlusion of a major vessel are not normally referred for barium investigation. Subacute ischemia of a small bowel segment produces changes described as the "picket-fence" or "stacked-coin" appearance of straightened, thickened folds.[105] Contour defects (thumbprints) are often seen and occur mostly along the mesenteric border (Fig. 11-66A). These changes may best be shown in the single contrast phase of the SBE and may become less obvious during subsequent lumen distention. An important feature is the transient nature of these appearances, which may either progress to necrosis or stricture or, more often, return to normal (Fig. 11-66B). Since this feature helps to distinguish ischemia from radiation enteropathy and some forms of inflammatory involvement, a repeat barium study approximately 3 weeks later should always be recommended.

Intramural Hemorrhage

Intramural hemorrhage may develop spontaneously in patients on anticoagulants or in those suffering from a bleeding diathesis. Blunt trauma is another cause. The hemorrhage may be localized or diffuse. The former is likely to be caused by trauma and presents as a mass effect associated with thickening of folds. The more diffuse, usually spontaneous intramural bleed closely resembles an ischemic bowel segment (Fig. 11-67).

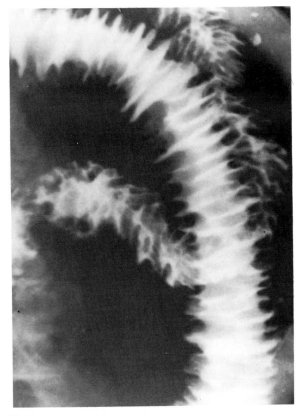

FIGURE 11-67

INTRAMURAL BLEEDING. A typical "stacked-coin" appearance is due to intramural bleeding in a patient with thrombocytopenia.

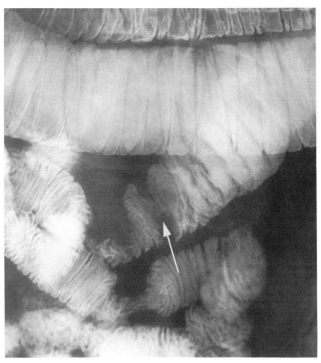

FIGURE 11–68

ADHESIVE BAND CAUSING PARTIAL SMALL BOWEL OBSTRUCTION. There is an abrupt change of caliber at the site of compression by an adhesive band *(arrow)*. Mucosal folds in this segment are preserved, and the lumen is dilated proximally. (From Herlinger, H., and Maglinte, D.D.T.: Small bowel obstruction. *In* Herlinger, H., and Maglinte, D.D.T. (eds.): Clinical Radiology of the Small Intestine. Philadelphia, W.B. Saunders, 1989, p. 486, with permission.)

Computed tomography can be most useful in blunt trauma-related bowel injuries. Mural hematoma can be distinguished from injury to the mesentery, and exploratory laparotomy can often be avoided.[106]

Gastrointestinal Bleeding

SBE for Suspected Bleeding From the Small Intestine. Only patients in whom examinations of the upper gastrointestinal tract and colon have been unrewarding should be referred for an SBE for suspected gastrointestinal (GI) bleeding. There is a low, over 10% yield of positive information that includes Meckel's diverticula, Crohn's disease, and benign and malignant tumors.[107] The more common causes of bleeding from the small bowel, however, seem to be arteriovenous malformations, which cannot be demonstrated by an SBE but can be shown by rarely done angiography or enteroscopy.[108]

SMALL BOWEL OBSTRUCTION

Small bowel obstruction (SBO) has become a major indication for SBE. The majority of obstructions are caused by adhesions following surgery; less fre-

quently they are the result of inflammation. About 15% of obstructions are caused by a malignancy, usually metastases. Hernias, intussusceptions, volvulus, gallstones, and other conditions are responsible for a remaining small group of SBO.

Technique Modification

The SBE can be carried out by the routine method of intubation or by using an already inserted long decompression tube. Depending on the quantity of retained fluid, an increased amount of barium will have to be infused. Whenever possible, barium should be taken close to the site of obstruction, usually identified as the site of an abrupt change from a dilated lumen proximally to a collapsed lumen beyond. MC is then infused for double contrast detail to identify the imprint of the causative lesion. If an excessive amount of retained fluid is found, the infusion of MC may have to be avoided.

Adhesive Bands

With single adhesive band obstructions, dilated bowel with stretched mucosal folds is seen to extend to the edge of a sharply demarcated lumen reduction.

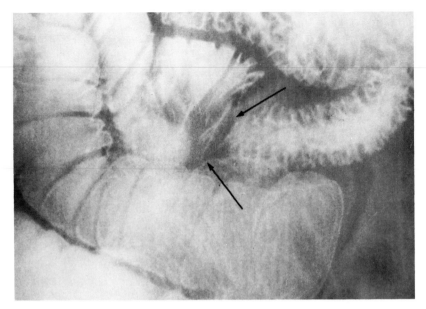

FIGURE 11–69

Adhesive band in an asymptomatic patient with a history of intermittent partial small bowel obstruction. Abrupt caliber change can be clearly identified (arrows). The distention produced by the SBE facilitates the detection of this feature.

A short, narrowed segment with compressed folds marks the site of the adhesive band (Fig. 11–68).[109] The distention associated with the SBE can draw attention to minimal compression, even at a time when patients are asymptomatic (Fig. 11–69). Closed-loop obstructions, implying compression of the afferent and efferent limbs of a loop of bowel protruding under an adhesive band, are not a rare complication. Diagnosis by SBE is possible before significant vascular compromise has occurred.[110]

Differential Diagnosis

A very important differential diagnosis, especially in patients with a prior history of laparotomy for abdominal malignancy, is the distinction between SBO caused by metastases and that caused by adhesions. The SBE, by illustrating outline and fold pattern changes at the site of obstruction (as previously described), can make this distinction with high reliability (Fig. 11–70).[111]

Hernias

Small bowel obstruction due to external hernia is usually diagnosed by clinical examination. However, the SBE may be able to demonstrate clinically unsuspected hernial obstruction in obese patients.[111] Para-ileostomy hernias (Fig. 11–71) and rarer forms of external and internal hernias may also be discovered by SBE (Fig. 11–72).[111]

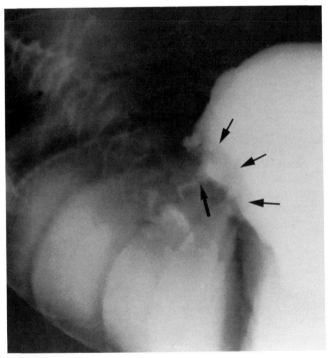

FIGURE 11–70

METASTATIC LESION CAUSING SMALL BOWEL OBSTRUCTION. The frayed outline of the narrow stricture (single arrow) and a pronounced irregularity of the rounded proximal contour (multiple arrows) favor a metastatic deposit. Past history of sigmoid colon carcinoma.

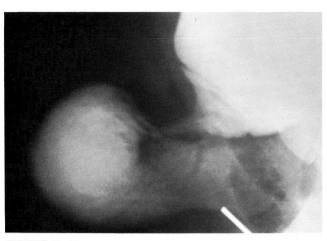

FIGURE 11–71

PARTIAL OBSTRUCTION BY A PARA-ILEOSTOMY HERNIA.
Such hernias may not be clinically evident, especially in a
patient with increased subcutaneous fat. (From Herlinger, H., and
Maglinte, D.D.T.: Small bowel obstruction. *In* Herlinger, H., and
Maglinte, D.D.T. (eds.): Clinical Radiology of the Small Intestine.
Philadelphia, W.B. Saunders, 1989, p. 494, with permission.)

MISCELLANEOUS DISORDERS

Edema

Edema is probably the most common abnormality of
the small intestine. However, it is usually submerged
in the primary symptomatology of a patient and is
not investigated radiologically as such. Hypoalbuminemia is the most common cause, related to protein
loss from the gastrointestinal tract, or to malabsorption, cirrhosis, or nephrosis. Protein loss may also be
associated with congestive heart failure, constrictive
pericarditis, and allergic states.

Interstitial fluid increase affects all layers of the
bowel wall, but especially the submucosal space with
its extensions into the core of the mucosal folds.
Barium studies therefore show diffuse thickening of
the folds with some degree of thickening and separation of loops (Fig. 11–73). There may be an increase
of intraluminal fluid.

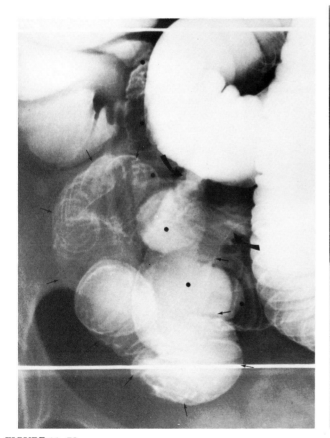

FIGURE 11–72

Internal hernia causing intermittent partial closed loop
obstruction. A loop of distal ileum *(small arrows)* is seen to be in
constant position with afferent and efferent limbs in close
approximation *(large arrows)*. *Dots* mark the superimposed
terminal ileum. Laparotomy revealed an internal hernia that had
passed through an opening in the mesentery of the appendix.

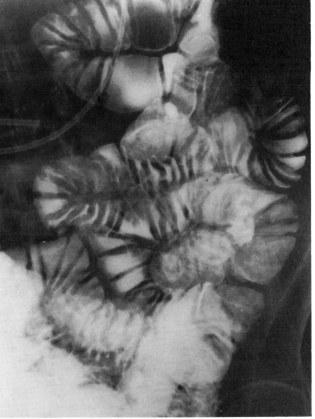

FIGURE 11–73

SMALL BOWEL ENEMA. Patient with celiac disease and
hypoalbuminemia. Folds are uniformly thickened, and slight wall
thickening is evident. Folds in the distended proximal jejunum
are widely separated, a sign typical of celiac disease.

AIDS

AIDS is an epidemic disease of the immune system that can affect most organs of the body.[112] A significant proportion of secondary infections and neoplasms involves the abdomen, and especially the gastrointestinal tract.

Cryptosporidiosis and *isosporiasis* are caused by protozoa that produce severe opportunistic infections in AIDS patients. Barium studies show fluid increase and pronounced fold thickening, mostly in the proximal small bowel (Fig. 11–74).

Cytomegalovirus, a member of the herpes virus group, can cause extensive intestinal and extraintestinal disease. Ulcers are a characteristic manifestation and may bleed or perforate (Fig. 11–75).

Mycobacterium avium intracellulare can infect most body systems. In the jejunum it can produce an appearance resembling Whipple's disease, nodules due to thickened villi, and enlarged, often matted mesenteric and retroperitoneal nodes.

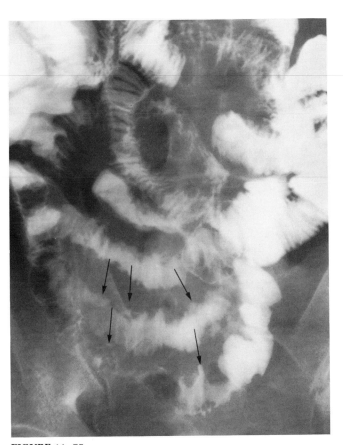

FIGURE 11–75

CYTOMEGALOVIRUS ENTERITIS IN AIDS. Distal ileal loops show fold thickening and increased separation, indicating thickening of the bowel wall. In addition, several penetrating ulcers are seen (*arrows*).

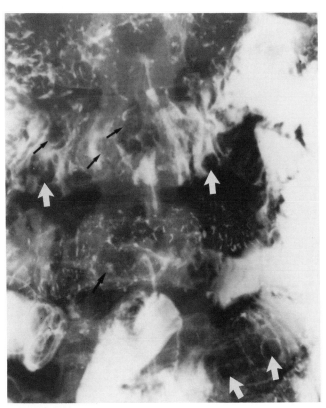

FIGURE 11–74

AIDS WITH CRYPTOSPORIDIOSIS AND KAPOSI'S SARCOMA. Follow-through examination shows barium flocculation with thickened folds in the jejunum due to cryptosporidiosis. Rounded filling defects, some with central ulceration (*arrows*), were due to Kaposi's sarcoma, which was also present in the stomach and duodenum. (Courtesy of R. Goren, M.D., Philadelphia, Pennsylvania.)

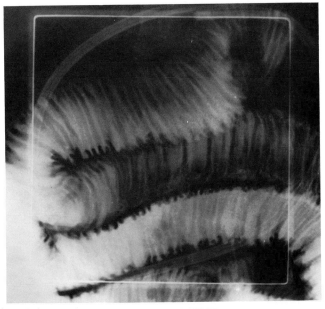

FIGURE 11–76

EOSINOPHILIC ENTERITIS. A 19-year-old female with a history of intermittent diarrheal illnesses. Endoscopic biopsy showed eosinophilic infiltration of the antral mucosa. Small bowel enema shows extensive thickening of straightened folds in much of the jejunum. Patient responded to steroid treatment.

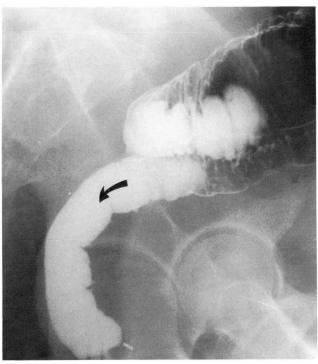

FIGURE 11–77

**ILEOANAL RESERVOIR AFTER COLECTOMY FOR
ULCERATIVE COLITIS.** An ileostomy enema was performed
before closure of the protective ileostomy. The ileal reservoir and
the efferent segment of ileum *(arrow)* were outlined, and the
integrity of the ileoanal anastomosis was confirmed. Anal
sphincter control could be assessed. (From Herlinger, H., and
Maglinte, D.D.T.: Miscellaneous disorders. *In* Herlinger, H., and
Maglinte, D.D.T. (eds.): Clinical Radiology of the Small Intestine.
Philadelphia, W.B. Saunders, 1989, p. 535, with permission.)

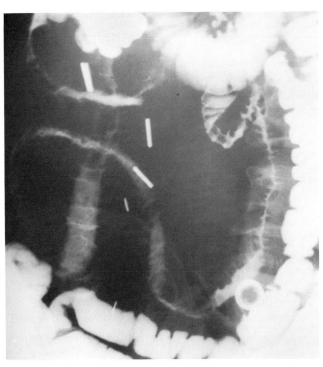

FIGURE 11–78

Hepatic artery infusion of fluorinated pyrimidine in patient with
liver metastases from colon carcinoma. Reversible toxic effect is
shown by ileal narrowing, fold thickening, and loop separation.
(From Herlinger, H., and Maglinte, D.D.T.: Miscellaneous
disorders. *In* Herlinger, H., and Maglinte, D.D.T. (eds.): Clinical
Radiology of the Small Intestine. Philadelphia, W.B. Saunders,
1989, p. 537, with permission.)

Kaposi's sarcoma may be responsible for multiple
cutaneous and visceral lesions, the latter showing a
typical radiologic appearance of submucosal elevations with central umbilication (see Fig. 11–74).
There may be extensive lymph node enlargement.

AIDS-related lymphoma is aggressive and may
involve the gastrointestinal tract and its lymph nodes.

Eosinophilic Enteritis

Eosinophilic enteritis is a self-limited disease that
presents with diarrhea, abdominal pain, and eosino-
philia. Barium studies show segmental or extensive
thickening of mucosal folds and of the bowel wall
(Fig. 11–76). There are also often nodular changes of
the mucosa in the gastric antrum.[113] Return to a
normal appearance either spontaneously or after cor-
ticosteroid therapy supports the diagnosis.

Ileo-anal Reservoir

Colectomy for ulcerative colitis or familial polyposis
can be combined with rectal mucosectomy, the formation of a distal ileal reservoir, and the introduction
of its efferent segment through the rectal cuff for

anastomosis at the anal verge. Continence is thus
provided in a natural way by the anal sphincter.[114] A
protective ileostomy is constructed and closed after
6 to 8 weeks.

A barium examination should be done before closure of the ileostomy to insure that a competent ileoanal anastomosis has been achieved (Fig. 11–77). For
this purpose, a low-density barium suspension (30%
to 40% w/v) can be injected antegrade through the
ileostomy and followed by air to propel the barium
to the anal canal.

Fluorinated Pyrimidine
Toxicity

5-FUDR (5-fluorouracil deoxyribonucleoside) and 5-
FU (5-fluorouracil) are frequently used in chemotherapy. Adverse effects are not unexpected, and, if severe, may force interruption of treatment. If the patient is referred to a barium study at that time,
narrowed and separated loops of distal ileum with
thickened or effaced folds may be demonstrated (Fig.
11–78).[115] Cessation of treatment leads to rapid improvement.

Nonsteroidal Anti-Inflammatory Drugs (NSAIDs)

Episodes of subacute small bowel obstruction have followed prolonged treatment with NSAIDs. In some cases multiple diaphragm-like strictures could be demonstrated by SBE.[116]

CONCLUSION

It is the author's belief that the SBE represents the most reliable method of investigating the small intestine and should be used whenever sound clinical indications exist. However, patient discomfort is associated with this method and should be mitigated by sedation and good technique. Only a high-quality study and a careful evaluation of its imaging result justify subjecting a patient to the examination.

In departments where small bowel examinations are undertaken on demand and for whatever reasons, the need to provide a follow-through examination remains. Even in these circumstances the follow-through should be predominantly a fluoroscopic examination and should be combined with a peroral pneumocolon if ileal pathology appears likely.

The SBE can be expected to make a useful contribution to diagnosis in the following clinical circumstances:

1. All forms of *malabsorption*. Adult celiac disease, bacterial overgrowth syndrome, adult cystic fibrosis, Zollinger-Ellison syndrome, amyloidosis, Whipple's disease, lymphangiectasia, and the short bowel syndrome are among the causes of a malabsorption state in which characteristic findings can be demonstrated by the SBE.

2. *Small bowel obstruction*. Whether done by routine intubation or through a decompression tube, the SBE can be accurate in determining the site and nature of the lesion responsible for obstruction. This can be of particular value in patients who have a history of laparotomy for malignancy.

3. *Crohn's disease*. SBE is not always required to demonstrate Crohn's disease. The follow-through examination aided by the peroral pneumocolon is a satisfactory method in the follow-up of patients with known terminal ileal disease. The more accurate determination of the proximal extent of the disease, the exclusion of early skip lesions, and the evaluation of strictures and fistulae are among the indications for SBE.

4. *Tumors*. Benign or malignant tumors are more accurately demonstrated by SBE as long as both the single and double contrast phases of the examination are used.

5. *Secondary malignancy and radiation damage*. The SBE is the most precise method available in differentiating between secondary malignancy and radiation damage, but it requires careful and experienced evaluation.

6. *Occult blood loss* after studies of the upper and lower digestive tracts have been reported negative. The low positive yield of the SBE in this indication is increased somewhat if there is also a history of abdominal pain.

7. *Determination of morphologic normality*. Only the SBE is capable of documenting those measurable parameters upon which a diagnosis of normality can be based.

Additional imaging methods, especially CT, can be of synergistic value. Its use is strongly recommended in tumors like carcinoids or lymphoma, with transmural extensions of inflammatory processes as in Crohn's disease, for the demonstration of nodal masses as in Whipple's disease, secondary lymphangiectasia, Kaposi's sarcoma, or mycobacterial infection, to mention only a few of the indications.

REFERENCES

1. Losowsky, M.S., Walker, B.E., and Kelleher, J.: Malabsorption in Clinical Practice. Edinburgh, Churchill-Livingstone, 1974.
2. Creamer, B.: Loss from the small intestine. J.R. Coll. Phys. (Engl), 5:323, 1971.
3. Creamer, B.: The Small Intestine. London, William Heinemann, 1974.
4. Laws, J.W., Booth, C.C., Shawdon, H., et al.: Correlation of radiological and histological findings in idiopathic steatorrhoea. Br. Med. J. 1:1311, 1963.
5. Frik, W.: Small bowel. In Schinz, H.R. (ed.): Roentgen Diagnosis. Vol. 5, 6th ed. London, William Heinemann, 1965.
6. Kreel, L.: Pharmacoradiology in barium examinations with special reference to glucagon. Br. J. Radiol. 48:691, 1975.
7. Ratcliffe, J.F.: The small bowel enema in children: A description of a technique. Clin. Radiol. 34:287, 1983.
8. Maglinte, D.D.T., Burney, B.T., and Miller, R.E.: Lesions missed on small bowel follow-through: Analysis and recommendations. Radiology 144:737, 1982.
9. Schulze-Delrieu, K.: Metoclopramide. In Koch-Weser, J. (ed.): Drug Therapy. N. Engl. J. Med. 305:28, 1981.
10. Kelvin, F.M., Gedgaudas, R.K., Thompson, W.M., and Rice, R.P.: The peroral pneumocolon examination of the ileocecal region. AJR 39:115, 1982.
11. Kressel, H.Y., Evers, K.A., Glick, S.N., et al.: Peroral pneumocolon examination: Technique and indications. Radiology 144:414, 1982.
12. Fitzgerald, T.J., Thompson, G.T., Sommers, S.S., and Frank, S.S.: Pneumocolon as an aid to small bowel studies. Clin. Radiol. 36:633, 1985.
13. Herlinger, H.: Small bowel. In Laufer, I. (ed.): Double Contrast Gastrointestinal Radiology: With Endoscopic Correlation, pp. 423–494. Philadelphia, W.B. Saunders, 1979.
14. Cole, L.G.: Artificial dilatation of the duodenum for radiographic examination. AJR 3:204, 1911.
15. Einhorn, M.: The Duodenal Tube and Its Possibilities, 2nd ed. Philadelphia, F.A. Davis, 1926.
16. Pribram, B.O., and Kleiber, N.: Ein Neuer Weg zur roentgenologischen Darstellung des Duodenums (Pneumoduodenum). Fortschr. Geb. Roentgenstr. 36:739, 1927.

17. Pesquera, G.S.: A method for the direct visualization of lesions in the small intestine. AJR 22:254, 1929.
18. Gershon-Cohen, J., and Shay, H.: Barium enteroclysis. AJR 42:456, 1939.
19. Schatzki, R.: Small intestine enema. AJR 30:743, 1943.
20. Lura, A.: Enema of the small intestine with special emphasis on the diagnosis of tumors. Br. J. Radiol. 24:264, 1951.
21. Scott-Harden, W.G.: Examination of the small bowel. In McLaren, J.W. (ed.): Modern Trends in Diagnostic Radiology, 3rd series, pp. 84–87. London, Butterworth & Co., 1960.
22. Pygott, F., Street, D.F., Shellshear, M.F., et al.: Radiological investigation of the small intestine. Gut 1:366, 1960.
23. Scott-Harden, W.G., Hamilton, H.A.R., and McCall-Smith, S.: Radiological investigation of the small intestine. Gut 2:316, 1961.
24. Gianturco, C.: Rapid fluoroscopic duodenal intubation. Radiology 88:1165, 1967.
25. Bilbao, M.K., Frische, L.H., Dotter, C.T., et al.: Hypotonic duodenography. Radiology 89:438, 1967.
26. Sellink, J.L.: Examination of the small intestine by means of duodenal intubation. Leiden, HE, Stenfert Kroese, BV, 1971.
27. Sellink, J.L.: Examination of a small intestine by duodenal intubation. Acta Radiol. 15:318, 1974.
28. Sellink, J.L., and Miller, R.E.: Radiology of the small bowel. Modern Enteroclysis Technique and Atlas. The Hague, Martinus Nijhoff, 1982.
29. Fleckenstein, P., and Pedersen, G.: The value of the duodenal intubation method (Sellink modification) for the radiological visualization of the small bowel. Scand. J. Gastroenterol. 10:423, 1974.
30. Sanders, D.E., and Ho, C.S.: The small bowel enema: Experience with 150 examinations. AJR 127:743, 1976.
31. Ekberg, O.: Crohn's disease of the small bowel examined by double contrast technique: A comparison with oral technique. Gastrointest. Radiol. 1:355, 1977.
32. Taverne, P.P., and van der Jagt, E.J.: Small bowel radiography: A prospective comparison study of three techniques in 200 patients. Fortschr. Geb. Roentgenstr. 143:293, 1985.
33. Bret, P., Cuche, C., and Schmutz, G.: Radiology of the small intestine. Berlin, Springer-Verlag, 1989.
34. Shirakabe, H., and Kobayashi, S.: Air double contrast barium study of the small bowel. In Herlinger, H., and Maglinte, D.D.T. (eds.): Clinical Radiology of the Small Intestine. Philadelphia, W.B. Saunders, 1989.
35. Trickey, S.F., Halls, J., and Hodson, C.J.: A further development of the small bowel enema. Proc. R. Soc. Med. 56:1070, 1963.
36. Sinclair, D.J., and Buist, T.A.S.: Water contrast barium enema technique using methyl cellulose in solution. Br. J. Radiol. 39:228, 1966.
37. Gmuendner, U., and Wirth, W.: Duenndarmdoppelkontrastdarstellung. Schweiz. Med. Wochenschr. 100:1236, 1970.
38. Marriott, P.H., and John, E.G.: Influence of electrolytes on the hydration of methylcellulose in solution. J. Pharm. Pharmacol. 25:633, 1973.
39. Herlinger, H.: A modified technique for the double contrast small bowel enema. Gastrointest. Radiol. 3:201, 1987.
40. Christie, D.L., and Ament, M.E.: A double blind crossover study of metoclopramide versus placebo for facilitating passage of multipurpose biopsy tube. Gastroenterology 71:726, 1976.
41. Maglinte, D.D.T., and Herlinger, H.: Enteroclysis catheters, intubation and infusion. In Herlinger, H., and Maglinte, D.D.T. (eds.): Clinical Radiology of the Small Intestine. Philadelphia, W.B. Saunders, 1989.
42. Maglinte, D.D.T., and Herlinger, H.: Single contrast and biphasic enteroclysis: The small bowel enema with methylcellulose. In Herlinger, H., and Maglinte, D.D.T. (eds.): Clinical Radiology of the Small Intestine. Philadelphia, W.B. Saunders, 1989.
43. Maglinte, D.D.T., and Herlinger, H.: Congenital and developmental anomalies in adolescents and adults. In Herlinger, H., and Maglinte, D.D.T. (eds.): Clinical Radiology of the Small Intestine. Philadelphia, W.B. Saunders, 1989.

44. Stewart, J.S., Pollock, D.J., Hoffbrand, A.V., et al.: A study of proximal and distal intestinal structure and absorptive function in idiopathic steatorrhea. Q. J. Med. 36:425, 1967.
45. Thaysen, T.E.H.: Absorption of Fat and Protein: Non-tropical Sprue. Copenhagen, Levin and Munksgaard, 1932.
46. Nelson, S.W.: Abnormal small bowel fold patterns. In Categorical Course on Gastrointestinal Radiology. Reston, VA, Am. Roentgen Ray Soc., 1977.
47. Tully, T.E., and Feinberg, S.B.: Roentgenographic classification of diffuse diseases of the small intestine presenting with malabsorption. AJR 121:283, 1974.
48. Osborn, A.G., and Friedland, G.W.: A radiological approach to the diagnosis of small bowel disease. Clin. Radiol. 24:281, 1973.
49. Pare, P., Douville, P., Caron, D., Lagace, R.: Adult celiac sprue: Changes in the pattern of clinical recognition. J. Clin. Gastroenterol. 10:395, 1988.
50. Herlinger, H., and Maglinte, D.D.T.: Jejunal fold separation in adult celiac diseases: Relevance of enteroclysis. Radiology 158:605, 1986.
51. Bova, J.G., Friedman, A.C., Weser, E., et al.: Adaptation of the ileum in nontropical sprue: Reversal of the jejunoileal fold pattern. AJR 144:299, 1985.
52. Marshak, R.H., and Linder, A.E.: Malabsorption syndromes: Sprue. In Radiology of the Small Intestine, ed. 2. Philadelphia, W. B. Saunders, 1976.
53. Farthing, M.J., McLean, A.M., Bartram, C.I., et al.: Radiological features of the jejunum in hypoalbuminemia. AJR 136:883, 1981.
54. Cohen, M.D., and Lintott, D.J.: Transient small bowel intussusception in adult coeliac disease. Clin. Radiol. 29:529, 1978.
55. Stokes, P.L., and Holmes, G.K.T.: Malignancy in celiac disease. Clin. Gastroenterol. 3:159, 1974.
56. Collins, S.M., Hamilton, J.D., Lewis, T.D., et al.: Small bowel malabsorption and gastrointestinal malignancy. Radiology 126:603, 1978.
57. Scott, B.B., and Losowsky, M.S.: Depressed cell-mediated immunity in coeliac disease. Gut 17:900, 1976.
58. Horowitz, A.L., and Meyers, M.A.: The "hide-bound" small bowel of scleroderma: Characteristic mucosal fold pattern. AJR 119:332, 1973.
59. Golladay, L.S., and Byrne, W.J.: Intestinal pseudo-obstruction. Surg. Gynecol. Obstet. 153:257, 1981.
60. Rohrman, C.A., Jr., Ricci, M.T., Krisnamurthy, S., and Schuffler, M.D.: Radiologic and histologic differentiation of neuromuscular disorders of the gastrointestinal tract: Visceral myopathies, visceral neuropathies, and progressive systemic sclerosis. AJR 143:933, 1981.
61. Scott, P.P., Scott, W.W., and Siegelman, S.S.: Amyloidosis: An overview. Semin. Roentgenol. 21:103, 1986.
62. Scully, R.E. (ed.). Case records of the Massachusetts General Hospital: Case 3-1990. N. Engl. J. Med. 322:183, 1990.
63. Rosen, F.S., Cooper, M.D., and Wedgewood, R.J.P.: The primary immunodeficiencies. N. Engl. J. Med. 311:235, 1984.
64. Hermans, P.E.: Nodular lymphoid hyperplasia of the small intestine and hypogammaglobulinemia: Theoretical and practical considerations. Fed. Proc. 26:1606, 1967.
65. Brandon, J., Glick, S.N., and Teplick, S.K.: Intestinal giardiasis: Importance of serial filming. AJR 144:581, 1985.
66. Dobbins, W.O. III: Current concepts of Whipple's disease (Editorial). J. Clin. Gastroenterol. 4:205, 1982.
67. Davis, S.J., and Patel, A.: Case report: distinctive echogenic lymphadenopathy in Whipple's disease. Clin. Radiol. 42:60, 1990.
68. Herlinger, H., and Maglinte, D.D.T.: Malabsorption and immune deficiencies. In Herlinger, H., and Maglinte, D.D.T. (eds.). Clinical Radiology of the Small Intestine. Philadelphia, W.B. Saunders, 1989.
69. Cherner, J.A., Jensen, R.T., Dubois, A., et al.: Gastrointestinal dysfunction in systemic mastocytosis. Gastroenterology 95:657, 1988.
70. Clemmett, A.R., Fishbone, G., Levine, R.J., et al.: Gastrointestinal lesions in mastocytosis. AJR 103:405, 1968.
71. Miller, L.S., Vinayek, R., Frucht, H., et al.: Reflux esophagitis

in patients with Zollinger-Ellison syndrome. Gastroenterology *98*:341, 1990.

72. Matsui, T., Iida, M., Fujishima, M., et al.: Linear erosions on Kerkring's folds may be diagnostic of Zollinger-Ellison syndrome. J. Clin. Gastroenterol. *11*:278, 1989.

73. Cooke, W.T., Cox, E.U., Fone, D.J., et al.: The clinical and metabolic significance of jejunal diverticula. Gut *4*:115, 1963.

74. Scully R.E. (ed.): Case records of the Massachusetts General Hospital, Case 25-1990. N. Engl. J. Med. *322*:1796, 1990.

75. Smith, A.N., and Balfour, T.W.: Malabsorption in Crohn's disease. Clin. Gastroenterol. *1*:433, 1972.

76. Glick, S.N., and Teplick, S.K.: Crohn's disease of the small intestine: Diffuse mucosal granularity. Radiology *154*:313, 1985.

77. Morson, B.C.: Histopathology of regional enteritis (Crohn's disease). *In* Engel, A., and Larsen, T. (eds.): Skandia International Symposium on Regional Enteritis (Crohn's disease), pp. 15–33. Stockholm, Nordiska Bokhandelns Forlag, 1971.

78. Ekberg, O., Baath, L., Sjostrom, B., and Linghagen, T.: Are superficial lesions in the distal part of the ileum early indicators of Crohn's disease in adult patients with abdominal pain? A clinical and radiologic long-term investigation. Gut *25*:341, 1984.

79. Engelholm, L., DeToeuf, J., Herlinger, H., and Maglinte, D.D.T.: Crohn's disease of the small bowel. In Herlinger, H., and Maglinte, D.D.T. (eds.): Clinical Radiology of the Small Intestine. Philadelphia, W.B. Saunders, 1989.

80. Yamagata, S., Baba, S., Hosoda, S., et al.: Crohn's disease in Japan. Gastroenterol. Jpn. *14*:366, 1979.

81. Meyers, M.A.: Clinical involvement of mesenteric and antimesenteric borders of small bowel loops. Gastrointest. Radiol. *1*:49, 1976.

82. Nolan, D.J.: Radiology of Crohn's disease of the small intestine: a review. J. Roy. Soc. Med. *74*:294, 1981.

83. Herlinger, H., O'Riordan, D., Saul, S., and Levine, M.S.: Nonspecific involvement of bowel adjoining Crohn's disease. Radiology *159*:47, 1986.

84. Frick, M.P., Salomonowitz, E., and Gedgaudas, E.: The value of computerized tomography in Crohn's disease. Mt. Sinai J. Med. (NY) *51*:368, 1984.

85. Ekberg, O., Sjostrom, B., and Brahme, E.J.: Radiologic findings in *Yersinia* ileitis. Radiology *123*:15, 1977.

86. Palmer, K.R., Patil, D.H., Basran, G.S., et al.: Abdominal tuberculosis in urban Britain—a common disease. Gut *26*:1296, 1985.

87. Brombart, M., and Massion, J.: Radiologic differential diagnosis between ileocecal tuberculosis and Crohn's disease. Am. J. Dig. Dis. *6*:589, 1961.

88. Herlinger, H.: Angiography in the diagnosis of ileocecal tuberculosis. Gastrointest. Radiol. *2*:371, 1978.

89. Jeffrey, R.B., Laing, F.C., and Townsend, R.R.: Acute appendicitis: Sonographic criteria based on 250 cases. Radiology *167*:327, 1988.

90. Olmstead, W.W., Ros, P.R., Hjermstad, B.M., et al.: Tumors of the small intestine with little or no malignant predispositions: A review of the literature and report of 56 cases. Gastrointest. Radiol. *12*:231, 1987.

91. Megibow, A.J., Redman, P.E., Bosniak, M.A., and Horowitz, L.: Diagnosis of gastrointestinal lipomas by CT. AJR *133*:743, 1979.

92. Curcio, C.M., Feinstein, R.S., Humphrey, R.L., et al.: Computed tomography of enteroenteric intussusception. J. Comput. Assist. Tomogr. *6*:969, 1982.

93. Paivansalo, M., Siniluoto, T., and Jalovaara, P.: Radiological findings in small bowel tumors. Fortschr. Roentgenstr. *149*:615, 1988.

94. Linos, D.A., Dozios, R.R., Dahlin, D.C., and Bartholomew, L.G.: Does Peutz-Jegher's syndrome predispose to gastrointestinal malignancy? Arch. Surg. *116*:1182, 1981.

95. Herlinger, H., and Maglinte, D.D.T.: Tumors of the small intestine. *In* Herlinger, H., and Maglinte, D.D.T. (eds.). Clinical Radiology of the Small Intestine. Philadelphia, W.B. Saunders, 1989.

96. Dragosics, B., Bauer, P., and Radaszkiewicz, T.: Primary gastrointestinal non-Hodgkin's lymphomas: A retrospective clinicopathologic study of 150 cases. Cancer *55*:1060, 1985.

97. Bragg, D.G., Colby, T.V., and Ward, J.H.: New concepts in the non-Hodgkin's lymphomas: Radiologic implications. Radiology *159*:289, 1986.

98. Meyers, M.A.: Dynamic Radiology of the Abdomen: Normal and Pathologic Anatomy, 3rd ed. New York, Springer-Verlag, 1988.

99. Marshak, R.H., Khilnani, M.T., Eliasoph, J., and Wolf, B.S.: Metastatic carcinoma of the small bowel. AJR *94*:385, 1965.

100. Wittich, G., Salomonowitz, E., Szepesi, T., et al.: Small bowel double contrast enema in stage III ovarian cancer. AJR *142*:299, 1984.

101. Goldstein, H.M., Beydoun, M.T., and Dodd, G.D.: Radiologic spectrum of melanoma metastatic to the gastrointestinal tract. AJR *129*:605, 1977.

102. Fishman, E.K., Kuhlman, J.E., Schucter, L.M., et al.: CT of malignant melanoma in the chest, abdomen and musculoskeletal system. Radiographics *10*:603, 1990.

103. Mason, G.R., Dietrich, P., Friedland, G.W., et al.: The radiologic findings in radiation-induced enteritis and colitis: A review of 30 cases. Clin. Radiol. *21*:232, 1970.

104. Morgenstern L., Hart M., Lugo D., and Friedman, M.B.: Changing aspects of radiation enteropathy. Arch. Surg. *120*:1225, 1985.

105. Marshak, R.H., Linder, A.E., and Maklansky, D.: Ischemia of the small intestine. Am. J. Gastroenterol. *66*:390, 1976.

106. Rizzo, M.J., Federle, M.P., and Griffiths, G.B.: Bowel and mesenteric injury following blunt abdominal trauma: Evaluation with CT. Radiology *173*:143, 1989.

107. Rex, D.K., Lappas, J.C., Maglinte, D.D.T., et al.: Enteroclysis in the evaluation of suspected small intestinal bleeding. Gastroenterology *97*:58, 1989.

108. Lewis, B.S., and Waye, J.D.: Chronic gastrointestinal bleeding of obscure origin: Role of small bowel enteroscopy. Gastroenterology *94*:1117, 1988.

109. Caroline, D.F., Herlinger, H., Laufer, I., et al.: Small bowel enema in the diagnosis of adhesive obstruction. AJR *142*:1133, 1984.

110. Price, J., and Nolan, D.J.: Closed loop obstruction: Diagnosis by enteroclysis. Gastrointest. Radiol. *14*:251, 1989.

111. Herlinger, H., and Maglinte, D.D.T.: Small bowel obstruction. *In* Herlinger, H., and Maglinte, D.D.T. (eds.): Clinical Radiology of the Small Intestine. Philadelphia, W.B. Saunders, 1989.

112. Megibow, A.J., Wall, S.D., Balthazar, E.J., and Rybak, B.J.: Gastrointestinal radiology in AIDS patients. *In* Federle, M.P., Megibow, A.J., and Naidich, D.P. (eds.): Radiology of AIDS. New York, Raven Press, 1988.

113. Schulman, A., Morton, P.C.G., and Dietrich, B.E.: Eosinophilic gastroenteritis. Clin. Radiol. *31*:101, 1970.

114. Lycke, K.G.: Radiology of the ileal reservoirs. *In* Herlinger, H., and Megibow, A.J. (eds.): Advances in Gastrointestinal Radiology, vol. 1. Chicago, Mosby–Year Book, 1991.

115. Kelvin, F.M., Gramm, H.F., Gluck, W.L., and Lokich, J.J.: Radiologic manifestations of small bowel toxicity due to floxuridine therapy. AJR *146*:39, 1986.

116. Levi, S., deLacey, G., Price, A.B., et al.: "Diaphragm-like" strictures of the small bowel in patients treated with nonsteroidal anti-inflammatory drugs. Br. J. Radiol. *63*:186, 1990.

DOUBLE CONTRAST ENEMA: TECHNICAL ASPECTS

Igor Laufer, M.D.

12

INTRODUCTION

Despite the continuing controversy regarding its precise role in colonic diagnosis,[1] the double contrast enema has enjoyed a marked increase in popularity since 1976. Thoeni and Margulis,[2] in a survey of 175 leading medical centers around the world, found that only 6% used the double contrast enema routinely in 1976, whereas by 1987, the figure had increased to 56%. A survey of 500 hospitals and 200 office practices in the United States by Market Measures, Inc., indicates that the number of double contrast enemas increased by 35% between 1981 and 1987 at the same time that single contrast enemas decreased by over 30% (Fig. 12–1A). Thus, the proportion of double contrast enemas to the total number of radiologic examinations of the colon increased from 23% in 1981 to 39% in 1987 (Fig. 12–1B).

The basic diagnostic virtue of the double contrast enema is its ability to demonstrate small polypoid lesions and subtle surface alterations in the early stages of inflammatory bowel disease. We therefore feel that the double contrast enema should be the primary radiologic investigative tool for the colon in all patients over the age of 35 because of the high incidence of colonic polyps in this country. Wolf and co-workers[3] have shown that elderly patients are able to tolerate the double contrast enema. Furthermore, in most younger patients, the radiologic examination is being performed either because of rectal bleeding or because of the clinical suspicion of inflammatory bowel disease. We have therefore adopted the double contrast enema as our routine radiologic examination of the colon unless there are specific reasons for using an alternative technique.

CONTRAINDICATIONS

The double contrast enema is contraindicated in conditions that are also contraindications to the use of the single contrast enema. In patients with suspected colonic perforation, a water-soluble contrast material is used. Toxic megacolon is also a contraindication to barium study of the colon, although in patients in whom the clinical diagnosis is not clear, a small amount of dilute barium may be introduced. Contrast studies of the colon should not be performed immediately following colonic biopsy through the rigid sigmoidoscope since this has been shown to predispose to rectal perforation. In such cases, a delay of at least 5 days is advisable to allow the mucosa to heal. No such delay is required after endoscopic biopsy using fiberoptic instruments since these yield only a superficial biopsy.[4, 5]

In addition to the previously mentioned contraindications, there are certain conditions for which we prefer to use the single contrast enema. These are suspected Hirschsprung's disease, acute diverticulitis, high-grade colonic obstruction, or colonic fistula. In addition, in patients with ischemic colitis, the changes are best shown by single contrast technique, since the edema and thumbprinting may be obliterated by gaseous distention.[6]

PATIENT PREPARATION

Bowel Cleansing

Adequate cleansing of the colon is equally critical for all types of colonic examination: single contrast enema, colonoscopy, and double contrast enema. A wide variety of preparations has been recommended.[7, 8]

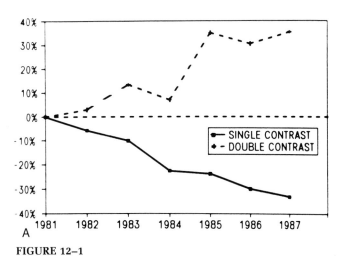

A

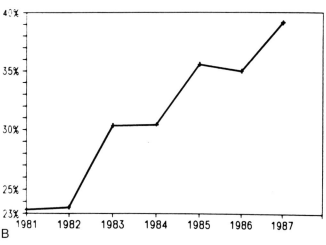

B

FIGURE 12–1

TRENDS IN RADIOLOGIC EXAMINATIONS OF THE COLON SINCE 1981. A, Single contrast enemas decreased by over 30% between 1981 and 1987, while double contrast enemas increased by 35%.

B, During this period, the proportion of double contrast enemas to total colon examinations rose from 23% to 39%. (Data provided by Market Measures, Inc., West Orange, NJ.)

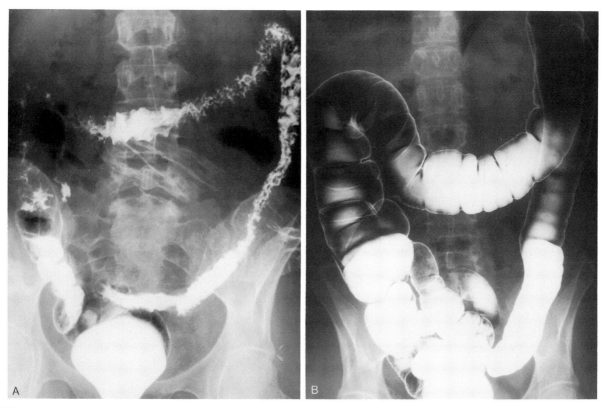

FIGURE 12–2

THE EFFECT OF GLUCAGON ON COLONIC SPASM. *A,* An overhead radiograph shows spasm throughout the colon, resulting in almost complete loss of barium and air.

B, After the intravenous injection of 1 mg glucagon and reinflation, the colon relaxes, and excellent radiographs are obtained. (From Laufer, I.: Barium contrast examination. *In* Berk, J.E., et al. (eds.): Bockus Gastroenterology, ed. 4, vol. 1. Philadelphia, W.B. Saunders, 1985, with permission.)

The principal components of adequate preparation include a clear liquid diet, laxatives, and a suppository. Our current preparation consists of the following:

1. The day before the examination
   a. clear liquids only by mouth
   b. At 5:00 P. M.—60 ml magnesium citrate
   c. At 10:00 P. M.—four tablets of bisacodyl
2. The morning of the examination—a bisacodyl suppository

This bowel cleansing preparation works reliably in all but the most debilitated patients, provided that instructions are followed. It is important to question patients upon arrival in the radiology department to determine whether the proper instructions were given and followed. If the patient reports that the last bowel movement was watery in nature, it can be assumed that adequate preparation has been achieved.

We no longer use cleansing enemas because they tend to leave a wet colon and prolong the patient's stay in the x-ray department. Rapid colonic lavage by the ingestion of electrolyte solutions such as Go-LYTELY (Braintree Laboratories, Braintree, MA) or Colyte (Reed & Carnrick, Piscataway, NJ) have been recommended for barium enema and colonoscopy.[9]

However, for the purpose of double contrast enemas, we find that these solutions leave too much residual fluid in the colon and degrade the quality of mucosal coating.[10]

Preliminary Film

The preliminary or scout film of the abdomen has been shown to be of little value prior to a barium enema.[11] We therefore use it routinely only in hospitalized patients. We also obtain a preliminary film in ambulatory patients whose history or symptoms suggest either inflammatory bowel disease or bowel obstruction. In addition, we obtain this film in cases in which we are uncertain about the adequacy of colonic cleansing. If the preliminary film shows definite fecal material in the colon, the patient is returned for an additional 24 hours of preparation with clear liquids and laxatives.

Hypotonic Drugs

Hypotonic drugs such as glucagon[12, 13] and Buscopan[14] have been shown to decrease patient discomfort during the double contrast enema. It is likely that they have no significant influence on the diagnostic accuracy of the examination.[15] We therefore do not use

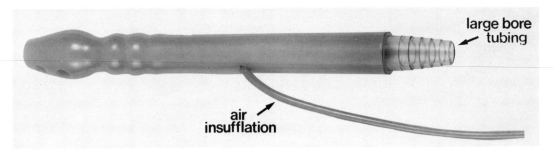

FIGURE 12–3

THE MILLER AIR TIP. The catheter for air insufflation emerges at the distal end of the enema tip. The enema tip is also available with a retention cuff. (Courtesy of E-Z-EM Company, Westbury, N.Y.)

glucagon routinely but only in selected cases. We inject 1 mg glucagon intravenously during the examination when the patient becomes very uncomfortable, when there is spasm resulting in pain, expulsion of the contrast material, or poor colonic distention (Fig. 12–2), or when an area of persistent narrowing is encountered. Glucagon may also be useful in cases in which it is important to visualize the terminal ileum.[16] However, it should be recognized that this may also promote air reflux into the small bowel and degrade the quality of the colon examination.[17] Therefore, in cases in which it is important to visualize the terminal ileum, it may be prudent to administer glucagon after the colon has been adequately examined and there is still no reflux into the terminal ileum.

Variations in Preparation

There are several exceptions to the foregoing bowel preparation. Patients who are suspected of having small bowel obstruction receive no laxative. In patients with active inflammatory bowel disease a milder laxative such as mineral oil may be administered. In patients with severe inflammatory bowel disease an "instant enema" may be undertaken with no preparation (see Chapter 17). The purpose of such a study is to document the presence of inflammatory bowel disease and to gain a general impression of its overall extent and severity.

MATERIALS

Several products and devices are available that greatly simplify and facilitate performance of the double contrast enema. These include large-bore tubing to allow relatively rapid instillation of high-density barium;[18] a specifically designed enema tip that allows separate instillation of barium and air (Fig. 12–3);[19] a simple apparatus for performing decubitus films with a horizontal beam;[20] and wedge filters for the decubitus radiographs to even out the exposure between the dependent and nondependent surfaces.[21, 22]

A barium suspension with good mucosal coating properties is essential. It has been shown by Schwartz and co-workers[23] that there is no simple relationship between the physical properties of the barium suspension and its coating ability. We have had good results with Polibar Plus and E-Z AC (E-Z-EM Co., Westbury, NY) and HD 85 (Lafayette Pharmacal, Lafayette, IN). The concentration of the barium suspension depends on the viscosity, but good coating can be achieved with 80% to 95% w/v concentration.

PROCEDURE

1. With the patient lying in the left lateral position, the enema tip is inserted into the rectum and taped to the buttocks with one or two pieces of tape. Taping is particularly important, since the ½-inch tubing filled with high-density barium becomes very heavy and tends to pull out of the rectum if not secured.

2. With the patient in the prone position, barium is introduced until it is just seen to round the splenic flexure.

3. Air is insufflated immediately until the head of the barium column crosses the spine.

4. The patient is turned onto the right side, and additional air is insufflated until the head of the column rounds the hepatic flexure. The patient is turned onto the back and onto the left side, and additional air is insufflated. A spot film of the sigmoid is obtained in the left posterior oblique (LPO) position (Fig. 12–4A). At this time the cecum and terminal ileum have usually not filled, and therefore an unobscured view of the sigmoid is obtained.

5. The patient turns to the right and returns to the prone position while additional air is insufflated. The enema bag is dropped on the floor for drainage of barium from the rectum. Drainage may be facilitated by insufflation of air and by angulation of the enema tip.

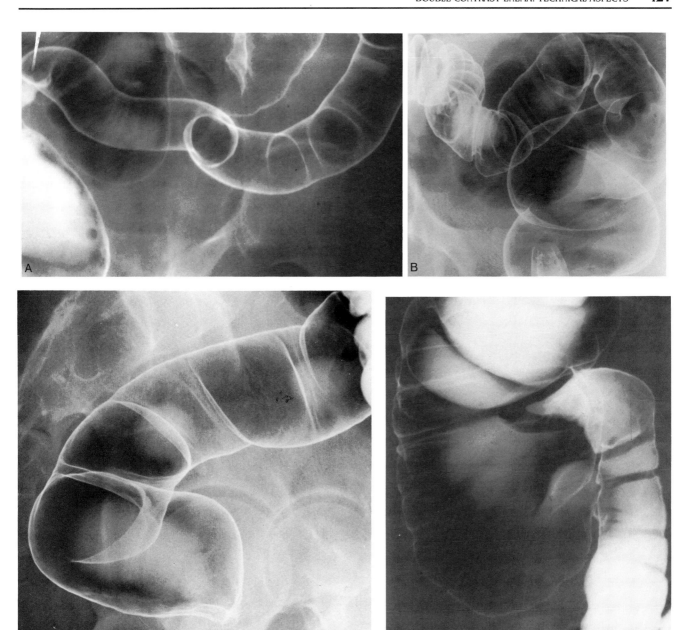

FIGURE 12–4

THE NORMAL ROUTINE DOUBLE CONTRAST ENEMA (films from various patients). *A,* Initial oblique spot film of the sigmoid in LPO projection.
    B, Prone spot film of the rectum after drainage of barium.
    C, Left lateral spot film of the rectum with enema tip removed.
    D, Supine spot film of the cecum, ileocecal valve, and terminal ileum.

Illustration continued on following page

6. When drainage is complete, the clamp is closed and additional air is insufflated to distend the rectum. A spot film of the rectosigmoid is exposed in the prone position (Fig. 12–4*B*).

7. Additional air is now insufflated until the entire colon is adequately distended.

8. The patient is turned into the left lateral position and a spot film of the rectum is obtained (Fig. 12–4*C*).

9. The patient returns to the supine position, and if the cecum and terminal ileum are filled, a spot film may be obtained with compression (Fig. 12–4*D*).

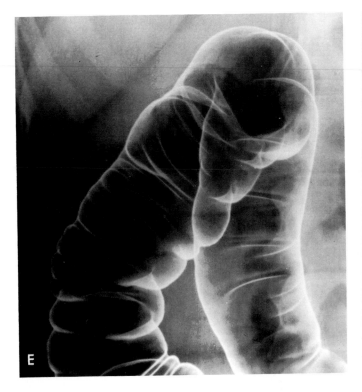

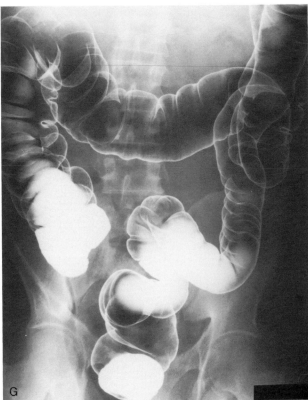

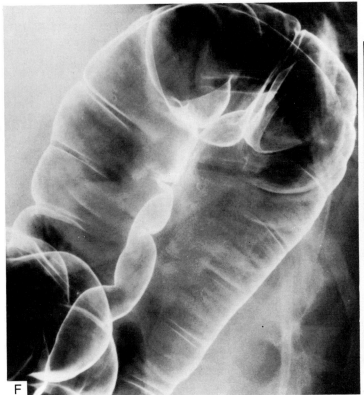

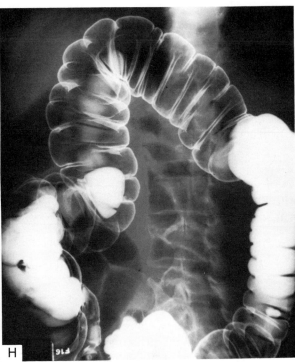

FIGURE 12–4 *Continued*

E, Upright spot film, hepatic flexure.
F, Upright spot film, splenic flexure.
G, Prone overhead film.
H, Supine, right posterior oblique film.

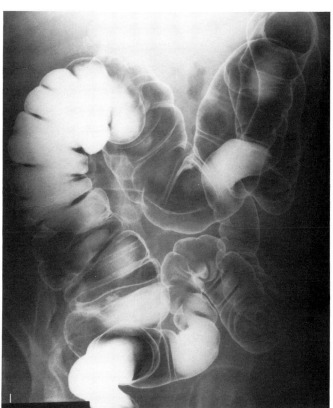

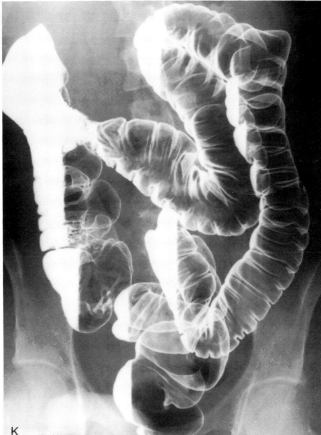

FIGURE 12–4 *Continued*

I, Supine, left posterior oblique film.
J, Prone, angled view of the rectosigmoid.
K, Right lateral decubitus.

Illustration continued on following page

10. The table is brought to the upright position for upright spot films of the flexures (Fig. 12–4E and F). In this position, barium fills the cecum.

11. The table is returned to the horizontal position, and additional views of the cecum and terminal ileum are obtained, if necessary. The head of the table may be lowered farther, and the patient turned from side to side to drain the cecum of barium and to distend it with air.

12. Routine overhead radiographs are obtained in the posteroanterior (PA) (Fig. 12–4G), right posterior oblique (RPO) (Fig. 12–4H), and LPO (Fig. 12–4I) positions. In patients over the age of 35 we also include a prone film of the rectosigmoid with the tube angled 35 degrees toward the feet (Fig. 12–4J).[24] Several puffs of air are insufflated into the colon before each of these films.

13. The enema tip is then removed and three films are obtained with the horizontal beam. These are the right (Fig. 12–4K) and left lateral decubitus (Fig. 12–

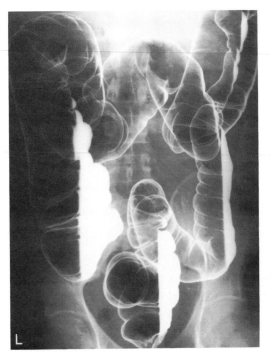

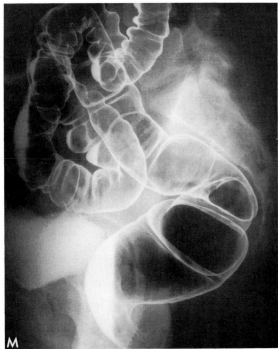

FIGURE 12–4 *Continued*

L, Left lateral decubitus.
M, Prone, cross-table lateral view of the rectosigmoid.

4L) films and the prone cross-table lateral of the rectosigmoid (Fig. 12–4M).[25]

The procedure just described is our routine complete examination of the colon. We do not include a postevacuation film routinely, since it has been shown to be of little diagnostic value except to document appendiceal filling.[26] We also include it when mucosal coating is poor and there is clinical suspicion of inflammatory bowel disease.

The routine study requires six spot films and seven overhead radiographs. In some instances the study can be shortened considerably and it is very likely that limiting the number of overhead radiographs to four does not diminish the diagnostic accuracy provided that good spot films are obtained.[27] The average normal study can be completed by the fluoroscopist in 5 minutes with 2 to 3 minutes of fluoroscopy time. The overhead radiographs can be completed in an additional 10 to 15 minutes. However, in problem patients additional time may need to be spent and additional radiographs exposed as indicated.

VARIATIONS IN TECHNIQUE

Remote Control

We have had some experience with the use of remote control apparatus for performing double contrast enemas but prefer tableside fluoroscopy. However, other authors[28, 29] have examined large numbers of patients with such equipment with excellent results.

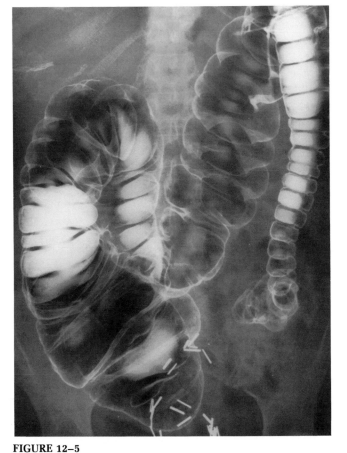

FIGURE 12–5

COLOSTOMY ENEMA. Excellent visualization of the residual colon following colostomy.

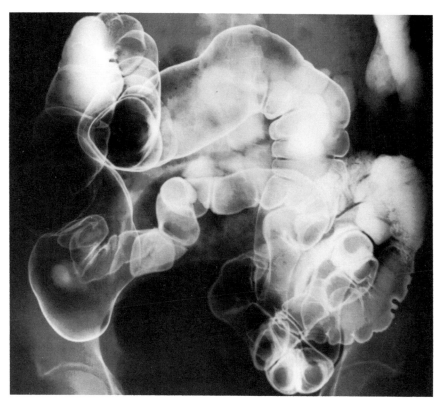

FIGURE 12–6

PERORAL PNEUMOCOLON. Excellent visualization of the right colon and distal small bowel.

Technologist Fluoroscopy

The use of fluoroscopy in the double contrast enema is mainly for monitoring the flow of barium and air and for positioning and timing spot films. Diagnostic fluoroscopy is minimized. Therefore, this examination is ideally suited for performance by a trained technologist.[30] We have evaluated technician performance of the double contrast enema and it appears that fluoroscopic studies with radiologist supervision and interpretation result in no loss of diagnostic accuracy.[31]

Colostomy Study

A double contrast enema can be performed in patients with a colostomy (Fig. 12–5). This is facilitated by the colostomy device described by Goldstein.[32] This device consists basically of a Foley catheter, which is passed through a feeding nipple. The catheter is then advanced into the colon until the nipple occludes the colostomy. A modification of this technique has been described by Pochaczevsky.[33] Accurate examination of the residual colon following colostomy may be particularly important because of the increased incidence of synchronous and meta-

chronous carcinomas in patients with previous resection of a colorectal carcinoma.[14]

Peroral Pneumocolon

In some patients an adequate examination of the right colon is not achieved either because of poor patient cooperation, retained fluid, or fecal residue, or because of technical reasons. In these patients as well as in those in whom the radiologic findings in the right colon and terminal ileum require further study, the peroral pneumocolon (PNC) can be used.[35, 36]

The PNC examination is basically designed to examine the distal small bowel and right colon following a small bowel study. It is important that the colon be cleansed. We use the same preparation as that for the colonic examination. A small bowel follow-through study is performed in the usual fashion, using barium sulfate (Entrobar, Lafayette Pharmacal, Lafayette, IN). When the terminal ileum and right colon are opacified to the midtransverse colon, a small rectal catheter is inserted and air is insufflated to obtain double contrast views. Glucagon in a dose of 1 mg may also be injected intravenously. Surprisingly good views of the right colon and terminal ileum can

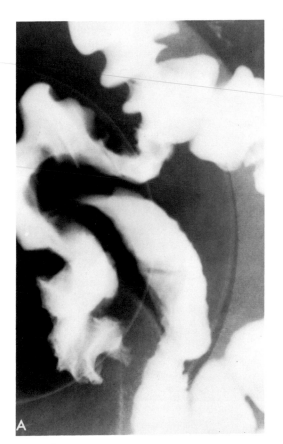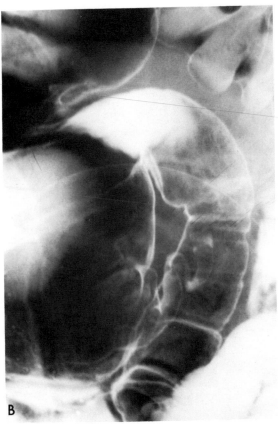

FIGURE 12–7

A, Suspicion of an abnormal cecum and terminal ileum on barium study.
B, Peroral pneumocolon technique shows a normal cecum and terminal ileum.

be obtained in this way (Figs. 12–6 and 12–7). It must be emphasized that it is important to use a barium suspension that does not flocculate or otherwise lose its coating properties during its passage through the small bowel.

PITFALLS

Prior Endoscopy

There is continuing debate regarding the advisability of performing double contrast enemas immediately following sigmoidoscopy or colonoscopy. It is clear that prior endoscopy increases the amount of air in the colon.[37] Our feeling is that this air makes the double contrast examination more difficult and more uncomfortable and results in less than optimal mucosal coating. Ideally, we therefore prefer not to perform these studies immediately following endoscopy. However, as a matter of logistics and convenience for patients, it is frequently done. In such cases, we obtain a preliminary film to evaluate the amount of bowel gas present. If it appears to be excessive, we ask the patient to wait, walk around, and try to expel as much of the gas as possible before we proceed with the examination.

In patients who have had endoscopy immediately prior to x-ray examination, it is of critical importance to ascertain whether a biopsy has been performed. The x-ray examination should never be done immediately following sigmoidoscopic biopsy through a rigid sigmoidoscope.[4, 5]

Uncooperative Patients

Occasionally, it may be important to examine the colon in patients who are uncooperative. In such cases, it has been demonstrated that intravenous sedation with drugs such as meperidine, diazepam, or fentanyl may be helpful and may allow for a successful examination.[38]

Colonic Spasm

Colonic spasm may be either diffuse or focal. If it is diffuse, it results in suboptimal visualization of the entire colon. In most cases, an injection of a hypotonic drug such as glucagon relaxes the colon and allows for adequate visualization (see Fig. 12–2). Focal colonic spasm may simulate a lesion and may prevent filling of the proximal colon. In most cases, such spasm responds to intravenous glucagon, but in rare

cases it does not. In cases of spasm, it may be helpful to have the patient evacuate and to attempt to fill the colon with single contrast barium to demonstrate that the colon distends completely.[39]

Nonfilling of the Right Colon

The right colon may not fill if an inadequate volume of high-density barium has been introduced. In such cases, Maglinte and Miller[40] have suggested that the addition of single contrast barium will push the high-density barium around to the right colon and salvage the examination. In other cases, we proceed to obtain radiographs of the coated and distended portions of the bowel, and the postevacuation film may demonstrate filling of the right colon that was not filled initially (Fig. 12–8). If the right colon has not filled by means of all of these maneuvers, it is suggested to

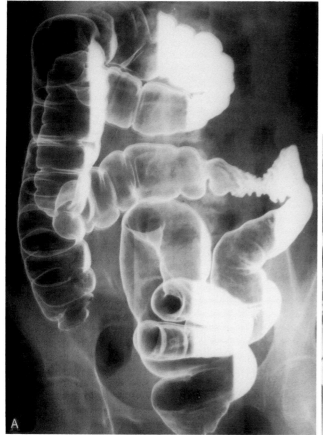

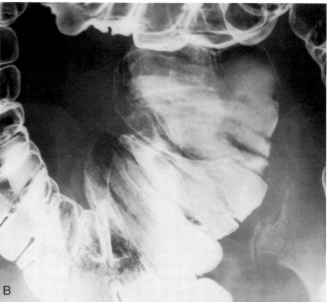

FIGURE 12–8

NONFILLING OF THE COLON because of redundancy. *A*, On the initial film, it is not clear whether the entire right colon has filled.
  B, The postevacuation film shows that the medially located cecum had not been filled previously. (From Margulis, A.R.: Alimentary Tract Radiology, No. 4. St. Louis, C.V. Mosby, 1989, with permission.)

convert to a single contrast examination and attempt to fill the entire colon with thin barium (Fig. 12–9).

Diverticulosis

It has been shown that most errors on barium enema examinations occur in the sigmoid colon and usually the source of error is severe diverticulosis.[41] This is a particular problem on double contrast studies because of the multiple ring shadows due to diverticula, which may be difficult to distinguish from polyps. Lappas and co-workers[42] have suggested that after the double contrast study, in patients with severe diverticulosis, a limited re-examination with an enema of water or very dilute barium may yield additional good views of the sigmoid colon (Fig. 12–10). Other authors have also found such a technique to be valuable.[43, 44]

COMPLICATIONS

Gas Pains

The most common "complication" of double contrast enema is residual abdominal pain. This is due to the air that remains within the colon after the examination is completed. Coblentz and co-workers[45] have reported that 50% of patients complained of such abdominal pain. In an attempt to reduce the incidence of this pain, they[46] and other authors[47, 48] have suggested that carbon dioxide be used for gaseous distention instead of room air. Carbon dioxide is absorbed more rapidly from the GI tract and therefore reduces the incidence and severity of postexamination pain.

Perforation

The serious complication of perforation is common to both single and double contrast enema examina-

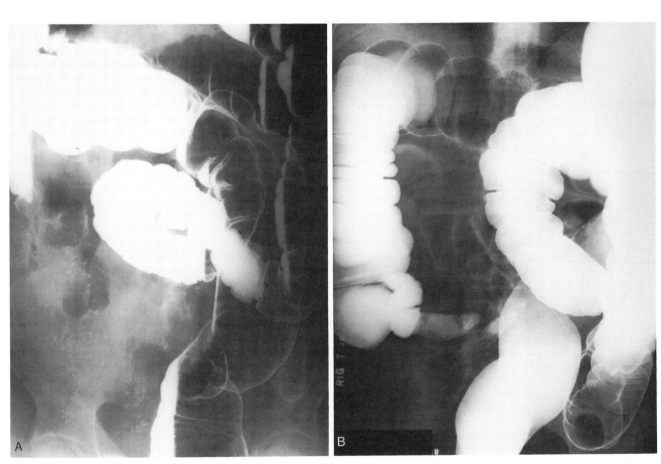

FIGURE 12–9

NONFILLING OF THE RIGHT COLON, salvaged by single contrast. *A,* On the initial films, the right colon could not be filled.
B, The right colon was then filled with thin barium, which allowed visualization of the cecum and terminal ileum.

tions.[49] There is no evidence that double contrast enemas have a higher complication rate than single contrast studies. Diner and colleagues[50] have shown that similar intracolonic pressures are generated by both types of examination.

There are basically two types of perforation that may occur. Rectal perforation or laceration results in the extravasation of barium into the wall of the rectum or into the perirectal or retroperitoneal tissues. This type of perforation occurs almost exclusively in cases in which the retention balloon is inflated in a patient with rectal pathology. It is particularly important to avoid inflation of such balloons in patients who have had a recent deep rectal biopsy or who have radiation proctitis or other forms of proctitis. When rectal perforation occurs, barium is seen either in the wall

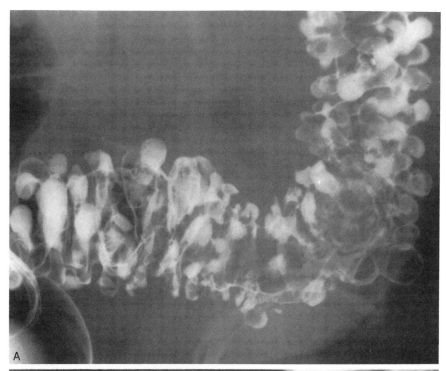

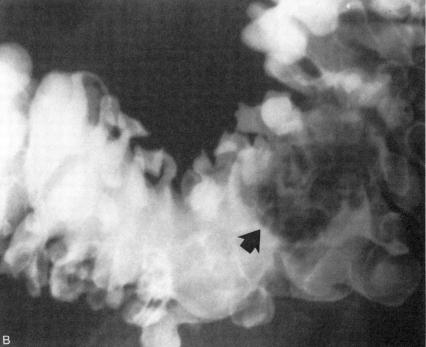

FIGURE 12–10

DIVERTICULOSIS WITH SIGMOID FLUSH. *A*, On the double contrast film, the diverticula are obvious, but a polypoid cancer cannot be identified.

B, Following refilling with single contrast barium, the polypoid cancer (*arrow*) is seen.

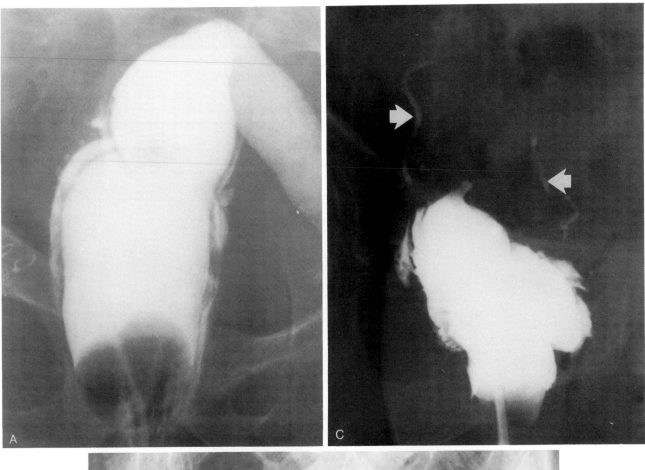

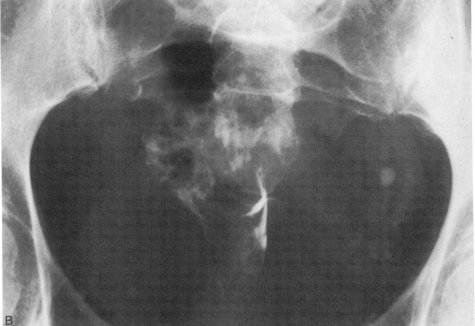

FIGURE 12–11

RECTAL TEAR COMPLICATING BARIUM ENEMA. *A,* During barium filling, barium is seen within the wall of the rectum. (From Laufer, I.: Barium contrast examination. *In* Berk, J.E., et al. (eds.): Bockus Gastroenterology, ed. 4, vol. 1. Philadelphia, W.B. Saunders, 1985, with permission.)

   B, Intramural barium may often be seen years after the trauma has occurred.

   C, Intravasation of barium into perirectal veins *(arrows)* in a patient with severe ulcerative colitis.

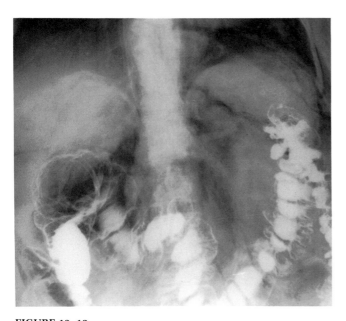

FIGURE 12–12

RETROPERITONEAL AIR AND PNEUMOMEDIASTINUM AS A COMPLICATION OF DOUBLE CONTRAST ENEMA. This complication is rare but usually occurs in patients with diverticulosis. (From Laufer, I.: Barium contrast examination. *In* Berk, J.E., et al. (eds.): Bockus Gastroenterology, ed. 4, vol. 1. Philadelphia, W.B. Saunders, 1985, with permission.)

of the rectum or as linear strands in the retroperitoneal tissues (Fig. 12–11A and B). Occasionally, barium may even enter the venous system and embolize to the liver or lungs (Fig. 12–11C). This complication is frequently fatal although recovery has been reported.[49]

Intraperitoneal rupture of the colon is almost always due to an underlying pathologic process that weakens the bowel wall. This complication should be recognized fluoroscopically by the appearance of barium in the paracolic gutters or barium outlining loops of bowel. A unique complication of double contrast as opposed to single contrast enemas is the

development of pneumoperitoneum,[51] pneumoretroperitoneum, and even pneumomediastinum without barium extravasation (Fig. 12–12).[52] It appears that this is more likely to occur in the presence of diverticulosis and that surgery may not be necessary when air alone escapes into the peritoneal cavity.

Portal Venous Gas

Air may enter the wall of the bowel either because of traumatic laceration or because of inflammatory or ischemic disease. In such cases, the air may also gain access to the venous system and be seen as portal venous air. Portal venous gas may be encountered as a complication of both single and double contrast enemas and patients usually recover uneventfully.[53, 54]

Other Complications

Other complications related to various aspects of the double contrast enema procedure are rare. These may include complications from the preparation,[55, 56] allergic reactions to barium or glucagon,[57] and occasional episodes of myocardial ischemia or infarction that are temporally related to the performance of a barium enema.[58]

Recently there have been reports of allergic reactions such as fatal anaphylaxis to the latex content of the retention balloon on enema tips. This complication has resulted in a recall of enema tips made of latex and new enema tips with retention balloons made of silicone rubber have recently become available.[59]

There is considerable debate about the need for antibiotic prophylaxis in certain patients undergoing x-ray examination of the colon. There is conflicting evidence regarding the occurrence of bacteremia in association with barium enemas.[60, 61] However, it is clear that endocarditis or septicemia as a complication of barium enema is extraordinarily rare. Therefore, routine antibiotic prophylaxis is in general not recommended except in patients with susceptible cardiac lesions who either have a prior history of endocarditis or have a prosthetic valve.

NORMAL APPEARANCES

Transverse Folds

In evaluating a double contrast enema examination it is necessary to assess the mucosal line as seen in profile as well as the en face appearance of the colonic mucosa. In profile the mucosal line should be thin, smooth, and straight. When viewed en face the normal mucosa is flat and featureless except for the haustral markings (see Fig. 12–4). In some patients a series of tightly spaced circular folds may be seen as a transient phenomenon (Fig. 12–13). This most likely represents intermittent contraction of the muscularis mucosae and is of no pathologic significance.

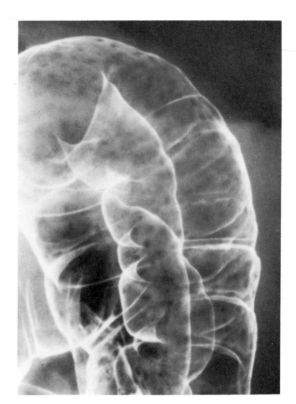

FIGURE 12–14

LYMPHOID FOLLICLES. Multiple tiny filling defects in the colon, representing the lymphoid follicular pattern in a child.

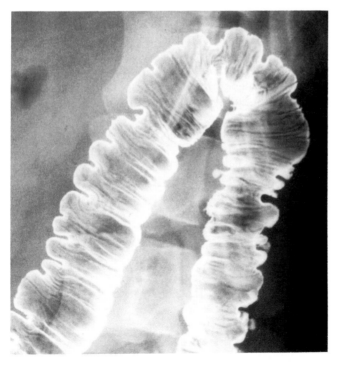

FIGURE 12–13

FINE TRANSVERSE FOLDS IN THE COLON AS A NORMAL VARIANT. Such folds may be caused by contraction of the muscularis mucosae.

Lymph Follicles

In some patients the mucosa may be studded with tiny nodules measuring 1 to 2 mm in diameter. This appearance is seen particularly frequently in children under the age of 5 years and has been termed *lymphoid hyperplasia* (Fig. 12–14).[62–64] This pattern corresponds precisely to the anatomic description of the distribution of lymphoid follicles in the human colon.[65] We believe these lymph follicles represent a normal feature of the pediatric colon,[66] although in some patients they may become hyperplastic in response to infection, allergy, or immunologic deficiency states.[67] In such cases the lymph follicles may be larger, and the typical umbilicated appearance is more easily seen.[62]

The normal lymphoid follicular pattern is seen regularly in children, but we have seen it only occasionally in adults (Fig. 12–15). Other authors have found this pattern in 13% to 63% of double contrast enemas in adults.[68, 69] These nodules are most commonly seen in the right colon and their incidence is probably related to the nature of the mucosal coating. They are easier to appreciate on good quality double contrast radiographs than on endoscopic examination of the colon. Burbige and associates[70] described the endoscopic appearance of colonic lymphoid nodules as a normal variant. In their case they postulated that the follicles were visible as 1-mm white spots because their patient had melanosis coli.

The normal lymphoid reticular pattern has a typical radiographic appearance. However, occasionally, when the lymph follicles are slightly enlarged they may appear to be umbilicated (Fig. 12–15B) and it may be difficult to distinguish the normal from the abnormal conditions. Glick and associates[71] have described small colonic nodules in a variety of conditions including lymphoma, Crohn's disease (Fig. 12–15C) and various forms of polyposis. In some of these cases, the distinction from normal may be difficult. Bronen and co-workers[72] have suggested that some cases of colonic cancer may be associated with lymphoid follicles scattered diffusely throughout the colon. This is in contrast to the frequently segmental distribution of lymphoid follicles in the normal patient. They therefore suggest that whenever lymphoid follicles are seen diffusely throughout the colon in a patient over the age of 60, a very careful search should be made for an underlying colonic neoplasm.

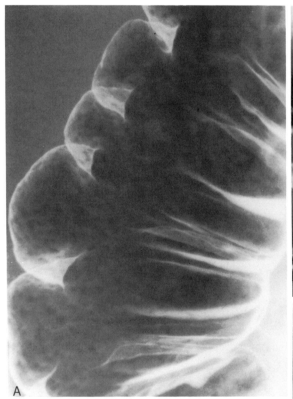

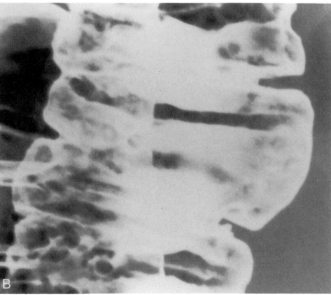

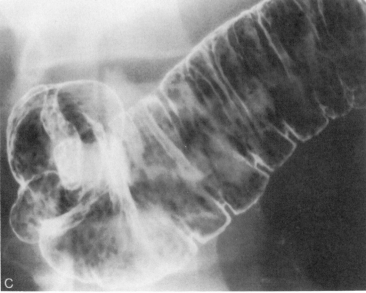

FIGURE 12–15

LYMPHOID FOLLICULAR PATTERNS IN ADULTS.

A, Normal adult demonstrating a lymphoid follicular pattern.

B, Prominent lymphoid follicles having an umbilicated appearance in a normal adult.

C, Prominent lymphoid follicles in a patient with Crohn's disease.

Surface Pattern

The colon has a fine surface pattern consisting of innominate lines (Fig. 12–16A and B) analogous to the areae gastricae (see Chapter 7). Several patterns have been described by Matsuura and co-workers.[73]

These include linear, network, and mixed patterns. These lines are rarely seen on our double contrast enemas because of the high density and viscosity of our barium suspensions. In some cases the lines are best seen with single contrast, especially when the bowel is partially collapsed (Fig. 12–16C).

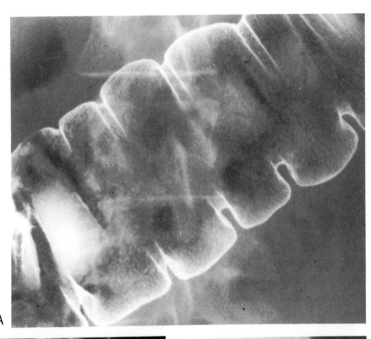

FIGURE 12–16

INNOMINATE LINES IN THE COLON. *A* and *B*, Two examples showing the innominate lines. (*B*, From Laufer, I.: Double contrast examination. *In* Margulis, A.R., and Burhenne, H.J. (eds.): Alimentary Tract Radiology, No. 4. St. Louis, C.V. Mosby, 1989, with permission.)
  C, A single contrast film shows the profile appearance of the innominate lines. These lines should not be mistaken for ulcers.

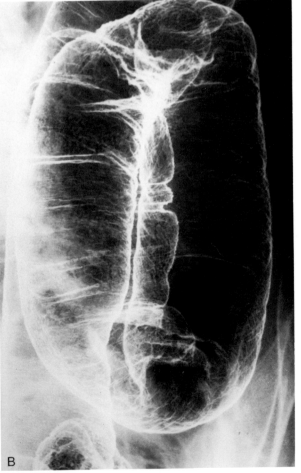

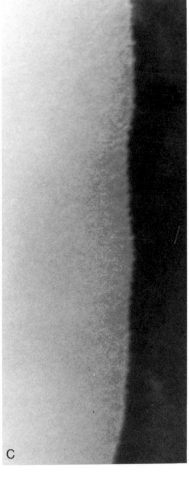

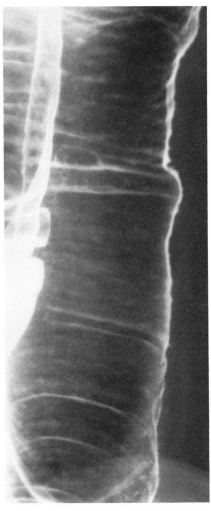

FIGURE 12–17

SURFACE PATTERN in a normal adult showing pinpoint barium collections en face and in profile.

Innominate lines may result in spiculation of the contour of the colon. Occasionally pinpoint collections of barium are seen en face and in profile (Fig. 12–17). These collections probably represent points of intersection of innominate lines[74] and should not be mistaken for ulceration.[75]

Terminal Ileum

Depending on the degree of distention, the terminal ileum may have either a smooth surface (see Fig. 12–6) or prominent circular folds (Fig. 12–18A). Lymph follicles are frequently seen in the terminal ileum (Fig. 12–18B), particularly in young patients, but they may occasionally be seen in older patients and are probably of no pathologic significance.

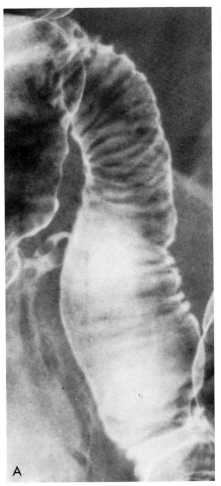
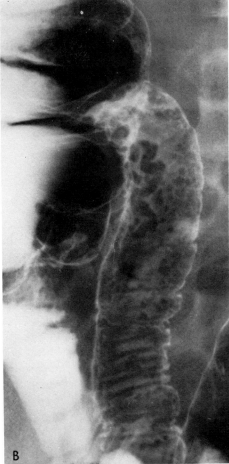

FIGURE 12–18

NORMAL TERMINAL ILEUM. A, Normal transverse folds in the terminal ileum. (From Laufer, I., and Costopoulos, L.: Early lesions of Crohn's disease. AJR 130:307, 1978. Reproduced by permission.)

B, Normal terminal ileum with tiny filling defects due to lymph follicles. (From Laufer, I.: Double contrast enema: Myths and misconceptions. Gastrointest. Radiol. 1:19, 1976. Reproduced by permission.)

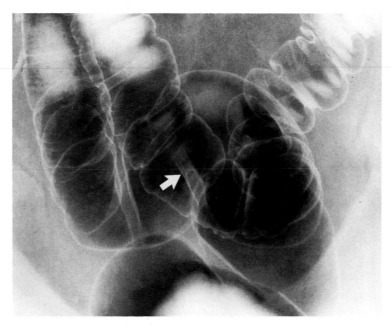

FIGURE 12–19

Folding of the colon, producing a linear filling defect *(arrow)*, which could be mistaken for the stalk of a polyp.

ARTIFACTS

The artifacts[76] related to poor barium suspension have been discussed in Chapter 2. Artifacts produced by precipitation or flaking of the barium may closely simulate the appearance of inflammatory bowel disease.[77]

Sharp angulation of the bowel may result in a long filling defect that may resemble the stalk of a polyp (Fig. 12–19). A similar appearance is often produced by a strand of mucus (Fig. 12–20). In other patients thick tenacious mucus may form a relatively solid, constant, polypoid mass. The case illustrated in Figure 12–21 was highly suggestive of polypoid carcinoma, but colonoscopy showed only tenacious mucus. A repeat double contrast enema showed no abnormality in this region. Although it is generally considered that a meticulously clean colon is a prerequisite for performing a double contrast enema, our experience has been that the double contrast tech-

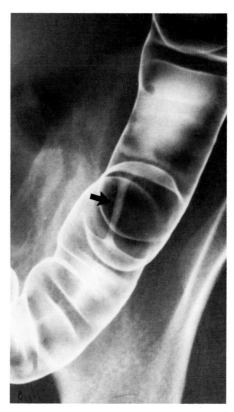

FIGURE 12–20

MUCUS STRAND *(arrow).*

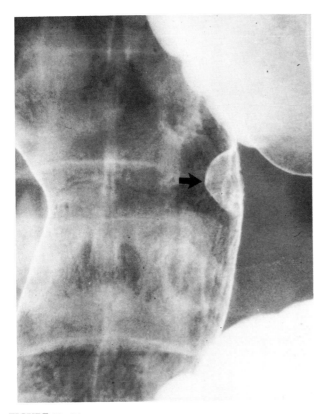

nique is even more valuable in patients whose colon is imperfectly prepared.[78] Solid fecal material and other extraneous material can frequently be definitively diagnosed by virtue of their mobility on horizontal-beam films (Fig. 12–22). Although solid fecal material is easily differentiated from polyps, smaller fecal residue and debris may adhere to the colonic mucosa and produce an appearance indistinguishable from that seen in familial polyposis or inflammatory bowel disease.

A variety of other shadows may overlap the colon and produce polypoid appearances on the double contrast enema. These shadows include the greater trochanter projected over the rectum, hemorrhoids, an inverted appendiceal stump, the tip of the appendix projected over the rectosigmoid, renal calculi, phleboliths, and calcified lymph nodes. Most of these potential errors can be avoided by reference to a preliminary film and by careful study of the radiographs.

FIGURE 12–21

TENACIOUS MUCUS RESEMBLING A POLYPOID LESION.
Colonoscopy showed only tenacious mucus and no evidence of a polypoid lesion. A repeat double contrast enema showed no abnormality.

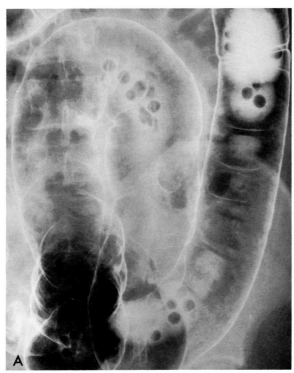

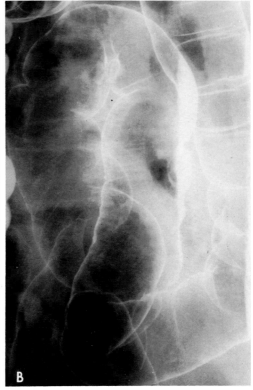

FIGURE 12–22

FILLING DEFECTS DUE TO EXTRANEOUS MATERIAL. *A,* Multiple filling defects in the colon due to undigested peas.

B, In the lateral decubitus view, the peas settle into the barium puddle, and the colonic mucosa can be seen to good advantage. (From Laufer, I.: Double contrast enema: Myths and misconceptions. Gastrointest. Radiol. 1:19, 1976. Reproduced by permission.)

REFERENCES

1. Margulis, A.R., and Thoeni R.F.: The present status of the radiologic examination of the colon. Radiology 167:1, 1988.
2. Thoeni, R.F., and Margulis, A.R.: The state of radiographic technique in the examination of the colon: A survey in 1987. Radiology 167:7, 1988.
3. Wolf, E.L., Frager, D., and Beneventano, T.C.: Feasibility of double-contrast barium enema in the elderly. AJR 145:47, 1985.
4. Maglinte, D.D.T., Strong, R.C., Strate R.W., et al.: Barium enema after colorectal biopsies: Experimental data. AJR 139:693, 1982.
5. Harned, R.K., Consigny, P.M., and Cooper, N.B.: Barium enema examination following biopsy of the rectum or colon. Radiology 145:11, 1982.
6. Bartram, C.I.: Obliteration of thumbprinting with double contrast enemas in acute ischemic colitis. Gastrointest. Radiol. 4:85, 1979.
7. Dodds, W.J., Scanlon, G.T., Shaw, D.K., et al.: An evaluation of colon cleansing regimens. AJR 128:57, 1977.
8. Fork, F.T., Ekberg, O., Nilsson, G., et al.: Colon cleansing regimens. Gastrointest. Radiol. 7:383, 1982.
9. Chan, C.H., Diner, W.C., Fontenot, E., et al.: Randomized single-blind clinical trial of a rapid colonic lavage solution (Golytely) vs. standard preparation for barium enema and colonoscopy. Gastrointest. Radiol. 10:378, 1985.
10. Bakran, A., Bradley, J.A., Breshnihan, E., et al.: Whole gut irrigation: An inadequate preparation for double contrast barium enema examination. Gastroenterology 73:28, 1977.
11. Eisenberg, R.L., and Hedgcock, M.W.: Preliminary radiograph for barium enema examination: Is it necessary? AJR 136:115, 1981.
12. Miller, R.E., Chernish, S.M., Skucas, J., et al.: Hypotonic colon examination with glucagon. Radiology 113:555, 1974.
13. Gohel, V.K., Dalinka, M.K., and Coren, G.S.: Hypotonic examination of the colon with glucagon. Radiology 115:1, 1975.
14. Lee, J.R.: Routine use of hyoscine N butylbromide (Buscopan) in double contrast barium enema examinations. Clin. Radiol. 33:273, 1982.
15. Thoeni, R.F., Vandeman, F., and Wall, S.D.: Effect of glucagon on the diagnostic accuracy of double-contrast barium enema examinations. AJR 142:111, 1984.
16. Violon, D., Steppe, R., and Potvliege, R.: Improved retrograde ileography with Glucagon. AJR 136:833, 1981.
17. Stone, E.E., and Conte, F.A.: Glucagon-induced small bowel air reflux: Degrading effects on double-contrast colon examination. Gastrointest. Radiol. 13:212, 1988.
18. Miller, R.E.: Barium enema examination with large-bore tubing and drainage. Radiology 82:905, 1964.
19. Miller, R.E.: A new enema tip. Radiology 92:1492, 1969.
20. Miller, R.E.: Simple apparatus for decubitus films with horizontal beam. Radiology 97:682, 1970.
21. De Lacey, G., Wignall, B., Ambrose, J., et al.: The double contrast barium enema: Improvements to lateral decubitus views including the use of a wedge filter. Clin. Radiol. 29:197, 1978.
22. Olson, D.L., Dodds, W.J., Stewart, E.T., et al.: Efficacy of an intracassette filter for improved pneumocolon decubitus radiographs. AJR 148:547, 1987.
23. Schwartz, S.C., Fischer, H.W., and House, A.J.: Studies in adherence of contrast media to mucosal surfaces. Radiology 112:727, 1974.
24. Dysart, D.N., and Stewart, H.R.: Special angled roentgenography for lesions of the rectosigmoid. AJR 96:285, 1966.
25. Niizuma, S., and Kobayashi, S.: Rectosigmoid double contrast examination in the prone position with a horizontal beam. AJR 128:519, 1977.
26. Smith, C., and Gardiner, R.: Efficacy of postevacuation view after double-contrast barium enema. Gastrointest. Radiol. 12:268, 1987.
27. Feczko, P.J., and Halpert, R.D.: Limiting overhead views in double-contrast colon examinations does not affect diagnostic accuracy. Gastrointest. Radiol. 12:175, 1987.
28. Hamelin, L., and Hurtubise, M.: Remote control technique in double contrast study of the colon. AJR 119:382, 1973.
29. Gelfand, D.W.: Gastrointestinal Radiology, pp. 95–104. New York, Churchill Livingstone, 1984.
30. Miller, R.E., and Maglinte, D.D.T.: Barium pneumocolon: Technologist-performed "7 Pump" method. AJR 139:1230, 1982.
31. Somers, S., Stevenson, G.W., Laufer, I., et al.: Evaluation of double contrast barium enemas performed by radiographic technologists. J. Can. Assoc. Radiol. 32:227, 1981.
32. Goldstein, H.M., and Miller, M.H.: Air contrast colon examination in patients with colostomies. AJR 127:607, 1976.
33. Pochaczevsky, R.: A colostomy device for barium enema examinations. Radiology 143:565, 1982.
34. Enker, W.E., and Dragacevic, S.: Multiple carcinomas of large bowel—natural experiment in etiology and pathogenesis. Ann. Surg. 187:8, 1978.
35. Kellett, M.J., Zboralske, F.F., and Margulis, A.R.: Per oral pneumocolon examination of the ileocecal region. Gastrointest. Radiol. 1:361, 1977.
36. Kressel, H.Y., Evers, K.A., Glick, S.N., et al.: The peroral pneumocolon examination: Technique and indications. Radiology 144:414, 1982.
37. Rodney, W.M., Randolph, J.F., and Peterson, D.W.: Cancellation rates and gas scores for air contrast barium enema immediately after 65-CM flexible sigmoidoscopy: A randomized clinical trial. J. Clin. Gastroenterol. 10:311, 1988.
38. Young, J.W.R., and Sanchez, F.: The use of sedation in the barium enema examination of uncooperative patients. AJR 141:340, 1983.
39. Levine, M.S., and Gasparaitis, A.E.: Barium filling for Glucagon-resistent spasm on double-contrast barium enema examinations. Radiology 160:264, 1986.
40. Maglinte, D.D.T., and Miller, R.E.: Salvaging the failed pneumocolon: A simple maneuver. AJR 142:719, 1984.
41. Ott, D.J., Gelfand, D.W., and Ramquist, N.A.: Causes of error in gastrointestinal radiology. Gastrointest. Radiol. 5:99, 1980.
42. Lappas, J.C., Maglinte, D.D.T., Kopecky, K.K., et al.: Diverticular disease: Imaging with post-double-contrast sigmoid flush. Radiology 168:35, 1988.
43. Demas, B.E., and Margulis, A.R.: Combined use of double and single contrast barium enema in the evaluation of suspected colonic disease. Gastrointest. Radiol. 9:241, 1984.
44. de Roos, A., Hermans, J., and Op den Orth, J.O.: Polypoid lesions of the sigmoid colon: A comparison of single-contrast, double-contrast, and biphasic examinations. Radiology 151:597, 1984.
45. Coblentz, C.L., Frost, R.A., Molinaro, V., et al.: Pain after barium enema: Effect of CO_2 and air on double-contrast study. Radiology 157:35, 1985.
46. Bernier, P., and Coblentz, C.: CO_2 delivery system for double-contrast barium enema examinations. Radiology 159:264, 1986.
47. Pochaczevsky, R.: Double-contrast examination of the colon with carbon dioxide: The use of effervescent powder. AJR 149:502, 1987.
48. Bessette, J.R., and Maglinte, D.D.T.: Double-contrast barium enema study: Simple conversion to CO_2. Radiology 162:274, 1987.
49. Gelfand, D.W.: Complications of gastrointestinal radiologic procedures: I. Complications of routine fluoroscopic studies. Gastrointest. Radiol. 5:293, 1980.
50. Diner, W.C., Patel, G., Texter, E.C., Jr., et al.: Intraluminal pressure measurements during barium enema: Full column vs. air contrast. AJR 137:217, 1981.
51. Gelfand, D.W., Ott, D.J., and Ramquist, N.A.: Pneumoperitoneum occurring during double-contrast enema. Gastrointest. Radiol. 4:307, 1979.
52. Beerman, P.J., Gelfand, D.W., and Ott, D.J.: Pneumomediastinum after double-contrast barium enema examination: A sign of colonic perforation. AJR 136:197, 1981.
53. Stein, M.G., Crues, J.V., III, and Hamlin, J.A.: Portal venous air associated with barium enema. AJR 140:1171, 1983.
54. Kees, C.J., and Hester, C.L.: Portal vein gas following barium enema examination. Radiology 102:525, 1972.
55. Galloway, D., Burns, H.J.G., Moffat, L.E.F., et al.: Faecal peritonitis after laxative preparation for barium enema. Br. Med. J. 284:472, 1982.

56. Zeligman, B.E., Feinberg, L.E., and Johnson, E.D.: A complication of cleansing enema: Retained protective shield of the enema tip. Gastrointest. Radiol. 11:372, 1986.
57. Schwartz, E.E., Glick, S.N., Foggs, M.B., et al.: Hypersensitivity reactions after barium enema examination. AJR 143:103, 1984.
58. Smith, H.J.: Performance of barium examinations after acute myocardial infarction: Report of a survey. AJR 149:63, 1987.
59. Gelfand, D.W.: Barium enemas, latex balloons and anaphylactic reactions. AJR 156:1, 1991.
60. Butt, J., Hentges, D., Pelican, G., et al.: Bacteremia during barium enema study. AJR 130:715, 1978.
61. Schimmel, D.H., Hanelin, L.G., Cohen, S., et al.: Bacteremia and the barium enema. AJR 128:207, 1977.
62. Capitanio, M.A., and Kirkpatrick, J.A.: Lymphoid hyperplasia of the colon in children. Radiology 94:323, 1970.
63. Franken, E.A. Jr.: Lymphoid hyperplasia of the colon. Radiology 94:329, 1970.
64. Theander, G., and Tragardh, B.: Lymphoid hyperplasia of the colon in childhood. Acta Radiol. (Diagn.) 17:631, 1976.
65. Dukes, C., and Bussey, H.J.R.: The number of lymphoid follicles of the human large intestine. J. Pathol. Bacteriol. 29:111, 1926.
66. Laufer, I., and deSa, D.: The lymphoid follicular pattern: A normal feature of the pediatric colon. AJR 130:51, 1978.
67. Riddlesberger, M.M. Jr., and Lebenthal, E.: Nodular colonic mucosa of childhood: Normal or pathologic? Gastroenterology 79:265, 1980.
68. Kelvin, F.M., Max, R.J., Norton, G.A., et al.: Lymphoid follicular pattern of the colon in adults. AJR 133:821, 1979.
69. Watanabe, H., Margulis, A.R., and Harter, L.: The occurrence of lymphoid nodules in the colon of adults. J. Clin. Gastroenterol. 5:535, 1983.
70. Burbige, E.J., and Sobyk, R.Z.F.: Endoscopic appearance of colonic lymphoid nodules: A normal variant. Gastroenterology 72:524, 1977.
71. Glick, S.N., Teplick, S.K., and Goren, R.A.: Small colonic nodularity and the double contrast barium enema. RadioGraphics 1:73, 1981.
72. Bronen, R.A., Glick, S.N., and Teplick, S.K.: Diffuse lymphoid follicles of the colon associated with colonic carcinoma. AJR 142:105, 1984.
73. Matsuura, K., Nakata, H., Takeda, N., et al.: Innominate lines of the colon. Radiology 123:581, 1977.
74. Williams, I.: Innominate grooves in the surface of the mucosa. Radiology 84:877, 1975.
75. Frank, D.F., Berk, R.N., and Goldstein, H.M.: Pseudoulcerations of the colon on barium enema examination. Gastrointest. Radiol. 2:129, 1977.
76. Gohel, V.K., Kressel, H.Y., and Laufer, I.: Double contrast artifacts. Gastrointest. Radiol. 3:139, 1978.
77. Laufer, I.: Air contrast studies of the colon in inflammatory bowel disease. C.R.C. Crit. Rev. Diagn. Imaging 9:421, 1977.
78. Laufer, I.: Double contrast enema: Myths and misconceptions. Gastrointest. Radiol. 1:19, 1976.

TUMORS OF THE COLON

Igor Laufer, M.D.

13

INTRODUCTION

Epidemiology

It is estimated that there are approximately 150,000 new cases of colorectal carcinoma in the United States each year with more than 60,000 deaths annually. In 1985, colorectal carcinoma accounted for 2.7% of all deaths in this country. Stated in other terms, 1 in 25 Americans will eventually develop colorectal cancer, and 1 in 37 will die of this disease.[1, 2] The magnitude of this problem is also illustrated in a recent review of medical malpractice claims against diagnostic radiology. Thirty percent of these claims were allegations of failure to diagnose malignancy, and most of these consisted of carcinomas of the lung and colon.[3] This finding emphasizes the radiologist's responsibility in ensuring the highest quality both in performance and in interpretation of radiologic examinations of the colon.

Although the evidence is not conclusive, it is widely believed that most colonic carcinomas arise in benign polyps.[4–7] This belief is based on the frequent coexistence of benign and malignant lesions in the same colon, the high incidence of malignant change in benign polyps, the invariable development of carcinoma in patients with familial polyposis, and the increasing incidence of cellular atypia as polyps increase in size.[2] There is also evidence that the systematic removal of benign polyps during routine proctosigmoidoscopy results in a lower incidence of rectal carcinoma.[8, 9]

Decreasing the mortality rate from this disease depends on detection and treatment of early carcinomas or premalignant lesions in asymptomatic patients. For practical purposes, almost all of these lesions are small polypoid lesions. Some lesions are found to be established carcinomas, many of them Dukes A, which carries an excellent prognosis.[10] The majority are benign polyps that can be removed endoscopically. It is to be hoped that the systematic removal of these benign polyps will decrease the likelihood of subsequent development of colorectal cancer. Semelka and MacEwan have suggested that the increased use of double contrast enema and colonoscopy over the last 20 years has resulted in a decrease in the diagnostic delay in patients with colorectal cancer and improved survival rates, particularly in women.[11]

Screening for Colorectal Cancer

Asymptomatic lesions may be discovered in patients who present for radiologic examinations of the colon because of symptoms due to other conditions such as diverticular disease, abdominal or pelvic masses, or functional disorders. Other patients with asymptomatic lesions may present for radiologic study because of positive findings in mass screening programs. The American Cancer Society has recommended the following screening program for asymptomatic persons with none of the risk factors for developing colorectal cancer:[12]

1. Starting at age 40, an annual digital rectal examination

2. Starting at age 50, an annual fecal occult blood test

3. Also starting at age 50, two annual proctosigmoidoscopies and, if negative, every 3 to 5 years thereafter.

These recommendations are based on the observation that a significant number of colorectal tumors can be detected by digital rectal examination with negligible additional cost. Most left-sided tumors can be detected by proctosigmoidoscopy, particularly if a flexible sigmoidoscope is used. It is expected that many right-sided tumors will be detected by the presence of fecal occult blood. Patients who have positive findings on the screening tests or patients who have any of the risk factors described in the next section require examination of the entire colon. This can be performed either by colonoscopy or by double contrast enema. Although there has been considerable discussion as to which diagnostic method is preferable, Eddy and co-workers, using a mathematical model, have concluded that colonoscopy and double contrast enema are equally effective but that the lower cost of the radiologic examination makes it a more cost-effective strategy.[13] This conclusion, based on theoretic considerations, has been confirmed by the work of Feczko and Halpert[14] and the calculations reported by Bressler.[15]

It should be emphasized that the program just described is intended to represent an individual screening program undertaken by physicians for their patients. Other authors have advocated a mass screening program for the detection of early colon cancer or premalignant lesions of the colon and rectum.[16–18] This is a program of multiple stool testing for occult blood and is based on the finding that early tumors in the large bowel tend to bleed intermittently. The incidence of false-positive tests for occult blood is decreased by removing meat from the diet, and sensitivity is increased by adding roughage to irritate the tumor, causing it to bleed.[19] Multiple stool samples are tested for occult blood, and all patients with positive reactions are followed up by x-ray study and appropriate endoscopy.

In these mass screening programs, colorectal cancers have been detected in between 1 in 450 and 1 in 1000 patients.[17, 18] In addition, large numbers of premalignant lesions (adenomas) have been found and removed. It has been found that patients with asymptomatic carcinomas discovered on screening pro-

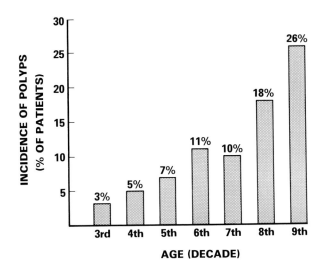

FIGURE 13–1

Incidence of colonic polyps related to age (based on 800 consecutive double contrast enemas). There is an increasing incidence of colonic polyps, ranging from 3% in the third decade of life to 26% in the ninth decade. (From Laufer, I.: The double contrast enema: Myths and misconceptions. Gastrointest. Radiol. 1:19, 1976, with permission.)

grams frequently have a Dukes A tumor and that a cure rate of 80% to 90% can be anticipated.[20]

Risk Factors

The program just described is for persons at normal risk for developing colorectal cancer. There are, however, a group of conditions in which the risk of developing colorectal cancer is increased. This group includes patients with ulcerative colitis,[21] previous polyps or carcinomas,[22] a family history of colon cancer,[23, 24] Peutz-Jeghers syndrome,[25] ureterosigmoidostomy,[26] and, possibly, pelvic irradiation.[27] In such patients, a more aggressive screening and surveillance program should be undertaken with examinations starting at an earlier age. In addition, double contrast enema or colonoscopy should be incorporated into their screening program.

Of course, patients with familial polyposis or Gardner's syndrome have a very high risk of developing colorectal cancer (see Chapter 15). However, in those conditions, total colectomy is usually carried out as soon as the diagnosis is established and therefore there is no opportunity for screening or follow-up studies. Some patients may have a subtotal colectomy with ileorectal anastomosis. In those patients early lesions may be detected on follow-up studies of the residual rectum.

In summation, it is likely that most colorectal carcinomas begin as benign polypoid lesions. The best hope for decreasing mortality from this disease

lies in the detection of early carcinoma or the precursors of carcinoma, that is, adenomas, in asymptomatic patients. These lesions are most likely to be detected in patients investigated for occult blood in the stool but they may also be detected by serendipity, by regular survey of high-risk patients, or by a mass screening program.

BENIGN TUMORS

Epithelial Polyps

Incidence

Benign tumors of the colon are extremely common and, in most patients, do not produce symptoms. Several authors have reported polyp detection rates ranging from 10% to 12.5%, using the double contrast enema.[28–32] There is a dramatic rise in polyp incidence with increasing age, as illustrated in Figure 13–1.[31, 33] Polyps are most frequently detected in the rectosigmoid and the left colon. Figure 13–2 illustrates the distribution of 108 consecutive polyps detected by double contrast enema. Bernstein and co-workers found that with increasing age, there was a shift of polyps to the right side of the colon.[34] This coincides with a shift in distribution in colonic carcinoma to the right side as the population ages.[35]

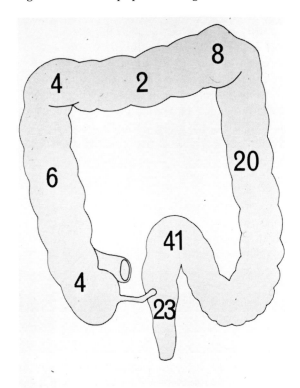

FIGURE 13–2

Distribution of colorectal polyps (based on 108 consecutive polyps). Approximately 60% of the polyps are in the rectum and sigmoid.

Pathology

Epithelial polyps of the colon can be considered to be either nonneoplastic or neoplastic. Most of the nonneoplastic polyps are hyperplastic polyps that have no malignant potential. Neoplastic polyps or adenomas are further classified on the basis of the proportion of villous change. Those with little or no villous component are referred to as tubular adenomas, whereas those with a predominantly villous appearance are called villous adenomas. Those polyps with a villous component ranging from 25% to 75% are referred to as tubulovillous adenomas. The incidence of malignancy rises with increase in the villous component of the adenoma.[36]

Diminutive Polyps

There has been considerable controversy regarding the pathologic nature of diminutive colonic polyps, that is, polyps under 5 mm in diameter. Some authors have suggested that only about one third of such small polyps are neoplastic in nature, whereas others have found that almost 75% are adenomas.[37, 38] Tedesco and colleagues pointed out that hyperplastic polyps were found predominantly in the distal portion of the large bowel, whereas adenomas were distributed evenly throughout the colon.[39] The situation has been reviewed by Bernstein and co-workers, who point out the importance of the size of the polyp and its location.[40] Colonic polyps in the 1 to 3 mm range are almost entirely hyperplastic, whereas the proportion of adenomas rises in the 4 to 5 mm range. Thus, from a clinical point of view, polyps in the 1 to 3 mm range can be considered to be hyperplastic, particularly if they are seen in the left side of the colon. Polyps in the 4 to 5 mm range have approximately a 50% probability of being adenomas in the left colon and are more likely to be adenomas when they are in the right colon. A significant number of hyperplastic polyps are found to have an atypical radiographic appearance; that is, they are larger than expected and have a lobulated surface. This emphasizes the importance of histologic examination of these polypoid lesions.[41]

The implications of these findings for radiology are clear. Our radiologic technique must be capable of finding lesions 5 mm or larger because the majority of these lesions represent adenomas and therefore have a significant, but small, malignant potential. It is probably not worthwhile trying to diagnose polyps under 5 mm radiologically because the majority of these are hyperplastic polyps. Furthermore, the incidence of radiologic false positives increases as we try to diagnose smaller and smaller lesions. Young patients who harbor any of the risk factors for colorectal carcinoma represent an exception to this rule. In these patients, we should attempt to diagnose even the smallest of colorectal polyps.

Diagnostic Methods

Single Versus Double Contrast

It is surprising that there continues to be controversy regarding the relative value of single and double contrast in diagnosing colorectal polyps since the single contrast method has never been shown to be equal or superior to double contrast. As summarized by Fork and colleagues, many studies with double contrast have shown that polyps can be demonstrated in 10% to 13% of all patients.[42] This correlates well with the typical 12.5% postmortem incidence of colonic polyps.[10] Even in the best of hands using single contrast technique, polyps are demonstrated in only 7% of patients. Most of the shortfall is explained by the poor sensitivity of the single contrast enema in diagnosing rectal lesions.[43] Nevertheless, when performed with care, the single contrast enema has been shown to be reasonably accurate for the diagnosis of larger polyps (greater than 1 cm), and it seems reasonable to use this technique in patients who are elderly or infirm.[44] However, for the average population in whom the object is to find premalignant or small malignant lesions, the double contrast technique is clearly the radiologic examination of choice.[45, 46]

Double Contrast Versus Colonoscopy

Considerable energy has been devoted to the discussion of the relative merits of double contrast enema and colonoscopy. Many of these studies have compared examinations done by operators of widely varying degrees of experience and interest. In comparing results, it is important to compare results achieved when both examinations are performed to the level of the state of the art.

First of all, it is important to realize that there is an error rate inherent in colonoscopy. This is due in part to the fact that the cecum is not reached in a significant proportion of colonoscopies.[47] In addition, there are significant endoscopic blind spots in the colon.[32, 48] In general, these blind spots are found at areas of sharp angulation of the bowel or behind prominent folds (Fig. 13–3). Polypoid lesions on a long stalk are particularly apt to be missed since, because of their mobility, they may escape from the

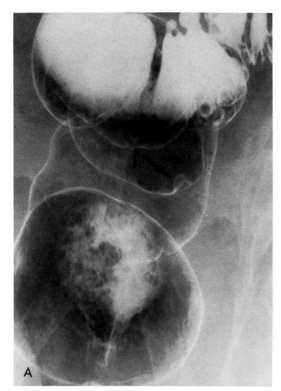

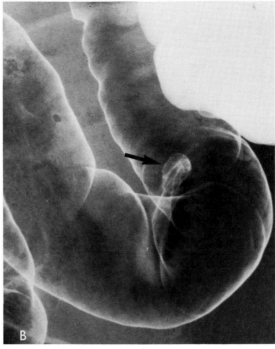

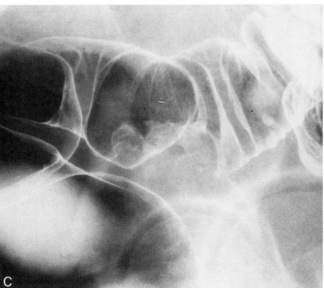

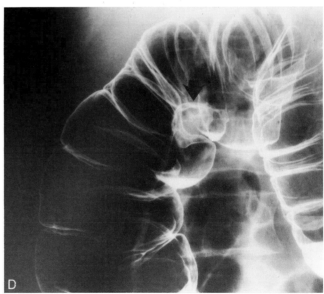

FIGURE 13–3

LESIONS MISSED AT ENDOSCOPY. *A,* There is a small sessile polyp behind a fold at the rectosigmoid junction. This lesion was missed twice on sigmoidoscopy and was finally detected at the third sigmoidoscopy.

B, A small polyp situated behind a fold at an area of angulation at the junction of the sigmoid and the descending colon. This polyp was missed on two colonoscopic examinations and was found on the third. (From Laufer, I., et al.: The radiologic demonstration of colorectal polyps undetected by endoscopy. Gastroenterology 70:167, 1976, with permission.)

C, Polypoid carcinoma just proximal to the rectosigmoid junction. This lesion was missed on several sigmoidoscopic and colonoscopic examinations and was confirmed only at surgery.

D, Polypoid carcinoma at the hepatic flexure missed on initial colonoscopy.

examining endoscope (Fig. 13–4). Thus, discrepancies between radiologic and endoscopic findings are not infrequent. It should not be assumed that the endoscopic findings are correct. Weyman and co-workers found that in over 40% of such discrepancies, the radiologic diagnosis was confirmed.[49] Therefore, when such discrepancies arise, one of the examinations must be repeated until the discrepancy is resolved.

Although some authors have found that radiology is superior to endoscopy in some cases,[50, 51] it is clear that generally the results achieved with good quality colonoscopy and double contrast enemas are comparable, especially when considering polyps greater than 1 cm in diameter.[52, 53] Fork found that double contrast enema detected 90% of all polypoid lesions, whereas colonoscopy detected 91%.[54] Beggs and colleagues reported that both colonoscopy and double

contrast enema detected between 95% and 97% of all colonic cancers.[55]

Since it is clear that the sensitivity of radiology and colonoscopy is very similar, it is appropriate to consider the cost and complications of each. The cost of colonoscopy generally runs 2 to 3 times higher than that of the radiologic study, and it carries approximately a fivefold higher complication rate.[56] Therefore, we agree with the conclusion reached by Eddy and co-workers that barium enemas and colonoscopies appear to be equally effective in reducing mortality but that the lower cost of the barium enema makes it a more cost-effective strategy.[13]

At this point, it is well to reiterate that poorly done double contrast enemas may be very inaccurate, whereas poorly performed colonoscopy not only may be inaccurate, but may carry a significant rate of complications and even mortality.

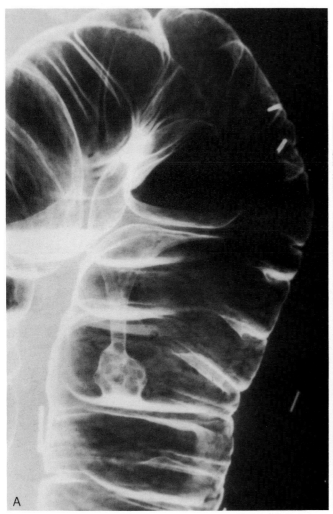

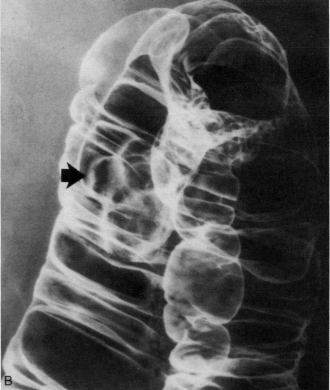

FIGURE 13–4

ELUSIVENESS OF POLYPS ON A LONG STALK. *A,* Double contrast study through a colostomy shows a polyp on a long stalk at the splenic flexure.

B, A later film from the examination shows that the polyp *(arrow)* has flipped up into the transverse colon. Such polyps may be difficult to detect by colonoscopy because of their mobility.

Radiography

It is obvious that a clean colon is essential for the detection of polyps. However, good mucosal coating is equally important. It has been amply demonstrated that in the presence of poor coating even large tumors can be missed (Fig. 13–5).[57] An adequate number of projections must be obtained, since it is not unusual for a lesion to be demonstrated on only one of the entire series of films (Fig. 13–6). Another important prerequisite is adequate colonic distention. The col- lapsed colon can hide sizable lesions (Fig. 13–7). Unraveling loops of bowel is not as important in double contrast enema as in single contrast, since even small lesions may be seen through overlapping loops. However, in some cases very careful study of the films may be necessary to detect these lesions (Fig. 13–8). Because of this see-through effect it may be difficult to determine which of the overlapping loops contains the polyp (Fig. 13–9).

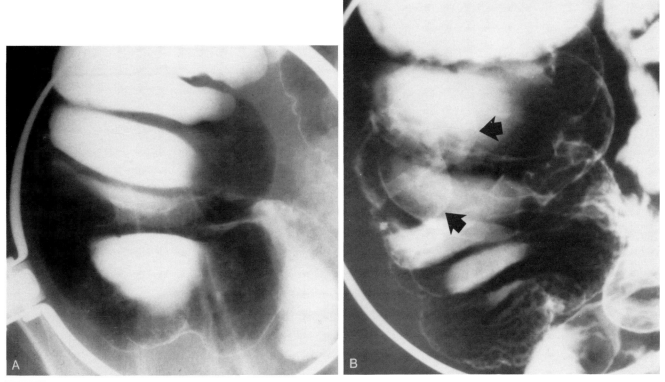

FIGURE 13–5

RISK OF POOR COATING. *A,* The initial film with poor coating in the right colon shows no evidence of a carcinoma.
  B, A later film with improvement in the mucosal coating shows a large polypoid carcinoma *(arrows)* on the anterior wall.

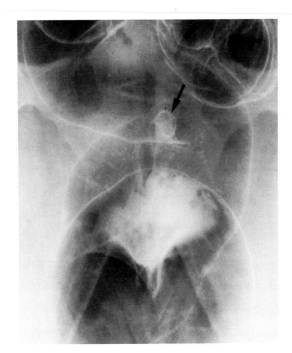

FIGURE 13–6

Small polyp *(arrow)* at the rectosigmoid junction behind a fold. This polyp was seen only on this prone-angled view and was not visible on any of the other radiographs. (From Laufer, I., et al.: The radiologic demonstration of colorectal polyps undetected by endoscopy. Gastroenterology *70*:167, 1976, with permission.)

FIGURE 13–7

IMPORTANCE OF ADEQUATE COLONIC DISTENTION. *A*, Poor distention of the colon. Only diverticula are seen.
    B, With adequate distention, a pedunculated polyp is clearly seen in addition to the diverticula.

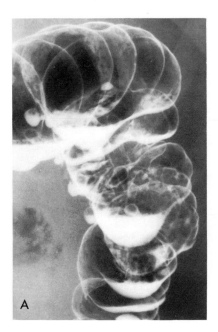

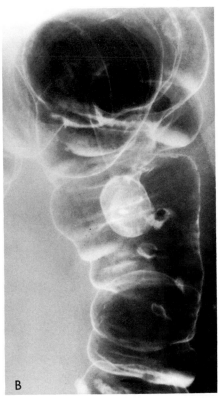

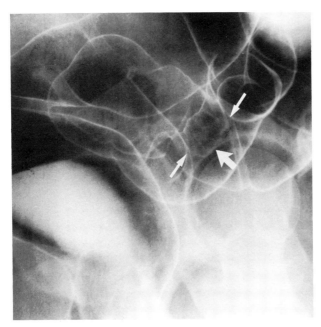

FIGURE 13–8

Sigmoid polyp (*arrows*) seen through overlapping loops of bowel.

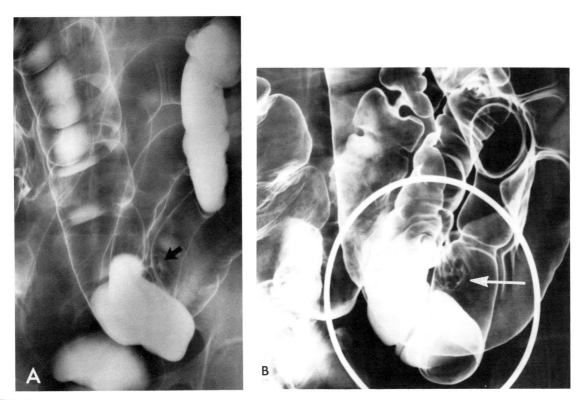

FIGURE 13–9

A, There are overlapping loops in the left lower quadrant. The lobulated polyp (*arrow*) at first was thought to be in the sigmoid colon, but was not detected at colonoscopy.

B, A repeat study showed that the polyp (*arrow*) is actually in the descending colon. Because of the flat nature of the polyp, it was removed at surgery and proved to be a benign tumor.

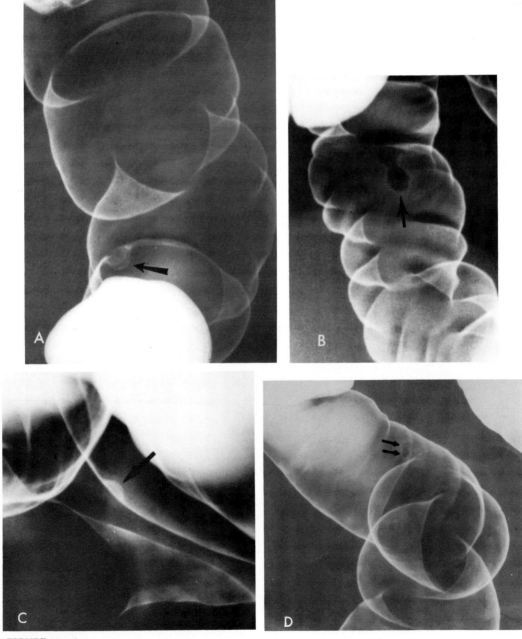

FIGURE 13–10

A VARIETY OF VERY SMALL POLYPS. *A*, Sessile polyp.
   B, Pedunculated polyp.
   C, Flat sessile polyp.
   D, Two very small polyps (*arrows*) in the sigmoid. These were confirmed by endoscopy.

In most instances small polyps (Fig. 13–10) can be distinguished from fecal residue by the mobility and irregular coating of solid fecal material. However, true polyps may exhibit several other radiologic features that are helpful. Demonstration of a stalk is conclusive proof of the presence of a polyp. The stalk may be demonstrated in profile particularly in horizontal beam films in the decubitus or upright position (see Fig. 13–4). Occasionally, mucus threads that resemble the stalk may be seen, but without a polyp at the end (Fig. 13–11). The stalk may also be seen on end through the head of the polyp, producing the appearance of a target or a "Mexican hat" (Fig. 13–12).

Another sign has been called the "bowler hat" sign by Youker and Welin.[58] This sign consists of two circular shadows, one representing barium caught in the angle between the polyp and the bowel wall and the other representing the head of the polyp. When the polyp is seen in profile, the combination of these two shadows resembles a bowler hat (Fig. 13–13).

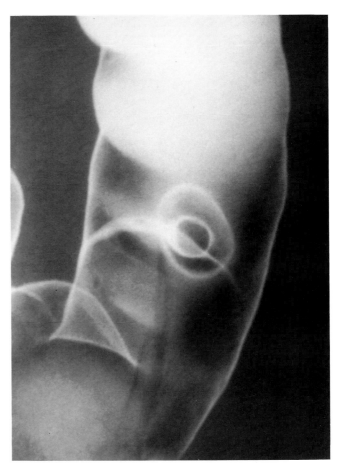

FIGURE 13–12

MEXICAN HAT SIGN. This is the typical appearance of a pedunculated polyp seen end-on. The outer ring represents the head of the polyp and the inner ring represents the stalk.

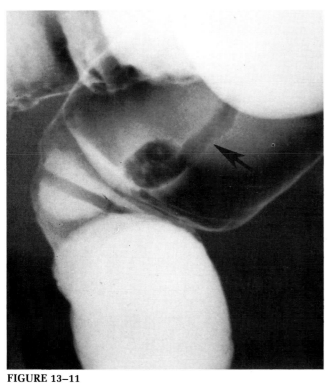

FIGURE 13–11

A coiled strand of mucus resembling a pedunculated polyp.

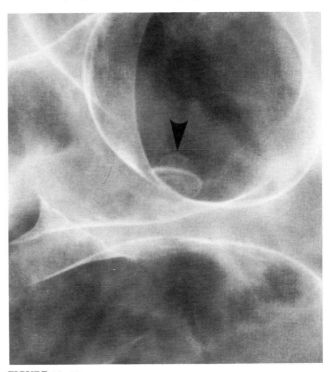

FIGURE 13–13

The bowler hat sign due to a sessile polyp.

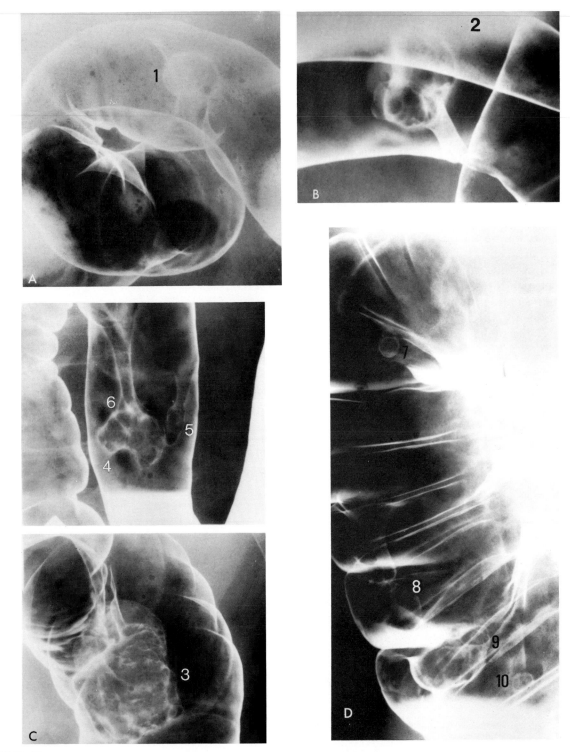

FIGURE 13–14

A through D, Ten polyps scattered throughout the colon. (B, From Laufer, I. Double contrast radiology in the diagnosis of gastrointestinal cancer. In Glass, G.B.J. (ed.): Progress in Gastroenterology. New York, Grune & Stratton, 1977. C, From Laufer, I.: The double contrast enema: myths and misconceptions. Gastrointest. Radiol. 1:19, 1976, with permission.)

Although the bowler hat sign can also be produced by diverticulum, the direction of the dome of the bowler hat distinguishes it as either a polyp or a diverticulum. When the dome of the hat points away from the axis of the bowel, it is a diverticulum, whereas when the dome of the polyp points toward the lumen of the bowel, it is a polyp.[58] This sign is discussed in detail in Chapter 2 (Fig. 2–18). A variation of the bowler hat sign called the "figure 8" sign has been described by Ament and Alfidi.[60]

The majority of polyps greater than 5 mm are adenomatous lesions. In our experience, approximately 25% of patients with one polyp have multiple polyps. The number may range anywhere from two to one dozen or more (Fig. 13–14). In the extreme case of familial polyposis the mucosal surface may be studded with polyps of varying sizes (Fig. 13–15).

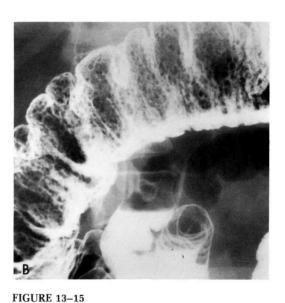

FIGURE 13–15

FAMILIAL POLYPOSIS. A to C, The colon is carpeted with tiny polyps, although they are relatively sparse in the rectum.

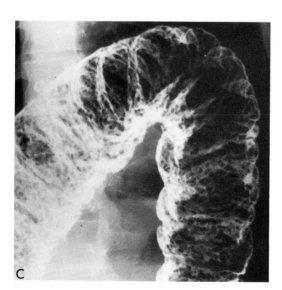

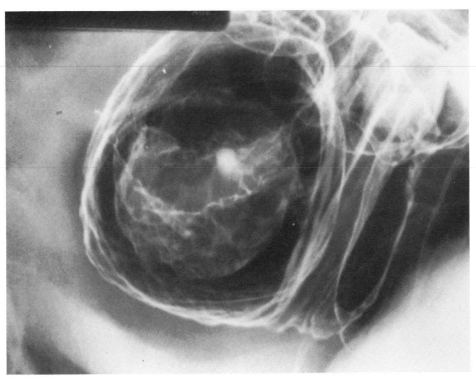

FIGURE 13–16

TYPICAL VILLOUS TUMOR IN THE SIGMOID. This tumor exhibits the typical, irregular, frond-like surface of a villous tumor. It was a malignant villous adenoma.

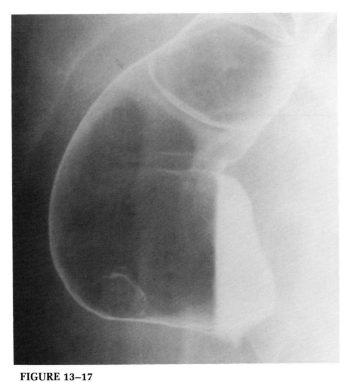

FIGURE 13–17

VILLOUS ADENOCARCINOMA OF THE RECTUM. There is a 1-cm polypoid lesion on the posterior wall of the rectum. This has none of the characteristic features of a villous adenoma, although on pathologic examination it was a carcinoma arising in a villous adenoma.

Villous adenomas are less common and have a higher malignant potential than tubular adenomas. According to the classic description, villous adenomas are characterized by a reticular, granular, or frond-like surface; they may be associated with symptoms of diarrhea and hypokalemia (Fig. 13–16). Delamarre and colleagues observed this characteristic radiologic appearance in two thirds of patients with villous lesions.[61] Iida and colleagues found that the presence of a granular mucosal surface on a polypoid lesion correlated well with the proportion of villous change and that this appearance was usually present

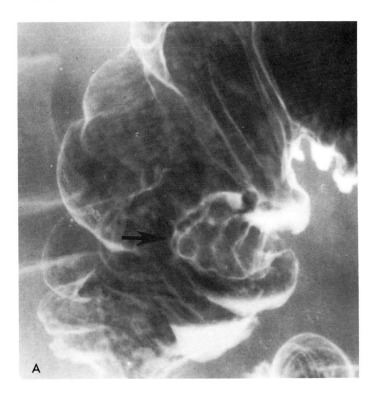

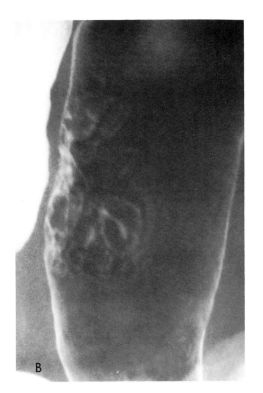

FIGURE 13–18

A, A flat, lobulated tumor at the hepatic flexure. This was an adenomatous polyp.

B, A flat tumor in the descending colon, with an irregular surface suggestive of a villous adenoma. This was a villoglandular polyp.

when villous elements consisted of more than 75% of the whole tumor.[62] However, small villous tumors are often indistinguishable roentgenographically from tubular adenomas (Fig. 13–17). As in other polypoid lesions of the colon, it may be very difficult to make a definitive diagnosis of malignancy in villous tumors. However, the majority of villous tumors greater than 2 cm in diameter are malignant.[61] It should also be noted that in some cases, a polypoid lesion may have a flat, lobulated appearance suggestive of a villous adenoma, but histologic study shows a tubular or tubulovillous adenoma (Fig. 13–18).

Rubesin and co-workers have used the term "carpet lesions" to describe flat, lobulated lesions causing primarily an alteration in the surface texture of the bowel (Fig. 13–19).[63] In a collection of 14 such cases, most were tubular adenomas with varying degrees of villous change. Only 3 of the 14 were frank villous adenomas and malignant change was observed in only one of the cases although 11 of the 14 adenomas were greater than 2 cm in diameter. It is of interest that in this series, carpet lesions were found only in the rectum and the right colon. We have also seen cases in which obvious polypoid carcinomas appear to have arisen on a background of a benign carpet lesion (Fig. 13–20).

Other nonneoplastic polyps may also occur in the colon. These include juvenile polyps, which may be single or multiple. These polyps may be found in children and adults (Fig. 13–21). Hamartomatous polyps are found in those with Peutz-Jeghers syndrome and inflammatory polyps in those with Cronkhite-Canada syndrome. The polyposis syndromes are considered in detail in Chapter 15.

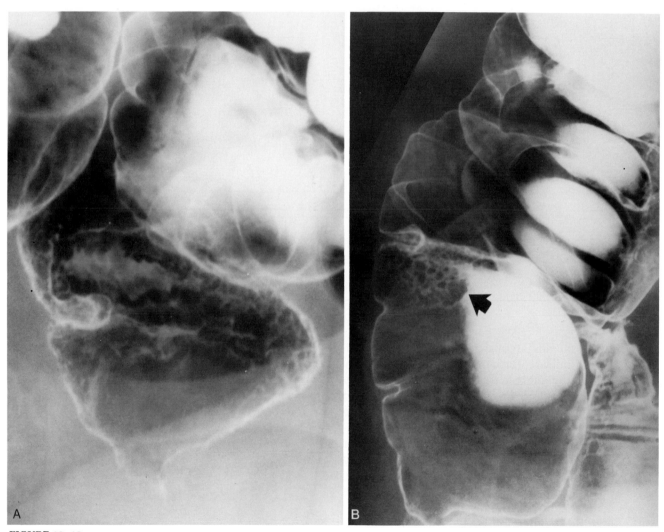

FIGURE 13–19

CARPET LESIONS. A, Typical appearance of a carpet lesion in the rectum. B, Typical carpet lesion (arrow) in the cecum.

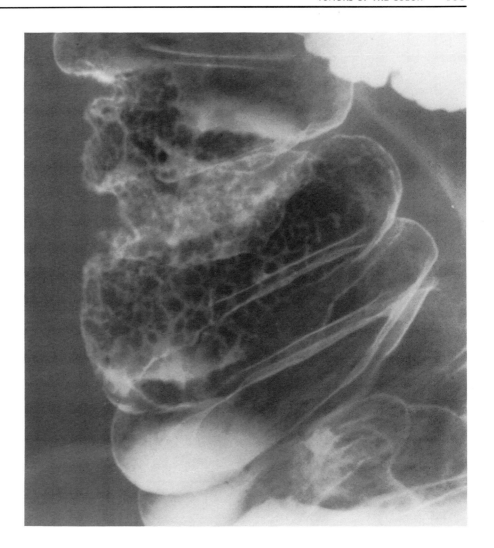

FIGURE 13–20

MALIGNANT TRANSFORMATION IN A CARPET LESION. There is an obvious polypoid carcinoma in the ascending colon. Surrounding the polypoid lesion is the mucosal change representing the underlying adenoma.

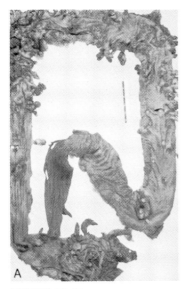

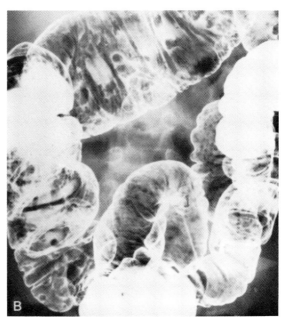

FIGURE 13–21

A and *B*, Juvenile colonic polyposis in an 8-year-old girl.

In most cases, when a polyp is detected radiologically, further studies consist of the appropriate endoscopic examination—either proctosigmoidoscopy or colonoscopy. Most polyps can be removed from any part of the colon, particularly if the polyp is pedunculated.[64, 65] The sequence of events is illustrated in Figures 13–22 and 13–23. In general, we tend to ignore polyps under 5 mm in diameter since they are usually predominantly hyperplastic polyps.

In addition, the attempt to diagnose such small polyps results in a higher radiologic false-positive rate. In the absence of any contraindications, we also believe that for polyps greater than 5 mm in diameter, an attempt should be made at endoscopic polypectomy.

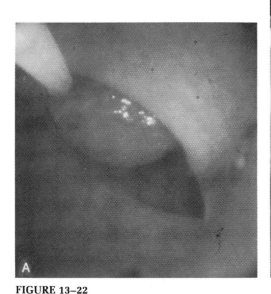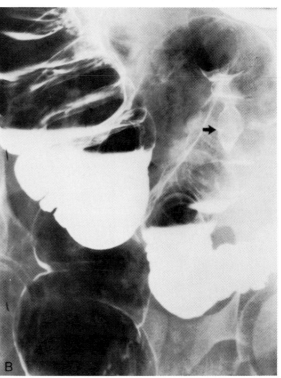

FIGURE 13–22

A and *B*, Pedunculated sigmoid polyp. The sheath containing the snare is seen advancing toward the polyp.

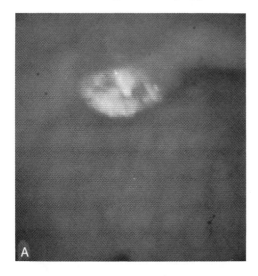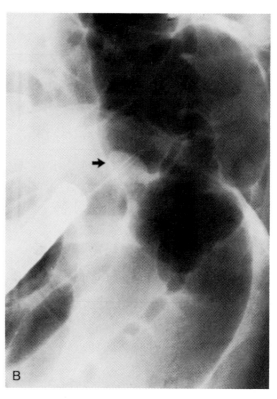

FIGURE 13–23

A and *B*, The snare is looped around the stalk of the polyp. The appearance of the transected stalk is shown.

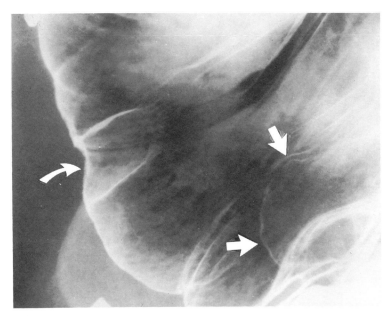

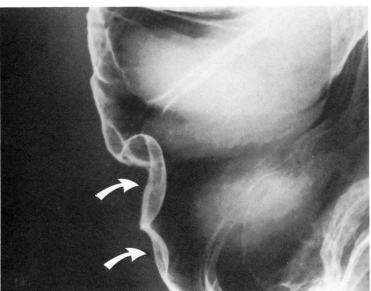

FIGURE 13–24

Bi-lobed lipoma of the ascending colon seen en face and in profile
(*curved arrows*). There is also a polypoid carcinoma of the cecum
(*straight arrows*). (From Laufer, I.: The double contrast enema: Myths and
misconceptions. Gastrointest. Radiol. 1:19, 1976, with permission.)

Benign Submucosal Tumors

Lipomas are the most common submucosal tumors in
the colon.[66, 67] They are found most frequently in the
cecum and the ascending colon (Fig. 13–24) and must
be differentiated from a prominent ileocecal valve
(Fig. 13–25). They frequently exhibit the characteristic findings of a submucosal mass. In addition, when
seen en face they may have a typically elliptical
shape. They are also characterized by their pliability
and ability to change in shape with change in position. As lipomas grow larger and extend intralumi-
nally, they appear to develop a pedicle and may be
seen to move freely at fluoroscopy. The specific diagnosis of a lipoma can be confirmed by CT scanning,
since these lesions have a low CT number corresponding to fat density (Fig. 13–26).[68] Malignant change is
virtually never encountered in these lesions.

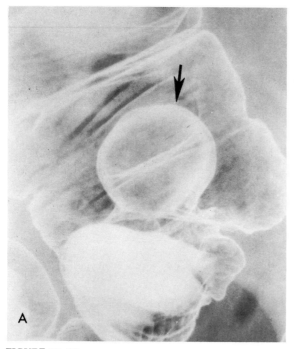
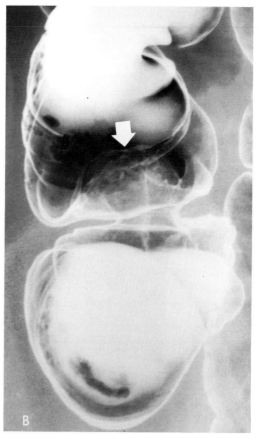

FIGURE 13–25

A and B, A lipoma arising from the superior lip of the ileocecal valve (A). This is to be distinguished from fatty infiltration causing diffuse enlargement of the ileocecal valve (B).

Other submucosal tumors, such as leiomyomas, may be indistinguishable from other polyps when they are small (Fig. 13–27). When they become larger, they exhibit the typical features of a submucosal tumor, and they may form the leading point of an intussusception (Fig. 13–27). Hemangiomas are unusual benign lesions of the large bowel. Patients usually present with recurrent episodes of rectal bleeding. On plain films, calcification within phleboliths may be the clue to the diagnosis. On double contrast examination of the colon, hemangiomas produce serpiginous filling defects simulating varices throughout the gastrointestinal tract (Fig. 13–28C).[69]

FIGURE 13–26

LIPOMA IN THE TRANSVERSE COLON. *A,* The double contrast study shows the typical appearance of a submucosal tumor. Note the elliptical shape.

B, The CT scan shows that the tumor is of fat density.

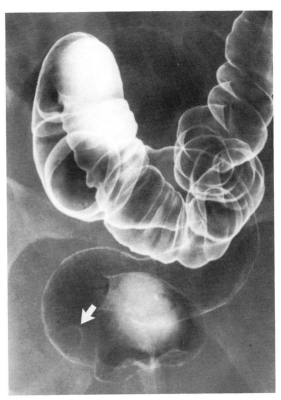

FIGURE 13–27

Leiomyoma of the rectum, presenting as a polypoid tumor *(arrow)* indistinguishable from other rectal polyps.

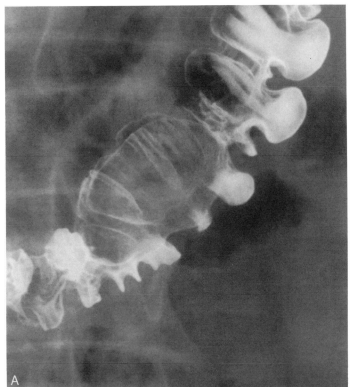

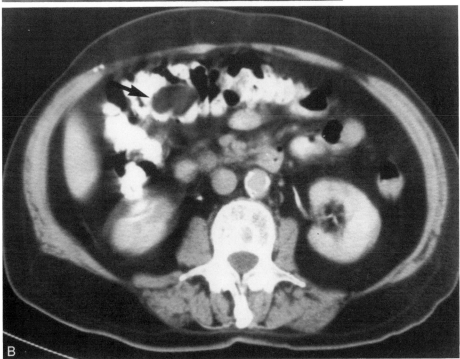

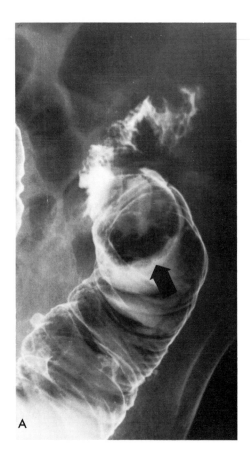

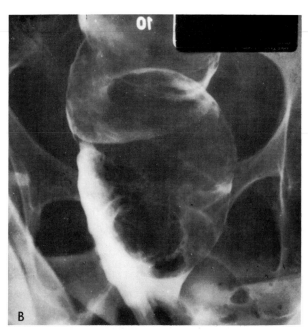

FIGURE 13–28

SUBMUCOSAL TUMORS. *A*, Leiomyoma causing colocolic intussusception, which was reduced spontaneously.

B, At a later date, the patient was readmitted with large bowel obstruction, with the intussusception presenting in the rectum.

C, Hemangioma of the sigmoid in another patient. Note the undulating contour of the sigmoid colon, characteristic of a hemangioma.

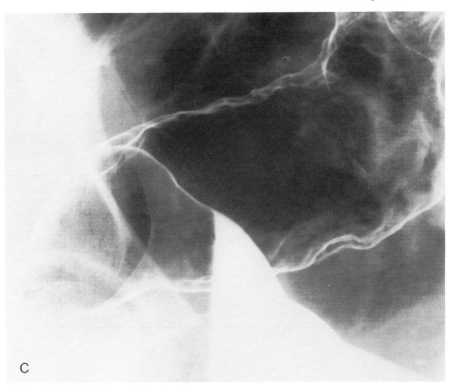

Polypoid Artifacts

As discussed and illustrated in Chapters 2 and 12, a variety of artifactual appearances may simulate a colonic polypoid lesion.[70] These include normal variants, such as a prominent ileocecal valve, folding of the intestinal wall, and lymphoid hyperplasia; nonpolypoid lesions, such as diverticula or an inverted appendiceal stump; extraneous material, including stool, air bubbles, oil droplets, pills, and undigested vegetables[71]; and calcified and skeletal structures seen through the colon.

MALIGNANT TUMORS

Early Cancer

There is little doubt that advanced cancers start as small polypoid lesions (Fig. 13–29).[72] Thus the radiologic detection of early colorectal cancer is basically an exercise in the detection of small polyps. Occasionally an early plaque-like carcinoma may be found (Fig. 13–30), and even more rarely carcinoma may start as a flat ulcer with no surrounding mass (see Chapter 14, Fig. 14–38).[73] Shinya and Wolff found an overall 6.5% rate of malignancy in polyps greater than 5 mm in size removed at colonoscopy.[74] The incidence of malignancy depended to a large extent on the pathologic nature of the benign polyp. There was no malignancy in hyperplastic polyps. Adenomatous polyps had malignancy in 3.3% of cases, whereas villous adenomas had a 12.6% incidence of malignancy (Fig. 13–31).

A number of radiologic criteria for the diagnosis of malignancy in polyps have been suggested.[75]

Size of the Polyp

Carcinoma is virtually nonexistent in polyps under 5 mm. In polyps measuring 5 to 10 mm, there is approximately a 1% incidence of carcinoma, whereas polyps over 2 cm have an incidence of malignancy approaching 50%.[4]

Rate of Growth

Malignant polyps tend to grow more quickly than benign polyps, although there is considerable overlap between the two groups.[76] For practical purposes, if there is definite evidence of growth on serial follow-up examinations of a polyp, malignancy should be suspected.

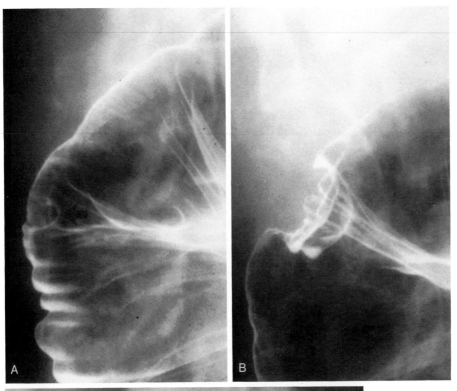

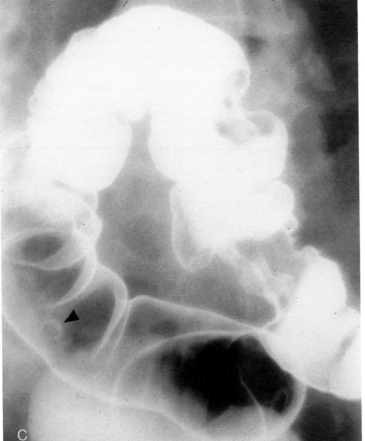

FIGURE 13–29

THE EVOLUTION OF COLON CANCER.
A, A 5 mm polyp (arrow) was demonstrated in the hepatic flexure. At colonoscopy, this region could not be reached because of a stricture in the sigmoid from radiation enteritis.

B, Five years later an invasive carcinoma is demonstrated at this site.

C, In another patient, the evolution of colon cancer is demonstrated with adenomas in the distal sigmoid (arrowhead), a polypoid carcinoma near the apex of the sigmoid, and an annular carcinoma more proximally in the sigmoid colon.

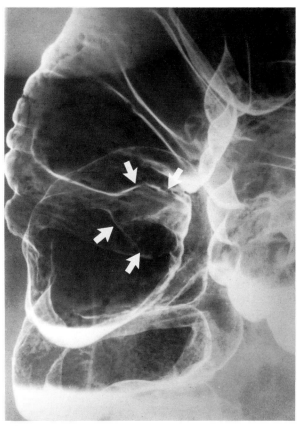

FIGURE 13–30

Plaque-like carcinoma of the ascending colon.

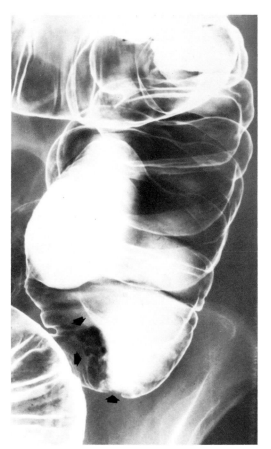

FIGURE 13–31

VILLOUS TUMOR OF THE CECUM WITH MUCOSAL CARCINOMA. A finely nodular lesion at the tip of the cecum represents the villous adenoma with mucosal carcinoma found on histologic examination.

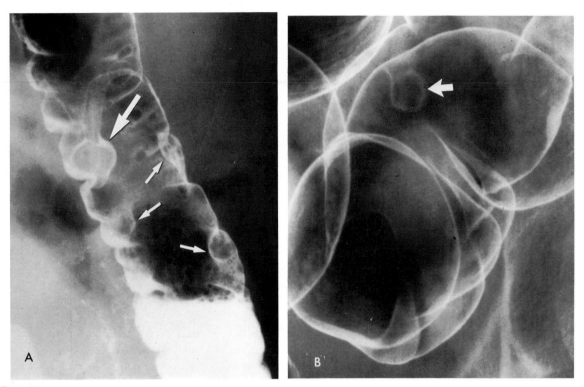

FIGURE 13–32

A, Polypoid carcinoma with a pedicle in a 29-year-old male with rectal bleeding. There is a pedunculated polyp in the descending colon *(large arrow)*, with a typically benign appearance. This was removed at colonoscopy and was found to be a carcinoma with invasion of the stalk. The smaller lesions *(small arrows)* were hyperplastic polyps. (From Laufer, I.: The double contrast enema: Myths and misconceptions. Gastrointest. Radiol. 1:19, 1976, with permission.)

B, Early carcinoma with a short, thick stalk.

Pedicle

A long, thin pedicle is highly suggestive of a benign polyp. Nevertheless, Smith has reported on several polypoid lesions with long, thin pedicles that turned out to harbor a malignancy.[77] As a rule, these are early carcinomas with no invasion of the stalk.[78] However, we have seen one case in which there was carcinoma in the head of the polyp, with invasion of the stalk (Fig. 13–32A). As a rule, the stalk associated with carcinoma is short and thick (Fig. 13–32B).

Irregularity of the Head of the Polyp

If the head of the polyp is irregular or lobulated the frequency of malignancy is increased (Fig. 13–33). This is certainly not invariable, since some benign polyps have very irregular and lobulated heads (Fig. 13–34).

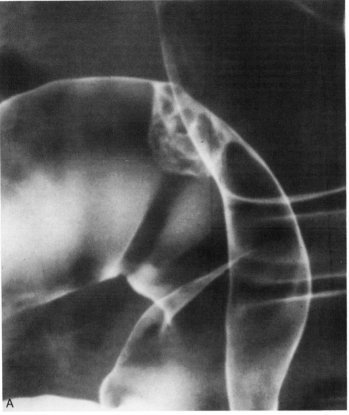

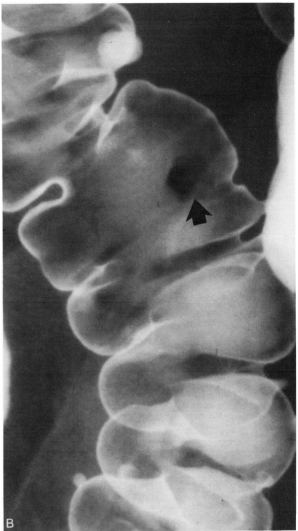

FIGURE 13–33

EARLY COLON CANCERS. *A,* Early carcinoma in the sigmoid. Note the sessile base and irregular surface of the polyp.

B, Early cancer near the splenic flexure. Note the lobulation of the surface of the polyp.

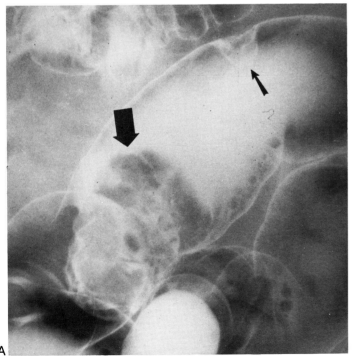

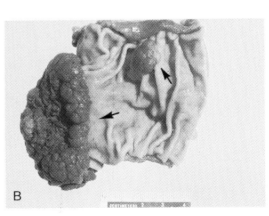

FIGURE 13–34

A and *B,* There are two polypoid tumors in the sigmoid. The distal lesion (*large arrow* in *A*) measures 4 cm in diameter, while the proximal lesion measures 1 cm in diameter and has an irregular puckered base. The radiologic findings suggest that the distal lesion is malignant because of its size, while the proximal lesion might be malignant because of its irregular base. The patient had a segmental resection of the sigmoid, and both lesions were benign adenomatous polyps.

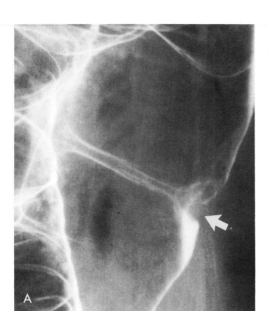

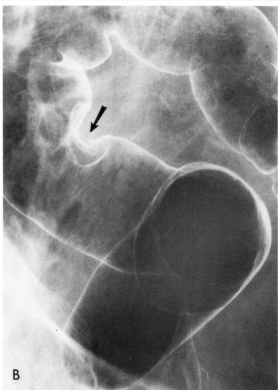

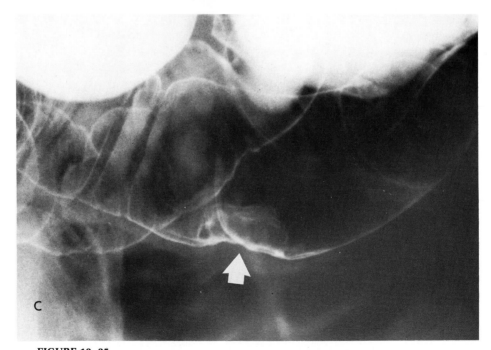

FIGURE 13–35

A to *C*, Three examples of early polypoid carcinomas with indentation of the base.

Indentation of the Base

Indentation or puckering of the base of the polyp was thought to be a reliable sign of malignancy (Fig. 13–35). Nevertheless, we have seen this sign in several polyps that proved to be benign (Fig. 13–36). Ament and co-workers have pointed out that basal indentation is a function of geometry rather than a true sign of malignancy.[79] In general, the larger the polyp, the greater the proportion of the circumference of the bowel that it occupies and thus the greater the likelihood of basal indentation. Of course, the larger the polyp, the greater is the chance of malignancy; therefore, it is understandable that basal indentation has been associated with malignancy.

Thus, although there is a general correlation between some of the signs previously mentioned and the presence of malignancy,[80] a definitive radiologic diagnosis of malignancy in a small polyp can rarely be made.[81] In a review of 30 early colon cancers in our hospital, there were three lesions that were 5 to 10 mm in maximal diameter. Three of the lesions had a stalk. Thus, we agree with Skucas,[82] Gabrielsson,[83] and their colleagues that the primary role of radiology is the detection of the lesion and that the histologic nature of all polyps greater than 5 mm should be determined after removal by endoscopic polypectomy.

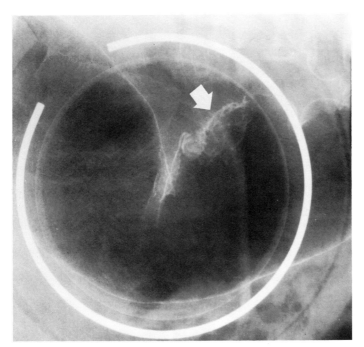

FIGURE 13–36

Polypoid lesion in the descending colon with an irregular indented base. The lesion was resected and was a benign adenomatous polyp.

Advanced Cancer

Over the past 20 years, it appears that there has been a shift to the right in the distribution of large bowel cancer such that at least 34% to 40% of the tumors are beyond the reach of even the 60 cm flexible sigmoidoscope.[84, 85] This shift is probably related to the aging of the population and the finding of colonic cancers in patients of increasing age.[35] The burden of the radiologist in detecting colonic cancers is compounded, since these right-sided lesions cannot be found by digital rectal examination or by sigmoidoscopy.

The majority of patients who present with symptomatic colorectal carcinoma have advanced lesions. These lesions are generally large annular (Fig. 13–37A) or polypoid (Fig. 13–37B) tumors that present no diagnostic problem, provided that the colon is reasonably clean and an adequate number of projections is obtained. The particular advantage of the double contrast technique in these lesions lies in the ability to see through overlapping loops of the bowel. Thus these lesions may be seen not only in profile, but also en face (Fig. 13–38). However, as illustrated in these figures, it may take some experience to recognize these tumors en face and through overlapping loops. Advanced cancers are frequently associated with adjacent "sentinel" polyps (Fig. 13–39A) or additional polyps elsewhere in the colon (Fig. 13–39B). In addition, approximately 5% of patients have multiple synchronous carcinomas of the colon (Fig. 13–40).[86] Therefore, an attempt should be made to examine the entire colon whenever possible.

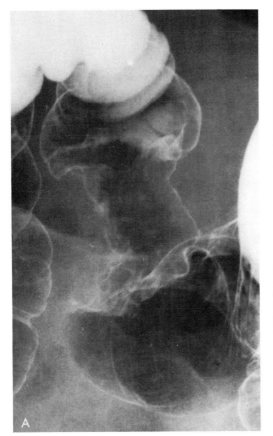
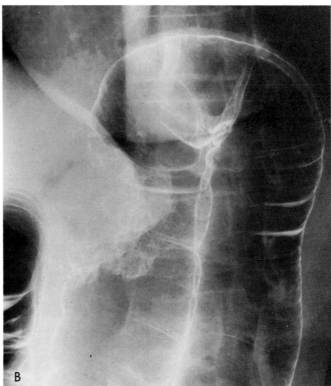

FIGURE 13–37

TYPICAL ADVANCED COLONIC CARCINOMA. *A,* Annular, apple-core lesion.
B, Large polypoid carcinoma at the splenic flexure.

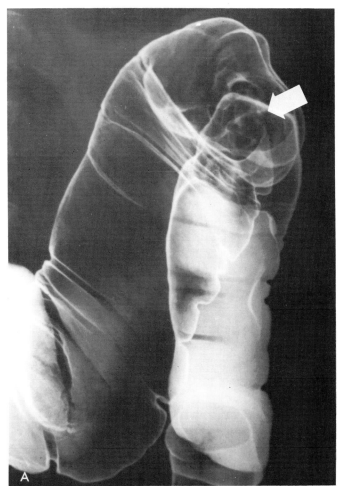

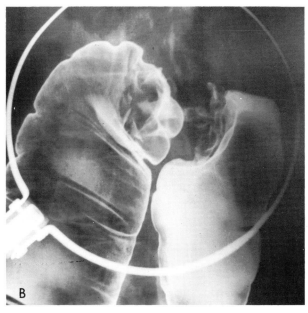

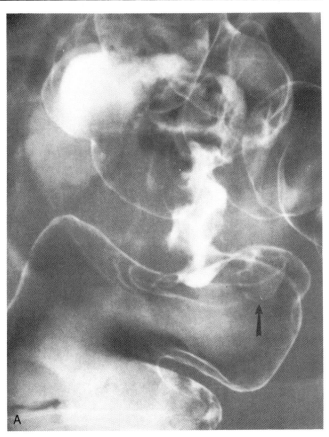

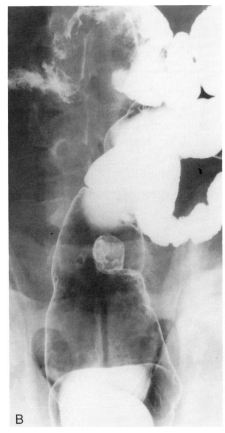

FIGURE 13–38

Annular carcinoma of the splenic flexure seen en face (A) and in profile (B).

FIGURE 13–39

CARCINOMA WITH ADDITIONAL POLYPS. A, Annular carcinoma of the rectosigmoid junction with a sentinel polyp (arrow).

B, There is a nearly obstructing polypoid carcinoid in the transverse colon and a second adenoma is seen in the sigmoid.

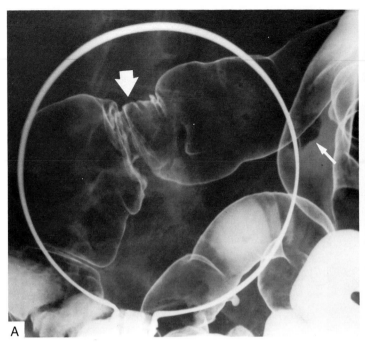
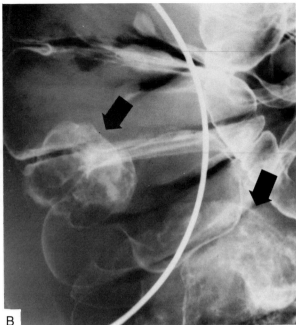

FIGURE 13–40

MULTIPLE SYNCHRONOUS CARCINOMAS. *A*, There is a polypoid tumor at the hepatic flexure with circumferential extension *(large arrow).* There is a smaller polypoid carcinoma in the descending colon *(small arrow).*

    B, Multiple polypoid carcinomas in the ascending colon.

Several authors have examined the nature and causes of errors in the diagnosis of colonic tumors. Ott and co-workers found that most missed lesions were in the sigmoid colon.[87] Baker and Alterman found that the proportion of missed lesions increased dramatically in patients who had more than 15 diverticula in the sigmoid colon (Fig. 13–41A).[88] Dreyfuss and Benacerraf reported that plaque-like and "saddle cancers" were highly likely to be missed on barium enema unless careful attention is paid to the contour of the bowel (Fig. 13–41B).[89] Kelvin and colleagues reviewed the radiologic errors in six institutions and found that 90% of the radiologic misses were due to a combination of perceptive and technical errors.[90] In only 10% of cases the lesion was "invisible" on films of adequate quality. All these studies

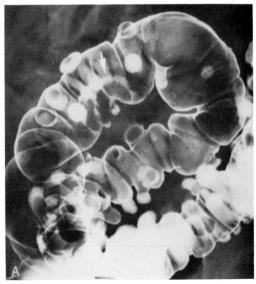
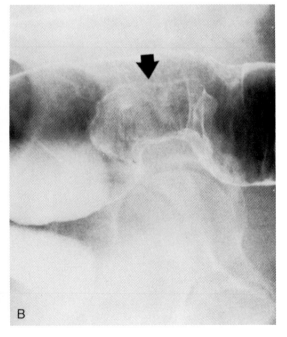

FIGURE 13–41

A, Carcinoma in a patient with diverticulosis. The polypoid carcinoma *(arrow)* is more difficult to recognize in the presence of extensive diverticulosis.

    B, Saddle cancer in the sigmoid colon.

emphasize the critical importance of careful attention to technical detail and to painstaking review of the radiographs. It is also important to emphasize that the sigmoid colon must be examined in particular detail, especially in the presence of diverticulosis.

Nevertheless, some advanced lesions are very difficult to detect. Figure 13–42A to C illustrates three views of a normal-appearing cecum with filling of the appendix. However, Figure 13–42D, which was obtained with the patient prone and the table tilted head-down, shows the annular carcinoma, which was located on the anterior wall of the cecum. Occasion-

ally, when the double contrast study remains inconclusive, we ask the patient to evacuate and we perform a single contrast study immediately thereafter.

In some cases advanced carcinoma may have an atypical appearance. An example is the linitis plastica type of carcinoma with predominant submucosal in-

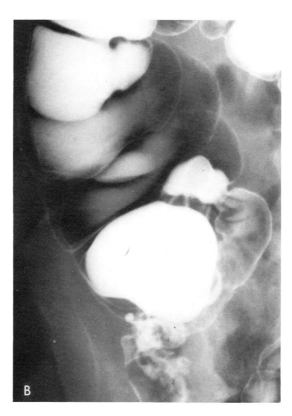

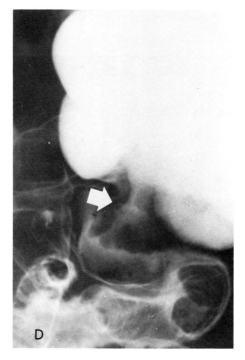

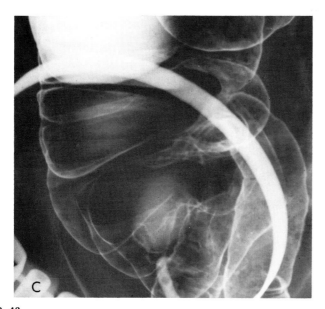

FIGURE 13–42

A and B, Apparently normal cecum with a small barium pool.

C, Apparently normal cecum, although there is small bowel overlapping the tip of the cecum.

D, With the patient in the prone position and tilted head-down to drain barium from the cecum, the annular carcinoma (arrow) is seen. This case illustrates the difficulty in demonstrating some advanced carcinomas.

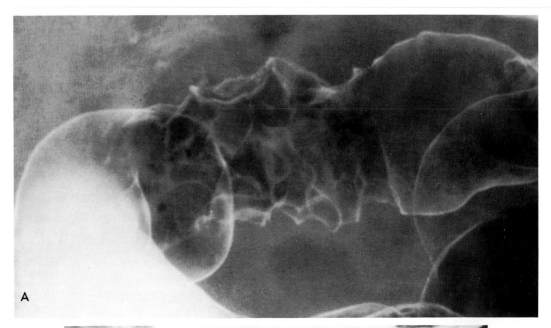

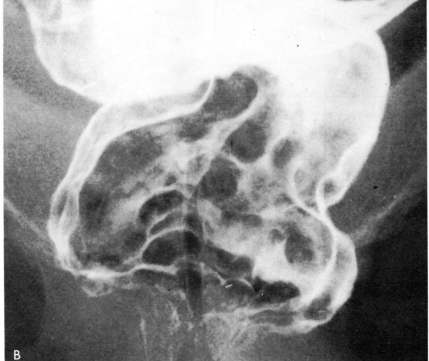

FIGURE 13–43

COLONIC LYMPHOMA. *A,* There is involvement of a short segment of
sigmoid colon by a mass lesion characterized by small nodules. This was due to
colonic involvement by disseminated lymphosarcoma.

    B, Diffuse submucosal nodularity due to non-Hodgkin's lymphoma. (Courtesy of
J. O. Op den Orth, M.D., Haarlem, Holland.)

filtration.[91] The radiologic picture may be suggestive of an inflammatory stricture due to Crohn's disease, diverticulitis, or ischemia. This type of carcinoma is particularly likely to develop in patients with ulcerative colitis (see Chapter 17).[92] A similar picture may be produced by a perforated carcinoma, in which the radiologic picture is dominated by the pericolic inflammatory reaction.[93]

Other Malignant Tumors

Submucosal Tumors

Other types of malignant tumors involving the colon are relatively uncommon. Primary colonic lymphoma most often involves the cecum or rectosigmoid and may produce either large ulcerated lesions or diffuse submucosal nodularity (Fig. 13–43).[94] CT scanning is useful for the demonstration of lymphadenopathy and for staging. Kaposi's sarcoma complicating AIDS may affect the colon. It usually manifests as small nodules with or without central umbilication (Fig. 13–44).[95] Leiomyosarcoma of the colon is a rare lesion. Two thirds of cases involve the rectum. The lesion usually grows as a bulky exophytic mass.[96] It may be impossible to distinguish radiologically between leiomyoma and leiomyosarcoma.

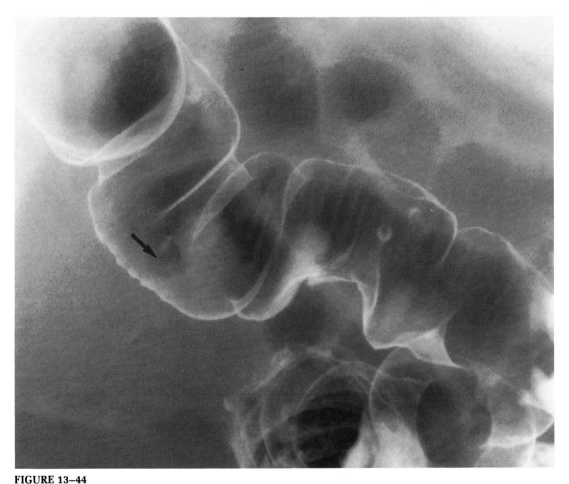

FIGURE 13–44

KAPOSI'S SARCOMA OF THE COLON. In a patient with AIDS, there are two submucosal lesions. The larger mass is seen distally whereas the smaller lesion (*arrow*) is umbilicated.

Metastatic Tumors

Metastatic lesions of the colon are being seen with increasing frequency as more aggressive treatment with radiotherapy and chemotherapy prolongs the life of patients with disseminated carcinoma. The most common lesions that involve the colon are carcinomas of the breast, stomach, lung, pancreas, kidney, and female genital tract.[97] The colon may be involved by direct spread, hematogenous metastases, or peritoneal seeding. With direct extension of an extracolonic mass, there is stretching of a loop of bowel, followed by spiculation and nodularity (Fig. 13–45A),[98] which may progress to ulceration and obstruction (Fig. 13–45B). Hematogenous metastases start as intramural filling defects (Fig. 13–46), which

may progress to infiltrate the entire circumference of the colonic wall. In some cases the radiologic appearance very closely mimics an inflammatory condition, particularly granulomatous colitis (Fig. 13–47).[99, 100] The classic description of peritoneal spread of tumor has been given by Meyers.[101] These metastases are particularly likely to drop into the pouch of Douglas and are seen as extrinsic or intramural filling defects on the anterior wall of the rectosigmoid junction (Fig. 13–48). A similar appearance may be produced by a pelvic abscess (Fig. 13–49). Peritoneal seeding may also classically affect the sigmoid colon, the ileocecal area, and the right paracolic gutter (Fig. 13–50).

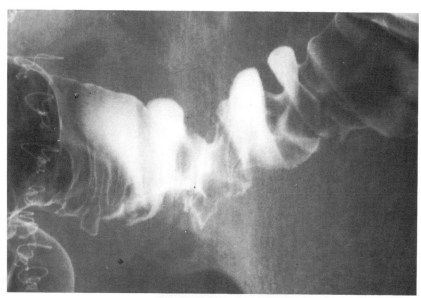

A

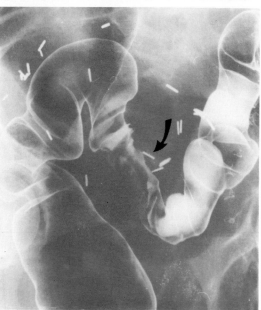

B

FIGURE 13–45

METASTATIC DISEASE INVOLVING THE SIGMOID COLON BY DIRECT EXTENSION. *A*, Carcinoma of the cervix with involvement of the inferior aspect of the sigmoid colon.

B, Another patient with carcinoma of the cervix with annular involvement of the sigmoid colon.

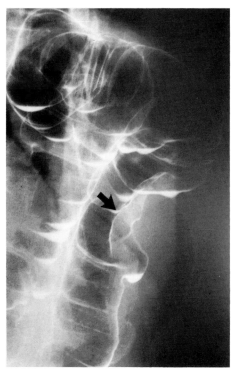

FIGURE 13–46

Submucosal mass involving the proximal descending colon due to a metastatic lesion from carcinoma of the ovary.

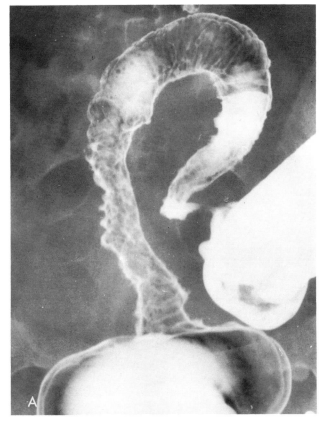

FIGURE 13–47

METASTATIC DISEASE TO THE COLON FROM CARCINOMA OF THE BREAST, SIMULATING INFLAMMATORY BOWEL DISEASE. *A,* There is marked narrowing, with mucosal irregularity of the sigmoid colon. The appearance of the mucosa is suggestive of an inflammatory lesion, particularly granulomatous colitis.

B, The lateral view shows the narrowing of the sigmoid, with an increase in the retrorectal soft tissues.

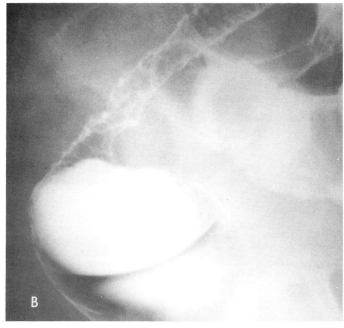

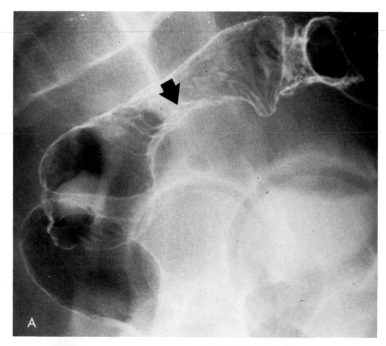

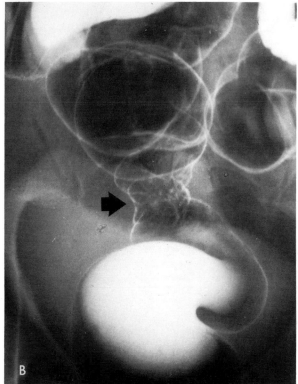

FIGURE 13–48

METASTASIS TO THE POUCH OF DOUGLAS FROM CARCINOMA OF THE COLON. A. There is an intramural filling defect on the anterior wall at the rectosigmoid junction. This is characteristic of peritoneal carcinomatosis involving the pouch of Douglas.

B, Frontal projection also shows evidence of compression at the rectosigmoid junction.

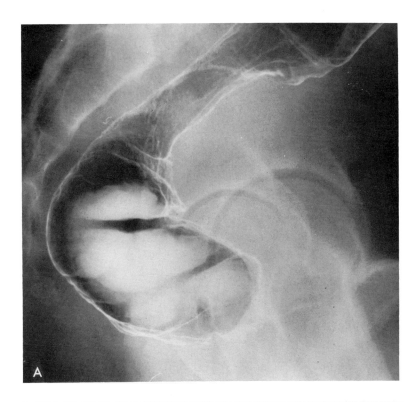

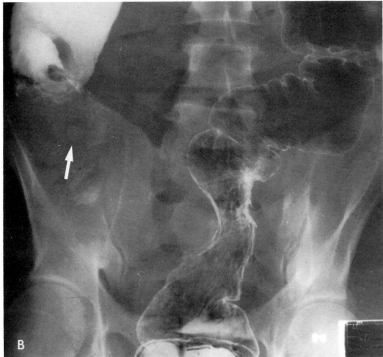

FIGURE 13–49

A and *B,* An identical appearance due to pelvic abscess in a patient with a
ruptured appendix. Note the soft tissue mass in the region of the cecum and
the appendicolith *(arrow).*

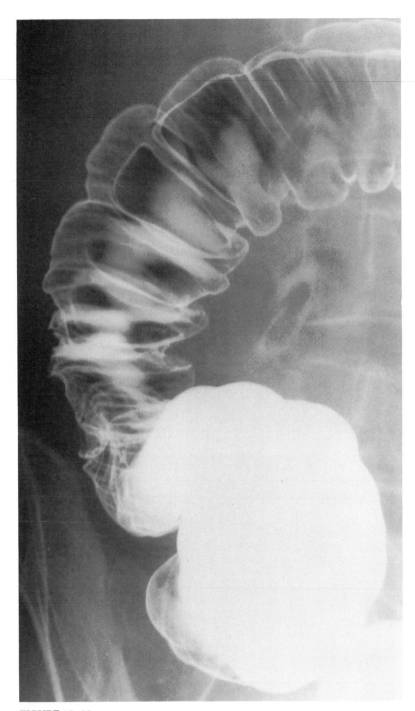

FIGURE 13–50

In a patient with ovarian carcinoma, there is metastatic seeding to the right paracolic gutter and ascending colon.

Diffuse peritoneal seeding frequently involves the transverse colon producing "omental cakes" of tumor. Rubesin and Levine have described the typical appearance of involvement of the transverse colon by these omental cakes.[102] There is predominant involvement of the superior border of the transverse colon with a mass effect, nodularity, and tethering of the mucosal folds. This may be associated with focal areas of narrowing. In these cases, the "striped colon sign," representing the en face appearance of tethered mucosal folds, is frequently seen (Fig. 13–51).[103]

Extrinsic involvement of the colon may arise from a variety of other organs including the kidney, pancreas, and gallbladder. This involvement may be due not only to neoplasms but also to inflammatory conditions such as pancreatitis (Fig. 13–52).

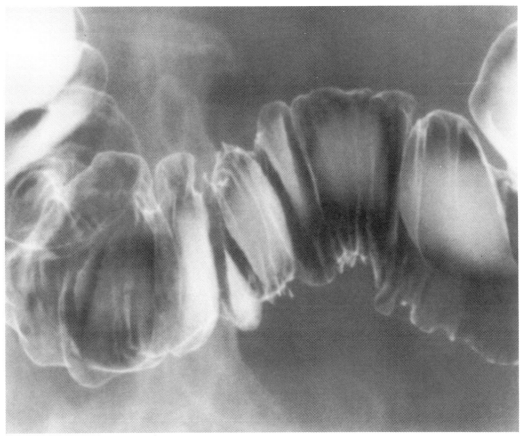

FIGURE 13–51

OMENTAL CAKE INVOLVING THE TRANSVERSE COLON. In this patient with metastatic ovarian carcinoma there is an omental cake involving the transverse colon. The striped colon sign is clearly demonstrated.

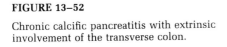

FIGURE 13–52

Chronic calcific pancreatitis with extrinsic involvement of the transverse colon.

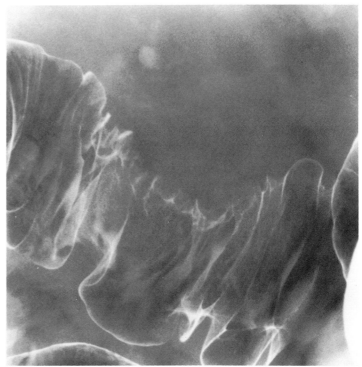

THE POSTOPERATIVE COLON

Patients who have had previous surgery for colorectal carcinoma undergo frequent postoperative examinations because of their relatively high risk for developing a second metachronous carcinoma,[104] and because of the need to assess postoperative symptoms. Ileocolic (Fig. 13–53A and B) and colocolic (Fig. 13–53C) anastomoses can be demonstrated in great detail with the double contrast enema, particularly with the use of intravenous glucagon. Plication defects are frequently identified. In some patients a filling defect due to a stitch granuloma may be seen in the early postoperative period (Fig. 13–53D). However, this defect regresses and becomes less prominent on follow-up studies.[105] It is important to obtain an early postoperative study within approximately 3 months of surgery to establish the baseline appearance of the anastomosis for comparison with subsequent studies.

With the availability of modern surgical staple guns, low anterior resections are being performed with increasing frequency.[106] The surgical anastomoses are beautifully demonstrated by double contrast technique (Fig. 13–54).

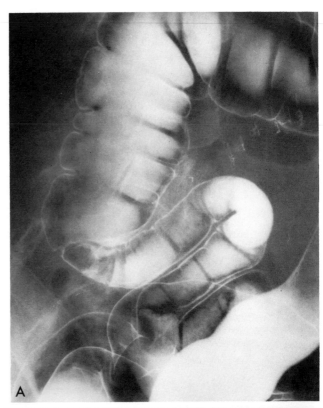

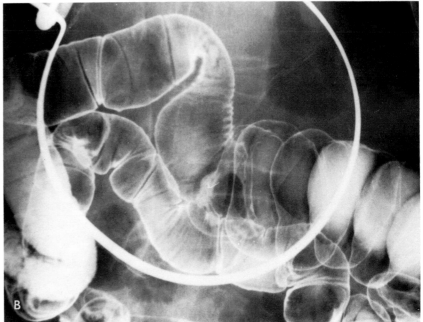

FIGURE 13–53

A, Normal ileocolic anastomosis in the ascending colon.

B, Normal ileocolic anastomosis in the transverse colon.

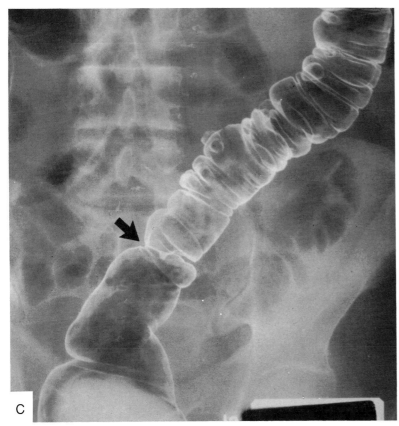

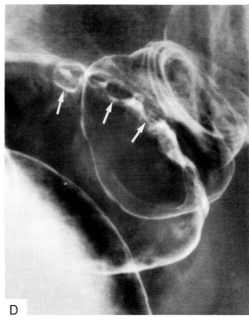

FIGURE 13–53 *Continued*

C, An example of a normal colocolic anastomosis.

D, Colocolic anastomosis with identifiable plication defects due to sutures *(arrows)*.

FIGURE 13–54

LOW ANTERIOR RESECTION. A double contrast examination shows the normal appearance of a low anterior resection using the staple gun.

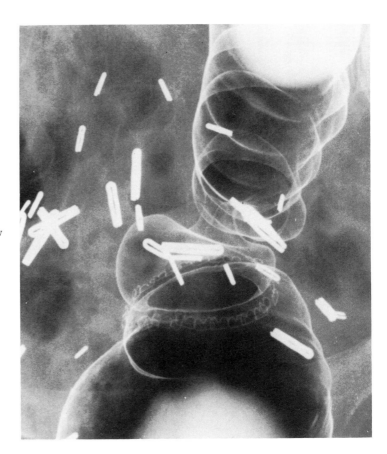

Follow-up for Colorectal Cancer

Patients who have been treated for colorectal cancer undergo follow-up study for the detection of recurrent disease and of metachronous tumors. CT is the examination of choice for the detection of recurrence remote from the anastomotic line and for the detection of distant metastases.[107, 108] However, the double contrast enema is the primary diagnostic procedure for the detection of local and anastomotic recurrences as well as metachronous lesions (Fig. 13–55). It is particularly important to examine the anastomotic site, since metastatic deposits tend to implant at the

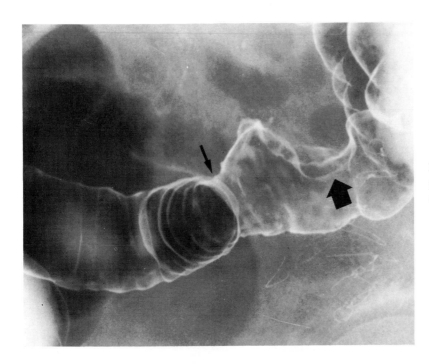

FIGURE 13–55

Recurrent carcinoma *(large arrow)* proximal to the anastomosis *(small arrow)*.

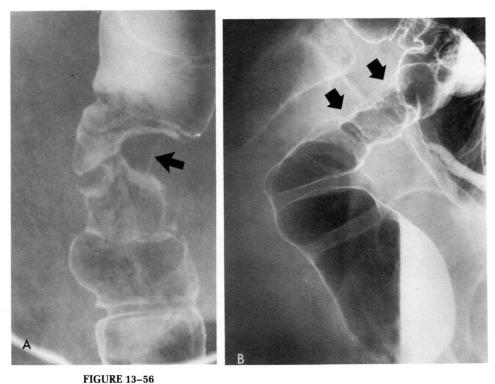

FIGURE 13–56

A and *B,* Two patients with recurrent carcinoma at the anastomosis.

anastomosis.[109, 110] Welch and Donaldson have shown that 20% of recurrences after colonic resection and anastomosis were found at the anastomotic site.[111] When the anastomotic site appears eccentric or irregular (Fig. 13–56) or has nodular filling defects (Fig. 13–57), recurrent tumor should be suspected. Colonoscopy may be helpful in such patients, although in some instances it may be misleading, since recurrent tumor may be submucosal and biopsy findings may be negative for malignancy. CT and CT-guided biopsy may be useful to document the presence and nature of an extracolonic mass.[112] Occasionally, a tumor recurrence may be found adjacent to but not at the anastomotic site (Fig. 13–55).

Patients who have undergone abdominoperineal resection with colostomy must also undergo regular examination because of the possibility of developing a second tumor. Double contrast examination of the residual colon can usually be performed through the colostomy (see Fig. 13–4; also Chapter 12; Fig. 12–5). CT and MRI are of particular value for the detection of pelvic recurrence of tumor in patients who have had abdominoperineal resection.[113, 114]

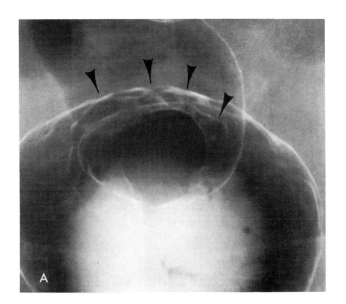

FIGURE 13–57

RECURRENT CARCINOMA AND FIVE VILLOUS ADENOMAS AT A COLORECTAL ANASTOMOSIS. *A,* Frontal view shows the anastomosis en face with the villous adenomas *(arrows)* arranged along the superior aspect.

B, Lateral view shows the recurrent carcinoma and the villous adenomas, which were confirmed at surgery.

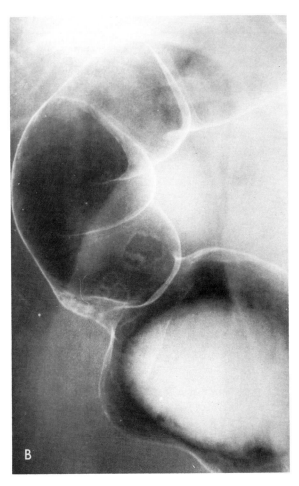

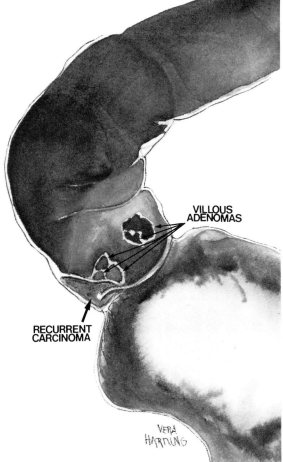

VILLOUS ADENOMAS

RECURRENT CARCINOMA

VERA HARTUNG

REFERENCES

1. Silverberg, E., and Lubera, J.A.: Cancer statistics, 1988. Cancer 38:5, 1988.
2. Winawer, S.J., Sherlock, P., Schottenfeld, D., et al.: Screening for colon cancer. Gastroenterology 70:783, 1976.
3. Hamer, M.M., Morlock, L.L.M., Foley, H.T., et al.: Medical malpractice in diagnostic radiology: Claims, compensations, and patient injury. Radiology 164:263, 1987.
4. Morson, B.C.: The polyp-cancer sequence in the large bowel. Proc. R. Soc. Med. 67:451, 1974.
5. Lane, N., and Fenoglio, C.M.: The adenoma-carcinoma sequence in the stomach and colon. I. Observations on the adenoma as precursor to ordinary large bowel carcinoma. Gastrointest. Radiol. 1:111, 1976.
6. Waye, J.D.: The development of carcinoma of the colon. Am. J. Gastroenterol. 67:427, 1977.
7. Ott, D.J., and Gelfand, D.W.: Colorectal tumors: Pathology and detection. AJR 131:691, 1978.
8. Dales, L.G., Friedman, G.D., Ramcharan, S., et al.: Multiphasic checkup evaluation study. 3. Outpatient clinic utilization, hospitalization and mortality experience after seven years. Prevent. Med. 2:221, 1973.
9. Gilbertsen, V.A.: Procto-sigmoidoscopy and polypectomy in reducing the incidence of rectal cancer. Cancer 34:936, 1974.
10. Berge, T., Ekelund, G., Mellner, C., et al.: Carcinoma of the colon and rectum in a defined population. Acta Chir. Scand. 438(Suppl.):1973.
11. Semelka, R.C., and MacEwan, D.W.: Changes in diagnostic investigation and improved detection of colon cancer, Manitoba 1964–1984. J. Can. Assoc. Radiol. 38:251, 1987.
12. Eddy, D.: Cancer of the colon and rectum. Cancer 30:208, 1980.
13. Eddy, D.M., Nugent, F.W., Eddy, J.F., et al.: Screening for colorectal cancer in a high-risk population. Gastroenterology 92:682, 1987.
14. Feczko, P.J., and Halpert, R.D.: Reassessing the role of radiology in hemoccult screening. AJR 146:697, 1986.
15. Bressler, E.L.: Comparison costs for hemoccult tests. AJR 147:644, 1986.
16. Greegor, D.H.: Occult blood testing for detection of asymptomatic colon cancer. Cancer 28:131, 1971.
17. Hastings, J.B.: Mass screening for colorectal cancer. Am. J. Surg. 127:228, 1974.
18. Miller, M.P., and Stanley, T.V.: Results of a mass screening program for colorectal cancer. Arch. Surg. 123:63, 1988.
19. Ostrow, J.D., Mulvaney, C.A., Hansel, J.R., et al.: Sensitivity and reproducibility of chemical tests for fecal occult blood with an emphasis on false-positive reactions. Am. J. Digest. Dis. 18:930, 1973.
20. Nivatvongs, S., Gilbertsen, V.A., Goldberg, S.M., et al.: Distribution of large-bowel cancers detected by occult blood test in asymptomatic patients. Dis. Colon Rectum 25:420, 1982.
21. Ransohoff, D.F.: Colon cancer and ulcerative colitis. Gastroenterology 94:1089, 1988.
22. Winawer, S.J., and Sherlock, P.: Surveillance for colorectal cancer in average-risk patients, familial high-risk groups, and patients with adenomas. Cancer 50:2609, 1982.
23. Dodd, G.D.: Genetics and cancer of the gastrointestinal system. Radiology 123:263, 1977.
24. Swaroop, V.S., Winawer, S.J., Kurtz, R.C., et al.: Multiple primary malignant tumors. Gastroenterology 93:779, 1987.
25. Dodds, W.J., Schulte, W.J., Hensley, G.T., et al.: Peutz-Jeghers syndrome and gastrointestinal malignancy. AJR 115:374, 1972.
26. Stewart, M., Macrae, F.A., and Williams, C.B.: Neoplasia and ureterosigmoidostomy: A colonoscopy survey. Br. J. Surg. 69:414, 1982.
27. Sandler, R.S., and Sandler, D.P.: Radiation-induced cancers of the colon and rectum: Assessing the risk. Gastroenterology 84:51, 1983.
28. Young, A.C.: Radiology of the colon and rectum. In Irvine, W.I. (ed.): Modern Trends in Surgery, pp. 35–53. London, Butterworth & Co., 1966.
29. Welin, S.: Results of the Malmö technique of colon examination. JAMA 199:119, 1967.
30. Hamelin, L., and Hurtubise, M.: Remote control technique in double contrast study of the colon. AJR 119:382, 1973.
31. Laufer, I.: The double contrast enema: Myths and misconceptions. Gastrointest. Radiol. 1:19, 1976.
32. Laufer, I., Smith, N.C.W., and Mullens, J.E.: The radiologic demonstration of colorectal polyps undetected by endoscopy. Gastroenterology 70:167, 1976.
33. Andren, L., and Frieberg, S.: Frequency of polyps of rectum and colon according to age and relation to cancer. Gastroenterology 36:631, 1959.
34. Bernstein, M.A., Feczko, P.J., Halpert, R.D., et al.: Distribution of colonic polyps: Increased incidence of proximal lesions in older patients. Radiology 155:35, 1985.
35. Schub, R., and Steinheber, F.U.: Rightward shift of colon cancer. J. Clin. Gastroenterol. 8(6):630, 1986.
36. Shinya, H., and Wolff, W.I.: Morphology, anatomic distribution and cancer potential of colonic polyps. Ann. Surg. 190:679, 1979.
37. Granqvist, S., Gabrielsson, N., and Sundelin, P.: Diminutive colonic polyps—clinical significance and management. Endoscopy 1:36, 1979.
38. Feczko, P.J., Bernstein, M.A., Halpert, R.D., et al.: Small colonic polyps: A reappraisal of their significance. Radiology 152:301, 1984.
39. Tedesco, F.J., Hendrix, J.C., Pickens, C.A., et al.: Diminutive polyps: Histopathology, spatial distribution, and clinical significance. Gastrointest. Endosc. 28:1, 1982.
40. Bernstein, M.A., and Feczko, P.J.: Changing concepts of colonic polyps: Clinical and radiographic implications. CRC Crit. Rev. Diagn. Imaging 26:177, 1986.
41. Levine, M.S., Barnes, M.J., Bronner, M.P., et al.: Atypical hyperplastic polyps at double-contrast barium enema examination. Radiology 175:691, 1990.
42. Fork, F.T., Lindstrom, C., and Ekelund, G.R.: Reliability of routine double-contrast examination (DCE) of the large bowel in polyp detection: A prospective clinical study. Gastrointest. Radiol. 8:163, 1983.
43. Teefey, S.A., and Carlson, H.C.: The fluoroscopic barium enema in colonic polyp detection. AJR 141:1279, 1983.
44. Gelfand, D.W., Chen, Y.M., and Ott, D.J.: Detection of colonic polyps on single-contrast barium enema study: Emphasis on the elderly. Radiology 164:333. 1987.
45. de Roos, A., Hermans, J., Chandie Shaw, P., et al.: Colon polyps and carcinomas: Prospective comparison of the single- and double-contrast examination in the same patients. Radiology 154:11, 1985.
46. Ott, D.J., Chen, Y.M., Gelfand, D.W., et al.: Single-contrast vs double-contrast barium enema in the detection of colonic polyps. AJR 146:993, 1986.
47. Obrecht, W.F., Jr., Wu, W.C., Gelfand, D.W., et al.: The extent of successful colonoscopy: A second assessment using modern equipment. Gastrointest. Radiol. 9:161, 1984.
48. Miller, R.E., and Lehman, G.: Polypoid colonic lesions undetected by endoscopy. Radiology 129:295, 1978.
49. Weyman, P.J., Koehler, R.E., and Zuckerman, G.R.: Resolution of radiographic-endoscopic discrepancies in colon neoplasms. J. Clin. Gastroenterol. 3:89, 1981.
50. Thoeni, R.F., and Petras, A.: Double-contrast barium-enema examination and endoscopy in the detection of polypoid lesions in the cecum and ascending colon. Radiology 144:257, 1982.
51. Evers, K., Laufer, I., Gordon, R.L., et al.: Double-contrast enema examination for detection of rectal carcinoma. Radiology 140:635, 1981.
52. Rex, D.K., Lehman, G.A., Lappas, J.C., et al.: Sensitivity of double-contrast barium study for left-colon polyps. Radiology 158:69, 1986.
53. Leinicke, J.L., Dodds, W.J., Hogan, W.J., et al.: A comparison of colonoscopy and roentgenography for detecting polypoid lesions of the colon. Gastrointest. Radiol. 2:125, 1977.
54. Fork, F.T.: Double contrast enema and colonoscopy in polyp detection. Gut 22:971, 1981.
55. Beggs, I., and Thomas, B.M.: Diagnosis of carcinoma of the colon by barium enema. Clin. Radiol. 34:423, 1983.
56. Ott, D.J., Gelfand, D.W., Chen, Y.M., et al.: Colonoscopy and

the barium enema: A radiologic viewpoint. South. Med. J. 78:1033, 1985.

57. Hartzell, H.V.: To err with air. JAMA 187:455, 1964.

58. Youker, J.E., and Welin, S.: Differentiation of true polypoid tumors of the colon from extraneous material: A new roentgen sign. Radiology 84:610, 1965.

59. Miller, W.T., Jr., Levine, M.S., Rubesin, S.E., and Laufer, I.: Bowler hat sign: A simple principle for differentiating polyps from diverticula. Radiology 173:615, 1989.

60. Ament, A.E., and Alfidi, R.J.: Sessile polyps: Analysis of radiographic projections with the aid of a double-contrast phantom. AJR 139:111, 1982.

61. Delamarre, J., Descombes, P., Marti, R., et al.: Villous tumors of the colon and rectum: Double-contrast study of 47 cases. Gastrointest. Radiol. 5:69, 1980.

62. Iida, M., Iwashita, A., Tsuneyoshi, Y., et al.: Villous tumor of the colon: Correlation of histologic, macroscopic, and radiographic features. Radiology 167:673, 1988.

63. Rubesin, S.E., Saul, S.H., Laufer, I., et al.: Carpet lesions of the colon. Radiographics 5:537, 1985.

64. Williams, C.B., Hunt, R.D., and Loose, H.: Colonoscopy in the management of colon polyps. Br. J. Surg. 61:673, 1974.

65. Wolff, W.I., and Shinya, H.: Endoscopic polypectomy: Therapeutic and clinicopathologic aspects. Cancer 36:683, 1975.

66. Margulis, A.R., and Jovanovich, A.: The roentgen diagnosis of submucous lipomas of the colon. AJR 84:1114, 1960.

67. Taylor, A.J., Stewart, E.T., and Dodds, W.J.: Gastrointestinal lipomas: A radiologic and pathologic review. AJR 155:1205, 1990.

68. Heiken, J.P., Forde, K.A., and Gold, R.P.: Computed tomography as a definitive method for diagnosing gastrointestinal lipomas. Radiology 142:409, 1982.

69. Dachman, A.H., Ros, P.R., Shekitka, K.M., et al.: Colorectal hemangioma: Radiologic findings. Radiology 167:31, 1988.

70. Gohel, V.K., Kressel, H.Y., and Laufer, I.: Double contrast artifacts. Gastrointest. Radiol. 3:139, 1978.

71. Press, H.C., and Davis, T.W.: Ingested foreign bodies simulating polyposis: Report of six cases. AJR 127:1040, 1976.

72. Ekelund, G., Lindstrom, C., and Rosengren, J.E.: Appearance and growth of early carcinomas of the colon-rectum. Acta Radiol. 15:670, 1974.

73. Spratt, J.S., and Ackerman, L.V.: Small primary adenocarcinomas of the colon and rectum. JAMA 179:337, 1962.

74. Shinya, H., and Wolff, W.: Flexible colonoscopy. Cancer 37:416, 1976.

75. Youker, J.E., Welin, S., and Main, G.: Computer analysis in the differentiation of benign and malignant polypoid lesions of the colon. Radiology 90:794, 1968.

76. Welin, S., Youker, J., and Spratt, J.S., Jr.: The rates and patterns of growth of 375 tumors of the large intestine and rectum observed serially by double contrast enema study (Malmö technique). AJR 90:673, 1963.

77. Smith, T.R.: Pedunculated malignant colonic polyps with superficial invasion of the stalk. Radiology 115:593, 1975.

78. Maruyama, M.: Radiologic Diagnosis of Polyps and Carcinoma of the Large Bowel. Tokyo, Igaku-Shoin, 1978.

79. Ament, A.E., Alfidi, R.J., and Rao, P.S.: Basal identation of sessile polypoid lesions: A function of geometry rather than a sign of malignancy. Radiology 143:341, 1982.

80. Ott, D.J., Gelfand, D.W., Wu, W.C., et al.: Colon polyp morphology on double-contrast barium enema: Its pathologic predictive value. AJR 141:965, 1983.

81. Kariya, A., Mayama, S., Nishizawa, M., et al.: Radiologic diagnosis of early cancer of the colon. Stomach Intest. 15:357, 1980.

82. Skucas, J., Spataro, R.F., and Cannucciara, D.P.: The radiographic features of small colon cancers. Radiology 143:335, 1982.

83. Gabrielsson, N., Granqvist, S., Ohlsen, H., et al.: Malignancy of colonic polyps: Diagnosis and management. Acta Radiol. [Diagn] 19:479, 1978.

84. Maglinte, D.D.T., Keller, K.J., Miller, R.E., et al.: Colon and rectal carcinoma: Spatial distribution and detection. Radiology 147:669, 1983.

85. Morgenstern, L., and Lee, S.E.: Spatial distribution of colonic carcinoma. Arch. Surg. 113:1142, 1978.

86. Fischel, R.E., and Dermer, R.: Multifocal carcinoma of the large intestine. Clin. Radiol. 26:495, 1975.

87. Ott, D.J., Gelfand, D.W., and Ramquist, N.A.: Causes of error in gastrointestinal radiology. Gastrointest. Radiol. 5:99, 1980.

88. Baker, S.R., and Alterman, D.D.: False-negative barium enema in patients with sigmoid cancer and coexistent diverticula. Gastrointest. Radiol. 10:171, 1985.

89. Dreyfuss, J.R., and Benacerraf, B.: Saddle cancers of the colon and their progression to annular carcinomas. Radiology 129:289, 1978.

90. Kelvin, F.M., Gardiner, R., Vas, W., et al.: Colorectal carcinoma missed on double contrast barium enema study: A problem in perception. AJR 137:307, 1981.

91. Raskin, M.M., Viamonte, M., and Viamonte, M., Jr.: Primary linitis plastica carcinoma of the colon. Radiology 113:17, 1974.

92. Hodgson, J.R., and Sauer, W.G.: The roentgenologic features of carcinoma in chronic ulcerative colitis. AJR 86:91, 1961.

93. Laufer, I., and Joffe, N.: Roentgen aspects of chronic perforating carcinoma of the colon. Dis. Colon Rectum 16:127, 1973.

94. Williams, S.M., Berk, R.N., and Harned, R.K.: Radiologic features of multinodular lymphoma of the colon. AJR 143:87–91, 1984.

95. Wall, S.F., Ominsky, S., Alteman, D.F., et al.: Multifocal abnormalities of the gastrointestinal tract in AIDS. AJR 146:1, 1986.

96. Marshak, R.H., and Lindner, A.E.: Leiomyosarcoma of the colon. Am. J. Gastroenterol. 54:155, 1970.

97. Khilnani, M.T., Marshak, R.H., Eliasaph, J., et al.: Roentgen features of metastases to the colon. AJR 96:302, 1966.

98. Gedgaudas, R.K., Kelvin, F.M., Thompson, W.M., et al.: The value of the preoperative barium enema in the assessment of pelvic masses. Radiology 146:609, 1983.

99. Meyers, M.A., Aliphant, N., Teixidor, H., et al.: Metastatic carcinoma simulating inflammatory colitis. AJR 123:74, 1975.

100. Lammer, J., Dirschmid, K., and Hugel, H.: Carcinomatous metastases to the colon simulating Crohn's disease. Gastrointest. Radiol. 6:89, 1981.

101. Meyers, M.A.: Distribution of intra-abdominal malignant seeding: Dependency on dynamics of flow of ascitic fluid. AJR 119:198, 1973.

102. Rubesin, S.E., and Levine, M.S.: Omental cakes: Colonic involvement by omental metastases. Radiology 154:593, 1985.

103. Ginaldi, S., Lindell, M.M., and Zornoza, J.: The striped colon: A new radiographic observation in metastatic serosal implants. AJR 134:453, .

104. Enker, W.E., and Dragacevic, S.: Multiple carcinomas of the large bowel: A natural experiment in etiology and pathogenesis. Ann. Surg. 187:8, 1978.

105. Shauffer, I.A., and Sequeira, J.: Suture granuloma simulating recurrent carcinoma. AJR 128:856, 1977.

106. Daly, B.D., and Crowley, B.M.: Radiological appearances of colonic ring staple anastomoses. Br. J. Radiol. 62:256, 1989.

107. Chen, Y.M., Ott, D.J., Wolfman, N.T., et al.: Recurrent colorectal carcinoma: Evaluation with barium enema examination and CT. Radiology 163:307, 1987.

108. McCarthy, S.M., Barnes, D., Deveney, K., et al.: Detection of recurrent rectosigmoid carcinoma: Prospective evaluation of CT and clinical factors. AJR 144:577, 1985.

109. Sharpe, M., and Golden, R.: End-to-end anastomosis of the colon following resection: A roentgen study of 42 cases. AJR 64:769, 1950.

110. Fleischner, F.G., and Berenberg, A.L.: Recurrent carcinoma of the colon at the site of anastomosis. Radiology 66:540, 1956.

111. Welch, J.P., and Donaldson, G.A.: Detection and treatment of recurrent cancer of the colon and rectum. Am. J. Surg. 135:505, 1978.

112. Freeny, P.C., Marks, W.M., Ryan, J.A., et al.: Colorectal carcinoma evaluation with CT: Preoperative staging and detection of postoperative recurrence. Radiology 158:347, 1986.

113. Moss, A.A.: Imaging of colorectal carcinoma. Radiology 170:308, 1989.

114. Balzarini, L., Ceglia, E., D'Ippolito, G.D., et al.: Local recurrence of rectosigmoid cancer: What about the choice of MRI for diagnosis? Gastrointest. Radiol. 15:338, 1990.

EARLY DIAGNOSIS OF GASTROINTESTINAL CANCER

Masakazu Maruyama, M.D.

14

INTRODUCTION

Radiologists seem to have abandoned their responsibility for gastrointestinal diagnosis by their loss of enthusiasm for the classic barium contrast methods of examination. Consequently, there has been a decline in barium studies of the gastrointestinal tract; at the same time, an overreliance on endoscopy and biopsy has developed. These tendencies have interfered with the sound progress and development of both radiology and endoscopy.

However, it must be remembered that the barium study, particularly with the use of double contrast, presents the most reliable opportunity for routine diagnosis of early cancer in the gastrointestinal tract. For this reason, the tradition of classic barium radiology should be developed and enhanced and should be passed on to succeeding generations by contemporary radiologists. This chapter deals with the present status and limitations of double contrast radiography and the results that have been achieved in the detection and diagnosis of early gastrointestinal cancer.

DEFINITION OF EARLY GASTROINTESTINAL CANCER

Our clinical interest lies in the diagnosis of carcinomas limited to the mucosa and submucosa. Theoretically, it would also be of value to be able to specify whether lymph node or distant metastases are present. However, in practice, this cannot be reliably achieved. Therefore, for gastric and colorectal carcinoma, the term *early* is used for those carcinomas in which invasion is limited to the mucosa and submucosa without regard to the presence of lymph node or distant metastases.[1] For historical reasons, in the case of esophageal cancer, the term *superficial* is used to refer to these same lesions and the term early is used only in cases without lymph node or distant metastases. Strictly speaking, the term "early esophageal cancer" should not be used preoperatively because of the difficulty in ascertaining lymph node or distant metastases. Nevertheless, it may be used in cases of intramucosal cancer because of the rarity of lymph node or distant metastases.

CLASSIFICATION OF EARLY GASTROINTESTINAL CANCER

Early cancers can be classified either according to the depth of invasion or according to the morphologic appearance of the lesion.

Classification according to depth of invasion is illustrated in Figure 14–1 in early esophageal cancer. Cancer confined to the epithelium is referred to as ep-cancer; cancer remaining within the muscularis mucosae is referred to as mm-cancer, and cancer involving the submucosa is referred to as sm-cancer.[2]

Classification according to morphology of the lesion has been best developed for early gastric cancer and is illustrated in Figure 14–2.[3] Essentially, early cancers can be classified as protruded lesions (type I), flat lesions (type II), or depressed lesions (type III).

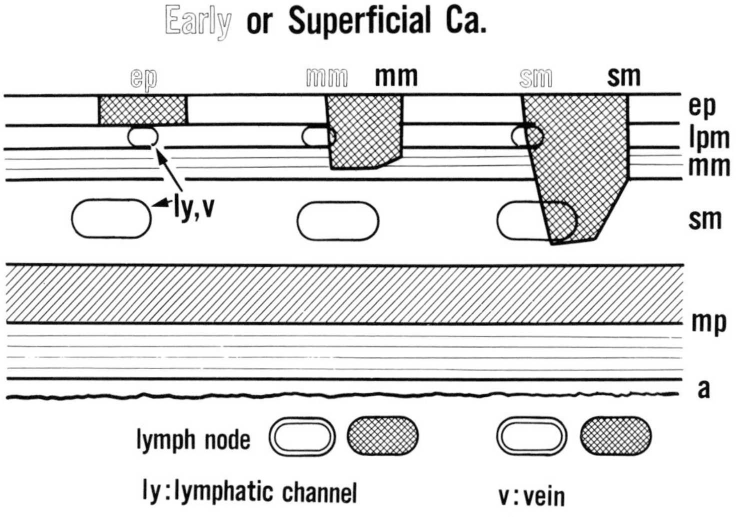

FIGURE 14–1

Schematic representation of the classification of depth of invasion by esophageal cancer.

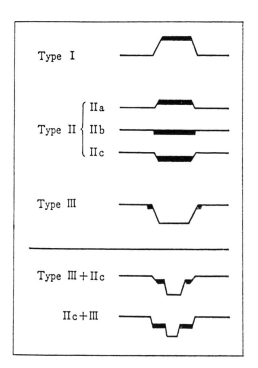

FIGURE 14–2

Schematic representation of the morphologic classification of early gastric cancer. (From Japanese Society for Gastric Cancer: The General Rules for the Gastric Cancer Study, ed. 11. Tokyo, Kanehara Shuppan, 1985, with permission.)

EARLY ESOPHAGEAL CANCER

Classification

There has been no definite macroscopic classification of early or superficial esophageal cancer. The radiologic and endoscopic classification for superficial cancer had been used independently until 1987 when a new macroscopic classification of superficial esophageal cancer was proposed in the 41st Annual Meeting of Japanese Society of Esophageal Diseases (Table 14–1).[4] This new classification has been in tentative use. Basically following the macroscopic classification of early gastric cancer, it was made in order to unify the macroscopic classification of early cancer throughout the gastrointestinal tract.

In this new classification, an elevation is diagnosed as type O-I if its height is over 2 or 3 mm. An elevation of approximately 1 mm is diagnosed as type O-IIa. Type O-IIc is a lesion that consists of a very shallow erosion with a depression of more or less 0.5 mm, and a lesion with deeper and more distinct depression is diagnosed as type O-III.

Characteristically about 50% of early or superficial esophageal cancers show a mixture of the basic macroscopic types mentioned in the new classification. Intraepithelial spread is a prominent feature in many

TABLE 14–1. New Macroscopic Classification of Superficial Esophageal Carcinoma*
Type O-I: Superficial and Protruded Type (>0.3 mm in height)
Type O-II: Superficial and Flat Type IIa slightly elevated IIb flat IIc slightly depressed
Type O-III: Superficial and Excavated

*In accordance with Japanese Society of Esophageal Diseases, June 1987.

cases of mixed type. Superficial spreading carcinoma is defined as a superficial cancer with no conspicuous elevation or depression whose spread along the longitudinal axis is over 5 cm.

Prognosis

The prognosis of early esophageal cancer is related both to depth of invasion and to the presence of distant spread. The influence of lymph node metastases is illustrated in Figure 14–3. The 5-year survival rate of patients with superficial esophageal cancer with lymph node metastases is substantially worse than the survival rate of patients with early esophageal cancer without lymph node metastases. Figure

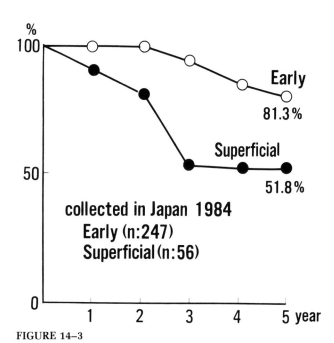

FIGURE 14–3

The 5-year survival rate of early (no lymph node metastases) esophageal cancer is substantially better than the survival rate of patients with superficial (with lymph node metastases) esophageal cancer.

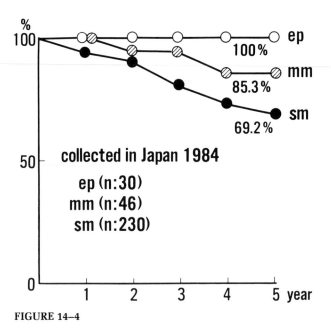

FIGURE 14-4

CORRELATION OF 5-YEAR SURVIVAL RATE TO DEPTH OF INVASION OF EARLY OR SUPERFICIAL ESOPHAGEAL CANCER. The decreased survival rate of patients with sm-cancer is due to the high incidence of lymph node metastases.

14–4 shows that survival rate is also related to the depth of invasion and that a marked deterioration is found in prognosis of patients with sm-cancer. This is due to the abundant lymphatic channels within the lamina propria mucosae leading to a higher incidence of lymph node metastases in sm-cancer. To achieve results comparable to those achieved with early gastric cancer, it is necessary to detect esophageal cancer when it is confined to the epithelium or muscularis mucosae (ep-cancer or mm-cancer) and not to the submucosa.

Endoscopic Correlation

In 1987 Shirakabe and colleagues reported that all ep-cancers were missed by radiology and detected by endoscopy, whereas 9 of 11 cases of mm-cancer were detected by radiology.[5] They also reported that all sm-cancers were detected by radiology. In 1984 Nishizawa and co-workers reported four cases, including three ep-cancers and one mm-cancer, missed by radiology and detected by the following endoscopy.[6] Based on this experience, they emphasized the superiority of endoscopy in the detection of ep- and mm-cancer. The Chinese team has shown that cytology is an extremely effective method of detecting invisible lesions through the use of endoscopy.[7]

Radiologic Features

The efforts to detect ep- and mm-cancer radiologically have recently been started by Shirakabe and col-

leagues.[8] They proposed characteristic macroscopic findings of ep- and mm-cancer, consisting of granularity for elevated lesions and irregular surface depression and irregular grooves for depressed lesions (Fig. 14–5). They tried to correlate those characteristics with radiologic images. They encountered no cases of sm-cancer that showed irregular grooves.

The protruded type of early esophageal cancer (type O-I) is visualized rather distinctly because of its height.[9] Sometimes, intraepithelial spread is seen with this type of cancer (Fig. 14–6). The granularity of flat, elevated lesions (type O-IIa) may be delineated so faintly that the extent of the cancer can only be defined with difficulty. However, very slight marginal

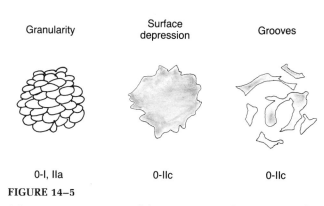

FIGURE 14-5

Schematic representation of the macroscopic characteristics of ep- and mm-cancer.

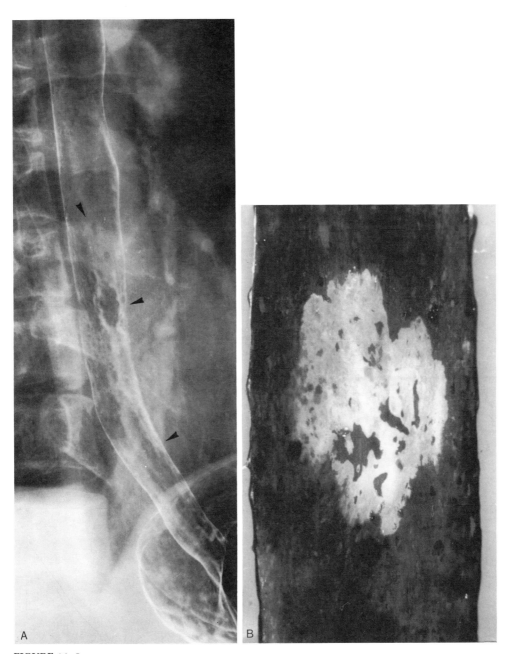

FIGURE 14–6

EARLY POLYPOID ESOPHAGEAL CANCER (TYPE O-I). *A*, Preoperative double contrast radiograph shows the polypoid early cancer. Invasion was limited to the muscularis mucosae. There is evidence of intraepithelial spread proximally and distally *(arrowheads)*.

B, Photograph of the resected specimen shows the lesion unstained with 3% Lugol's solution. The lesion measured 55 × 50 mm in diameter.

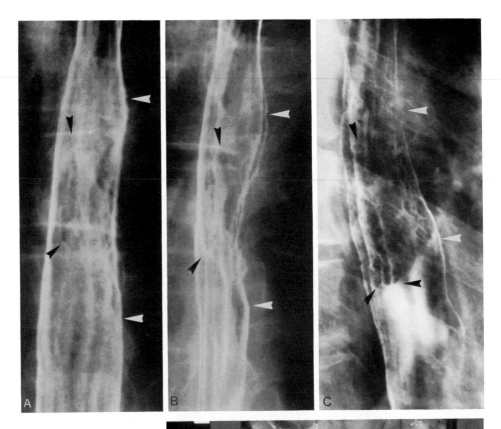

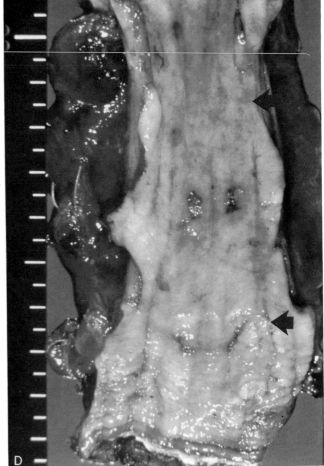

FIGURE 14–7

EARLY ESOPHAGEAL CANCER (TYPE O-IIa) WITH INVASION LIMITED TO THE EPITHELIUM. *A,* There is a granular surface in the midesophagus with marginal irregularity.

B shows a granular surface as well as wall stiffness.

C, Frontal view shows the margins of the lesion with its surface.

D, Resected specimen shows the approximate extent of the lesion (*arrows*). Note the difficulty in delineating the extent of the tumor.

stiffness and irregularity are visualized in Figure 14–7A to C, which were taken with moderate distention of the esophagus. These abnormalities become prominent with mild distention. Macroscopically, the lesion is recognized as granularity with subtle alteration in elevation or depression from the normal surrounding mucosa without clear demarcation of its border (Fig. 14–7D).

As illustrated in Figure 14–5, type IIc lesions consist of two subgroups: lesions characterized by depression and lesions consisting of irregular grooves. The surface depression of ep-cancer (Fig. 14–8) is difficult to recognize even on a double contrast specimen radiograph (Fig. 14–8A), and the extent of its margin is not defined totally on a preoperative double contrast image (Fig. 14–8B and C). The surface depression of mm-cancer is recognized much more easily than that of ep-cancer on a preoperative double contrast image, and slight wall stiffness is visualized

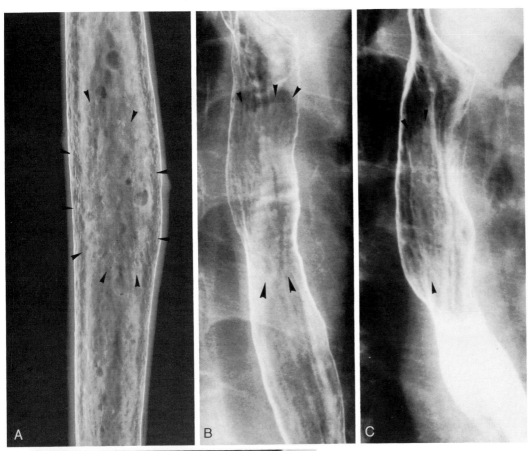

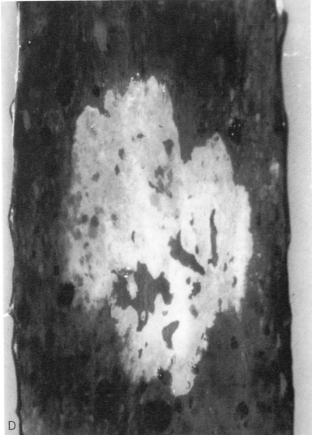

FIGURE 14–8

EARLY ESOPHAGEAL CANCER, SLIGHTLY DEPRESSED TYPE (O-IIc) WITH INVASION LIMITED TO THE EPITHELIUM. *A,* The specimen radiograph shows the extent of the surface depression *(arrowheads).* (Courtesy of G. Yamaki, M.D., Toranomon Hospital, Japan). The lesion is very difficult to recognize on the preoperative radiographs *(B* and *C).*

D, Photograph of the resected specimen shows the lesion measuring 60 × 32 mm unstained with 3% Lugol's solution.

when a part of the lesion comes to the margin (Fig. 14–9). The surface depression and wall stiffness of sm-cancer become more prominent than those seen in mm-cancer (Fig. 14–10).

An ep-cancer (Fig. 14–11) consisting of irregular grooves is clearly demonstrated as serpiginous ero-

sions on specimen double contrast radiographs (Fig. 14–11A). It is extremely difficult to demonstrate such erosions of ep-cancer on a preoperative double contrast image with the same distention of the esophagus as in Figure 14–11A (Fig. 14–11B). The extent of the abnormality can be recognized roughly on a frontal

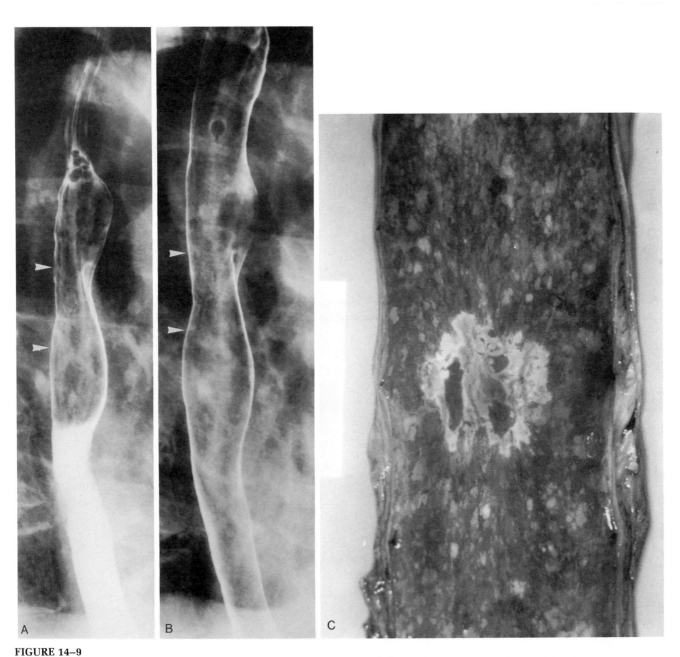

FIGURE 14–9

SLIGHTLY DEPRESSED EARLY ESOPHAGEAL CANCER (TYPE O-IIc) WITH INVASION TO THE MUSCULARIS MUCOSAE. With the esophagus in mild (A) and moderate (B) distention, irregular surface depression and slight wall stiffness are seen.

C, Photograph of the resected specimen shows the 23 × 23 mm lesion. (Courtesy of Dr. G. Yamaki, Toranomon Hospital, Japan).

view (Fig. 14–11C), and it is visualized as an irregular surface depression instead of grooves. There is only one point of correspondence (x) between pre- and postoperative double contrast images (Fig. 14–11C). Figure 14–11D and E shows a profile view of the lesion with the esophagus distended. The lesion is difficult to recognize on a specimen radiograph (Fig. 14–11D). The preoperative radiographs suggest wall thickening. The wall stiffness is distinctly seen on a preoperative double contrast image with a mild degree of esophageal distention (Fig. 14–11E).

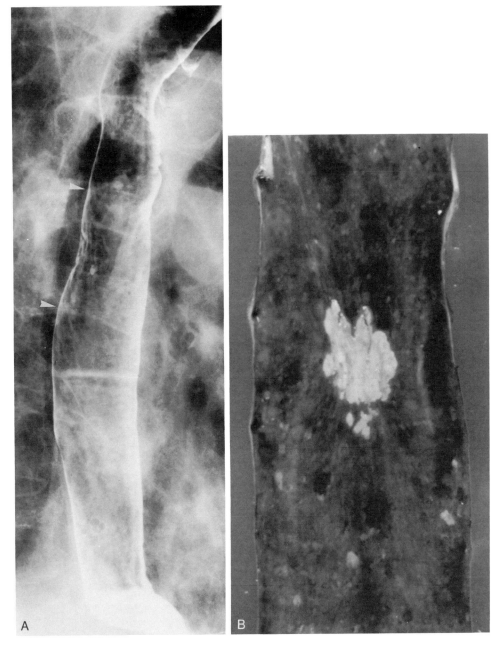

FIGURE 14–10

SLIGHTLY DEPRESSED SUPERFICIAL ESOPHAGEAL CANCER (TYPE O-IIc) WITH INVASION TO THE SUBMUCOSA. A, Double contrast radiograph shows prominent wall stiffness (*arrowheads*) and an irregular surface depression.

B, Photograph of the resected specimen shows a 25 × 14 mm lesion. (Courtesy of Dr. G. Yamaki, Toranomon Hospital, Japan).

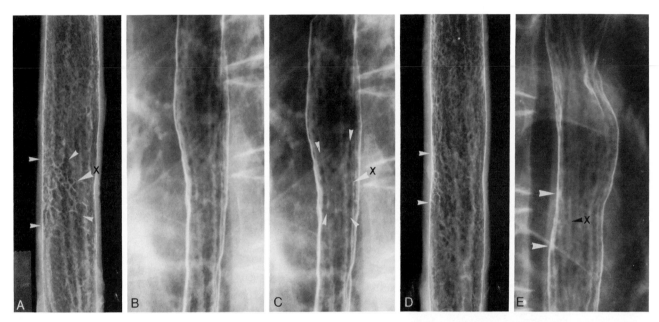

FIGURE 14–11

IRREGULAR GROOVE PATTERN, SLIGHTLY DEPRESSED EARLY ESOPHAGEAL CANCER WITH INVASION LIMITED TO THE EPITHELIUM. *A,* Specimen radiograph shows the en face appearance of irregular grooves representing serpiginous erosions. (From Shirakabe, H., et al.: A new proposal of macroscopic classification of superficial esophageal carcinoma (in Japanese). I to Cho (Stomach and Intestine) *22*:1349, 1987, with permission.)

B and *C,* On frontal views, the lesion is only faintly visualized as an irregular surface depression *(arrowheads).* There is only one point of precise correspondence between the specimen radiograph and the preoperative radiograph *(arrowhead X).*

D, Specimen radiograph with the lesion in profile shows no evidence of wall stiffness.

E, Preoperative radiograph with moderate distention shows thickening of the affected portion in the profile view. There is only one point of precise correspondence *(arrowhead X)* to the specimen radiograph in *A.*

F, The specimen photograph shows the resected lesion with its irregular grooves.

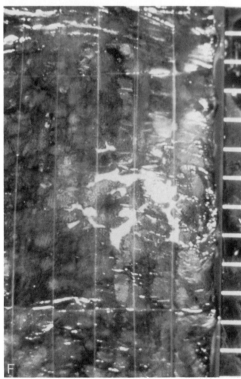

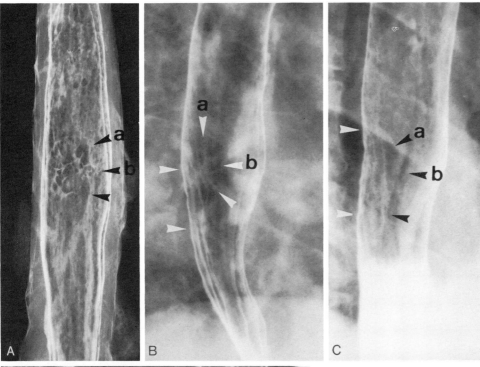

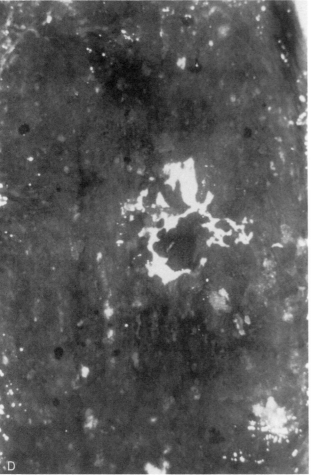

FIGURE 14–12

SLIGHTLY DEPRESSED EARLY CANCER (TYPE O-IIc) WITH INVASION TO THE MUSCULARIS MUCOSAE.
A, Specimen radiograph in frontal projection shows irregular grooves (arrowheads) due to serpiginous erosions with radiolucent halos. (From Shirakabe, H., et al.: A new proposal of macroscopic classification of superficial esophageal carcinoma (in Japanese). I to Cho (Stomach and Intestine) 22:1349, 1987, with permission.)
B, Preoperative double contrast radiograph shows the lesion only faintly. There are only two points of correspondence (arrowheads a and b) to the specimen radiograph.
C, With the lesion viewed in profile, wall stiffness is seen.
D, The resected specimen shows the lesion with serpiginous erosions.

The irregular grooves in mm-cancer are distinctly delineated as serpiginous erosions with radiolucent halos on a specimen double contrast image (Fig. 14–12A). The grooves are faintly delineated on a preoperative double contrast image with moderate distention of the esophagus (Fig. 14–12B). Actually only two corresponding points (black arrowheads a and b) can be indicated. The wall stiffness in mm-cancer may also be effaced on specimen double contrast radiographs. However, it is definitely visualized on a preoperative double contrast image even in a moderately distended esophagus (Fig. 14–12C). Moreover, it seems to be more pronounced than in ep-cancer (see Fig. 14–11E).

The excavated type of early esophageal cancer (type O-III) is detected easily in the initial radiologic examination. The majority of cases are sm-cancers. In the series of Shirakabe and colleagues, all sm-cancers except one could be detected in the initial radiologic examination.[5]

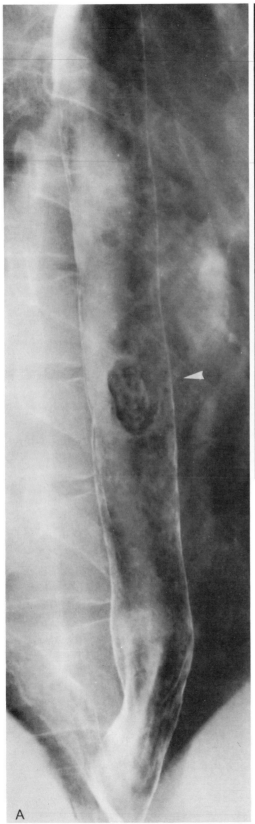

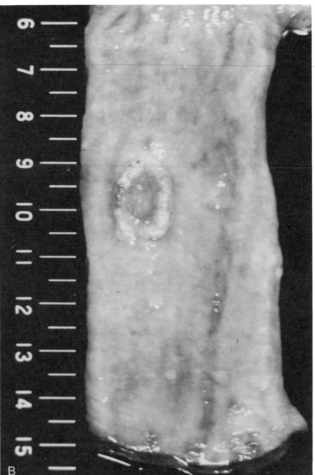

FIGURE 14–13

SUPERFICIAL ESOPHAGEAL CANCER, MIXED TYPE (TYPE O-IIa + IIc), INVASION TO THE SUBMUCOSA. *A,* Preoperative radiograph shows a filling defect *(arrowhead)* representing an elevated portion of the lesion. Collections of barium within the filling defect represent the depressed portions of the lesion.

B, Photograph of the resected specimen shows the slightly elevated lesion with a central depression.

Approximately 50% of early esophageal cancers consist of a mixture of the basic types (Fig. 14–13). In many of these cases, the dominant lesion is associated with a type IIb-like lesion due to intraepithelial spread (see Fig. 14–6A and B). Therefore, it is important to pay attention not only to the predominant lesion but also to search for evidence of intraepithelial spread in the detailed radiologic study.

Radiology must acknowledge its limitation in the diagnosis of early esophageal cancer, particularly for ep-cancer and mm-cancer. However, this may be ascribed to the relative lack of experience in the diagnosis of these conditions, and the accumulation of cases and experience may lead to improvements in diagnosis in the very near future. In fact, a retrospective view of the initial films in cases missed by radiology has shown that subtle signs of ep- or mm-cancer are present in most cases.[10]

EARLY GASTRIC CANCER

Definition

The definition and classification of early gastric cancer were first proposed at the annual meeting of the Japan Gastroenterological Endoscopy Society in 1962. Early gastric cancer was defined as carcinoma in which invasion is limited to the mucosa and submucosa, without regard for the presence of lymph node and distant metastases. In 1963, at the annual meeting of the Japanese Research Society for Gastric Cancer, this definition was temporarily modified to "carcinoma limited to the mucosa and submucosa without metastases." However, the original form was later adopted by both societies because the presence of metastases could not be detected prior to surgery.[3]

Classification

The macroscopic classification of early gastric cancer was proposed because Borrmann's classification of advanced cancer was not considered applicable to cancer that was limited to the mucosa and submucosa (Table 14–2; see Fig. 14–2). It should be stressed that this classification of early gastric cancer refers to macroscopic appearance. It can be used for radiologic and endoscopic diagnosis on the assumption that a one-to-one correspondence is possible among macroscopic, radiologic, and endoscopic findings under ideal conditions.

The Japanese classification of early gastric cancer seems to have been accepted internationally despite opposition raised because of its lack of reproducibility and its prognostic value.[11] In cases of intramucosal cancer of the stomach (m-cancer), it should be stressed that both polypoid and depressed forms reveal an almost identical prognosis despite the presence of lymph node metastasis in the depressed form. It is very important to note the risk of liver metastasis in the polypoid form, which is always a differentiated carcinoma histologically.[12]

Endoscopic Correlation

Gelfand and co-workers stress that most recent Western literature suggests that radiology is less accurate and misses more lesions than endoscopy.[13] Such

TABLE 14–2. Classification of Early Gastric Cancer
I. **Polypoid (>0.5 cm in height)**

II. **Superficial**
    a. Elevated (<0.5 cm in height)
    b. Flat—minimal or no alteration in height of mucosa
    c. Depressed—superficial ulceration, usually not extending beyond the muscularis mucosae

III. **Excavated—Prominent Depression, Usually Due to Ulceration**

reports are written by gastroenterologists expressing the endoscopic point of view. A criticism of most such studies is that endoscopy is used as a final arbiter by which radiology must always be judged to be less accurate, even though many of these communications do not deal with early gastric cancer.[14]

Maruyama illustrated the efficacy of radiology and endoscopy in the diagnosis of gastric cancer with computer-controlled processing of diagnostic data.[15] In 226 cases diagnosed as early cancer, 188 were submitted to endoscopy and 67 were positive for cancer by biopsy, accounting for 30.1% of all cases diagnosed as early cancer in the initial radiologic examination. Fifty of 68 cases were surgically resected, and 38 of these were proved histologically to be early cancer, accounting for 64.3% of the resected cases. From the 5630 cases diagnosed as normal, 730 were referred to endoscopy, and biopsy was positive for cancer in 11 cases. When the endoscopy group is regarded as a denominator, these 11 cases account for 1.5% (11/730) of cases diagnosed as normal in the initial radiologic examination. They account for 0.2% (11/5630) of all cases diagnosed as normal. In other words, these cases were missed by the initial radiologic examination (radiologic false negatives).

Sensitivity of the initial radiologic examination was 97.1%, specificity 32.3%, and accuracy 33.8%, whereas sensitivity of endoscopy was 99.8%, specificity 39.7%, and accuracy 46.2%. Only a minor difference was found in the sensitivity and specificity between radiology and endoscopy in the diagnosis of gastric cancer, including early and advanced cancers. A recent report by Hamada and co-workers stated that only 73.6% of all early cancer cases could be detected by initial radiologic examination, even when cases of vague abnormalities were included.

The question of whether radiology or endoscopy is the better method for screening for gastric cancer cannot be discussed without taking into account the incidence of complications and the reluctance of patients to undergo panendoscopy.[17]

Technical Considerations

There is little value in prolonged fluoroscopy. The sequence of exposures is designed to visualize the entire stomach by combination of the fixed number of films and positioning of the patient. For this reason fluoroscopy should be used only for positioning the patient for spot filming. Unnecessary positional change should be avoided.

Positional change is very important in double contrast radiography of the stomach. For delineation of a polypoid lesion, it is necessary to collect the barium around it. For delineation of a depressed lesion, it is necessary to pool the barium within it as much as possible. It is necessary to be aware of the outflow of the contrast medium from the depression (Fig. 14–14). Even a crater of advanced cancer is often missed by a careless change of position (Fig. 14–14A and B). This is particularly likely to happen with a depression on the posterior wall at the angle or distal body of the stomach when the patient is quickly turned from right to left decubitus or from the supine to the left lateral position. Therefore, a variety of positional changes should be performed when searching for a depressed lesion located in this area. At least one double contrast radiograph should be taken after the

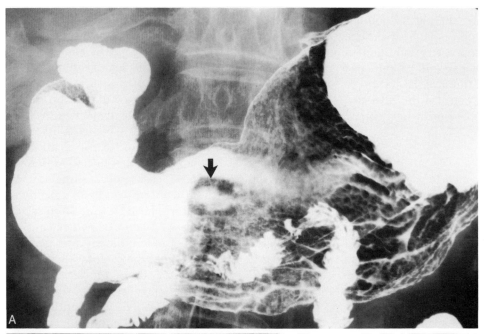

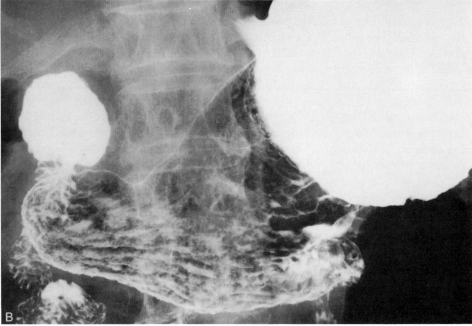

FIGURE 14–14

THE IMPORTANCE OF POSITIONING FOR DETECTION OF GASTRIC CANCER. *A,* The ulcerated cancer *(arrow)* is best demonstrated while turning the patient from right lateral decubitus toward the left posterior oblique position.

B, When the patient is turned from left lateral decubitus toward the supine position, there is insufficient barium to demonstrate the lesion.

FIGURE 14–15

EARLY GASTRIC CANCER (TYPE IIc).
A, The film with the patient in the supine position does not give an en face view of the lesion located on the posterior wall near the lesser curvature.

B, The film in the right posterior oblique position gives the best frontal view of the lesion. The radiolucent nodules within the depression consist of regenerative epithelium.

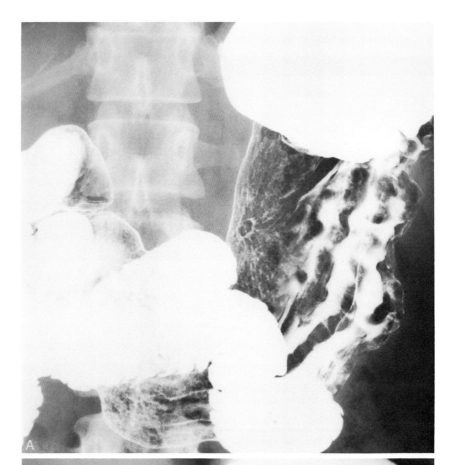

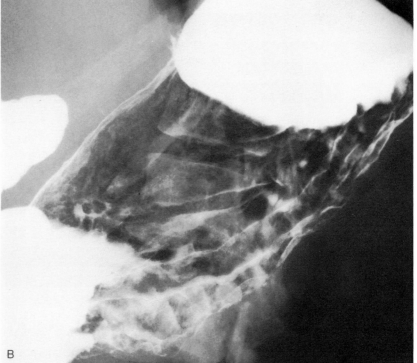

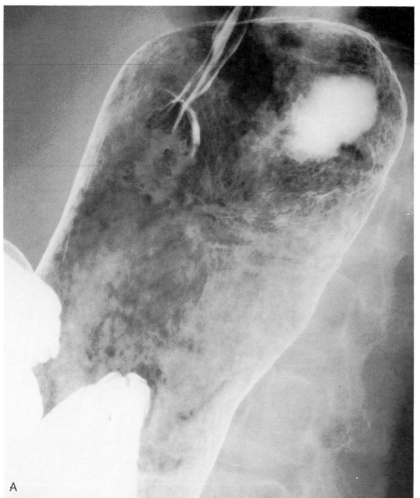

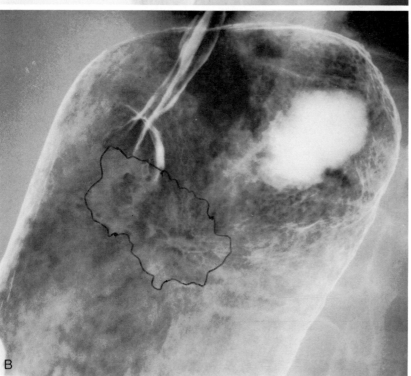

FIGURE 14–16

DEPRESSED EARLY GASTRIC CANCER NEAR THE GASTRIC CARDIA. *A,* In the right lateral position with considerable gastric distention, a type IIc lesion is demonstrated on the lesser curvature aspect of the gastric cardia.

B, A close-up view of the approximate extent of the lesion.

patient has been turned from the right decubitus to the supine position. By this procedure the contrast medium is retained in a depression (see Fig. 14–14A). The concept of allowing the barium to wash across the mucosal surface has been described in Chapter 2 as the "flow technique."

Visualization of a lesion en face is of utmost importance in the recognition of early gastric cancer by double contrast radiography. The en face view can be obtained by a standard sequence of exposures when the lesion is on the posterior wall of the stomach. As a general rule, the closer the lesion is to the lesser curvature, the more difficult it is to obtain an en face view. For this purpose, right posterior oblique (Fig. 14–15) or right lateral projections (Fig. 14–16) are useful, depending on the exact location of the lesion.

The compression method gives optimal views of lesions along the lesser curvature of the antrum when double contrast radiography has been unsuccessful.

A lesion located on the greater curvature of the gastric body or in its vicinity is adequately delineated by the left posterior oblique or left lateral position (Fig. 14–17). Even a lesion located just opposite the incisura angularis can be visualized en face by positional changes from the supine to the left lateral decubitus position (Fig. 14–18A and B). Compression should always be added to a lesion located on the greater curvature of the gastric antrum (Fig. 14–18C).

In the double contrast study of a depressed lesion, it is necessary to be aware of the changing appearance caused by changes in the volume of barium and air. In a detailed study air should be adjusted in three

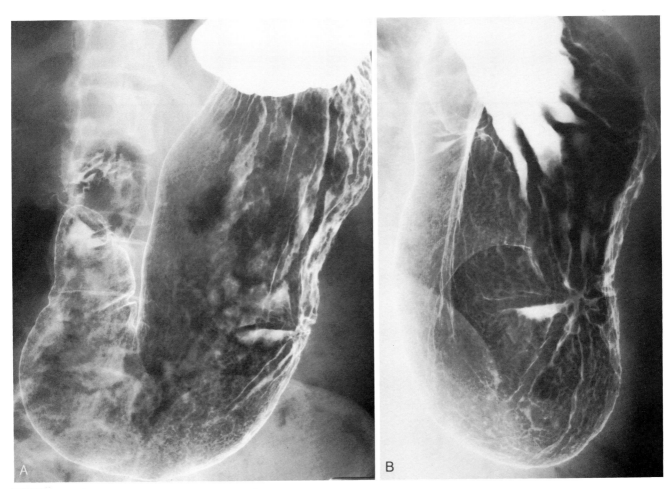

FIGURE 14–17

EARLY GASTRIC CANCER ON THE GREATER CURVATURE. A, The depressed early cancer (type IIc) on the greater curve is best demonstrated in the left posterior oblique position. (Courtesy of Dr. T. Hamada, Juntendo University, Tokyo, Japan). B, With the patient turned into the left lateral decubitus position, the lesion is seen en face.

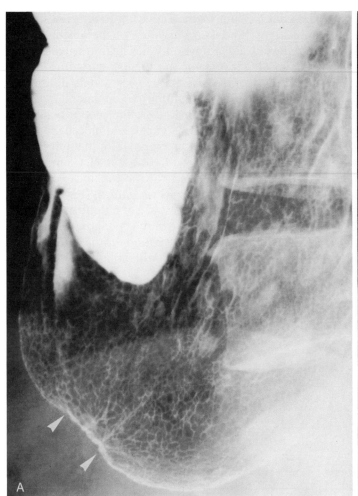

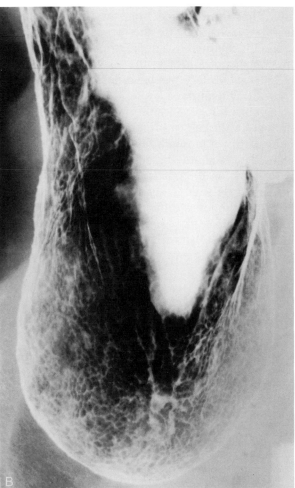

FIGURE 14–18

EARLY GASTRIC CANCER ON THE GREATER CURVATURE OPPOSITE THE INCISURA. *A*, With the patient in the RPO position, a profile view of the depressed early gastric cancer (type IIc; *arrowheads*) is obtained.

B, With the patient in the head-down, left lateral position, the lesion is seen en face.

C, A compression view of the same lesion.

steps; slight distention revealing the irregular barium collection in a depressed lesion and the prominent converging folds (Fig. 14–19A), optimal distention for demonstration of the lesion with clear relation to the converging folds (Fig. 14–19B), and overdistention effacing most of the converging folds (Fig. 14–19C). Such a dynamic observation of a lesion by changing the volume of air is essential for making the diagnosis of cancer, and the distinction between cancer limited to the mucosal membrane and cancer with submucosal involvement.

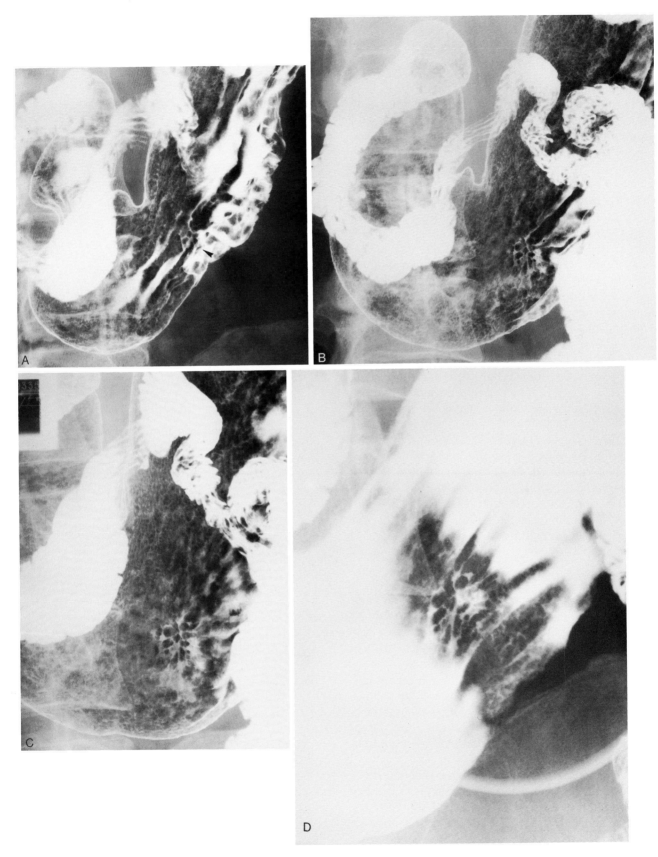

FIGURE 14–19

THE EFFECT OF INCREASING DISTENTION ON THE APPEARANCE OF AN EARLY GASTRIC CANCER. *A*, With modest distention, there is a depressed early cancer with radiating folds. However, the extent of the lesion is not adequately delineated.

B, With increasing distention, there is optimal delineation of the depression with the prominent mucosal folds.

C, With additional gaseous distention, converging folds are effaced.

D, Compression view of the same lesion with nodularity due to irregular proliferation of cancerous tissue.

Radiologic Diagnosis of Early Polypoid Cancer

General Considerations

The diagnosis of early polypoid cancer is based on a detailed analysis of the radiologic features that may suggest the histologic characteristics of a polypoid lesion.[18] The first object is to determine the size, shape, and surface pattern of a polypoid lesion. These lesions usually measure 1 to 4 cm in largest diameter except in unusual cases.

The height of a polypoid lesion is next estimated on compression or double contrast images. The surface pattern of the lesion plays the most important role for distinction between benignity and malignancy. A granular or lobulated appearance is characteristic of early cancer. This appearance, although irregular and enlarged, is similar to that of the surrounding mucosa bearing the lesion. This condition is recognized as a uniform granularity of the areae gastricae. The extent of granularity depends on the intensity of the intestinal metaplasia (Fig. 14–20).

A tendency to imitate the pattern of the areae gastricae is preserved in a polypoid cancer whose invasion is limited to the submucosal layer. The diagnosis of early polypoid cancer is based on this observation. Double contrast radiography is the method for visualization of the background where cancer has developed. Compression method is best suited for visualization of the lesion itself. As the cancerous infiltration extends deeper than the submucosal layer, the surface pattern disappears and usually is replaced by erosion or ulceration.

Types I and IIa

Type I lesion is less common than type IIa. The gross form of type I is usually a sessile polyp, with an irregular surface pattern simulating the areae gastricae (Fig. 14–21). In most cases type I is larger than 2 cm and is rarely pedunculated. Most pedunculated lesions are benign hyperplastic polyps with a smooth surface pattern. Subpedunculated lesions are primarily benign hyperplastic polyps with some unusual cases of malignancy. At present, endoscopic polypectomy is the first choice of treatment for pedunculated lesions.

A flat, mucosal elevation not higher than 0.5 cm is diagnosed as a type IIa lesion when the surface pattern mentioned above is visualized (Fig. 14–22). It has a somewhat irregular granularity compared with that of an adenoma.

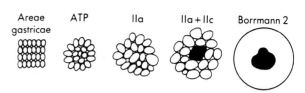

FIGURE 14–20

Schematic representation of the surface pattern of various polypoid lesions of the stomach. (ATP = atypical epithelium or adenomatous polyp). (From Shirakabe H., and Maruyama M.: Neoplastic diseases of the stomach. In Margulis, A.R., and Burhenne, H.J. (eds.): Alimentary Tract Radiology, ed. 4, St. Louis, C.V. Mosby, 1989, p. 600, with permission.)

Type IIa + IIc

A flat, mucosal elevation with a recognizable central depression is diagnosed as type IIa + IIc (Fig. 14–23). Its size ranges from 1 to 3 cm and is sometimes over 3 cm. The central depression is irregular. The depth of invasion is roughly estimated by the depth of the central depression. When a central depression is clearly seen, there is a risk that the invasion extends more deeply than the submucosal layer. The likelihood of lymph node and liver metastases is also high in this type of lesion.

Radiologic Diagnosis of Early Depressed Cancer

General Considerations

The invasion pattern in early depressed cancer can be regarded as two-dimensional and in advanced cancer as three-dimensional. This concept theoretically enables the radiologic diagnosis of early depressed cancer.[19] Practically, diagnosis is based on the analysis of a depression and converging folds. The various appearances of a depression and converging folds can be separated into differentiated and undifferentiated carcinoma and the difference between these two histologic types is discerned on well-documented double contrast images.[20]

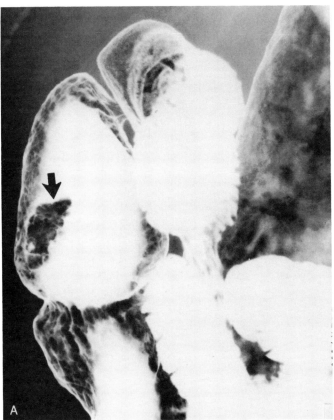

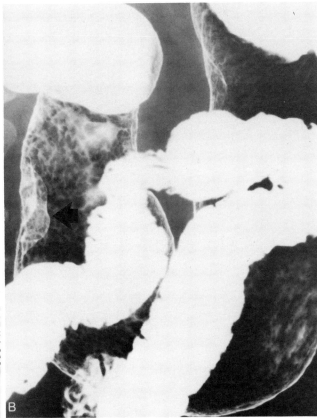

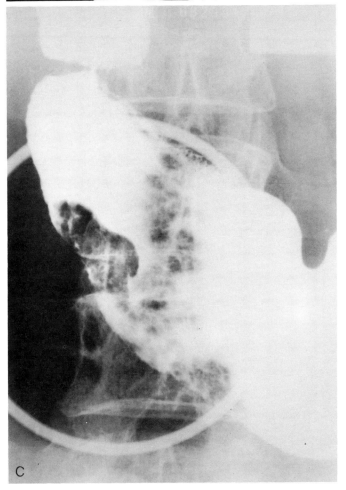

FIGURE 14–21

EARLY POLYPOID GASTRIC CANCER (TYPE I). *A*, With the patient in the RPO position, the lesion is seen en face *(arrow)*.

B, With the patient in the LPO position, the lesion is seen in profile *(arrow)*.

C, A prone compression view of the same lesion.

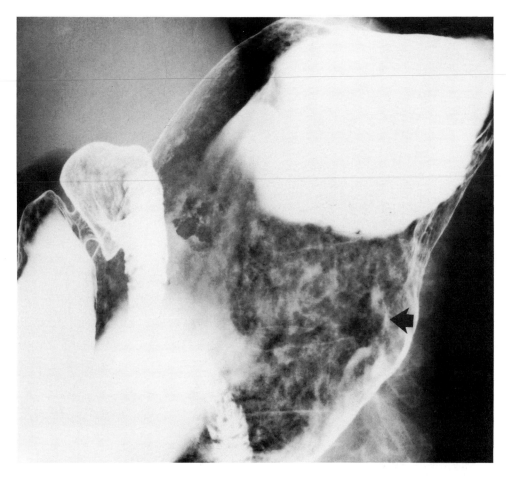

FIGURE 14–22

POLYPOID EARLY GASTRIC CANCER (TYPE IIa). The lesion on the posterior wall of the upper body *(arrow)* is best seen with the patient in the RPO position.

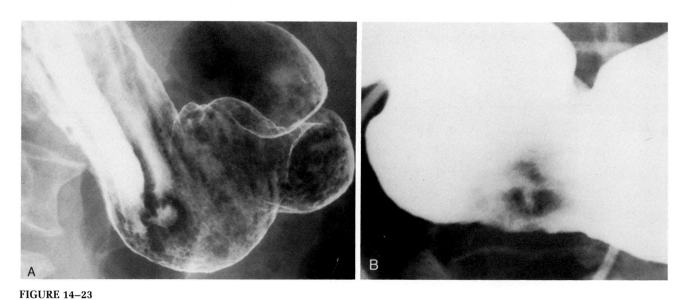

FIGURE 14–23

MIXED TYPE EARLY GASTRIC CANCER (TYPE IIa + IIc) ON THE ANTERIOR WALL IN THE REGION OF THE INCISURA. *A,* Double contrast examination of the anterior wall with the patient in the prone position shows the protrusion with a central depression.
   B, The same findings demonstrated on compression study.

The depression is analyzed in terms of its outline, surface, and depth. The depression is usually irregular and has a serrated or spiculated margin, whereas a benign ulcer usually has a sharp, straight margin. The depression is not always demarcated from the normal surrounding mucosa, and it may be difficult to define the precise extent of a lesion.

In most cases of depressed early cancer the surface of the depression is uneven due to an irregular proliferation of cancerous tissue. Sometimes an island-like nodule of regenerative epethelium remains in the depression and is more prominent than the irregularity of the cancerous depression. The depth of the depression varies, depending on the cancerous erosion and associated peptic ulceration. With regard to depth of invasion of depressed early cancer, Nishizawa reported that the more sharply demarcated a depressed lesion and the more prominent the converging folds, the deeper is the involvement.[21]

The converging folds also have characteristic abnormalities such as tapering, clubbing, interruption, and fusion (Fig. 14–24). The diagnosis of early depressed cancer can be made easily if these converging fold patterns are delineated by double contrast radiography, together with the characteristics of the depression mentioned above. Moreover, the converg-

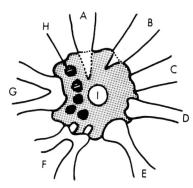

FIGURE 14–24

VARIOUS APPEARANCES OF CONVERGING FOLDS AND UNEVENNESS IN EARLY DEPRESSED CANCER. *A,* Gradual tapering.
  B, Abrupt tapering.
  C, Abrupt interruption.
  D and *E,* Clubbing.
  F, Fusion with abrupt tapering.
  G, Fusion (V-shaped deformity).
  H, Unevenness.
  I, Regenerative epithelium. (From Shirakabe, H., and Maruyama, M.: Neoplastic diseases of the stomach. *In* Margulis, A.R., and Burhenne, H.J. (eds.): Alimentary Tract Radiology, ed. 4, St. Louis, C.V. Mosby, 1989, p. 604, with permission.)

ing folds are a very reliable clue, leading to the detection of lesions in many cases. On the other hand, a cancerous erosion not accompanied by converging folds is discovered only with difficulty (Fig. 14–25).

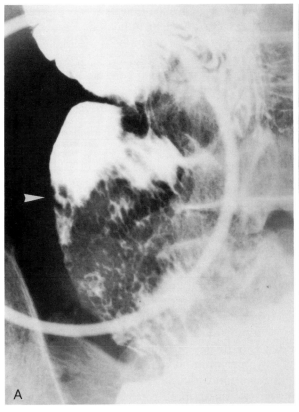

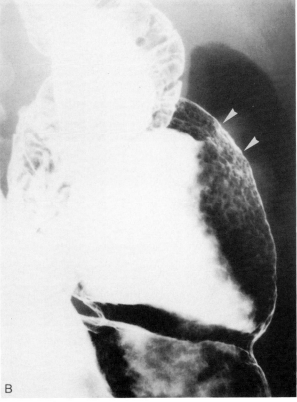

FIGURE 14–25

DEPRESSED EARLY GASTRIC CANCER (TYPE IIc) WITHOUT RADIATING FOLDS. *A,* The lesion is best demonstrated by compression.
  B, The prone double contrast view shows the lesion in profile as an area of localized wall stiffness.

Types IIc, IIc + III, and III

The distinction between type IIc and type III lesions is made by the depth of the collection of contrast medium retained in a depression. The depth of the contrast medium in a benign ulcer can be regarded as typical of type III. Type IIc lesions are characterized by a more shallow barium collection. In addition, type IIc lesions do not show uniform density of the contrast medium (see Figs. 14–15, 14–16, 14–18, and 14–19). Irregular proliferation of cancerous tissue (see Fig. 14–19D) or regenerative epithelium (see Fig. 14–15B) usually causes the uneven density.[22] In the superficial spreading type of early cancer it is difficult to distinguish the boundary between normal mucosa and the depression.

If the depression is variable in its depth, it is necessary to decide whether any portion of the depression is comparable to the depth of benign ulcer. In that case the lesion is classified as type IIc + III or type III + IIc, depending on which appearance predominates.

On the other hand, if an ulcer niche is prominent, one must be alert to the slightest suggestion of a type IIc lesion, especially in the profile view. The mistaken diagnosis of peptic ulcer is easily made unless attention is paid to the mucosa surrounding the niche. In such cases the type IIc lesion becomes clearer during the course of medical treatment as the niche decreases in size. This phenomenon is referred to as the "malignant cycle of ulceration" in early gastric cancer.[23]

In some cases the type III lesion is so predominant that the type IIc lesion can scarcely be recognized macroscopically as the slightest abnormality, either entirely or partially around the type III part. Close observation of the niche may lead to recognition of the partial irregularity of its margin. However, it is expected that the features of the lesion would evolve into type III + IIc or IIc + III in a few weeks, especially when treated medically. This tendency has been dramatically observed when H2-antagonists are used for treatment of the ulcer.

Type IIb-like Lesion

Type IIb was initially used to refer to a cancerous lesion in its incipient phase, in which there was no depression or elevation from the normal mucosal surface. Pure type IIb lesions have been incidentally discovered in the course of operating on the stomach for some other lesion, and all have been smaller than 0.5 cm.[24]

However, many clinical cases have not been classified as pure type IIb lesions, but rather as simulating IIb lesions on the basis of subtle differences in elevation or depression from the normal surrounding mucosa without clear distinction of their border.

These have been called IIb-simulating lesions or IIb-like lesions. This classification can be applied further to describe the border of a depressed lesion with IIb-like peripheral spread. It is important to pay attention to subtle differences in mucosal coating from the surrounding normal mucosa for recognition of IIb-like mucosal spread of cancer.

Carcinoma Less Than 1.0 cm

Most carcinomas less than 1.0 cm in diameter are not accompanied by ulceration. Consequently it is very difficult to discover the lesion, regardless of its nature. If a lesion is located in an area in which double contrast radiography gives good visualization of the mucosal detail, the diagnosis of malignancy can be made by following the general principles of radiologic diagnosis. Otherwise, the compression method should be applied whenever possible (see Fig. 14–25A and B). If a lesion is smaller than 0.5 cm in the largest diameter, the radiologic diagnosis of malignancy is not always possible, because the lesion is too small for the criteria of malignancy to be applied. Sometimes an irregular surrounding translucency, which is unusual in a benign ulcer, gives a strong suggestion of malignancy. In recent years endoscopic resection has been the first choice of treatment for a polypoid early cancer less than 1.0 cm. For an early depressed cancer not accompanied by ulceration, endoscopic resection is also indicated when submucosal involvement can be excluded radiologically and endoscopically.

EARLY COLORECTAL CANCER

Classification

The general classification can be applied to early colorectal cancer. It has been believed that in the colon and rectum almost all early cancers that are recognizable macroscopically are polypoid or elevated in their form. Recently, however, attention has been paid to a flat or depressed type of early cancer, which is detected only by endoscopy.[25] In most such cases, slight redness is a clue to detection. Its size ranges from 5 to 20 mm with a mean of 11 mm.

Early colorectal cancer has a much better prognosis than that of early gastric cancer. It has been confirmed that there is no lymph node metastasis in cases of intramucosal cancer, including cancer in an adenoma. Attention should be paid to the difference in terminology used for adenoma and early cancer of the colon and rectum. In the Western literature, intramucosal carcinoma, including cancer in an adenoma,

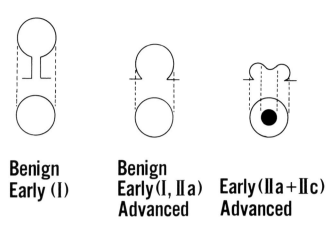

Benign
Early (I)

Benign
Early(I, IIa)
Advanced

Early(IIa+IIc)
Advanced

FIGURE 14–26

Correlation of macroscopic form with histology of polypoid lesions of adenoma and of early and advanced cancer of the colon and rectum.

is called not cancer but severe dysplasia. Early cancer corresponds to sm-cancer, which is usually named invasive carcinoma. Such specific terminology has been used only for cancer of the colon and rectum to avoid overly aggressive surgery for intramucosal cancer in which there is no lymph node metastasis.

Endoscopic Correlation

In 1988 Maruyama reported the result of a comparative study of radiology and endoscopy in the detection of early colorectal cancer based on 130 cases, including 73 cases in which radiology was followed by endoscopy and 57 cases in which endoscopy was followed by radiology.[26] In the group for which radiology was done first, radiology missed 16 cases (21.9%), and endoscopy missed four cases (5.5%). Two cases escaped detection by both radiology and endoscopy. On the other hand, in the group for which endoscopy was done first, radiology missed three cases (5.3%) and endoscopy missed five cases (8.7%). Sessile lesions were missed more frequently than pedunculated lesions by radiology. Lesions measuring 1 cm or less were likely to be missed.

It was shown that when radiology preceded endoscopy, more lesions were missed than when radiology followed endoscopy. In total, radiology missed twice as many lesions as endoscopy. Overall, 90% of the misses by radiology and endoscopy were in the rectum and sigmoid. Maruyama believes that both examinations should be done whenever possible for the detection of early cancer and that radiology should be preceded by endoscopy in order to keep the miss rate to a minimum.

General Considerations

The majority of early colorectal cancers are polypoid lesions and the diagnosis is made on the basis of the shape and size of the lesion.[27] As a basic concept it is necessary to note that there is no advanced cancer in pedunculated lesions and that there is no adenoma in centrally depressed lesions (Fig. 14–26). Moreover, advanced cancer is rare in polyps smaller than 2 cm in diameter.

In pedunculated lesions early cancer (type Ip = pedunculated) is by no means distinct from adenoma because the cancerous change in adenoma cannot be recognized macroscopically. Accordingly, only the presence of a stalk can be detected radiologically. Endoscopic resection is required to establish the histologic diagnosis. Generally, the larger the size of the pedunculated lesion, the higher the frequency of malignancy (early cancer). However, it must be remembered that most malignant lesions are more than 1 cm in size.

About 90% of sessile lesions without central depression could be diagnosed as early cancer (type Is = sessile) when their size was at the 1 cm level.[27] This observation goes back to the description of Weber in 1941.[28] However, in a recent study that included new data, Maruyama reported that the possibility of early cancer at this size level fell to 43% and ascribed such a change to the ambiguity of the histologic criteria for adenoma and cancer.

In 1985 Nakamura and colleagues claimed that a considerable number of adenomas diagnosed following the conventional criteria were regarded to be malignant by a computer-assisted morphometric study.[29] Based on this morphometric study, they also postulated that most lesions of colorectal cancer do not develop through the adenoma–carcinoma sequence, but develop de novo. Centrally depressed sessile lesions are always malignant with some exceptional cases. Most early cancers with this form (type IIa + IIc) are less than 2 cm in largest diameter.

Radiology of Early Colorectal Cancer

In the radiologic diagnosis of early cancer, the presence of depression and basal indentation plays an important role in the estimation of the depth of invasion,[27, 30–33] although there has been some disagreement with this concept.[34] Ushio and Maruyama correlated the depth of invasion with the presence of basal indentation (Fig. 14–27) and found that in general there was a correlation and that the greater the basal indentation, the deeper the invasion.[31]

DEPTH OF INVASION	GRADE OF BASAL INDENTATION				
	d1	d′ 1	d2	d3	d4
Mucosa (m)	▦				
Submucosa (sm)	▦				
Propria muscle (pm)	▨	▨	▨	▨	▨
Subserosa (ss)		▥	▥	▥	▥
Serosa (s)					

FIGURE 14–27

Correlation of depth of invasion with the degree of basal indentation.

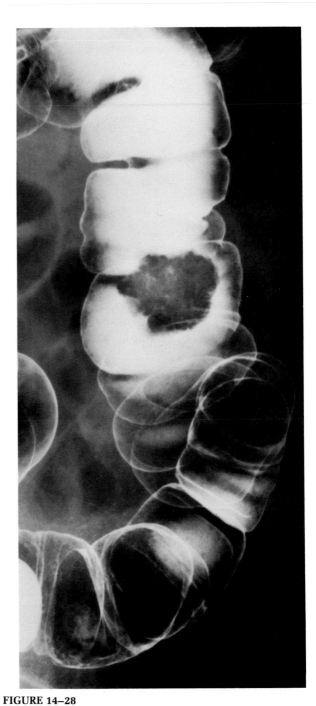

FIGURE 14–28

LARGE, SESSILE, EARLY POLYPOID CANCER (TYPE IS). A 30-mm polypoid lesion is in the mid-descending colon. The depth of invasion was limited to the submucosa.

Types Is and IIa

Sometimes a sessile lesion measuring 3 cm in the largest diameter is still limited to the submucosal layer (Fig. 14–28). A sessile lesion measuring 1 cm is most frequently type I early cancer (Fig. 14–29), but the histologic diagnosis remains ambiguous as long as the submucosal membrane is not involved. Type IIa usually reveals surface nodularity. However, there is always a problem in the histologic criteria for the diagnosis of adenoma (Fig. 14–30) and cancer (Fig. 14–31). Radiologically, the possibility of advanced cancer is excluded by the presence of only slight indentation (Fig. 14–31B). Rarely there is a lesion that reveals extensive stalk invasion in a pedunculated early cancer (Fig. 14–32).

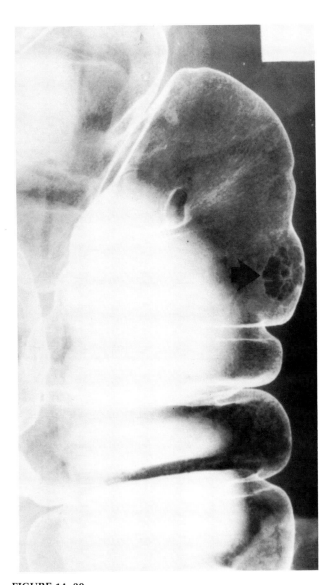

FIGURE 14–30

Sessile adenoma measuring 15 mm in diameter (arrow) in the ascending colon. Patient is in the prone position.

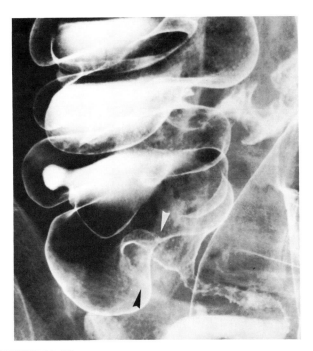

FIGURE 14–29

POLYPOID EARLY CANCER OF THE CECUM (TYPE IIa). A 12-mm early cancer (arrowheads) is in the cecum with invasion limited to the mucosa.

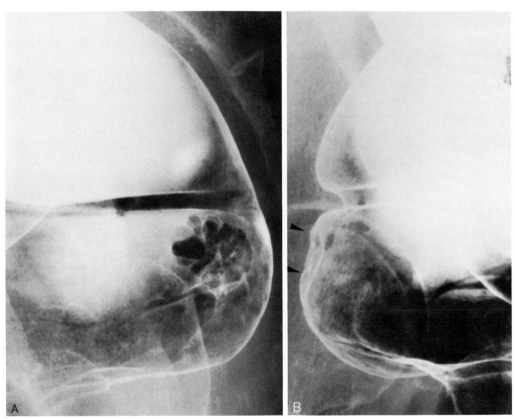

FIGURE 14–31

POLYPOID EARLY CANCER (TYPE IS) IN THE RECTUM. *A,* The 19-mm lesion is seen en face.

B, The profile view shows slight basal indentation, suggesting that the lesion is limited to the mucosa or submucosa.

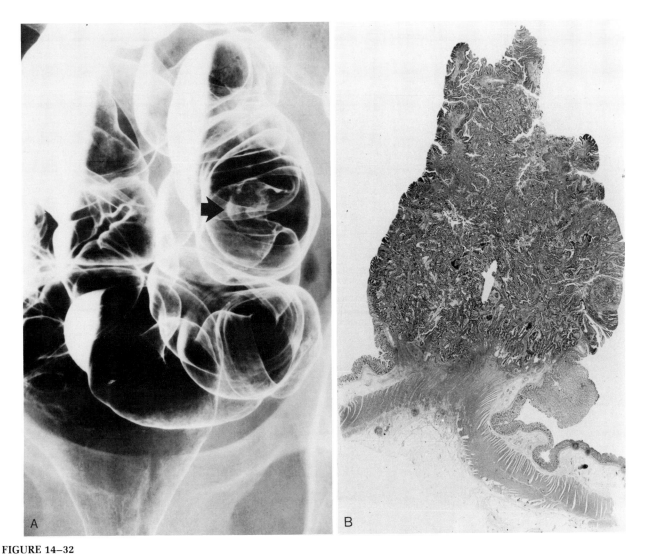

FIGURE 14–32

EXTENSIVE STALK INVASION IN A PEDUNCULATED EARLY CANCER. *A,* An early polypoid cancer is seen in the sigmoid colon *(arrow).* Invasion was into the submucosa.

   B, A cross section of the lesion shows that there is extensive invasion of the stalk in a pedunculated early cancer.

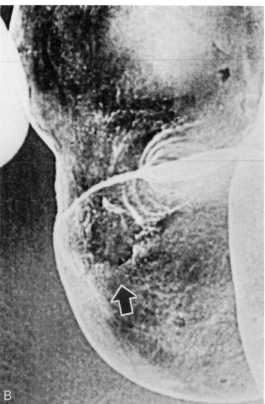

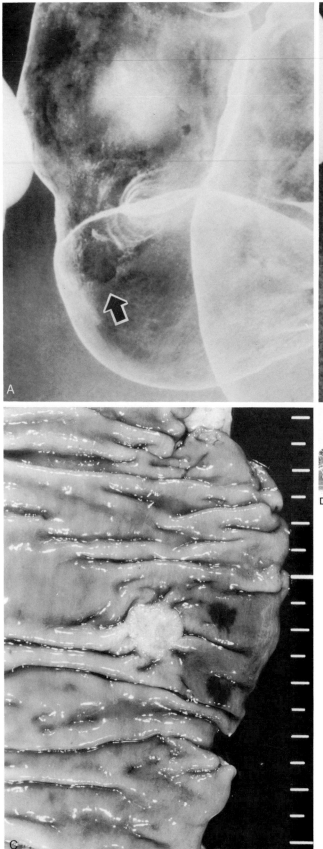

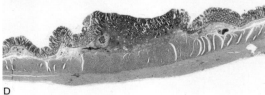

FIGURE 14–33

IMPACT OF IMAGE PROCESSING BY COMPUTED RADIOGRAPHY. *A,* A prone double contrast radiograph shows a small polypoid early cancer *(arrow).* The central depression is not clearly seen.

B, After image processing with computed radiography, the central depression *(arrow)* is clearly visualized.

C, Photograph of the resected specimen shows the polypoid lesion with slight central depression.

D, A cross section of the lesion shows extensive submucosal involvement and slight central depression.

Type IIa + IIc

Type IIa + IIc is most important in radiologic diagnosis because it is almost always a cancer with submucosal involvement. The difficulty arises in delineating a central depression in a lesion otherwise diagnosed as type Is (Fig. 14–33). The central depression becomes more visible by image processing of the original film (Fig. 14–33B). This suggests improvements in our diagnostic abilities with the use of computed radiography.

Usually, the depth of invasion should be estimated to be deeper than the submucosa when a central depression is prominent. However, slight indentation is a reliable indicator that invasion is limited to the submucosa (Fig. 14–34). In a lesion with a marked central depression the presence of slight indentation is decisive in the estimation of invasive depth. Even a lesion with deep central depression is most probably diagnosed as early cancer with massive submucosal involvement by the presence of slight indentation (Fig. 14–35).

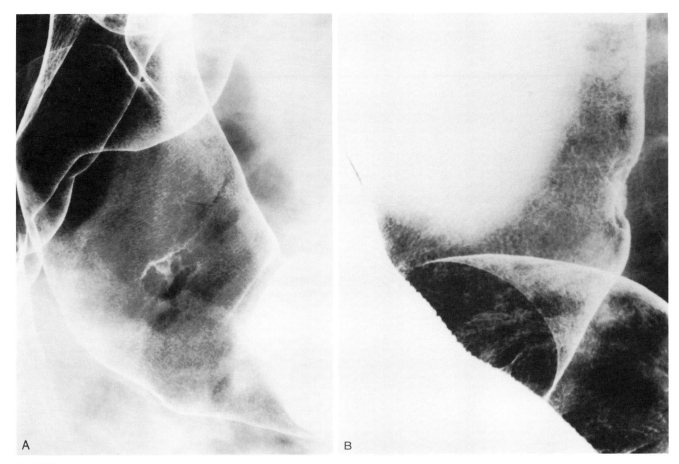

A

B

FIGURE 14–34

EARLY CANCER (TYPE IIa + IIc) WITH INVASION LIMITED TO THE SUBMUCOSA. *A,* The double contrast radiograph shows the polypoid lesion with a central depression.

B, The profile view shows only slight basal indentation, suggesting that invasion is limited to the submucosa.

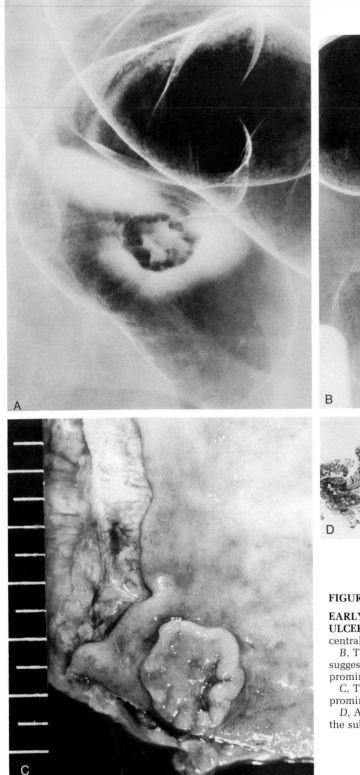

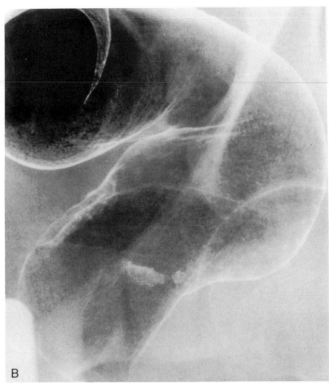

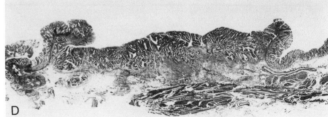

FIGURE 14–35

EARLY CANCER (TYPE IIa + IIc) WITH MARKED CENTRAL ULCERATION. *A,* The polypoid lesion is seen with prominent central depression.

B, The profile view shows only slight basal indentation, suggesting that the cancer is limited to the submucosa despite the prominent depressed area.

C, The specimen photograph shows the polypoid lesion with prominent central depression.

D, A cross section of the lesion shows invasion extending into the submucosa but not beyond.

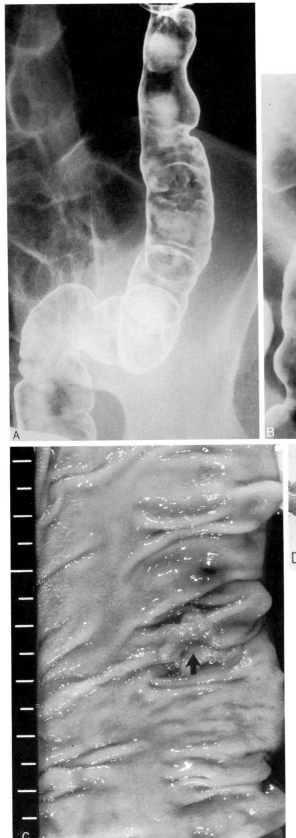

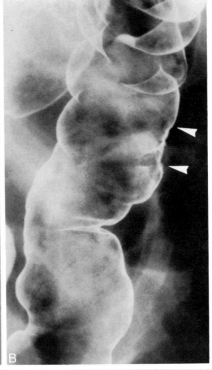

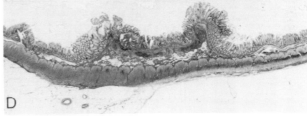

FIGURE 14–36

DEPRESSED EARLY COLON CANCER (TYPE IIc + IIa). *A,* The double contrast radiograph shows a central depression with raised margins.

B, A profile view shows slight basal indentation *(arrowheads)* suggesting that the cancer is limited to the submucosa.

C, The resected specimen shows the lesion *(arrow).*

D, A cross section of the lesion shows that it is primarily a depressed lesion and that invasion is limited to the mucosa.

Type IIc + IIa or Lesions With Predominant Depression

Lesions with predominant depression have attracted the attention of radiologists as well as endoscopists.[35] In some cases a depression is accompanied by slightly raised margins (Fig. 14–36). A lesion consisting of pure depression like a IIc early gastric cancer is rarely encountered (Fig. 14–37). We have also seen a case of depressed early cancer with a peculiar pattern of submucosal involvement (Fig. 14–38).

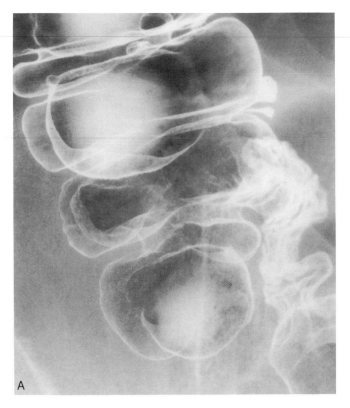

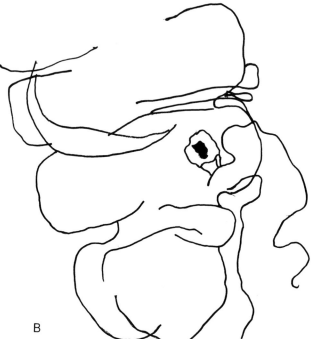

FIGURE 14–37

DEPRESSED EARLY COLON CANCER (TYPE IIc + IIa) AT THE ILEOCECAL VALVE. *A* and *B*, The radiograph and line drawing show the central depression very faintly. The surrounding raised margin is more clearly seen. (Courtesy of Dr. M. Matsukawa, Juntendo University, Tokyo, Japan.)

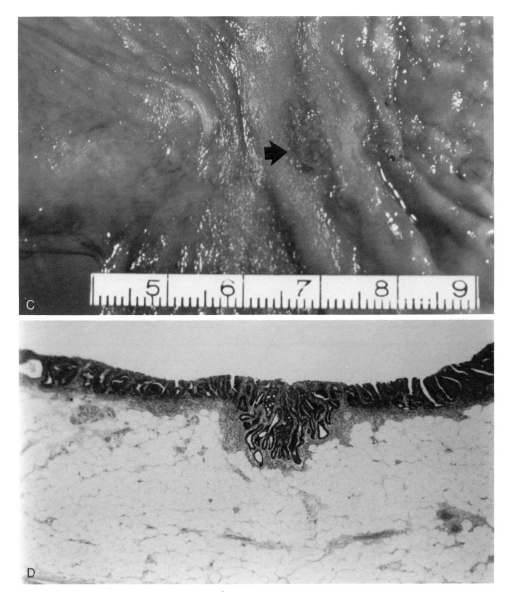

FIGURE 14–37 *Continued*

C, The resected specimen shows the lesion as a pure depression
(arrow).

D, A cross section of the lesion shows involvement of a
submucosa.

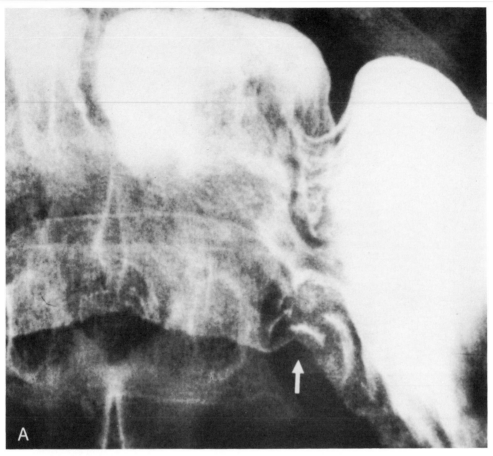

FIGURE 14–38

MINUTE DEPRESSED EARLY CANCER OF THE TRANSVERSE COLON (TYPE IIc). *A,* The compression radiograph shows a 7 mm depressed lesion *(arrow)* in the transverse colon. (Courtesy of Dr. N. Komatsubara, Kosei Hospital, Japan.)

CONCLUSION

Double contrast radiography is an excellent method for the detection of early cancer of the gastrointestinal tract. Detailed histopathologic analysis of resected specimens provides a theoretical framework for radiologic diagnosis. Radiologists should redouble their efforts to stem the decline of this classic method of examination, which is essential to supplement the drawbacks and limitations of endoscopy.

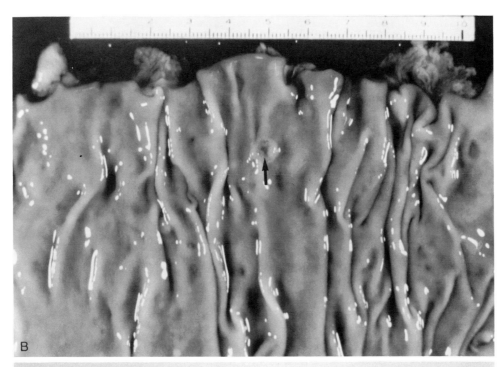

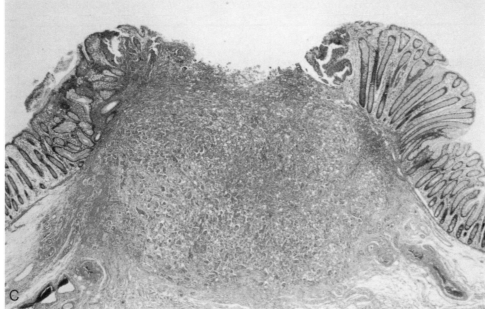

FIGURE 14–38 *Continued*

B, The resected specimen shows a tiny depressed lesion *(arrow).*

C, A cross section of the lesion shows the depression with extensive submucosal involvement.

REFERENCES

1. Japanese Society for Esophageal Diseases: Guidelines for the Clinical and Pathological Studies on Carcinoma of the Esophagus, October 1984, ed. 6. Tokyo, Kanehara Shuppan, 1984.
2. Japanese Research Society for Cancer of Colon and Rectum: General Rules for Clinical and Pathological Studies on Cancer of Colon, Rectum and Anus. 4th ed. Tokyo, Kanehara Shuppan, 1985.
3. Japanese Society for Gastric Cancer: The General Rules for the Gastric Cancer Study, ed. 11. Tokyo, Kanehara Shuppan, 1985.
4. Ide, H., Murata, Y., Okujima, N., et al.: New macroscopic classification of superficial esophageal carcinoma from pathologic standpoint (in Japanese). I to Cho (Stomach and Intestine) 22:1369, 1987.
5. Shirakabe, H., Yamaki, G., Nishizawa, M., and Maruyama, M.: Radiology of Superficial Carcinoma of the Esophagus. The Society of Gastrointestinal Radiologists, 16th Annual Meeting, Scottsdale, Arizona, 1987.
6. Nishizawa, M., Okada, T., Hosoi, T., et al.: Detecting early esophageal cancers with special reference to the intraepithelial stage. Endoscopy 16:92, 1984.
7. Yang, G., Huang, H., Qui, S., et al.: Endoscopic diagnosis of 115 cases of early esophageal carcinoma. Endoscopy 14:157, 1982.
8. Shirakabe, H., Yamaki, G., Maruyama, M., et al.: A new proposal of macroscopic classification of superficial esophageal carcinoma (in Japanese). I to Cho (Stomach and Intestine) 22:1349, 1987.
9. Sato, T., Sakai, Y., Kajita, A., et al.: Radiographic microstructures of early esophageal carcinoma: Correlation of specimen radiography with pathologic findings and clinical radiography. Gastrointest. Radiol. 11:12, 1986.
10. Yamaki, G., Shirakabe, H., Usui, Y., et al.: Retrospective radiographic study of esophageal carcinoma (in Japanese). I to Cho (Stomach and Intestine) 23:1187, 1988.
11. Hermanek, P., and Rösch, W.: Critical evaluation of the Japanese "early gastric cancer" classification. Endoscopy 5:220, 1973.
12. Nakamura, K., Sugano, H., Sugiyama, N., et al.: Clinical and histopathological features of scirrhous carcinoma of the stomach (in Japanese). I to Cho (Stomach and Intestine) 11:1275, 1976.
13. Gelfand, D.W., Otto, D.J., and Chen, Y.M.: Radiology and endoscopy: A radiologic viewpoint. Ann. Intern. Med. 101:550, 1984.
14. Fraser, G.M.: Radiology. Curr. Opinion Gastroenterol. 6:833, 1985.
15. Maruyama, M.: Comparison of radiology and endoscopy in the diagnosis of gastric cancer. In Preece, P.E., Cuschieri, A., and Wellwood, J.M. (eds.): Cancer of the Stomach, p. 123. Orlando, FL, Grune & Stratton, 1986.
16. Hamada, T., Kaji, F., Shirakabe, H.: Detectability of gastric cancer by radiology compared to endoscopy. In Maruyama, M., and Kimura, K. (eds.): Review of Clinical Research in Gastroenterology, pp. 35–56. Tokyo, Igaku-Shoin, 1988.
17. Nishizawa, M., Momoto, K., Hosoi, T., et al.: A comparison of x-ray and panendoscopy in the clinical routine of upper gastrointestinal tract (in Japanese). I to Cho (Stomach and Intestine) 19:185, 1984.
18. Maruyama, M., Yamada, T., and Matsue, H.: Theoretical basis for the radiographic diagnosis of polypoid early cancer. In Shirakabe, H., et al. (eds.): Atlas of X-ray Diagnosis of Early Gastric Cancer. Tokyo, Igaku-Shoin, 1982.
19. Maruyama, M., Sugiyama, N., Baba, Y., et al.: Radiodiagnostic possibility of gastric carcinoma involving the propria muscle layer (in Japanese). I to Cho (Stomach and Intestine) 11:855, 1976.
20. Baba, Y., Narui, T., Ninomiya, K., et al.: A comparative study between radiologic and macroscopic findings of early gastric carcinoma with lib-like intramucosal spread: With special reference to radiologic definition of proximal boundary (in Japanese). I to Cho (Stomach and Intestine) 12:1087, 1977.
21. Nishizawa, M.: Radiographic demonstration of depressed early cancer of the stomach (in Japanese). I to Cho (Stomach and Intestine) 6:221, 1971.
22. Murakami, T., Yasui, A., Takehara, H., et al.: Non-cancerous regenerative epithelium in the central portion of scar-carcinoma of the stomach (in Japanese). Nippon Byori Gakkai Zasshi (Trans. Soc. Pathol. Jpn.) 55:229, 1966.
23. Sakita, T., Oguro, Y., Takasu, S., et al.: Observations on the healing of ulcerations in early gastric cancer. Gastroenterology 60:835, 1971.
24. Nakamura, K., Sugano, H., and Takagi, K.: Carcinoma of the stomach in incipient phase: Its histogenesis and histological appearance. Gann 59:251, 1968.
25. Maruyama, M.: An introduction to depressed early cancer of the colon and rectum (in Japanese). I to Cho (Stomach and Intestine) 22:1369, 1987.
26. Maruyama, M.: Radiographic diagnosis of early colorectal cancer. J. Japan. Soc. Coloproctol. 41:873, 1988.
27. Maruyama, M.: Radiologic Diagnosis of Polyps and Carcinoma of the Large Bowel. Tokyo, Igaku-Shoin, 1978.
28. Weber, H.M.: The diagnosis of early intestinal cancer. AJR 64:929, 1950.
29. Nakamura, K., Shibuya, S., Nishizawa, M., et al.: Adenomacarcinoma sequence of colorectal carcinoma analyzed by use of objective indices of grade of atypicality and their growing processes in early phase. I to Cho (Stomach and Intestine) 20:877, 1985.
30. Welin, S., Youker, J., and Spratt, J.S., Jr.: The rates and patterns of growth of 375 tumors of the large intestine and rectum observed serially by double contrast enema study (Malmö technique). AJR 90:673, 1963.
31. Ushio, K., Goto, H., Muramatsu, Y., et al.: Significance of the profile view in the x-ray diagnosis of cancer of the digestive tract: Diagnosis of depth invasion by double contrast study. I to Cho (Stomach and Intestine) 21:27, 1986.
32. Bellomi, M., Castoldi, M.X., Gozzi, G., et al.: Radiologic diagnosis of invasive carcinoma on adenomatous polyps of the colon. Eur. J. Radiol. 6:199, 1986.
33. Ament, A.E., and Alfidi, R.J.: Sessile polyps analysis of radiographic projections with the aid of a double contrast phantom. AJR 135:111, 1982.
34. Skucas, J., Spataro, R.F., and Cannucciari, D.P.: The radiographic features of small colon cancers. Radiology 143:335, 1982.
35. Maruyama, M.: Recent trend in gross pathology of early colorectal cancer. I to Cho (Stomach and Intestine) 22:879, 883, 1987.

15

POLYPOSIS SYNDROMES

Clive I. Bartram
Igor Laufer, M.D.

Gastrointestinal polyposis refers to the presence of multiple polyps in part or all of the gastrointestinal tract. The large bowel is most often involved. A histologic classification is given in Table 15–1. Most of the polyposis syndromes have a solitary counterpart. Although determination of the exact nature of the polyposis is based mainly on histologic examination of one or more polyps,[1] detailed radiographic examination is required to show the extent of involvement, any local complication, or extraintestinal manifestation.

The polyposis syndromes are difficult to classify. This may be achieved either according to the predominant site of involvement—stomach, large bowel or diffuse throughout the GI tract[2]—or according to the histology of the polyp. However, in clinical practice, the significant factors are the mode of inheritance and the associated cancer risk.

TABLE 15–1. Histologic Classification of Polyposis Syndromes	
Classification	Syndrome(s)
Epithelial	
Neoplastic	Familial adenomatous polyposis
	Gardner's syndrome
	Recessive adenomatous polyposis
	Turcot's syndrome
	Torres's syndrome
Hamartomatous	Juvenile polyposis
	Peutz-Jeghers syndrome
	Cowden's syndrome
Inflammatory	Colitic polyposis
	Cronkhite-Canada syndrome
Miscellaneous	Metaplastic polyposis
Nonepithelial	Lipomas, lymphomas, neuromas, myomas, fibromas

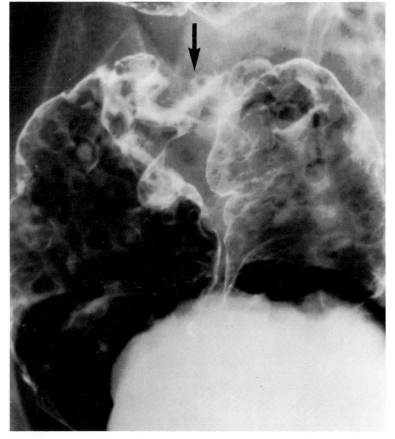

FIGURE 15–1

TYPICAL ANNULAR CARCINOMA IN THE SIGMOID COLON *(ARROW)* IN A 32-YEAR-OLD PATIENT WITH FAMILIAL ADENOMATOUS POLYPOSIS. Note that the mucosa proximal and distal to the carcinoma is carpeted with adenomatous polyps.

INHERITED POLYPOSIS SYNDROMES

There are three polyposis syndromes that have a dominant inheritance pattern and are associated with an increased incidence of cancer.[3] These are familial adenomatous polyposis including Gardner's syndrome, Peutz-Jegher's syndrome, and juvenile polyposis. Registries have been established to monitor members of affected families who require prolonged follow-up, genetic counseling, and prophylactic surgery to prevent cancer.

Familial Adenomatous Polyposis

Familial adenomatous polyposis (FAP) used to be termed "familial adenomatous polyposis coli," but the "coli" has been discarded because in almost every case adenomatous polyps could be found outside the large bowel. Its incidence is about 1 in every 7000 to 10,000 births. There is no family history in 20% of these cases, which are presumed to be spontaneous genetic mutations. Familial adenomatous polyposis is a hereditary condition of dominant character, in which numerous adenomas of the large bowel develop at an early age with a high risk of colonic cancer developing in early adult life.

Adenomas develop in the late teens. Symptoms of bleeding, diarrhea, pain, and discharge of mucus may occur when the patient is in the early 30's. Of the patients presenting with symptoms, two thirds will have cancer (Fig. 15–1).[4] The average age at which cancer develops is 39 years. The youngest cancer patient in the St. Mark's series is 19 years, but there are isolated reports of cancer appearing in the early teens. Multiple cancers are found in 47.6% of patients, compared with only 3.9% in the general population. The distribution of the tumor is similar in the two groups.[2]

In FAP the polyps are present throughout the colon and rectum. They may be more numerous distally, but the typical presence of about 1000 adenomas makes this difficult to appreciate. The polyps are usually sessile and more or less uniform in size (Figs. 15–2 and 15–3). When larger, they may become

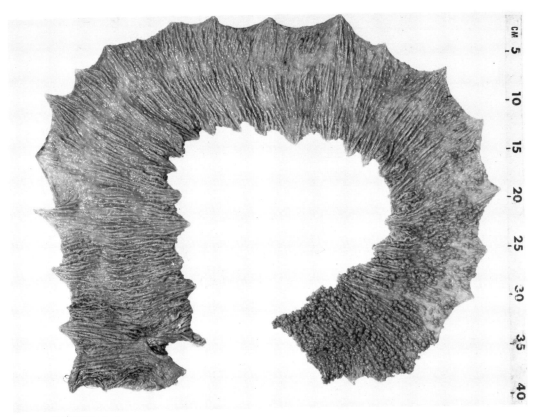

FIGURE 15–2

COLECTOMY SPECIMEN IN A PATIENT WITH FAMILIAL ADENOMATOUS POLYPOSIS.
There are innumerable small polyps throughout the colon, which are most prominent in the distal left colon.

pedunculated in the left side of the colon (Fig. 15–4). Umbilication has been reported but is rare.[5] Double contrast enema (DCE) in a symptomatic patient typically reveals numerous small polyps throughout the colon and rectum, an appearance seldom mimicked by any other condition. However, because the diagnosis commits the patient to colectomy, histologic confirmation is essential. The radiologic diagnosis becomes more difficult in asymptomatic members of a polyposis family. The age when the polyps develop, although mainly in the teens, varies considerably. In the early stages only a few polyps may be visible (Fig. 15–5), and a nodular surface pattern to the mucosa may be present with or without larger polyps (Fig. 15–6). This is highly suggestive of FAP.[6] Endoscopically it can be detected by dye spray techniques. Biopsy confirms that it is due to very small adenomas, and this appearance represents the earliest stage at which FAP can be diagnosed.

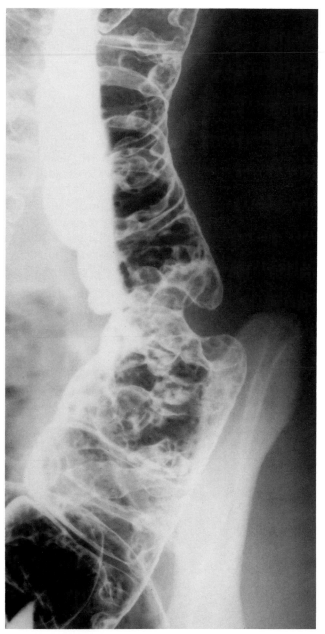

FIGURE 15–4

Familial adenomatous polyposis with a dual polyp population: small sessile lesions and larger pedunculated ones in the descending colon. An annular carcinoma is also present.

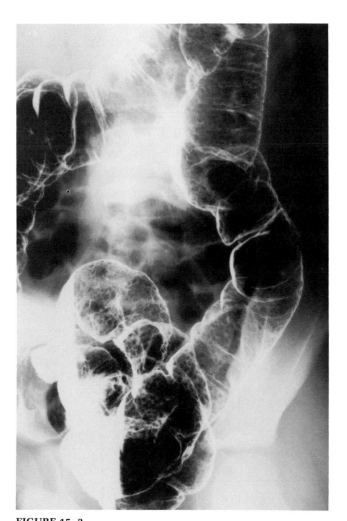

FIGURE 15–3

Typical FAP with numerous small sessile polyps, of roughly the same size extending throughout the colon and rectum.

FIGURE 15–5

FAMILIAL ADENOMATOUS POLYPOSIS. Patient was 23 years old. This was the only macroscopic polyp in the colon. At endoscopy dye spray showed a nodular pattern, which was not seen on DCE probably because the mucosal coating was too thick.

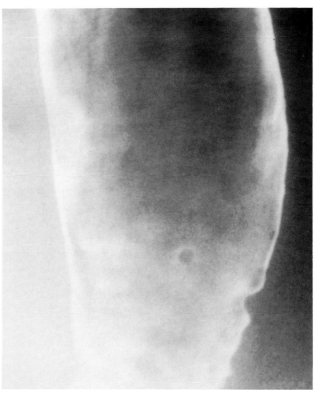

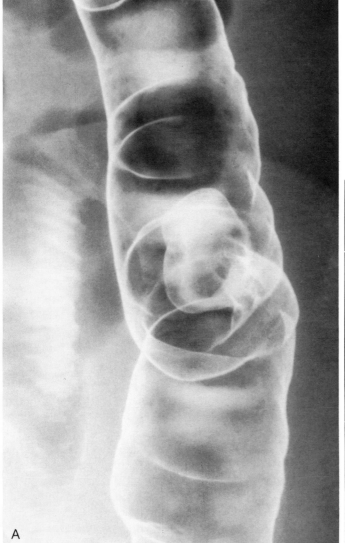

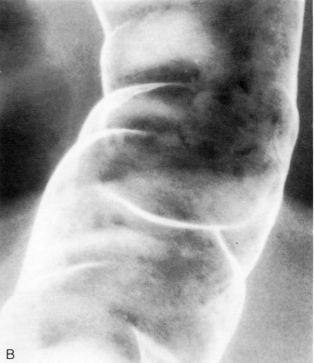

A

B

FIGURE 15–6

A, Familial adenomatous polyposis in a 32-year-old patient with one large pedunculated polyp as the sole obvious macroscopic abnormality.

B, Close inspection of the mucosa reveals a nodular pattern, with small filling defects in the mucosal coating that are not high enough to cause a meniscus and are about 2 mm in diameter. On resection these were shown to be small adenomas. (From Bartram, C.I., and Thornton, A.: Colonic polyp patterns in familial polyposis. AJR 142:305–308, 1984, with permission, © by American Roentgen Ray Society.)

Radiologically the nodular pattern of FAP is similar to that seen in lymphoid hyperplasia (Fig. 15–7). The elevations of only about 2 mm in diameter are too low to produce a meniscus. Lymphoid hyperplasia may be seen in association with colonic carcinoma,[7] is not as extensive as the nodular pattern in FAP, and is found in a different age group. When polyps develop in the colon, there is usually one or two found in the rectum, so that sigmoidoscopy may be used for routine surveillance.

One of the main functions of a Polyposis Registry is to monitor members of an affected family. Regular sigmoidoscopy, starting in the early teens and continuing into later middle age is required. All polyps must be excised and if any are found to be adenomas, it can be assumed that the colon is involved by FAP. Double contrast enema may be indicated

1. To demonstrate that polyps are present throughout the colon and that the appearance is typical of FAP.

2. To show any large polyp that might be malignant or an overt carcinoma.

3. To allow for delay in surgical treatment, for example, in a young adult who wishes to complete his education. The risk of developing cancer in the first 5 years after the diagnosis is established is 11.9%.[8] This figure includes all ages, so that the risk would be less for a young adult. Nevertheless, an annual DCE to exclude the development of any large polyps is justified.

4. To defer surgery in any patient who is unfit for colectomy. Such a patient should have a regular DCE.

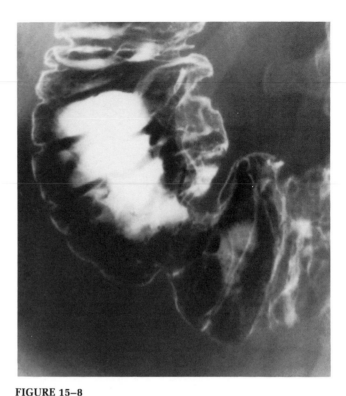

FIGURE 15–8

Hypotonic duodenogram in a patient with FAP showing irregular enlargement of the ampulla with a short slightly irregular stricture just inferior to this. Several polyps are also present. Histologically this was a villous adenoma of the ampulla with carcinomatous change just below, causing the narrowing.

The risk of cancer increases appreciably with delay. Cancer is found in 31.6% of patients after the diagnosis of polyposis has been established for 10 to 15 years, and in 100% of patients with a history of over 20 years.[8]

Treatment of FAP requires colectomy with either ileorectal anastomosis or rectal excision and ileal pouch. Because the retained rectum contains adenomas, regular follow-up with endoscopy and polypectomy is essential. A significant cancer risk remains over the long term, with 13% of FAP patients developing rectal cancer, mainly Dukes A, over a 25-year period. Because the mucosa is removed when an ileal pouch is formed, there is no further cancer risk at this site. As efforts at prevention of cancer in the large bowel succeed, these patients live longer and are more likely to develop cancers in other sites. Thus, removing the rectum does not totally prevent cancer deaths in this group of patients.

Invasive adenocarcinoma is found in the upper gastrointestinal tract in 4.5% of FAP patients (Fig. 15–8). The most common sites are the duodenum, the ampulla of Vater, and the stomach.[9] These carcinomas are related to the presence of adenomatous polyps that are found in the duodenum in at least

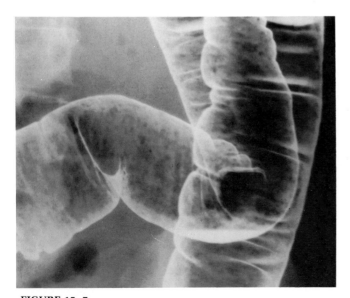

FIGURE 15–7

Lymphoid nodular hyperplasia of the colon in a 29-year-old.

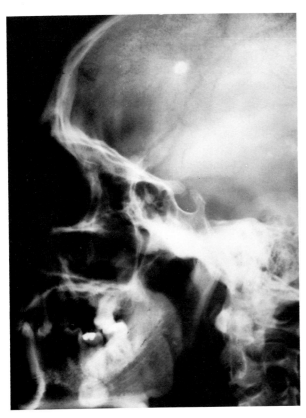

FIGURE 15–9

GARDNER'S SYNDROME. Osteomas of the cranial vault and mandible.

30% of FAP patients. Adenomas are seen less frequently in the stomach, where hamartomatous fundic gland polyps are more common. There is also a significantly increased risk of papillary thyroid cancer, mainly affecting women under the age of 35.[10]

Gardner's Syndrome

The combination of adenomatous polyps of the large bowel, multiple osteomas of the skull and mandible (Fig. 15–9), multiple epidermoid cysts, and soft tissue tumors of the skin was described in a family of seven members by Gardner and Richards.[11] Subsequently, abnormal dentition and desmoid tumor formation were added to the syndrome.[12]

In spite of extraintestinal manifestations in Gardner's syndrome, the colonic polyposis is precisely similar to that found in FAP, and it has the same cancer risk so that management of the colonic polyposis is similar to that of FAP.

Desmoid tumors may arise 1 to 3 years after surgery for polyposis.[13] In the St. Mark's series, this complication occurred in 8.6% of cases.[2] The tumors grow in the mesentery of the small bowel (Fig. 15–10) or in the anterior abdominal wall. Symptoms arise from obstruction to the gastrointestinal or urinary tract. The lesions are usually inoperable and are best left

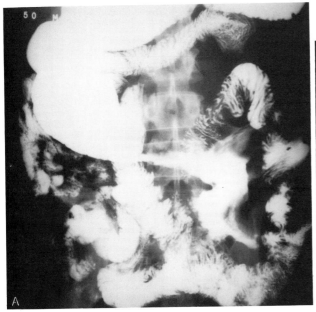

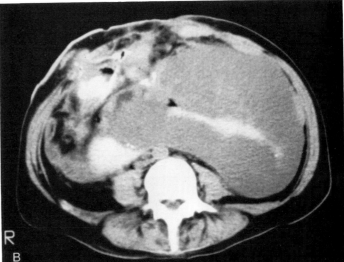

FIGURE 15–10

A, Patient with Gardner's syndrome and a large intra-abdominal desmoid. Barium follow-through reveals a large track of barium leading into the desmoid. This is probably the result of necrosis in the desmoid.
B, Computed tomography demonstrates the size of the desmoid and the communication with small bowel.

alone, since after a period of growth they remain static in size. Surgery is indicated when the lesions become very large or cause significant enteric compression or severe pain. Complete excision should be attempted. Other recorded associations with the syndrome are adrenal cancer,[14] adenomas of the small bowel (Fig. 15–11), carcinoid tumors,[15] skin hyperpigmentation, and lymphoid polyps of the ileum.[16] Skeletal lesions include osteomas of the vault, sinuses, and angle of the mandible, dental abnormalities such as hypercementosis and supernumerary teeth, and localized cortical thickening in long bones, osteomas, and exostosis. Sclerotic areas in the mandible and cortical thickening have been noted in FAP without other evidence of Gardner's syndrome.

The lack of clear distinction among these groups increases the need for complete double contrast studies of the upper gastrointestinal tract in all patients with FAP. If polyps are found in the duodenum, the high incidence of periampullary cancer must be considered and may justify repeat examination to detect early malignant transformation.

Minor (Recessive) Adenomatous Polyposis

Veale[17] has suggested that there are two genes controlling adenoma formation. P is dominant and responsible for FAP, whereas p is recessive, causing only a few polyps to develop. Patients with the recessive type usually have only one or a few adenomas, but can form up to 50 or 60. The minimum number found with FAP in a survey of 150 colectomies was 150, the average number being about 1000.[2] The dividing line would be about 100. To the radiologist a simple rule is that when the polyps can be counted, the recessive form is present, known as minor adenomatous polyposis (MAP), but when the polyps are too numerous to count, FAP is present. The only exception to this is that patients with FAP examined in early adult life, when the polyps are just developing, may have only a few polyps. However, the minor form should not be present in this age group, because the adenomas develop in middle age, in keeping with the age distribution of solitary adenomas.

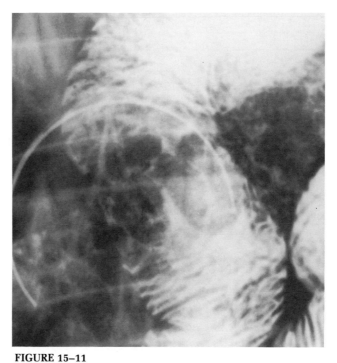

FIGURE 15–11

Barium follow-through with a compression spot film of a patient with Gardner's syndrome and numerous polyps in the small bowel. This one was a large villous adenoma.

Most patients with a colonic adenoma have only one or two polyps but 12% have more than three.[18] Multiplicity of adenomas becomes more common in old age and is associated with an increase in severe dysplasia and therefore cancer (Fig. 15–12). Multiple adenomas are therefore a definite marker for increased cancer risk, although not to the same extent as FAP. Multiple adenomatous polyposis is a different condition from FAP, being of recessive inheritance. The polyps develop at the same time as a solitary adenoma, not early in life as with FAP, and very rarely exceed 50 in number.

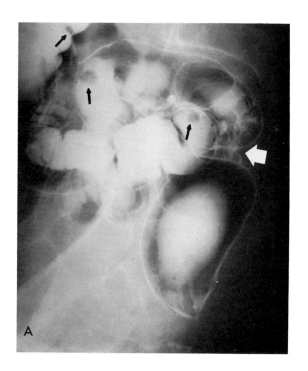

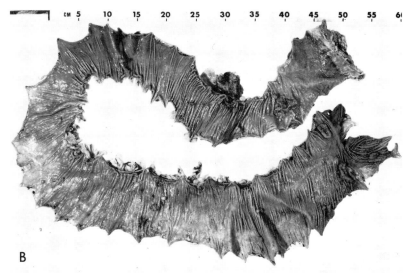

FIGURE 15–12

MINOR ADENOMATOUS POLYPOSIS WITH CARCINOMA. A, Lateral view shows a rectal carcinoma *(white arrow)* with several smaller polyps *(black arrows)*.

B, Resected specimen shows approximately 30 adenomas scattered throughout the colon. The carcinoma is not included in this specimen.

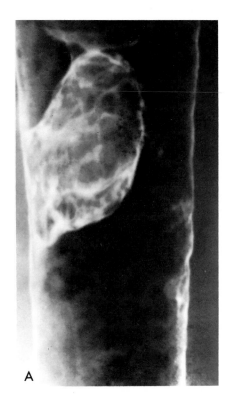

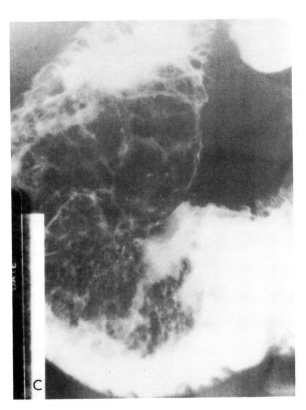

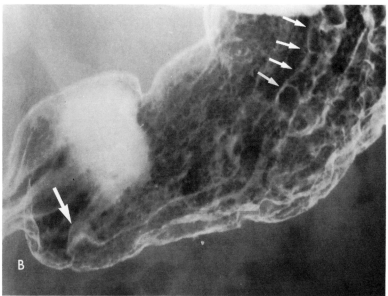

FIGURE 15–13

PEUTZ-JEGHERS SYNDROME. *A*, Large sessile and pedunculated polyps in the colon.

B and *C*, In another patient there are small polyps in the stomach *(arrows)* and a large hamartomatous polyp in the duodenum.

Peutz-Jeghers Syndrome

The association of polyposis and mucocutaneous hyperpigmentation was first described by Peutz in 1921,[19] and the dominant inheritance by Jeghers and co-workers in 1949.[20] The polyps are hamartomatous. Intussusception in the small bowel leads to recurrent bouts of colicky abdominal pain, and erosions on larger polyps cause bleeding. The esophagus is only rarely affected, the small bowel in almost 100%, with gastroduodenal polyps in 40% and colonic polyps in 30%. Gastroduodenal and small bowel polyps may be very numerous, but usually only a few polyps are seen in the colon (Fig. 15–13). These tend to be larger and pedunculated (Fig. 15–14). The heads of the polyps show irregular lobulation, and pedunculation is also common in the small bowel (Fig. 15–15). "Top and tail" endoscopy[21] at 3 to 4 yearly intervals can remove the larger polyps that might bleed. High-quality small bowel examinations are essential to show any large polyp (Fig. 15–16). Surgical removal of polyps by enterotomy would be considered in any symptomatic patient or when polyps larger than 1.5 cm were found radiologically. The small bowel should be examined at 3- to 4-year intervals or if the patient develops symptoms.

In Peutz-Jeghers syndrome, there is a 1% to 3% risk of malignancy, mainly in the duodenum,[22] but there is also an increased risk of colonic cancer. The Peutz-Jeghers hamartoma is not essentially premalignant, but there does appear to be a definite risk of epithelial dysplasia of the adenomatous type with the concomitant likelihood of invasive cancer. An increased incidence of ovarian tumors has also been reported.[23]

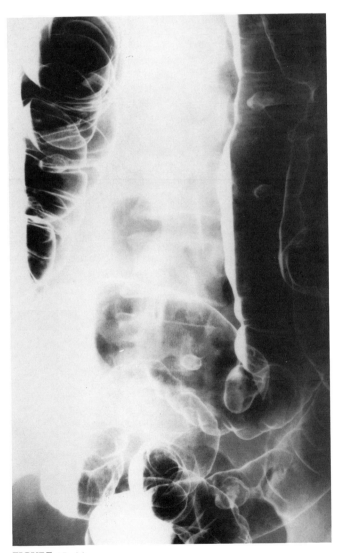

FIGURE 15–14

Double contrast enema in a 19-year-old girl with Peutz-Jeghers syndrome. Note that there are relatively few polyps; most are pedunculated and have lobulated heads.

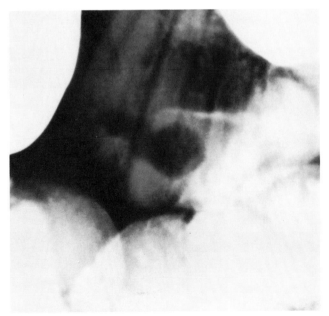

FIGURE 15–15

Compression view during a small bowel enema showing a 1.5 cm pedunculated polyp in the lower jejunum.

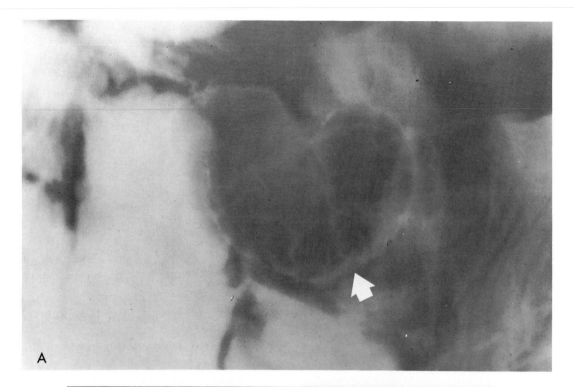

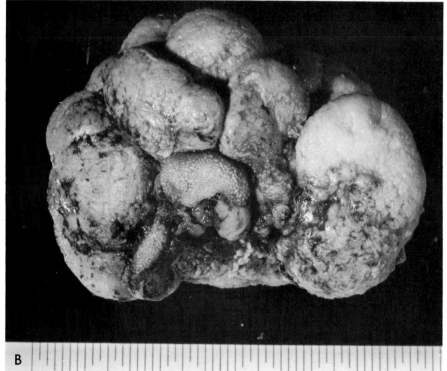

FIGURE 15–16

HAMARTOMATOUS POLYP IN THE SMALL BOWEL WITH REPEATED INTUSSUSCEPTION. *A*, There is a 4-cm lobulated polyp *(arrow)* in the jejunum.

B, Close-up view of the resected polyp, showing the typical lobulated surface.

Juvenile Polyposis

The solitary juvenile polyp is a well-known entity. Juvenile polyposis was only described by Veale and co-workers in 1966.[24] The polyps are found predominantly in the colon, and the condition appears to be of Mendelian dominant inheritance. Various congenital defects, such as cardiac abnormalities, malrotation of the bowel, extra digits, Meckel's diverticulum, mesenteric lymphangioma, and porphyria, may be associated with juvenile polyposis. Presentation with rectal bleeding, failure to thrive, and rectal prolapse is usually seen in a child under the age of 10 years. Throughout the colon there may be numerous polyps that are smooth (Fig. 15–17) and often pedunculated (Fig. 15–18). There is a significant increase in colorectal cancer before the age of 40. This may be due to adenomatous transformation of the polyps with dysplasia progressing to invasive cancer. Careful monitoring with DCE of affected and other members of juvenile polyposis families is recommended.

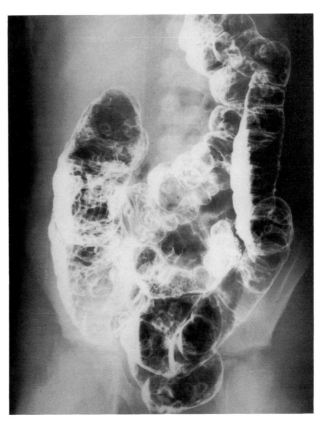

FIGURE 15–18

JUVENILE POLYPOSIS IN AN 11-YEAR-OLD GIRL. Note the large number of smooth pedunculated polyps throughout the colon and rectum.

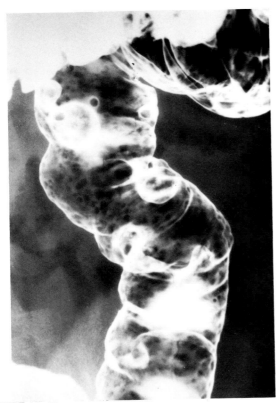

FIGURE 15–17

JUVENILE POLYPS. An 8-year-old girl with multiple colonic polyps due to juvenile polyposis.

Cowden's Syndrome

Cowden's syndrome, otherwise known as multiple hamartoma syndrome, was named after the first family described with this syndrome. It is transmitted as an autosomal dominant trait and characterized by cutaneous and oral verrucous papules and gastrointestinal polyposis. The gastrointestinal polyps are not adenomas and there appears to be little or no increased risk of colon cancer. There is, however, an increased risk of various other diseases and malignancies including carcinoma of the breast and thyroid, ovarian cysts, fibromas, angiomas, and lipomas.[25]

OTHER FORMS OF POLYPOSIS

There is an ill-defined group of other forms of polyposis, often rare, in which a familial tendency may or may not be present, but in which there is a documented increased cancer risk.

Neoplastic Polyposis

Turcot's Syndrome

Turcot and co-workers[26] in 1959 reported the case of a 15-year-old boy who died from a medulloblastoma 2 years after colectomy for polyposis and whose sister, also with polyposis, had died from a frontal glioma. The syndrome links malignant cerebral neoplasia, mainly gliomas, with colonic polyposis. It has been argued whether the syndrome is recessive or dominant and merely a phenotype of pleiotropia of FAP. Turcot's syndrome is very rare, and it is probably recessive in inheritance and not related to FAP.[27]

Torre Syndrome

Torre syndrome is another cutaneous marker for possible GI tract malignancy. Cutaneous sebaceous neoplasms with or without keratoacanthomas may be associated with multiple colonic adenomatous polyps.[28]

Lymphoma

Lymphoid follicles are scattered throughout the colon. These follicles can be involved diffusely by lymphoma, giving rise to a lymphomatous form of polyposis (Fig. 15–19).[29]

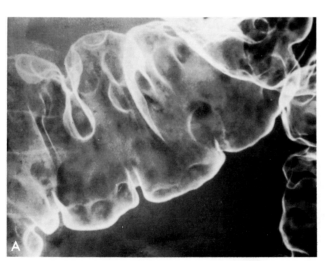
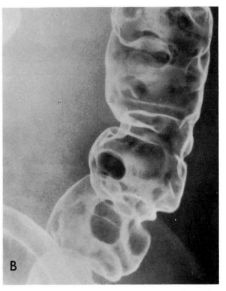
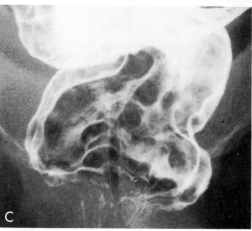

FIGURE 15–19

A to C, Polyposis due to colonic lymphoma. There are multiple polypoid lesions scattered throughout the colon owing to lymphoma. (Courtesy of J. O. Op den Orth, M.D., Haarlem, Holland.)

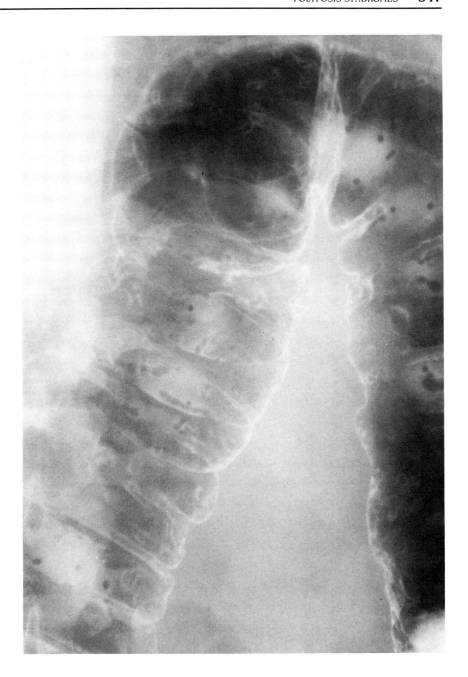

FIGURE 15–20

Postinflammatory polyposis in a patient with ulcerative colitis, showing sessile and frond-like lesions.

Inflammatory Polyposis

Colitic Polyposis

Inflammatory polyps (discussed in Chapter 17) are found in 10% to 20% of patients with ulcerative colitis. Invariably there is a history of a severe previous attack followed by remission. The lesions may be sessile or frond-like in appearance, and may be adherent in parts (Fig. 15–20). Filiform polyposis is associated with either ulcerative colitis or, less frequently, with Crohn's disease (Fig. 15–21).[30] In the latter, it may be seen occasionally in the small bowel or stomach (Fig. 15–22). Occasionally, inflammatory polyps may be associated with amebic colitis.[31] In areas in which schistosomiasis is endemic, bilharzial polyposis is common.[32]

Adenomatous polyps can be distinguished because they are usually rounded, not filiform, and never adherent. The distribution of the polyps is also different. Inflammatory polyps may occur in any part of the colon, but are most common on the left side because this area is most often ulcerated in an acute attack. In familial adenomatous polyposis the polyps are found throughout the colon and rectum. The double contrast enema allows these two conditions to be differentiated. This is important, because they may be confused on sigmoidoscopy. In all patients, histologic examination is indicated.

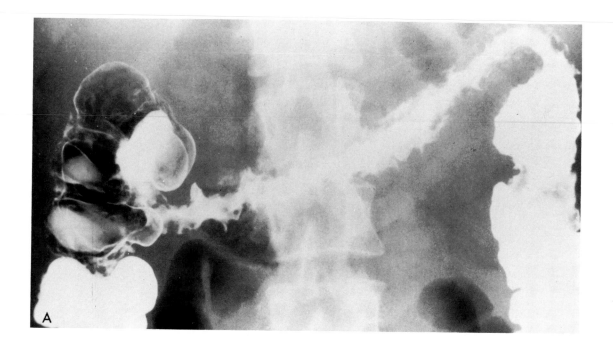

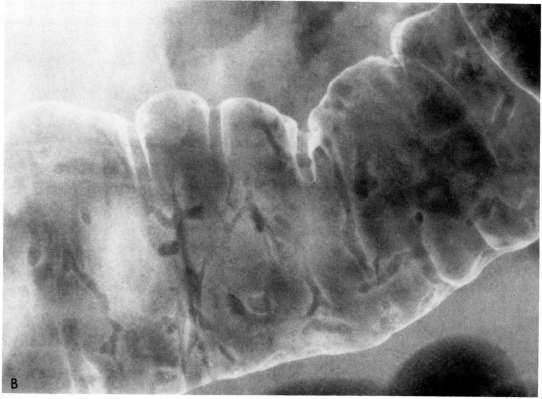

FIGURE 15–21

FILIFORM POLYPOSIS DEVELOPING IN A PATIENT WITH GRANULOMATOUS COLITIS. *A,* During the acute attack of colitis there is extensive ulceration in the transverse colon.

B, During remission there is marked improvement in the appearance of the transverse colon with a few linear filling defects representing filiform polyps. (From Zegel, H. G., and Laufer, I.: Filiform polyposis. Radiology *127*:615–619, 1978, with permission.)

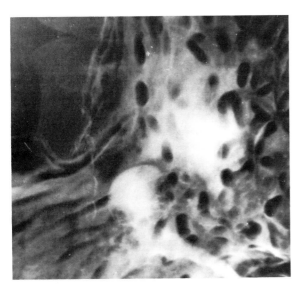

FIGURE 15–22

FILIFORM POLYPOSIS OF THE STOMACH IN A PATIENT WITH CROHN'S DISEASE. This patient had extensive involvement by Crohn's disease throughout the small bowel and in the stomach and duodenum. (From Zegel, H. G., and Laufer, I.: Filiform polyposis. Radiology 127:615–619, 1978, with permission.)

Cronkhite-Canada Syndrome

In 1955 Cronkhite and Canada[33] described two cases of nonfamilial gastrointestinal polyposis with cutaneous hyperpigmentation, alopecia, and nail dystrophy. The mean age of onset of Cronkhite-Canada syndrome is 60 years, mostly in males, presenting with lassitude, weight loss, and diarrhea. Malabsorption is profound. The mucous membrane is thickened with polypoid irregularity, edema of the lamina propria, and cystic dilatation of epithelial tubules. Polyps are present throughout the stomach and colon. These polyps are smooth, sessile, and rarely pedunculated (Fig. 15–23). Superficial erosions are common. The small bowel is involved in 75% of cases. There may be marked thickening of folds in the small bowel and the stomach, which may mimic Menetrier's syndrome. Colorectal cancer (14.5%) and gross gastrointestinal bleeding (27%) are the most common complications. Most patients die within 2 years of onset of the disease, although long-term survival and even remission have occurred.[34]

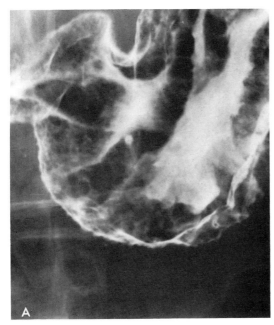
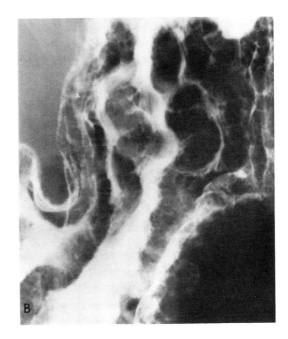

FIGURE 15–23

CRONKHITE-CANADA SYNDROME. A and B, Two views of the stomach show markedly thickened gastric folds with multiple polyps. There were also polyps in the small bowel and colon. Typical clinical features of the Cronkhite-Canada syndrome were present, and open biopsy of the stomach confirmed the diagnosis.

Lymphoid Polyposis

The colon is rich in lymphoid tissue. Follicular hyperplasia is a common normal variant, especially in children, in whom the follicles may appear umbilicated. In adults the nodules usually involve only part of the colon,[35] are about 2 mm in size and only very slightly elevated, so that a meniscus is not seen around the lesions (see Fig. 15–7). Very rarely hypertrophy of the follicles creates benign lymphoid polyposis (Fig. 15–24).[36]

Metaplastic (Hyperplastic) Polyposis

Small metaplastic polyps in the rectum are common, but it is rare for multiple polyps to be found in the

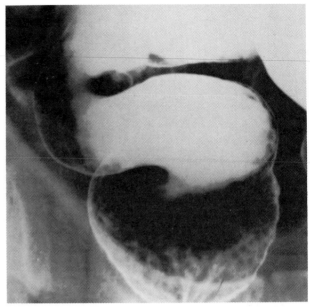

FIGURE 15–25

HYPERPLASTIC POLYPOSIS. There are multiple hyperplastic polyps in the rectum of a 31-year-old male.

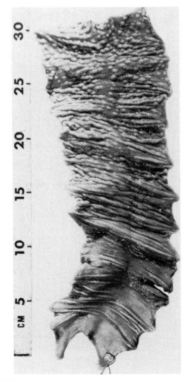

FIGURE 15–24

The resected specimen in a patient with benign lymphoid polyposis.

colorectum (Fig. 15–25). However, if this occurs, it may simulate familial polyposis radiologically,[37] emphasizing the need for careful histologic examination of the polyps in all cases. Although no risk of malignancy is associated with metaplastic polyps, so that colectomy is not indicated, detecting the development of any adenoma within a number of metaplastic polyps is difficult. More than 1% of metaplastic polyps are larger than 1 cm and tend to become pedunculated. Resection of polyps larger than 1 cm may be warranted.

Gastric Polyposis

Hyperplastic polyps in the stomach are usually smooth, larger than 1 cm, and randomly distributed (Fig. 15–26). Multiple hyperplastic polyps may result from regeneration of the epithelium in an area of chronic gastritis.[38] These polyps are not premalignant, but an increased incidence of malignancy in the surrounding mucosa has been reported, secondary to chronic gastritis.[39]

Gastric adenomas are rare. They are usually large solitary antral lesions (Fig. 15–27), but may be multiple in patients with pernicious anemia[40] and are liable to malignant change.

Numerous small hamartomatous polyps have been found in the body and fundus in patients with familial polyposis of the large bowel (Fig. 15–28).[41]

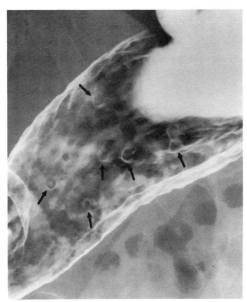

FIGURE 15–26

Multiple small hyperplastic polyps in the body of the stomach.

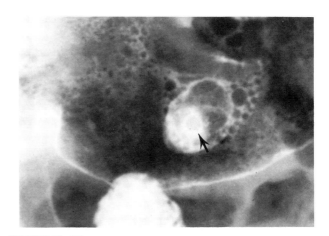

FIGURE 15–27

Pedunculated adenomatous polyp in the gastric antrum. The thin pedicle *(arrow)* is seen through the head of the polyp.

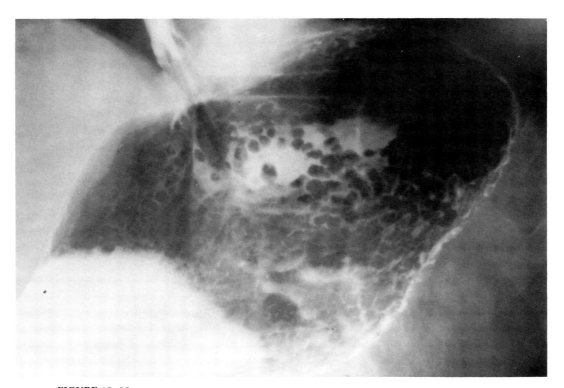

FIGURE 15–28

Multiple hamartomatous gastric polyps around the cardia and fundus in a patient with familial adenomatous polyposis.

Miscellaneous

Submucosal deposits due to malignant melanoma, metastatic carcinoma, or very rarely malacoplakia, may produce a diffuse polypoid change in the GI tract, which frequently shows umbilication.

Food residue in the small and large bowel should not be confused with polyposis,[42] since the particles move under compression revealing a normal underlying mucosa. Adherent residue in the colon has an irregular outline and meniscus and is usually easily differentiated from a polyp.

SUMMARY

Gastrointestinal polyposis may present by various means: clinically, as in the Peutz-Jeghers syndrome; on sigmoidoscopic examination; or fortuitously during radiologic investigation. In most patients the age, clinical features, and radiologic findings provide a likely diagnosis. This must always be confirmed by histologic examination, because the nature of the polyposis will have a profound effect on the management of the patient. All patients should have full double contrast studies of the upper and lower gastrointestinal tract to assess the extent of the polyposis and risk of overt malignancy. All require long-term follow-up. Particular consideration must be given to the possible development of periampullary carcinoma in patients with FAP, and to the risk of colonic carcinoma in early adult life for patients with juvenile polyposis. In the Peutz-Jeghers syndrome the small bowel must be carefully reviewed for large polyps every 3 to 4 years.

ACKNOWLEDGMENT

We are grateful to Dr. Basil C. Morson of the Department of Pathology, St. Mark's Hospital, London, for supplying the specimen photographs for this chapter.

REFERENCES

1. Morson, B.C.: Some peculiarities in the histology of intestinal polyps. Dis. Colon Rectum 5:337, 1962.
2. Bussey, H.J.R.: Gastrointestinal polyposis. Gut 11:970, 1970.
3. Bussey, H.J.R., Veale, A.M.O., and Morson, B.C.: Genetics of gastrointestinal polyposis. Gastroenterology 74:1325, 1978.
4. Bussey, H.J.R.: Familial Polyposis Coli: Family Studies, Histopathology. Differential Diagnosis and Results of Treatment. Baltimore, Johns Hopkins Press, 1975, pp. 47–48.
5. Smith, H.J., and Lee, E.L.: Umbilicated adenomas in familial polyposis coli: Radiologic and histologic correlation. AJR 147:61, 1986.
6. Bartram, C.I., and Thornton, A.: Colonic polyp patterns in familial polyposis. AJR 142:305, 1984.
7. Glick, S.N., Teplick, S.K., and Ross, W.M.: Colonic lymphoid follicles associated with colonic neoplasms. Radiology 168:630, 1988.
8. Muto, T., Bussey, H.J.R., and Morson, B.C.: The evolution of cancer of the colon and rectum. Cancer 36:2251, 1975.
9. Jagelman, D.G., DeCosse, J.J., and Bussey, H.J.R.: Upper gastrointestinal cancer in familial adenomatous polyposis. Lancet 21:1149, 1988.
10. Plail, R.O., Bussey, H.J.R., Glazer, G., and Thomson, J.P.S.: Adenomatous polyposis: An association with carcinoma of the thyroid. Br. J. Surg. 74:377, 1987.
11. Gardner, E.J., and Richards, R.C.: Multiple cutaneous and subcutaneous lesions occurring simultaneously with hereditary polyposis and osteomatosis. Am. J. Hum. Genet. 5:139, 1953.
12. Gardner, E.J.: Follow-up study of a family exhibiting dominant inheritance for a syndrome including intestinal polyps, osteomas, fibromas and epidermal cysts. Am. J. Hum. Genet. 14:376, 1962.
13. Simpson, R.D., Harrison, E.G., and Mayo, C.W.: Mesenteric fibromatosis in familial polyposis: A variant of Gardner's syndrome. Cancer 17:526, 1964.
14. Marshall, W.H., Martin, F.I.R., and Mackay, I.R.: Gardner's syndrome with adrenal carcinoma. Aust. Ann. Med. 16:242, 1967.
15. Heald, R.J.: Gardner's syndrome in association with two tumors in the ileum. Proc. R. Soc. Med. 60:914, 1967.
16. Thomford, N.R., and Greenberger, N.J.: Lymphoid polyps of the ileum associated with Gardner's syndrome. Arch. Surg. 96:289, 1968.
17. Veale, A.M.O.: Intestinal polyposis. Eugenics Laboratory Memoirs, Series 40. London, Cambridge University Press, 1965.
18. Morson, B.C., and Konishi, F.: Contribution of the pathologist to the radiology and management of colorectal polyps. Gastrointest. Radiol. 7:275, 1982.
19. Peutz, J.L.A.: Over een zeer merkwaardige gecombineerde familiaire polyposis van des slijmvliezen van den tractus intestinalis met die van de neuskeenlholte en gepaard met eigenaardige pigmentaties van huid en slijmvliezen. Ned. Maandschr. Geneeskd. 2:134, 1921.
20. Jeghers, H., McKusick, V.A., and Katz, K.H.: Generalized intestinal polyposis and melanin spots of the oral mucosa, lips and digits. N. Engl. J. Med. 241:993, 1949.
21. Williams, C.B., Goldblatt, M., and Delaney, P.V.: Top and tail endoscopy and follow-up in Peutz-Jeghers syndrome. Endoscopy 14:82, 1982.
22. Dodds, W.J.: Clinical and roentgen features of the intestinal polyposis syndromes. Gastrointest. Radiol. 1:127, 1976.
23. Christian, C.D., McLoughlin, T.G., Cathcart, E.R., et al.: Peutz-Jeghers syndrome associated with functioning ovarian tumor. JAMA 190:935, 1964.
24. Veale, A.M.O., McColl, L., Bussey, H.J.R., et al.: Juvenile polyposis coli. J. Med. Genet. 3:5, 1966.
25. Carlson, G.J., Nivatvongs, A.S., and Snover, D.C.: Colorectal polyps in Cowden's disease (multiple hamartoma syndrome). Am. J. Surg. Pathol. 8:763, 1984.
26. Turcot, J., Despres, J.P., and St. Pierre, F.: Malignant tumors of the central nervous system associated with familial polyposis of the colon. Dis. Colon Rectum 2:465, 1959.
27. Itoh, J., Ohsato, K., Yao, T., et al: Turcot's syndrome and its mode of inheritance. Gut 20:414, 1979.
28. Schartz, R.A., Flieger, D.N., and Saied, N.K.: The Torre syndrome with gastrointestinal polyposis. Arch. Dermatol. 116:312, 1980.
29. Davis, M., Maxwell, G., Gogel, H., et al.: Lymphomatous polyposis of the colon. Gastrointest. Radiol. 14:70, 1989.
30. Zegel, H.G., and Laufer, I.: Filiform polyposis. Radiology 127:615, 1978.
31. Berkowitz, D., and Bernstein, L.H.: Colonic pseudopolyps in association with amebic colitis. Gastroenterology 68:786, 1975.
32. Medina, J.T., Seaman, W.B., Guzman-Acosta, C., et al.: The roentgen appearances of schistosomiasis Mansoni involving the colon. Radiology 85:682, 1965.
33. Cronkhite, L.W., and Canada, W.J.: Generalized gastrointestinal polyposis: An unusual syndrome of polyposis, pigmentation, alopecia and onychotrophia. N. Engl. J. Med 252:1011, 1955.
34. Daniel, E.S., Ludwig, S.L., Lewin, K.J., et al.: The Cronkhite-

Canada syndrome: An analysis of clinical and pathologic features and therapy in 55 patients. Medicine *61*:293, 1987.

35. Kelvin, F.M., Max, R.J., Norton, G.A., et al.: Lymphoid follicular pattern of the colon in adults. AJR *133*:821, 1979.

36. Collins, J.O., Falk, M., and Gilbone, R.: Benign lymphoid polyposis of the colon. Pediatrics *38*:897, 1966.

37. Cohen, S.M., Brown, L., Janower, M.L., and McCready, F.J.: Multiple metaplastic (hyperplastic) polyposis of the colon. Gastrointest. Radiol. *6*:333, 1981.

38. Morson, B.C.: Intestinal metaplasia of the gastric mucosa. Br. J. Cancer *9*:365, 1955.

39. Ming, S.C., and Goldman, H.: Gastric polyps: A histogenetic classification and its relation to carcinoma. Cancer *18*:721, 1965.

40. Jorgensen, J.: The mortality among patients with pernicious anemia in Denmark and the incidence of gastric cancer among the same. Acta Med. Scand. *139*:472, 1951.

41. Parks, T.G., Bussey, H.J.R., and Lockhart-Mummery, H.E.: Familial polyposis coli associated with extra-colonic abnormalities. Gut *11*:323, 1970.

42. Press, H.C., Jr. and Davis, T.W.: Ingested foreign bodies simulating polyposis: Report of 6 cases. AJR *127*:1040, 1976.

DIVERTICULAR DISEASE

16

Clive I. Bartram, F.R.C.P., F.R.C.R.
Igor Laufer, M.D.

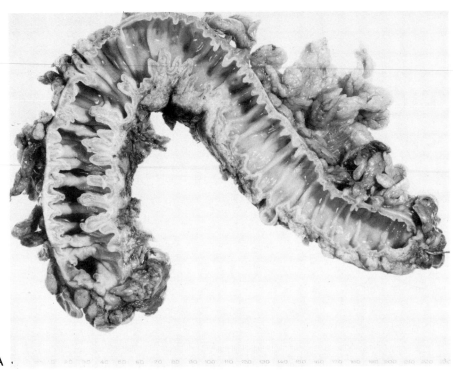

A

FIGURE 16–1

TYPICAL MUSCLE CHANGES OF DIVERTICULAR DISEASE. *A,* A surgical specimen shows muscle hypertrophy without inflammation.

B, A radiograph in another patient shows the typical sawtooth appearance of muscle hypertrophy.

Diverticular disease is common in the elderly in Western countries, affecting between 33% and 48% of the population over the age of 50.[1, 2] About 1 in 70 of this group require hospital treatment, and 1 in 200 need an operation.[3] Younger age groups are not exempt from this disease, and diverticula may be seen in about 10% of barium enemas in patients between the ages of 30 and 50. About 5% of patients presenting with symptoms from diverticular disease are less than 40 years of age.[4]

The term diverticular disease implies the presence of a characteristic muscle abnormality. Diverticula are often present, and there may be associated inflammatory changes.[5] The term diverticulosis refers only to the presence of diverticula, with or without a muscle abnormality. Diverticulitis indicates either macroscopic or microscopic inflammation affecting one or more diverticula, often accompanied by pericolic abscess formation.

RADIOLOGIC PATHOLOGY

The most consistent abnormality involves the muscle of the sigmoid colon.[5] Elastin deposits between the muscle cells of the teniae coli[6] result in contracture, so that in uncomplicated diverticular disease, the thickening of the circular muscle is secondary to the

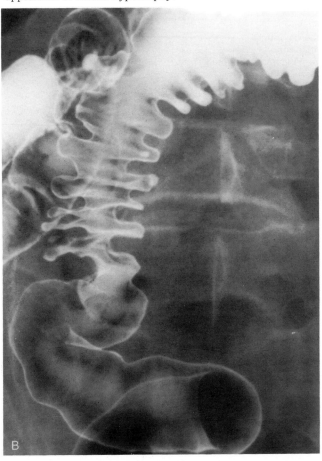

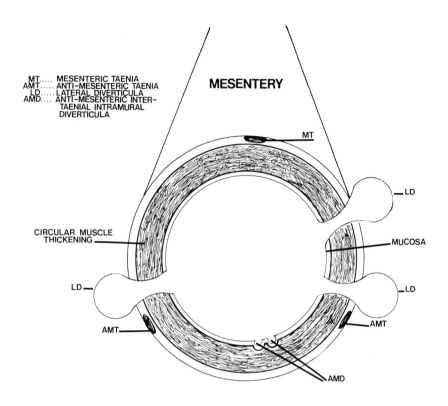

FIGURE 16–2

Schematic diagram of diverticular anatomy.

concertina effect from longitudinal shortening of the teniae. Similarly, the redundant mucosa becomes corrugated into transverse folds (Fig. 16–1A). The circular muscle thickening is commonly localized into two semicircular arcs between the mesenteric and antimesenteric teniae (Fig. 16–2), but it may be uniform.

The diverticula, composed of mucosa and muscularis mucosae, are of the false, pulsion type. They develop as outpouches through defects in the circular muscle at the sites of small penetrating arteries. Lateral diverticula arise between the mesenteric and antimesenteric teniae. They emerge from the convexity of the folded circular muscle, often in two lateral rows, their openings alternating with the opposite side (see Fig. 16–2).

Small diverticula are found in the antimesenteric intertenial area. They are usually associated with lateral diverticula and are of the small saccular, ridge, or intramural type.[7] Diverticula are most common in the sigmoid colon. In about 17% of cases, they are distributed throughout the colon.[8] Isolated diverticula in the cecum and ascending colon are found in 4% to 12% of patients.[2, 8, 9]

RADIOGRAPHIC CHANGES

Plain Film

Plain film radiography is of little value in the primary assessment of disease. A bubbly appearance due to air in the diverticula has been described.[10] Plain films are used mostly in the evaluation of diverticular disease complicated by an inflammatory mass, with or without intestinal obstruction.

Contrast Examinations

A double contrast enema (DCE) shows both the muscular and the diverticular components of the disease. The interdigitating clefts of the mucosal surface reflect the muscle change (Fig. 16–3A).[11] As this may not be uniform circumferentially, the appearances will vary with the angle at which the surface is viewed. Occasionally, a localized bar of thickened muscle may simulate a polyp (Fig. 16–3B). The muscle clefts and diverticula may be more apparent in the prone-angled view, which is nearer to the plane of the mesentery, than in the supine oblique view, which is more at right angles to the mesentery.

The diverticula vary in appearance with the angle at which they are viewed, and also with the amount of air and barium they contain (Fig. 16–4). To some extent, this is governed by whether the diverticulum is located on the dependent or nondependent wall. In about 20% of patients, a spiky, irregular outline along one side of the bowel wall is seen (Fig. 16–5). This irregular outline is caused by diverticula in the antimesenteric intertenial ridge.[7] This appearance has been referred to as prediverticular,[12] but use of this term is incorrect, as such an appearance has been shown to be the result of small diverticula. The usual large lateral diverticula may develop later, as shown by Welin and Welin,[13] but such a progression is not established. The appearance is perhaps best considered as part of the spectrum of diverticular disease.

Muscle change is usually associated with diverticula, but in about 8% of cases, only the muscle abnormality is present, and in 19%, only diverticula are present.[2] One should note that diverticula do not always fill, as contraction of the longitudinal muscle closes the necks of the diverticula. This phenomenon may be apparent during filling when the bowel has a palisade configuration. When the longitudinal muscle

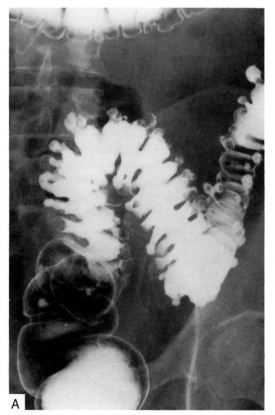

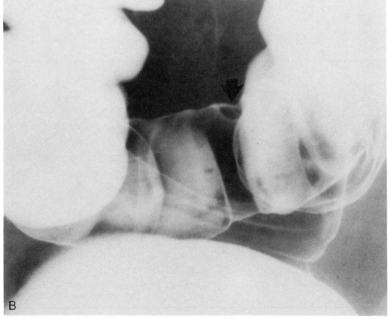

FIGURE 16–3

A, Diverticular disease with interdigitating muscle clefts and diverticula. *B*, Localized thickened muscle bar *(arrow)* simulating a polyp.

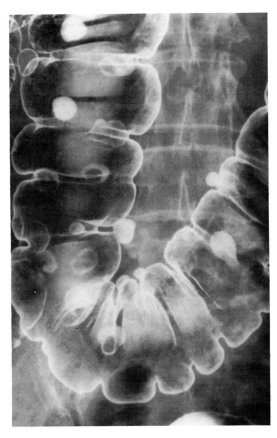

FIGURE 16–4

Diverticula containing varying amounts of air and barium.

relaxes, the palisade configuration disappears, and the diverticula fill.[14] Sometimes the converse occurs, and in 4% of patients, the diverticula seem transient,[15] being evident with muscle contraction but disappearing after smooth muscle relaxants have been given.

A post-DCE sigmoid flush in which 500 to 750 ml of a 1.5% barium suspension is used improves luminal distention, provides better filling of the diverticula, and widens the interhaustral space. The density of the flush leaves a thin coating of the thicker barium and reduces pooling of dense barium or pockets of gas, making the image much clearer.[16] This technique is recommended when neither double contrast nor compression views have been satisfactory. It may improve visualization of the sigmoid in up to 75% of studies, allowing greater confidence in polyp detection and the exclusion of artifacts.

Fecoliths within diverticula are common and may prevent complete filling or may create a ring with a clearly defined outer border and irregular inner edge as the barium tracks between the diverticulum and the fecolith. Inversion of diverticula has been reported as a result of endoscopy, but its recognition on the basis of radiologic examination is exceptionally rare.[17]

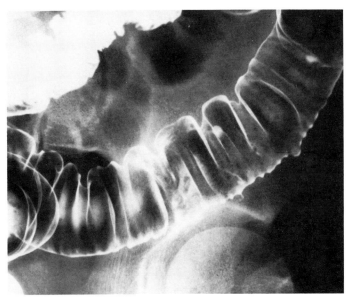

FIGURE 16–5

Small diverticula in the antimesenteric intertenial ridge.

COMPLICATIONS

Inflammation

Inspissated fecal material within a diverticulum may cause abrasion and lead to inflammation. Diverticula are extraluminal lesions outside the protective muscle layer. In most cases, diverticulitis is a consequence of perforation of a diverticulum. A minimal perforation or "microperforation" may cause only a local reaction in the pericolic or mesenteric fat (Fig. 16–6A). A larger perforation may produce more easily recognizable extravasation into the pericolic tissues (Fig. 16–6B). A pericolic abscess will then develop

(Fig. 16–6C). The affected diverticulum may not fill, so there may be no mucosal change seen on the DCE. If the inflammation is more massive and not localized, generalized peritonitis will result. Inflammatory changes will tend to spread longitudinally in the pericolic plain, and an abscess may dissect longitudinally as well as around the bowel (Fig. 16–6D).

The abscess may resolve spontaneously, with the bowel returning to its appearance prior to the episode of acute diverticulitis (Fig. 16–7). In other patients, resolution may leave slight narrowing of the lumen or deformity of a diverticulum as the only evidence of the previous episode of diverticulitis (Fig. 16–8).

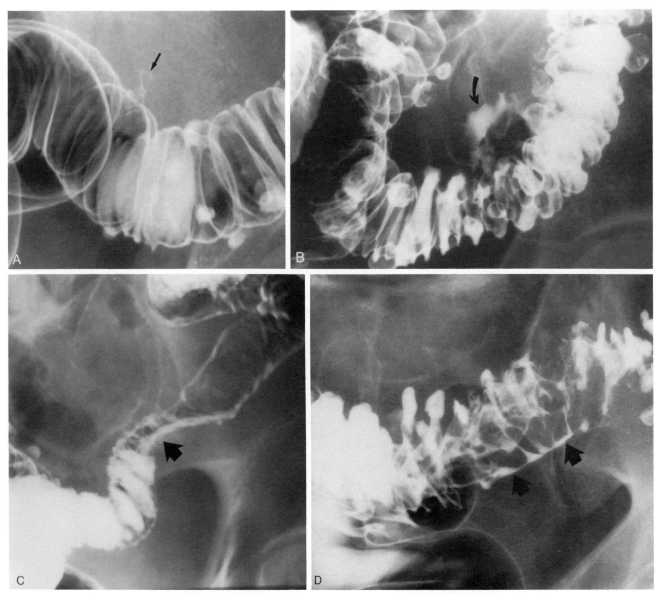

FIGURE 16–6

EVOLUTION OF CHANGES IN DIVERTICULITIS. A, A microperforation (arrow) from the superior aspect of the colon.
  B, More obvious extravasation into the pericolic tissue (arrow) from a perforated diverticulum.
  C, Extrinsic impression on the sigmoid colon (arrow) from a pericolic abscess.
  D, Intramural tracking (arrows) from dissection of a pericolic abscess with communication into adjacent diverticula.

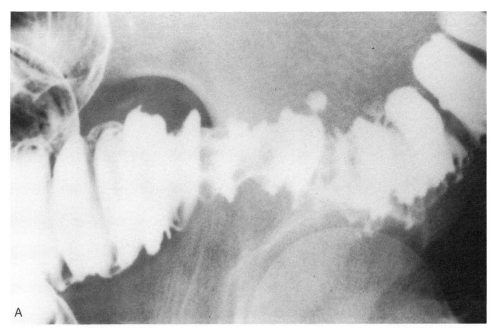

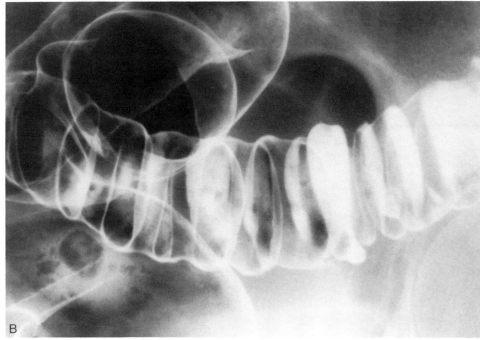

FIGURE 16–7

COMPLETE RESOLUTION OF DIVERTICULITIS. *A,* Irregular narrowing of the lumen with widened folds due to a localized pericolic abscess.

B, The same patient 3 months later showing complete resolution.

In addition, the abscess may discharge and drain via any of the adjacent organs, giving rise to a fistula (see the following section).

The diagnosis of diverticulitis can be made from a contrast enema only by the recognition of a perforated diverticulum or its sequela, a pericolic abscess. Barium may track through the perforated diverticulum into the abscess. The abscess itself causes an extrinsic deformity of the lumen (see Fig. 16–6C). Initially, this deformity should be on the mesenteric side, but it may spread to encircle the lumen. Any extrinsic defect originating on the lateral border between the antimesenteric teniae should be the result of other disease,[18] as only the lateral diverticula are perforated.

The abscess lies outside the muscle, and suppuration spreads easily within the pericolic fat, forming a dissecting abscess. The fat may outline the abscess mass on plain films.[19] Five diagnostic features of acute diverticulitis have been described:[20] (1) narrowing, deformity, or displacement of the bowel lumen, (2) altered mucosal pattern, (3) soft tissue mass, (4) gas or air–fluid levels within the mass, and (5) extraluminal barium due to barium tracking through the perforated diverticulum into the pericolic abscess.

The "drape sign," described by Marshak and associates,[21] refers to the bending of adjacent diverticula so that the bowel appears to be draped over the presumed site of an abscess. This sign may be a late

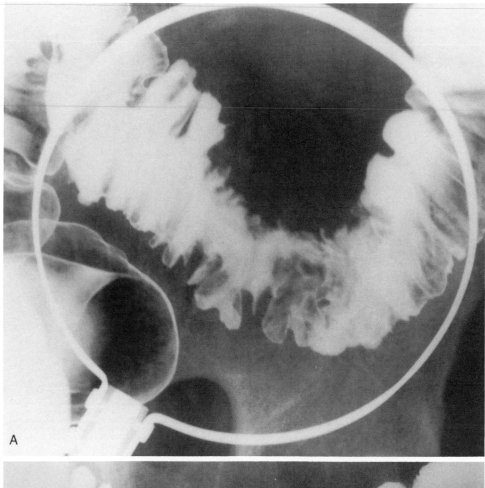

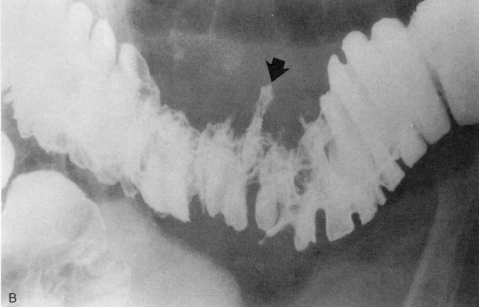

FIGURE 16–8

RESOLUTION OF DIVERTICULITIS WITH A DEFORMED DIVERTICULUM. *A,* In the acute stage, there is a diverticular abscess along the superior aspect of the sigmoid colon.

B, Several months later, after clinical resolution, there is a residual deformed diverticulum (*arrow*).

indication of inflammation and reflect fibrotic contracture.

Additional manifestations of pericolic abscess formation include the following:

1. Localized small bowel ileus.

2. Complete small bowel obstruction from kinking and edema of the bowel adjacent to the abscess (a less common occurrence).

3. A degree of large bowel obstruction. (This condition is quite common, but complete obstruction is rare.)

4. Free intraperitoneal air from the perforated diverticulum (a rare occurrence).

5. Fistula formation (relatively common).

Computed tomography (CT) has been considered the preferred examination in diverticulitis, because it allows imaging of the bowel wall thickness and the extraluminal components of what is essentially an extraluminal problem. However, a contrast enema still has a role in diagnosis. In 102 patients with diverticulitis, the contrast enema diagnosis was correct in 77%, compared with only 41% based on CT.[22] In about 11% of cases,[23] the wall thickening may be 1 to 3 cm, and the inflammation remains intramural. In addition, there is overlap with CT findings in patients with colon cancer. Small exudates may be missed, and intramural collections may appear isodense. A contrast enema remains a useful supplement to CT in those cases in which inflammation is not widespread, but localized, and helps reduce false-positive diagnoses.

Fistula

Spontaneous fistula may result from the spread of inflammation from a pericolic abscess to adjacent organs, notably the bladder (Fig. 16–9A), vagina (Fig. 16–9B), or small bowel. Sometimes the rupture of a

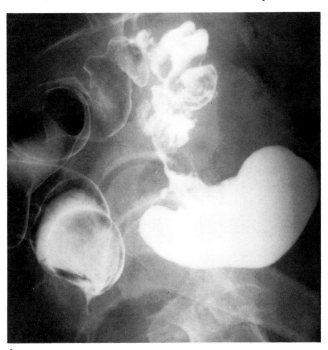

A

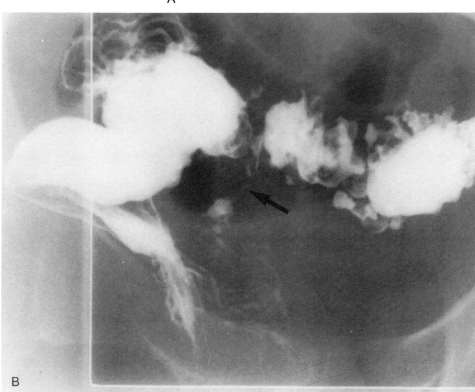

B

FIGURE 16–9

FISTULAS COMPLICATING DIVERTICULITIS. *A,* Colovesical fistula due to diverticular disease.

B, A colovaginal fistula complicating acute diverticulitis. The communication is from the sigmoid colon to the vagina *(arrow).*

diverticulum that has become adherent to an adjacent organ leads to a fistula. In such circumstances, the underlying disease may be minimal.

The bladder is most commonly involved. The communication is demonstrated by barium enema in about 30% of patients (see Fig. 16–9A), and by air in the bladder on a plain film radiograph in about another 30%. Taken in conjunction, plain film and contrast radiography reveal about 40% of colovesical fistula.[24]

Hemorrhage

Classically, the affected patient is elderly, obese, and hypertensive. Slight hypogastric pain is experienced, and a large volume of bright red blood is passed rectally. Angiography has shown that hemorrhage is twice as likely to arise in the right side of the colon as in the left side.[25] The vascular architecture has been studied by Meyers and colleagues.[26] The intramural branches of the marginal artery, the vasa recta, penetrate the colonic wall from serosa to submucosa and course over the domes of the diverticula in the serosa. Intimal thickening, with weakening of the

wall, can lead to eccentric rupture and massive bleeding.[26] The reason that this phenomenon is more common in the right side of the colon is unknown, but possibly, the wider necks of the diverticula may lead to greater exposure to the noxious agents in the colon.

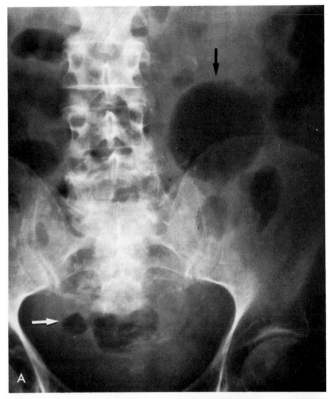

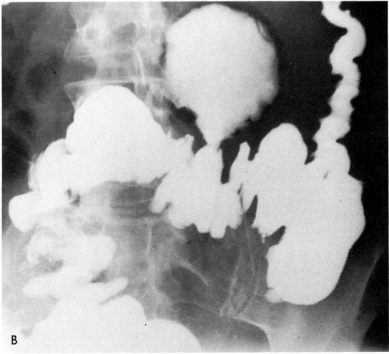

FIGURE 16–10

A, Plain abdominal film showing air in the giant sigmoid and rectal diverticula *(arrows).*

B, Giant sigmoid diverticulum (arrow) filled with barium.

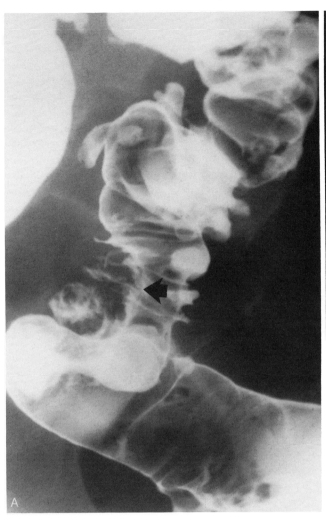

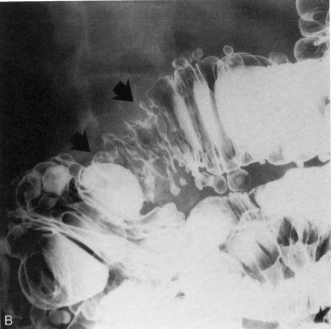

FIGURE 16–11

UNUSUAL LOCATIONS FOR DIVERTICULITIS. *A,* Diverticular abscess *(arrow)* in the descending colon.
B, Right-sided diverticulitis at the hepatic flexure *(arrows).*

UNUSUAL PRESENTATIONS

Cecal Diverticula

Isolated cecal diverticula may be seen in 4% to 12% of patients who have been found to have diverticula on radiologic examination.[2, 8] Often thought to be congenital, these diverticula have been shown to be false, pulsion diverticula similar to those in the sigmoid.[2] An association with solitary ulcers of the cecum has been suggested,[9] but a recent study showed no such relationship.[27]

Rectal Diverticula

Rectal diverticula are extremely rare (Fig. 16–10), because the teniae fuse to ensheath the rectum completely. When found, rectal diverticula tend to be large and associated with sigmoid diverticular disease.[28]

Giant Sigmoid Diverticula

On resection, giant sigmoid diverticula are found to be pseudocysts with a thin membranous lining and usually fibrous with a chronic inflammatory infiltrate and some mucosal remnants. If muscularis propria is present, the lesion is more likely to represent a communicating colonic duplication.

Several etiologic theories for these lesions have been suggested: intraluminal drainage of an abscess with peridiverticular adhesions preventing its collapse; gas formation from retention of gas-forming bacteria after the neck of the diverticulum has been occluded; and a ball-valve mechanism.[29]

Radiologically, a giant diverticulum appears initially as a large, smooth air-filled cavity in the left iliac fossa (see Fig. 16–10). An air–fluid level is seen in about 25% of cases; the cyst fills with barium in 60% and may be bilocular or multiple. The cyst may perforate, undergo volvulus, or very rarely, malignant change.[30] The diagnosis is based on the appearance of the smooth cyst wall with associated diverticular disease

Diverticulitis of the Right Side of the Colon

The vast majority of cases of acute diverticulitis involve the sigmoid colon. Less commonly, the descending colon may be affected (Fig. 16–11A). Even more rarely, diverticulitis may occur on the right side of the colon (Fig. 16–11B).[31] Because of this unusual location, it is often mistaken for a carcinoma.

COEXISTING LESIONS

Polyps

Diverticular disease complicates polyp detection, and as shown by colonoscopy, it is the commonest cause of missing polyps on the DCE.[32]

Viewed tangentially, the intraluminal location of a polyp compared with the extraluminal diverticulum is obvious. However, when viewed en face or obliquely, the images may be confusing. Both may appear as a ring shadow. According to the classic description of the meniscus within a diverticulum, the outer border is sharply defined and fades centrally (Fig. 16–12), as opposed to being well defined centrally and fading peripherally around a polyp.[33] The "bowler hat" sign may be seen with both polyps and diverticula when the diverticulum is coated with barium and filled with air. If the bowler hat points toward the center of the long axis of the bowel, the lesion should be intraluminal and a polyp; however, if it points away from this axis, it represents a diverticulum. This rule is useful, except when the lesion is in the midline or directly parallel to the long axis (see Chapters 2 and 13).[34] Fecoliths within diverticula create a special problem.[35] If the fecolith projects out of the diverticulum, there is a meniscus around its base and an intraluminal component (Fig. 16–13). Usually, barium enters at least part of the diverticulum, so that a ring with a clearly defined outer margin, but ragged inner edge, is visible (Fig. 16–12).

Other distinguishing features[36] are summarized in Figure 16–14. The head of a pedunculated polyp may be lost within a barium pool, but the stalk is visible

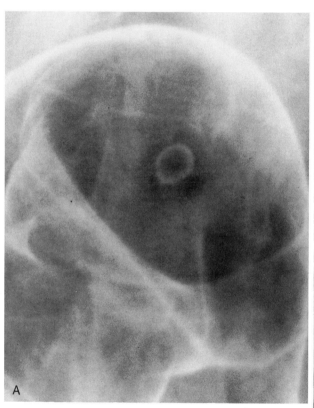

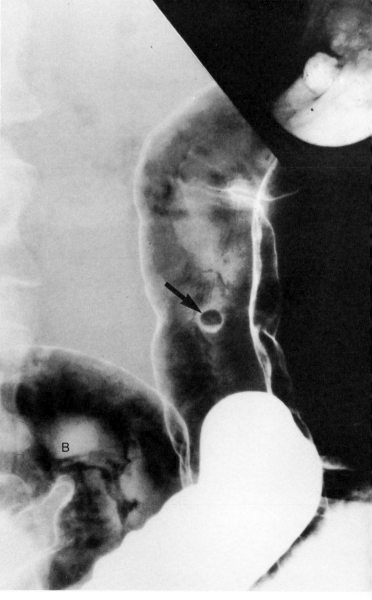

FIGURE 16–12

A, En face view showing the meniscus created by the thin layer of barium within the diverticulum, which is clearly defined outside and is fading inside as the layer is no longer imaged tangentially.

B, The ring shadow (arrow) could be mistaken for a polyp, but as the colonoscopic view shows (see inset, top right), this sign was due to a fecolith protruding from the diverticulum.

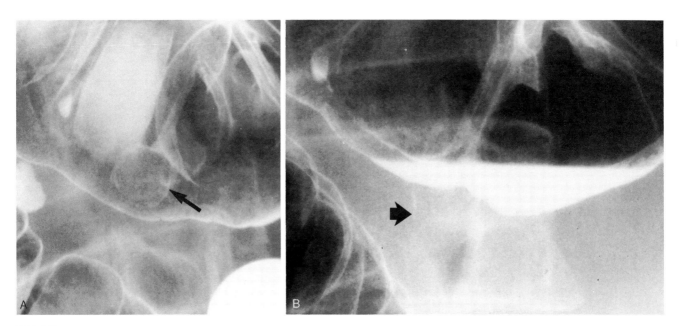

FIGURE 16–13

FECOLITH IN A DIVERTICULUM. *A*, The 1.5-cm ring shadow in the transverse colon *(arrow)* suggests a polyp, although the internal edge is irregular.

B, In an erect view (see also Fig. 16–12*B*), the diverticulum projects beyond the lumen, and a thin track of contrast is visible *(arrow)* between the diverticulum and the fecolith.

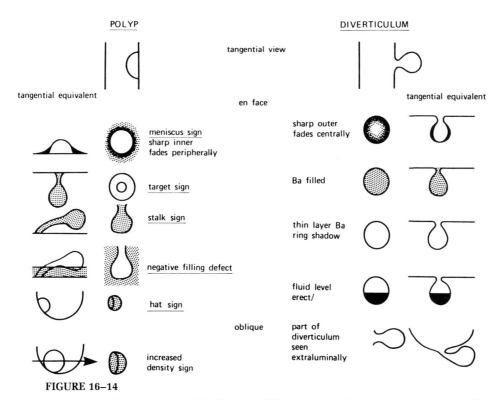

FIGURE 16–14

Diagrammatic Representation of the features distinguishing a diverticulum from a polyp. (From Htoo, A.M. and Bartram, C.I.: The radiological diagnosis of polyps in the presence of diverticular disease. Br. J. Radiol. 52:263, 1979, with permission.)

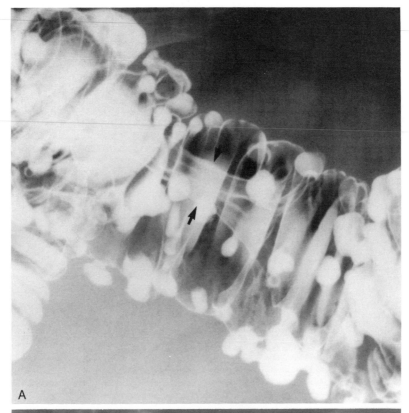

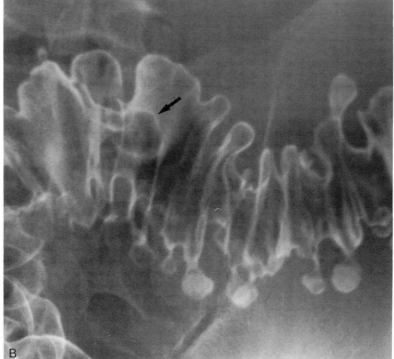

FIGURE 16–15

A, The parallel lines of the stalk of the pedunculated polyp, or "stalk sign," are visible *(arrows)*, although the head is obscured in the barium pool.

B, A pedunculated polyp *(arrow)* seen as a filling defect in the barium pool.

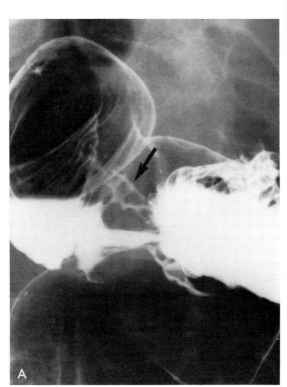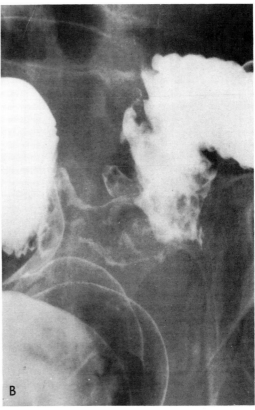

FIGURE 16–16

CARCINOMA IN DIVERTICULAR DISEASE AND THE VALUE OF RELAXANT DRUGS. *A,* Carcinomatous stricture in diverticular disease showing shouldered ends. The lesion is seen through overlapping loops of sigmoid.

B, Same examination after administration of relaxants, showing the lumen of the strictured segment in double contrast. Irregular pools of barium reflect the mucosal destruction due to malignancy.

as two parallel lines (Fig. 16–15*A*). The complete polyp may also be seen as a filling defect within the barium pool (Fig. 16–15*B*). This visualization is aided by compression, or by flushing of the sigmoid with dilute barium to improve luminal resolution. Smooth muscle relaxants should always be given to patients with diverticular disease to reduce muscle tone and maximize distention of the sigmoid.[36] Administration of muscle relaxants is particularly important in the evaluation of strictures in patients with diverticular disease to rule out coexisting carcinoma (Fig. 16–16).

Carcinoma

Approximately 10% of sigmoid carcinomas are associated with diverticular disease. However, the differentiation between a benign and a malignant stricture may be difficult (Figs. 16–17 and 16–18). Strictures in diverticular disease may result from a combination of inflammatory change, muscle thickening, and redundant mucosal folds narrowing the lumen. Such lesions have tapered ends with an intact mucosa. Within the strictured segment, a few diverticula may fill, or barium may enter the closed necks of divertic-

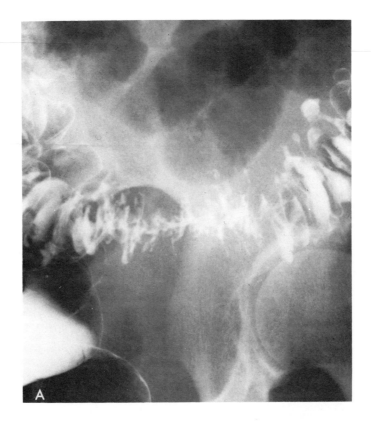

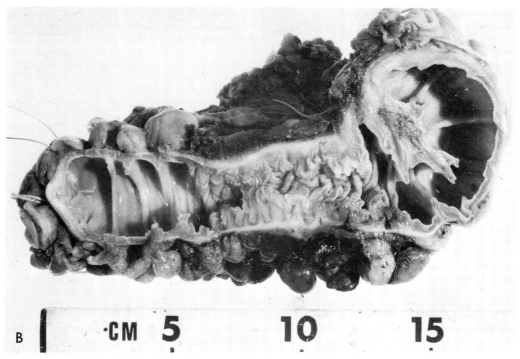

FIGURE 16–17

ACUTE DIVERTICULITIS. *A,* Stricture due to inflammatory changes.
 B, Resected specimen. The serosa is thickened from inflammatory changes. Muscle thickening and redundant mucosal folds contribute to the stricture.

ula, causing a spiky outline (Fig. 16–17). Carcinoma tends to cause a shorter stricture, with irregular, shouldered ends. The lumen of the stricture is irregular, with no normal mucosal fold pattern present.[37] The absence of a normal mucosal fold pattern or diverticular opening is always suspicious (Fig. 16–18C). Inflammatory changes superimposed on malignancy may obscure such distinguishing features. Relaxants are useful in obtaining some dilatation in benign strictures and a better definition of the ends of the stricture (see Fig. 16–16). In a series of patients with strictures in diverticular disease, the distinction between benignity and malignancy was impossible in 16% of patients with diverticular disease and in 4% of patients with carcinoma.[38] Even with good views, the distinction between benign and malignant lesions may be difficult, and flexible sigmoidoscopy is advised when any doubt exists.

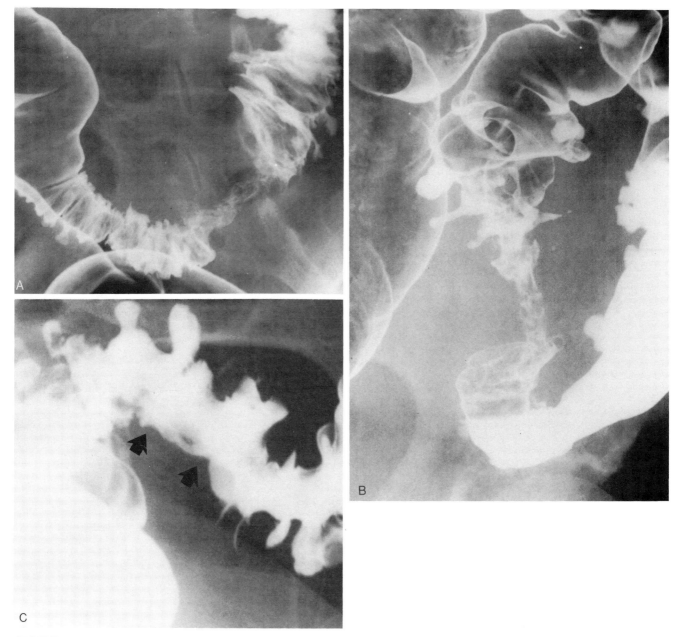

FIGURE 16–18

DIFFERENTIATION BETWEEN DIVERTICULITIS AND CARCINOMA. *A,* A typical benign stricture due to diverticulitis with intact mucosa and tapered margins. Note the extrinsic impression due to a diverticular abscess along the superior aspect of the sigmoid.

B, An example of acute diverticulitis simulating a carcinoma.

C, In another patient with diverticulosis, there is a 3-cm segment (*arrows*), which is raised and irregular and bears no diverticula. This finding was due to a plaque-like carcinoma.

Inflammatory Bowel Disease

Both ulcerative and Crohn's colitis have a second peak of frequency of presentation in the older (65 to 75 years) age group. Diverticular disease is also likely to be present, therefore, in some of these patients.

Ulcerative Colitis

The diagnosis of distal ulcerative colitis in the presence of diverticular disease has been considered difficult.[39] Provided that a double contrast view is obtained, however, the finding of a granular mucosa is sufficient radiologic evidence to establish the diagnosis of colitis. The smooth muscle changes and mucosal edema that accompany active colitis may modify the radiologic appearances of the diverticular disease. The mouths of the diverticula may be occluded, so that they do not fill when a barium enema is administered. Inflammatory involvement of the diverticula can alter their shape, so that they are conical or pointed.[39] This appearance can cause confusion with that of deep ulceration (Fig. 16–19). The muscle abnormality may not be so apparent, as deep interdigitating folds are not seen. Muscle changes have been considered partly responsible for fecal stasis.[40] With regression of the colitis, however, the underlying diverticula and muscle changes may revert to a typical appearance.

Complications from diverticulitis in the presence of ulcerative colitis are said to have a grave prognosis,[41] possibly because diagnosis is delayed and the symptoms are wrongly attributed to colitis.

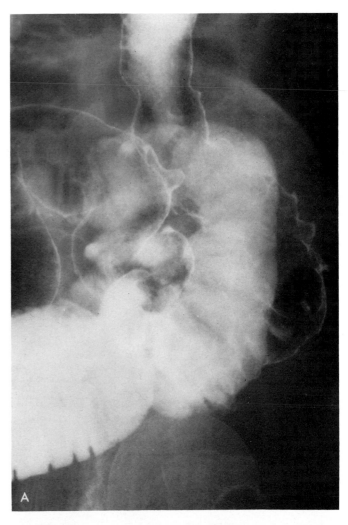

FIGURE 16–19

ULCERATIVE COLITIS WITH DIVERTICULAR DISEASE. A, Granular sigmoid mucosa with some interdigitating folds and several conical diverticula.

B, Part of resected specimen confirming muscle change of diverticular disease, with thickened folds and only a few patent ostia to diverticula.

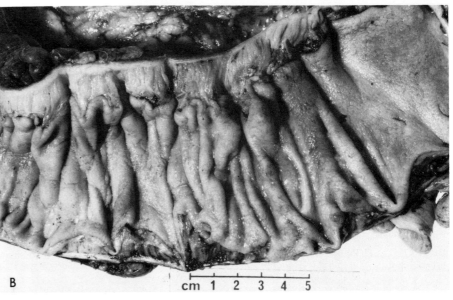

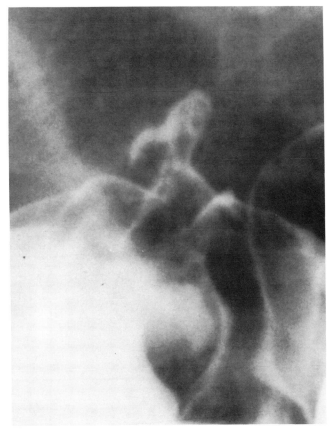

FIGURE 16–20

Crohn's ulcer in a diverticulum.

Crohn's Disease

Occasionally, the deep fissuring in Crohn's disease may suggest the muscle abnormality of diverticular disease. The ulceration of Crohn's disease is spiky and haphazard compared with the smooth interdigitating folds of the muscle abnormality.[42] Usually, other stigmata of Crohn's disease are present. Multiple anal fistulae are common, and the characteristic aphthoid ulceration may be seen in the rectal or sigmoid colonic mucosa.[43] However, this sign may be technically difficult to detect in the sigmoid with muscle changes, multiple diverticula, and a poor double contrast view. Ulceration within the diverticula may be visible (Fig. 16–20). Because the domes of the diverticula are in the pericolic tissue outside the muscle barrier, there is no protective barrier to ulceration and inflammation. A higher incidence of peridiverticulitis and dissecting abscess formation is found than would be expected in diverticular disease alone (Fig. 16–21).[44] Although long fissuring tracts of 10 cm or more are usually associated with Crohn's disease,[45] they may occasionally occur in its absence.[46, 47]

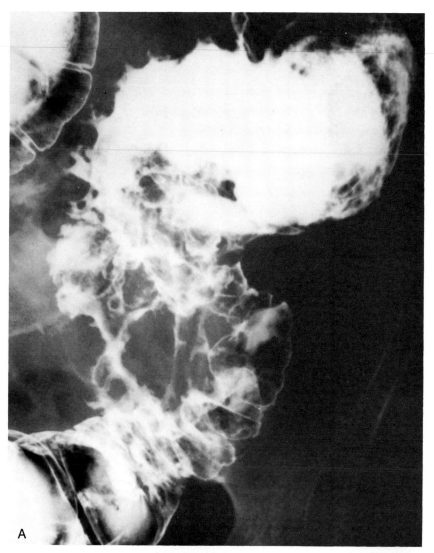

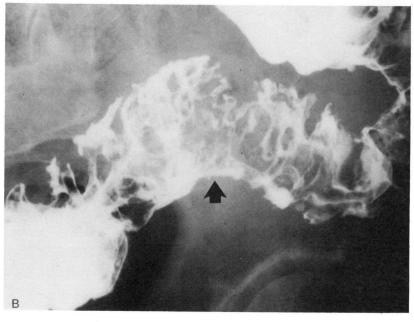

FIGURE 16–21

**CROHN'S COLITIS COMPLICATING
DIVERTICULAR DISEASE.** *A*, Multiple
dissecting fistulous tracts are present in the
sigmoid. Many of the diverticula show ulcers
and tracks, owing to involvement of their
mucosa by Crohn's disease.

B, A second example of intramural tracking
(arrow) in a patient with diverticulitis due to
Crohn's disease.

DIFFERENTIAL DIAGNOSIS

Polyps and Cancer

The main diagnostic difficulty in patients with diverticular disease lies in the differentiation between a polyp and a diverticulum and between a diverticular abscess and a carcinoma of the colon. These distinctions have been previously discussed.

Aphthoid Ulcers

When diverticula are extremely small and are seen en face, they may be difficult to distinguish from aphthoid ulcers in Crohn's disease (Fig. 16–22). In most instances, however, the distinction is not difficult, because the surrounding inflammatory reaction is lacking in patients with diverticular disease, so there is no halo around the barium pool, which is

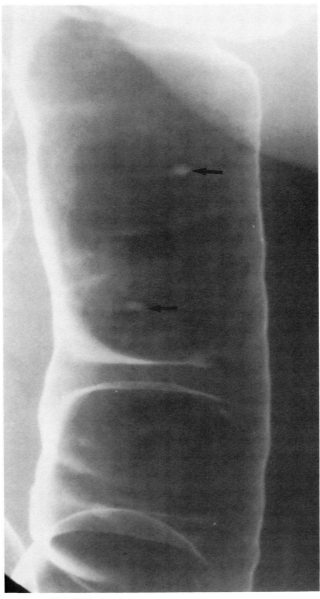

FIGURE 16–22

Tiny diverticula (arrows) simulating aphthoid ulcers.

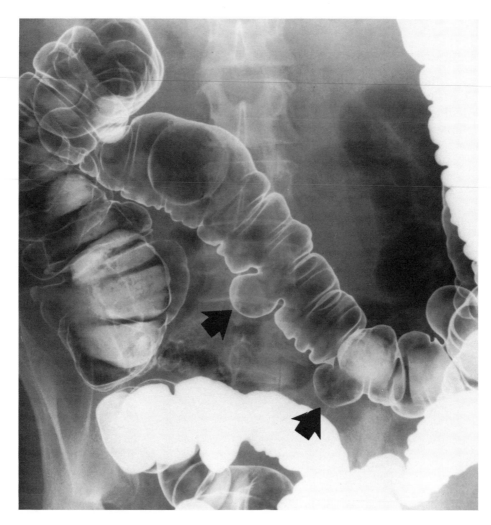

FIGURE 16–23

Wide-mouthed diverticula or sacculations (*arrows*) along the transverse colon in a patient with scleroderma.

also well defined compared with the irregular barium coating on the slough of an aphthoid ulcer.

Scleroderma

Involvement of the colon in scleroderma is characterized by wide-mouth diverticula or sacculations (Fig. 16–23).[48] These lesions are easily distinguished from those of ordinary diverticulosis because the lesions of scleroderma involve the colon proximal to the sigmoid colon and are not associated with narrowing or muscle hypertrophy.

ACKNOWLEDGMENT

We are grateful to Dr. Basil C. Morson of the Department of Pathology, St. Mark's Hospital, London, for supplying the specimen photographs for this chapter.

REFERENCES

1. Manousos, O.N., Truelove, S.C., and Lumsden, K.: Prevalence of colonic diverticulosis in the general population of Oxford area. Br. Med J. 3:762, 1967.
2. Hughes, L.E.: Postmortem survey of diverticular disease of the colon. Gut 10:336, 1969.
3. Hughes, L.E.: Complications of diverticular disease: Inflammation, obstruction and bleeding. Clin. Gastroenterol. 4:147, 1975.
4. Parks, T.G.: Natural history of diverticular disease of the colon. Clin. Gastroenterol. 4:53, 1975.
5. Morson, B.C.: The muscle abnormality in diverticular disease of the sigmoid colon. Br. J. Radiol. 36:385, 1963.
6. White-Way, J., and Morson, B.C.: Elastosis in diverticular disease of the sigmoid colon. Gut 26:258, 1985.
7. Marcus, R., and Watt, J.: The radiological appearances of diverticula in the anti-mesenteric intertaenial area of the pelvic colon. Clin. Radiol. 16:87, 1965.
8. Zollinger, R.W.: The prognosis of diverticulitis of the colon. Arch. Surg. 97:418, 1968.
9. Lloyd-Williams, K.: Acute solitary ulcers and acute diverticulitis of the cecum and ascending colon. Br. J. Surg. 47:351, 1960.
10. Massik, P., and Wheatley, F.E.: The recognition of air in

diverticula of the colon as a diagnostic aid. Radiology 64:417, 1955.

11. Williams, I.: Changing emphasis in diverticular disease of the colon. Br. J. Radiol. 36:393, 1963.

12. Spriggs, E.I., and Marter, O.A.: Intestinal diverticula. Q. J. Med. 19:1, 1925.

13. Welin, S., and Welin, G.: The Double Contrast Examination of the Colon: Experiences With the Welin Modification. Stuttgart, Georg Thieme Verlag, 1976.

14. Williams, I.: Diverticular disease of the colon without diverticula. Radiology 89:401, 1967.

15. Rawlinson, J., and Brunton, F.J.: Transient diverticula of the colon. Br. J. Radiol. 62:27, 1989.

16. Lappas, J.C., Maglinte, D.D.T., Kopecky, K.K., et al.: Diverticular disease: Imaging with post–double-contrast sigmoid flush. Radiology 168:35, 1988.

17. Freeny, P.C., and Walker, J.H.: Inverted diverticula of the gastrointestinal tract. Gastrointest. Radiol. 4:57, 1979.

18. Meyers, M.A.: Dynamic Radiology of the Abdomen: Normal and Pathologic Anatomy. New York, Springer-Verlag, 1988, p. 311.

19. Fleischer, F.G., and Ming, S.C.: Revised concepts on diverticular disease of the colon. II. So-called diverticulitis; diverticular sigmoiditis and perisigmoiditis; diverticular abscess, fistula, and frank peritonitis. Radiology 84:599, 1965.

20. Chennells, P.M., and Simpkins, K.C.: The barium enema diagnosis of pericolic abscess. Clin. Radiol. 32:73, 1981.

21. Marshak, R.H., Lindner, A.E., and Maklansky, D.: Diverticulosis and diverticulitis of the colon. Mt. Sinai J. Med. 46:261, 1979.

22. Johnson, C.D., Baker, M.E., Rice, R.P., et al.: Diagnosis of acute colonic diverticulitis: Comparison of barium enema and CT. AJR 148:541, 1987.

23. Balthazar, E.J., Megibow, A., Schinella, R.A., and Gordon, R.: Limitations in the CT diagnosis of acute diverticulitis: Comparison of CT, contrast enema, and pathologic findings in 16 patients. AJR 154:281, 1990.

24. Small, W.P., and Smith, A.N.: Fistula and conditions associated with diverticular disease of the colon. Clin. Gastroenterol. 4:176, 1975.

25. Casarella, W.J., Kantor, I.E., and Seaman, W.B.: Right-sided colonic diverticula as a cause of acute rectal hemorrhage. N. Engl. J. Med. 286:450, 1972.

26. Meyers, M.A., Alonso, D.R., Gray, G.F., et al.: Pathogenesis of bleeding colonic diverticulosis. Gastroenterology 71:577, 1976.

27. Brodey, P.A., Hill, R.P., and Baron, S.: Benign ulceration of the cecum. Radiology 122:323, 1977.

28. Dawson, J.R., Lieber, A., and Simmons, T.: Rectal diverticula. Radiology 84:610, 1976.

29. Muhletaler, C.A., Berger, J., and Robinette, C.L.: Pathogenesis of giant colonic diverticula. Gastrointest. Radiol. 6:217, 1981.

30. Kricun, R., Stark, J.J., Reither, R.D., and Dex, W.J.: Giant colonic diverticulum. AJR 135:507, 1980.

31. Wada, M., Kikuchi, Y., and Doy, M.: Uncomplicated acute diverticulitis of the cecum and ascending colon: Sonographic findings in 18 patients. AJR 155:283, 1990.

32. Williams, C.B., Hunt, R.H., and Loose, H.: Colonoscopy in the management of colon polyps. Br. J. Surg. 61:673, 1974.

33. Youker, J.E., and Welin, S.: Differentiation of true polypoid lesions of the colon from extraneous material, a new roentgen sign. Radiology 84:610, 1965.

34. Miller, W.T., Levine, M.S., Rubesin, S.E., and Laufer, I.: Bowler-hat sign: A simple principle for differentiating polyps from diverticula. Radiology 173:615, 1989.

35. Keller, K.C., Halpert, R.D., Feczko, P.J., and Simons, S.M.: Radiologic recognition of colonic diverticula simulating polyps. AJR 143:93, 1984.

36. Htoo, A.M., and Bartram, C.I.: The radiological diagnosis of polyps in the presence of diverticular disease. Br. J. Radiol. 52:263, 1979.

37. Schatzki, R.: The roentgenologic differential diagnosis between cancer and diverticulitis. Radiology 34:651, 1940.

38. Colcock, B.P., and Sass, R.E.: Diverticulitis and carcinoma of the colon: Differential diagnosis. Surg. Gynecol. Obstet. 99:627, 1954.

39. Beranbaum, S.L., Yaghmai, M., and Beranbaum, E.R.: Ulcerative colitis in association with diverticular disease of the colon. Radiology 85:880, 1965.

40. Jalan, K.N., Walker, R.J., Prescott, R.J., et al.: Fecal stasis and diverticular disease in ulcerative colitis. Gut 11:688, 1970.

41. Bates, T., and Kaminsky, V.: Diverticulitis and ulcerative colitis. Br. J. Surg. 61:293, 1974.

42. Schmidt, G.T., Lennard-Jones, J.E., and Morson, B.C.: Crohn's disease of the colon and its distinction from diverticulitis. Gut 9:7, 1968.

43. Laufer, I., and Costopoulos, L.: Early lesions of Crohn's disease. AJR 130:307, 1978.

44. Meyers, M.A., Alonso, D.R., Morson, B.C., et al.: Pathogenesis of diverticulitis complicating granulomatous colitis. Gastroenterology 74:24, 1978.

45. Marshak, R.H., Janowitz, H.D., and Present, D.H.: Granulomatous colitis in association with diverticula. N. Engl. J. Med. 283:1080, 1970.

46. Loeb, P.M., Berk, R.N., and Saltzstein, S.L.: Longitudinal fistula of the colon in diverticulitis. Gastroenterology 67:720, 1974.

47. Ferrucci, J.T., Ragsdale, B.D., and Barrett, P.J.: Double tracking of the sigmoid colon. Radiology 120:307, 1976.

48. Cohen, S., Laufer, I., Snape, W.J., et al.: The gastrointestinal manifestations of scleroderma: Pathogenesis and management. Gastroenterology 79:155, 1980.

INFLAMMATORY BOWEL DISEASE

17

Clive I. Bartram, F.R.C.P., F.R.C.R.
Igor Laufer, M.D.

The definitive diagnosis of colitis ultimately depends on the histologic findings, but the macroscopic view of the mucosa and the overall configuration of the bowel remain important for mapping the extent and severity of the colitis, for predicting the most likely cause, and for showing any complication.[1] The double contrast image provides the finest radiographic detail of the mucosal surface and has been clearly demonstrated to be superior to single contrast studies in the detection of early changes.[2] Distention pressures of single and double contrast examinations are the same, so that there is no contraindication to double contrast examination in patients with colitis. Gentleness and regard for patient comfort are particularly important in these patients. Depending on the activity of the disease, some modification of the bowel preparation may be required.

RADIOGRAPHIC TECHNIQUE

Double Contrast Enema (DCE)

Most patients with inflammatory bowel disease may be examined with the standard technique of double contrast enema (DCE), which is described in Chapter 12. It may be dangerous, however, and it is certainly most unpleasant for a patient with active colitis, and a bowel frequency of up to 20 times per day, to be given a routine full bowel preparation. This procedure should be modified according to the patient's clinical condition. The patient may be given clear fluids for a day and then may be given a cleansing tap water enema. Bisacodyl tannex (Clysodrast) should not be added to cleansing solution. Mild laxatives may be used if the patient has only a few bowel actions per day.[3]

Instant Enema

In many patients with active colitis, sufficient information may be obtained without resorting to any bowel preparation. The instant enema was developed by Young for just this purpose (Fig. 17–1).[4] The instant enema is a double contrast examination of the affected colon, obtained without bowel preparation or any modification to the patient's therapy. This procedure is possible because fecal residue does not build up adjacent to areas of active mucosal disease. The presence of exudate and spasm combined with the loss of normal reabsorptive capacity result in the clearance of fecal residue from the diseased colon. In ulcerative colitis, as the rectum and colon involved are in continuity, double contrast views of the affected bowel free from residue may be obtained.[6] Such images may not be obtainable in Crohn's disease, in which the colitis may be patchy.

Preliminary radiography may be performed initially to exclude perforation or toxic megacolon and to show the extent of the residue. The barium suspension, which is usually about 80%, is run into the splenic flexure or is run until fecal residue is encountered. The rectum is drained, and then gas, preferably carbon dioxide, is insufflated with rotation of the patient to coat and distend the involved colon. It is important to remember to fill the colon gently, particularly in patients with active distal disease and urgency, who are extremely intolerant of rectal filling. Smooth muscle relaxants improve distention, although they are not always required. There are references to smooth muscle relaxants precipitating toxic megacolon,[7] but these references are to long-acting atropine-like agents, and the current short-acting agents such as glucagon probably involve little danger.

Often, only a single prone view is required (see Fig. 17–1A). A lateral view of the rectum is useful in providing a more complete perspective of the rectal volume, particularly in patients in whom an ileorectal anastomosis may be considered. An erect view shows the transverse colon and flexures in double contrast (see Fig. 17–1B).

Advantages of the instant enema are its simplicity, comfort, and safety for the patient as well as its minimal radiation dose, allowing it to be repeated as necessary. About 10,000 such examinations have been performed at St. Mark's Hospital, and in only one or two isolated cases has there been the suggestion of clinical deterioration after the study. In the appropriate clinical setting, the instant enema provides a unique record of the colitis that is simple to refer to and easy to compare.[8] The decision to perform colectomy is often a difficult management issue, and the ability to discuss a case with the documentation provided by the instant enema can be most helpful.

Indications

The instant enema may be used in a variety of situations: when the upper limit of inflammation cannot be seen during sigmoidoscopy; when a patient has severe diarrhea; when a patient has acute bleeding that may be due to ischemia, and when a patient has Crohn's disease with severe anal involvement. The instant enema may provide sufficient information for diagnosis, but should it fail for technical reasons, the patient can simply be rescheduled for a formal DCE after suitable bowel preparation.

The main purposes of the instant enema apply to patients with known colitis, particularly ulcerative colitis, and are as follows:

1. To map the extent and severity of the colitis.

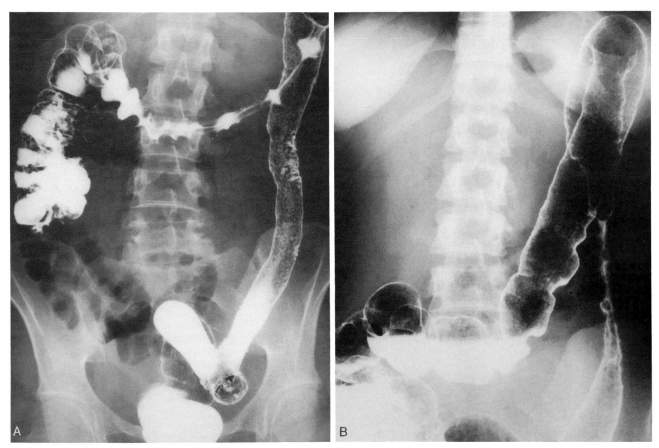

FIGURE 17–1

INSTANT ENEMA IN ULCERATIVE COLITIS. A, *In the prone view, the transverse colon is compressed and dependent, so that gaseous distention is poor. There is a granular mucosa in the descending colon with some areas of superficial ulceration, but the extent of the colitis is not clear.*

B, An erect view provides good double contrast images of the flexures and the transverse colon, confirming that the colitis is extensive.

2. To monitor the progress of the disease, for example, when the patient fails to respond to medical treatment.

3. To show the extent and severity of disease accurately in an acute attack in which the plain film is ambiguous.

Contraindications

Absolute contraindications to the instant enema include the following:

1. Toxic megacolon or perforation. The plain film should be diagnostic for these conditions. If for any reason a contrast examination is required, it should be a single contrast study in which a water-soluble contrast agent is used.

2. The search for complicating malignancy. Bowel preparation is essential to obtain the optimum overall view of the mucosa to detect early lesions.

Relative contraindications include the following:

1. Cases in which the information from the plain film is adequate for immediate clinical management.

2. Mild cases that involve diagnostic uncertainty regarding the presence of colitis or of its nature. In such mild cases, a full DCE after bowel preparation gives the maximal information regarding the state of the mucosa.

ULCERATIVE COLITIS

In the uncomplicated state, the inflammatory changes of ulcerative colitis are limited to the mucosa and are accompanied by a considerable increase in vascularity.[9] The disease invariably starts in the rectum, where it may remain as proctitis or may spread proximally to involve the colon to varying degrees. The mucosal disease is characterized by a granular mucosa with a confluent symmetric distribution.[10] Patients present with diarrhea, frequency, urgency, tenesmus, rectal bleeding, and general ill health of either sudden or gradual onset. The disease is often most severe during the first year, and approximately 5% to 10% of patients require urgent surgery during the initial attack. In an acute attack, the majority of the colon may be ulcerated, but with remission the colon may return to normal (Fig. 17–2), although histologic examination often shows a persistent abnormality with flat, chronic atrophic mucosa. The disease may be characterized by episodes of exacerbation and remission, or it may remain at a lower level of chronic activity.

The following terms are often used in the discussion of inflammatory bowel disease. *Proctitis* refers to inflammation limited to the rectum (Fig. 17–3A). *Proctosigmoiditis* refers to inflammation limited to the rectum and sigmoid. Approximately 10% of patients with proctitis or proctosigmoiditis develop more extensive disease.[11] *Distal colitis* refers to cases that involve the distal colon to the level of the left iliac crest (Fig. 17–3B). *Extensive colitis* refers to macroscopic involvement extending at least to the hepatic flexure. It has been found that in most such cases, the entire colon is involved histologically, and that this type of total colitis is a significant risk factor for the development of colitic carcinoma.[12]

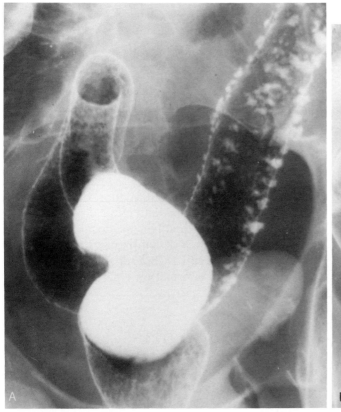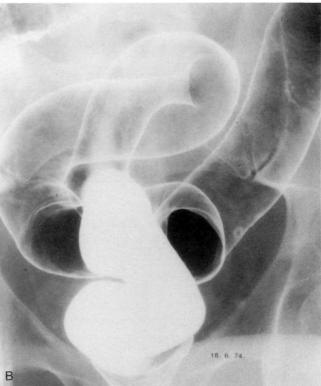

FIGURE 17–2

EXTENSIVE ULCERATION IN ULCERATIVE COLITIS WITH REMISSION. *A*, During the acute attack, there is a granular appearance of the sigmoid colon and deep ulceration in the descending colon.

B, Several months later, after medical treatment, there is complete remission with an apparently normal, flat mucosal surface.

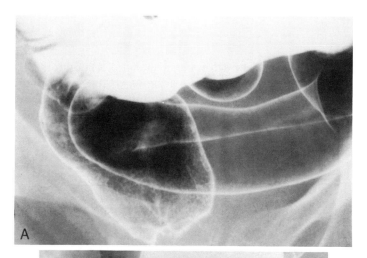

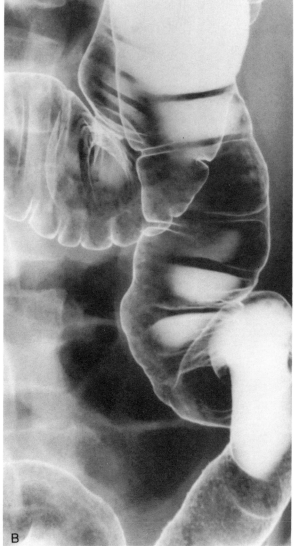

FIGURE 17–3

LOCALIZED FORMS OF COLITIS. *A*, Ulcerative proctitis with inflammation limited to the rectum. Note the normal appearance of the sigmoid.

B, Distal colitis with inflammation involving the sigmoid. Note the transition at the level of the left iliac crest from diseased sigmoid to normal descending colon.

Mucosal Changes

Granularity

The normal mucosal surface of the colon as seen with the DCE is smooth and featureless (Fig. 17–4A). The earliest change seen in ulcerative colitis is a fine granular appearance due to edema and hyperemia (Fig. 17–4B). As the disease progresses, the mucosal surface breaks down into superficial erosions. Barium adheres to these erosions, producing a stippled appearance (Fig. 17–4C). With healing of the mucosal surface, a coarse granular appearance is seen (Fig. 17–4D).[13, 14]

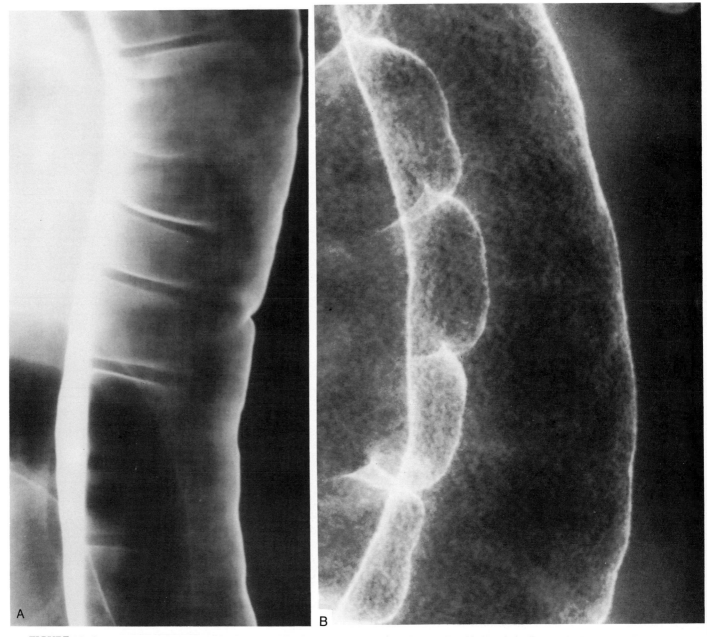

A

B

FIGURE 17–4

THE EVOLUTION OF MUCOSAL CHANGES IN ULCERATIVE COLITIS. *A,* The normal colonic mucosa with a smooth, featureless appearance.

B, The earliest change with fine granularity of the mucosal surface. (From Laufer, I., et al.: Correlation of endoscopy and double contrast radiography in the early stages of ulcerative and granulomatous colitis. Radiology *118:*1–6, 1976, with permission.)

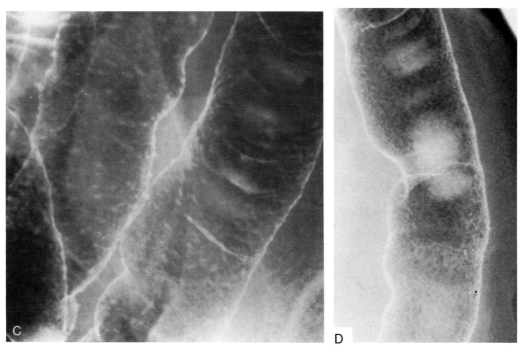

FIGURE 17–4 *Continued*

C, A stippled appearance due to superficial erosions.

D, Coarse granular appearance in chronic ulcerative colitis. *(D,* From Laufer, I.: Air contrast studies of the colon in inflammatory bowel disease. CRC Crit. Rev. Diagnost. Imaging 9:421, 1977, with permission.)

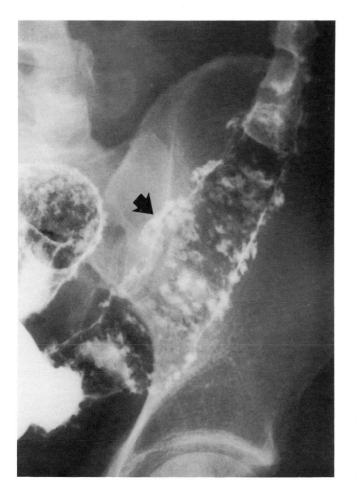

Ulceration

Ulceration develops as the result of patchy sloughing of the mucosal membrane. The ulcers may have a linear configuration that often follows the line of the teniae, forming a "collar stud" configuration (Fig. 17–5). Unlike granularity, ulceration is clearly defined in profile. Disruption of the mucosal line is the key to the presence of ulceration and allows its distinction from the en face appearance of coarse granularity.[13] Sometimes, the ulceration may extend longitudinally under the mucosa for several centimeters, creating the so-called double tracking sign (Fig. 17–5). The important point is that ulceration on a background of diffuse granularity is characteristic of ulcerative colitis (Fig. 17–6). This feature can be appreciated both on radiographs of the colon and on appropriately prepared surgical specimens (Fig. 17–7). The presence of ulceration is important, as it implies a severe attack both clinically and pathologically.

FIGURE 17–5

ULCERATION WITH DOUBLE TRACKING IN SEVERE ULCERATIVE COLITIS. An instant enema shows ulceration with "collar stud" ulcers and double tracking *(arrow)* in a patient with acute exacerbation of distal ulcerative colitis.

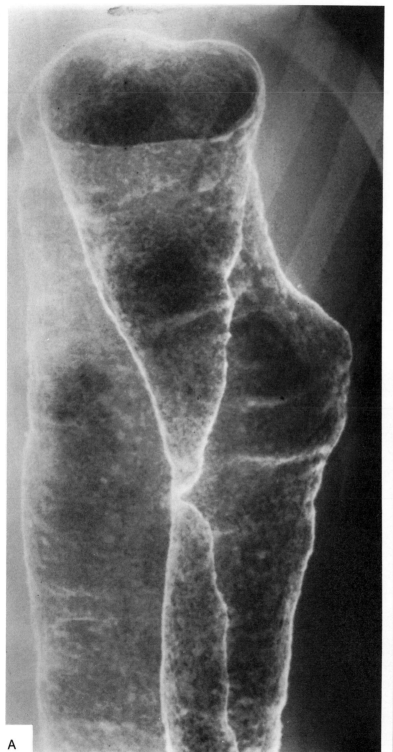

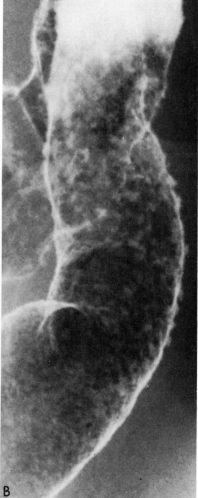

FIGURE 17–6

A through *C,* Three examples of ulceration on a background of granular mucosa. Although the appearance of the ulcers is nonspecific, the background granularity is characteristic of ulcerative as opposed to granulomatous colitis.

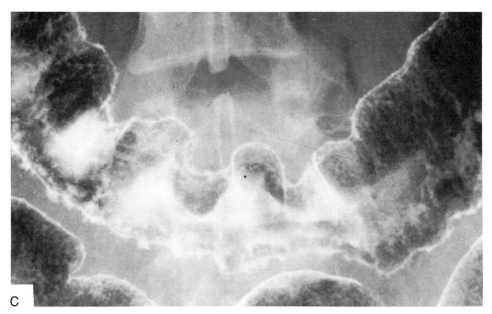

C

FIGURE 17–6 Continued

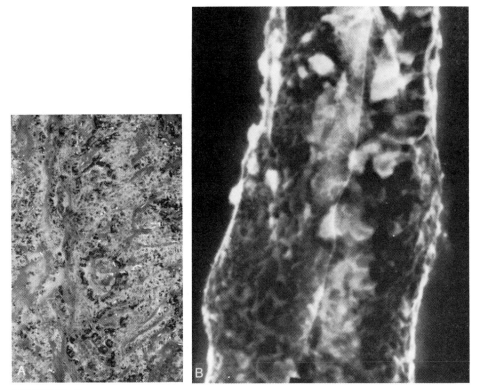

FIGURE 17–7

Pathologic photograph (A) and radiograph (B) of ulceration on a background of diffusely granular mucosa in ulcerative colitis. The ulcers are seen in profile and en face as amorphous collections of barium. The specimen has been lightly coated with barium to highlight the ulcers and the granularity of the mucosa.

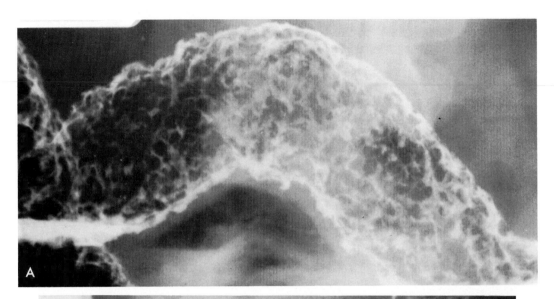

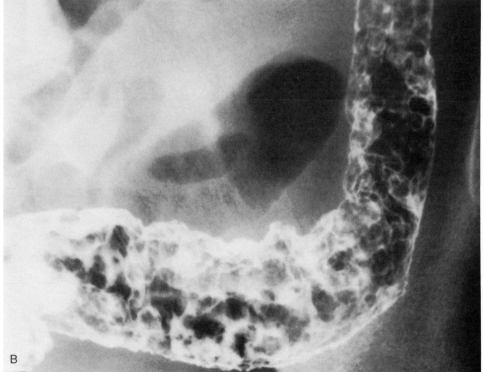

FIGURE 17–8

A and *B*, Extensive mucosal ulceration with inflamed mucosal remnants resulting in pseudopolyposis.

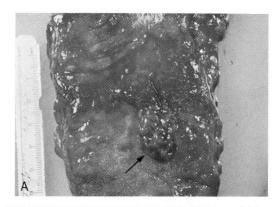

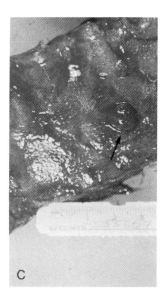

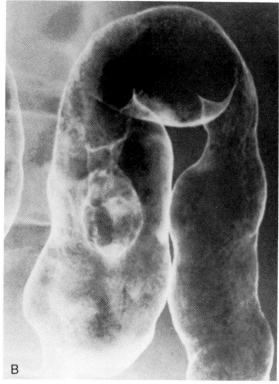

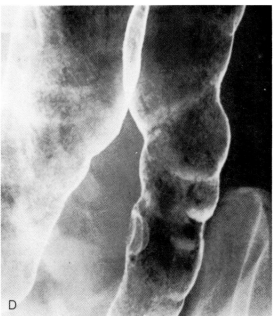

Polypoid Changes

There are three causes of polypoid change in ulcerative colitis, each of which is related to a different underlying pathologic process.

When ulceration is extensive, the mucosal remnants appear polypoid, and the "mucosal line" may be intact, but because so much mucosa has been lost, the mucosal line is formed not from the mucosal surface but from the muscle base, with swollen inflamed residual mucosa projecting above this. However, a polyp is by definition elevated above the mucosa, so that this condition is correctly termed *pseudopolyposis* (Fig. 17–8).[15]

Polypoid masses of inflammatory granulation tissue may develop with active disease. These *inflammatory polyps* can be solitary or multiple and are seen against a background of granular mucosa (Fig. 17–9).

FIGURE 17–9

Endoscopic photographs (A and C) and radiographs (B and D) of two inflammatory polyps in a patient with minimally active ulcerative colitis, as evidenced by the granular appearance of the mucosa.

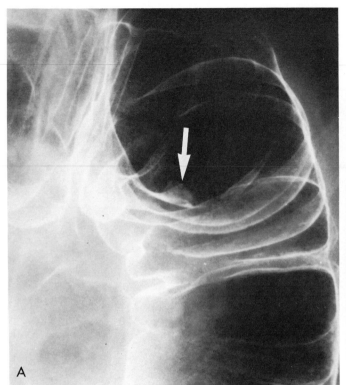

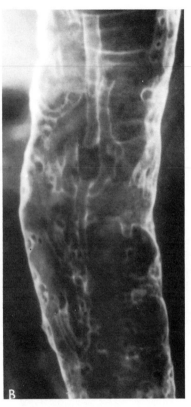

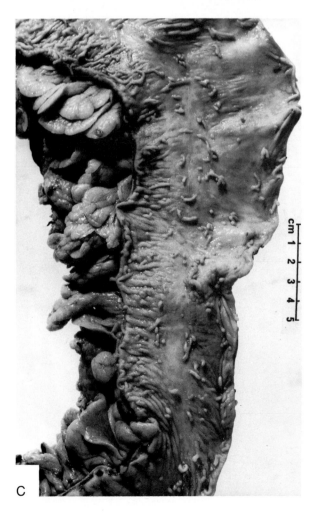

FIGURE 17–10

POSTINFLAMMATORY POLYPS. *A,* A small sessile polyp *(arrow)* at the splenic flexure in a patient with a history of acute ulcerative colitis. Note that the mucosa now has a smooth appearance, indicating that the disease is quiescent.

B, Filiform polyposis in a patient with a history of acute ulcerative colitis. (*A* and *B,* From Bartram, C.I.: Radiology in the current assessment of ulcerative colitis. Gastrointest. Radiol. 1:383, 1977, with permission.)

C, The resected specimen shows a normal mucosa with postinflammatory polyps.

During an acute attack, the undermining ulceration creates a flap of mucosa. This flap may persist as the ulcer base heals with granulation tissue. Although the mucosa may otherwise heal completely and the bowel may return to a normal configuration, these mucosal tags remain as markers of the sites of ulceration. The tags may be sessile or frond-like, reflecting the configuration of the ulceration (Fig. 17–10). This condition is most appropriately termed *postinflammatory polyposis,* and it is seen in about 10% to 20% of patients.[16] The tags may be single or multiple, segmental or diffuse. The polyps vary from small sessile lesions to long frond-like outgrowths, which are termed *filiform polyps* (Fig. 17–11).[17] This morphologic appearance is found only in postinflammatory polyposis and enables a confident radiologic diagnosis to be made. Where undercutting ulcers have

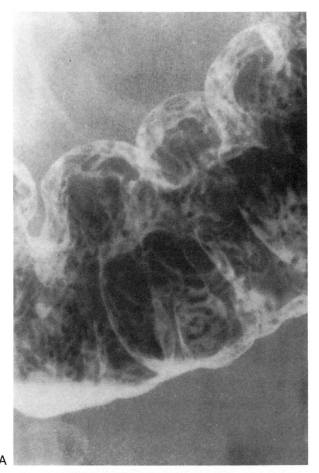

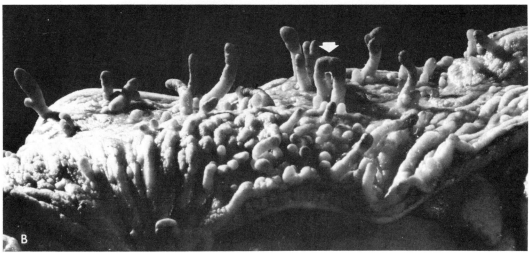

FIGURE 17–11

POSTINFLAMMATORY POLYPOSIS. *A,* A mass of frondlike inflammatory polyps on a background of normal mucosa. *B,* The resected specimen viewed tangentially shows the fronds, some of which are adherent to each other, forming mucosal bridges *(arrow).* (From Morson, B.C.: The Pathogenesis of Colorectal Cancer. Philadelphia, W.B. Saunders, 1978, with permission.)

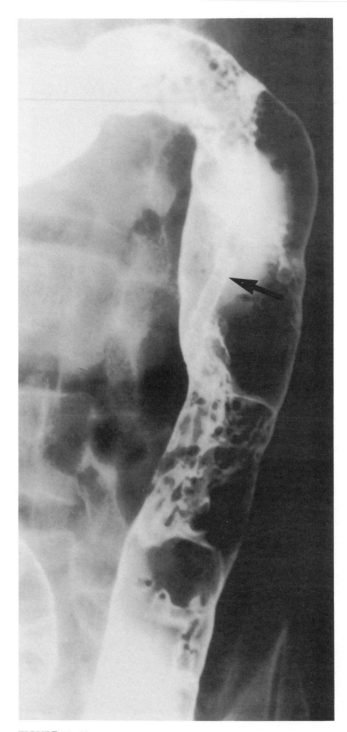

FIGURE 17–12

Mucosal bridging (*arrow*) in ulcerative colitis.

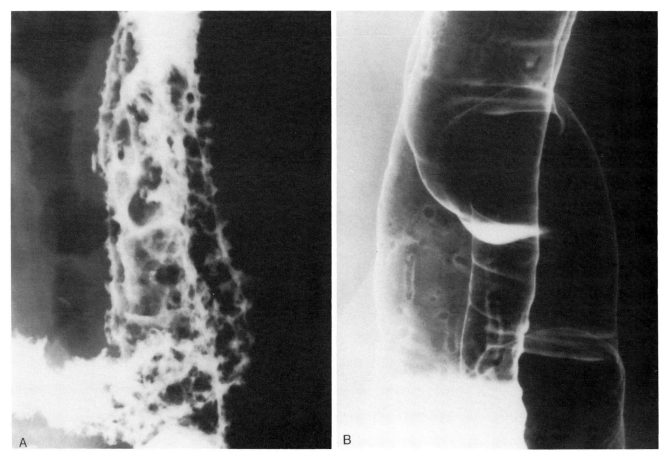

FIGURE 17–13

DEVELOPMENT OF FILIFORM POLYPOSIS. *A*, An acute episode of ulcerative colitis shows extensive, confluent ulceration in the region of the splenic flexure.

 B, Eight years later, the colitis is in remission, and multiple filiform polyps are seen at the site of the previous ulcers.

coalesced, a "mucosal bridge" may be left (Fig. 17–12).[18] Usually, these polyps are of no clinical significance other than being indicators of a previous severe attack.[19] Obstruction is rarely encountered, and these polyps are not premalignant. Figure 17–13 shows the transition from an acute episode of ulcerative colitis to filiform polyposis.

The only diagnostic problem is distinguishing isolated polyps (inflammatory or postinflammatory) from adenomas, or even carcinomas. Solitary large inflammatory polyps may cause diagnostic problems.[20] Recognition of a filiform component and of pliability of the lesion support an inflammatory origin. Adenomas may have a lobulated surface and a stalk, both of which are uncommon in inflammatory polyps. When doubt arises, endoscopic excision and histologic examination are required.

Rectum and Retrorectal Space

The rectum is almost always involved in the initial attack of ulcerative colitis, although the severity of rectal disease may be less than the severity of the proximal disease. In addition to the typical granular appearance (Fig. 17–14*A*), there may be thickening of the rectal folds, or valves of Houston, to greater than 7 mm (Fig. 17–14*B*).[21] With chronic disease, they become obliterated.[22] These changes are associated with widening of the retrorectal space to greater than 1 cm when measured at the level of S4 (Fig. 17–14).[23]

Following treatment, or with multiple episodes of exacerbation and remission of the disease, the rectum may appear normal despite evidence of proximal disease. This normal appearance reflects the variation in the rate of healing of various parts of the colon (Fig. 17–15). With chronic disease, the rectum may

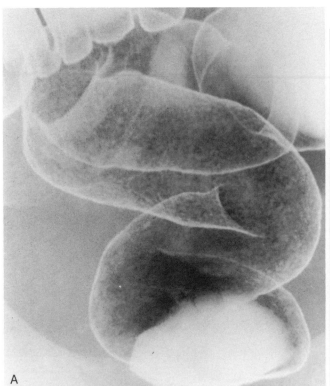

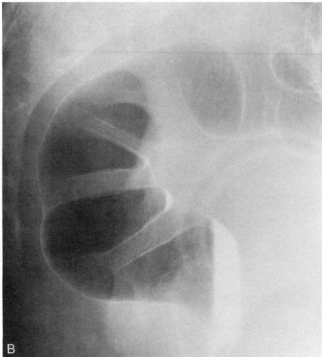

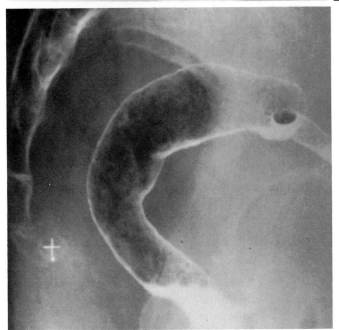

FIGURE 17–14

THE RECTUM IN ULCERATIVE COLITIS. A, Typical appearance with granular mucosa.

B, Thickening of the valves of Houston in active proctitis.

C, Chronic ulcerative colitis with narrowing of the rectum, obliteration of the valves of Houston, and an increase in the retrorectal space. (From Laufer, I.: Air contrast studies of the colon in inflammatory bowel disease. CRC Crit. Rev. Diagnost. Imaging 9:421, 1977, with permission.)

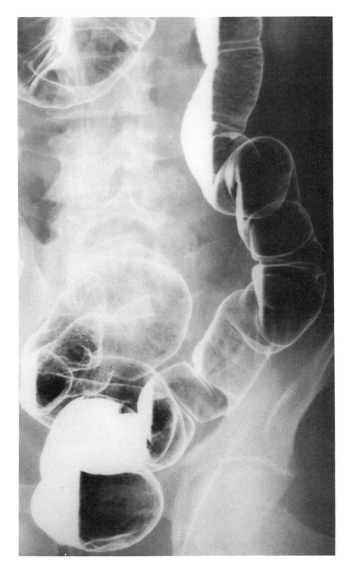

FIGURE 17–15

RECTAL SPARING AND THE APPEARANCE OF A SKIP LESION DUE TO ASYMMETRIC HEALING. In this patient with ulcerative colitis, granular mucosa is seen in the rectum and in the proximal descending colon. The rectum appears spared, and the distal descending colon appears normal. The appearance of rectal sparing and a skip lesion are due to variations in healing in various segments of the bowel.

become narrowed with a reduced volume. Functionally, this change is important because these patients suffer from urgency and frequency.

Terminal Ileum

The terminal ileum is normal in the large majority of patients with ulcerative colitis (Fig. 17–16). However, involvement of the terminal ileum has been found in 10% of colectomies for ulcerative colitis (Fig. 17–

17).[24] Involvement is confined to a range of 5 to 25 cm of the terminal ileum. Characteristic features are dilatation, absent peristalsis, and a granular mucosa (Fig. 17–18). Discrete ulceration is not seen in "backwash ileitis" that is due to ulcerative colitis. When present, it usually indicates that the abnormalities are the result of Crohn's disease.

The ileocecal valve is usually dilated and incompetent. The exact reason for this change is unknown. It may be due to backwash of colonic contents through

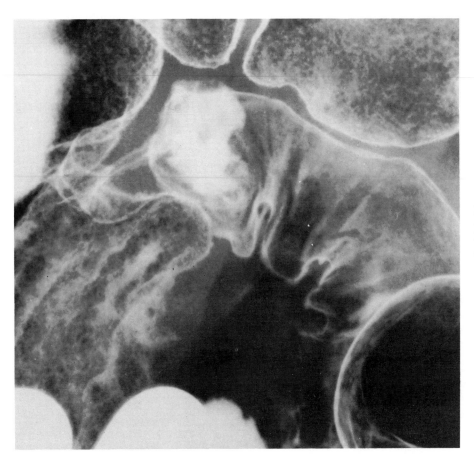

FIGURE 17–16

Normal terminal ileum in a patient with extensive involvement of the entire colon by ulcerative colitis.

FIGURE 17–17

CHRONIC ULCERATIVE COLITIS WITH "BACKWASH" ILEITIS. There are changes of long-standing total colitis with granular mucosa and loss of haustration. There are a few inflammatory polyps in the distal descending colon. The ileocecal valve is patulous, and the terminal ileum is dilated.

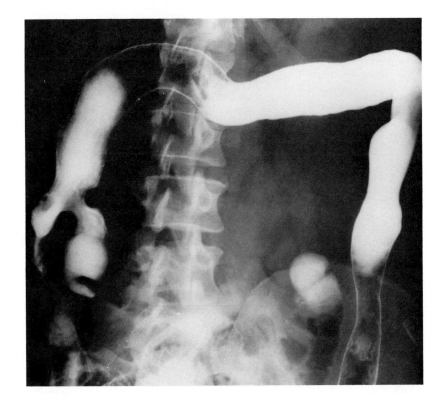

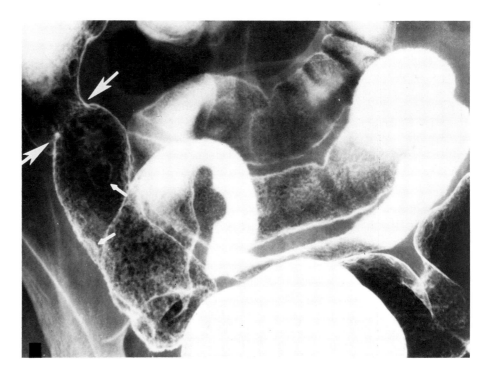

FIGURE 17-18

EXTENSIVE BACKWASH ILEITIS.
The ileocecal valve *(large arrows)* is patulous, and the mucosa of the distal small bowel has the granular appearance characteristic of the colon in ulcerative colitis. In addition, there are inflammatory polyps *(small arrows)* in the terminal ileum.

an incompetent valve. However, pathologic changes in the ileum have been found to precede incompetence of the valve.[24] Reflux ileitis is always associated with total colitis, which is usually of long-standing, low-grade activity. Clinically, reflux ileitis is of little significance except that it confirms the presence of total colitis. Ileostomies may be fashioned from the ileum, and mucosal changes rapidly revert to normal once the colon has been removed.

Reflux ileitis tends to be overdiagnosed when the single contrast enema is used. Reflux of colonic contents into the terminal ileum may produce an indistinct mucosal outline, which may be mistaken for mucosal inflammation. Sellink has shown that with the small bowel enteroclysis technique, the terminal ileum can be washed out, and a normal appearance can be produced.[25]

These secondary changes are useful indicators of the presence of ulcerative colitis in patients who have been treated with steroid enemas resulting in rectal healing.

SECONDARY CHANGES

Haustration

As with the rectal folds, blunting of the haustra is an early change with inflammation. The haustra are normally seen as thin parallel lines that are about 2 mm apart. Broadening of the haustra is a useful supplementary sign of active disease should the mucosal coating be equivocal (Fig. 17-19). With more active colitis, the haustra become obliterated and are

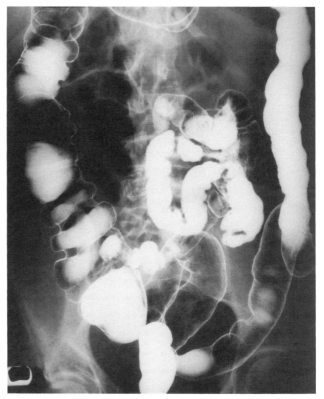

FIGURE 17-19

HAUSTRAL CHANGES. In this patient with minimally active ulcerative colitis, the haustral folds on the right side of the colon are abnormally widened and blunted.

never present in ulcerative colitis with ulceration. It is important to remember that the left hemicolon may be devoid of haustration normally, so that as an isolated finding, loss of haustration in the descending colon is not evidence of colitis. If haustration alone is considered, only changes in the colon proximal to the mid–transverse colon can therefore be considered abnormal. In practice, when the mucosal changes are minimal, loss of haustration in the proximal colon is useful supplementary evidence in confirming that the patient has total active colitis.

Configurational Change

The configuration of the colon also undergoes a generalized change, becoming narrowed and shortened with depression of the flexures. Typically, such a colon is also without haustration or has a widened postrectal space and a minimally granular mucosa, giving it a "pipe stem" appearance. These characteristic changes are found in long-standing total colitis of chronic activity (see Fig. 17–18A). The secondary changes mirror the primary mucosal abnormality, so that with regression of the disease, the colon can revert to an entirely normal appearance (Fig. 17–20).

Diagnostic Accuracy

The accuracy of the examination refers to its ability to show the extent and severity of the mucosal abnormality. In general, the radiologic findings have correlated closely with the gross appearance of the resected specimen.[3] However, radiology tends to underestimate the extent of involvement as judged by histology. Total colitis was found histologically in almost every case in which the disease appeared radiographically to extend only to the hepatic flexure.[13] This finding supports the use of the term extensive colitis to describe colitis that extends radiologically to the hepatic flexure, implying that the whole colon is affected histologically.[12] The reason for this underestimation is probably twofold. First, in the unprepared colon, any residue is pushed into the proximal colon and obscures mucosal detail. Second, the transition from abnormal to normal is usually not abrupt, but gradual.

Microscopic, Collagenous, and Minimal Change Colitis

In the relatively rare disorders of microscopic, collagenous, and minimal change colitis, patients present

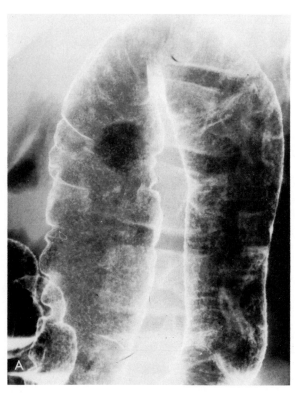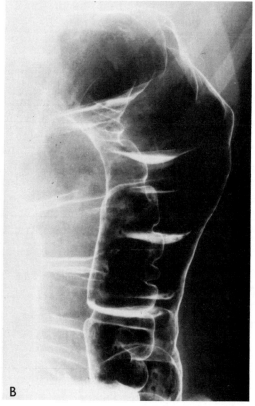

FIGURE 17–20

REVERSIBILITY OF THE HAUSTRAL CHANGES. A, Active ulcerative colitis, with stippling of the mucosa and loss of haustration.
  B, In remission, the mucosa is flat, and the haustra have returned.

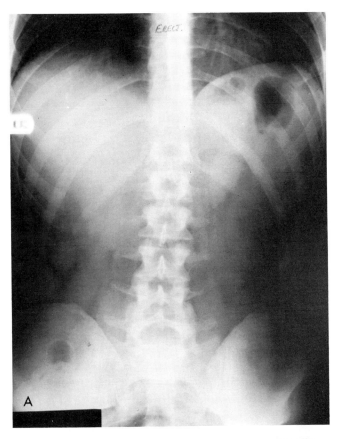

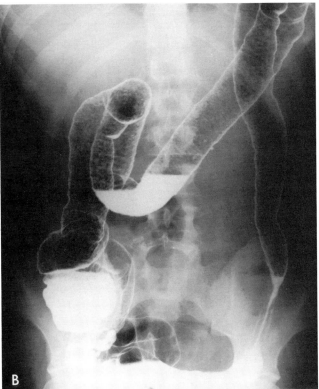

FIGURE 17–21

TOTAL COLITIS. A, On the plain film, there is no evidence of fecal residue, which suggests total colitis.

B, This diagnosis is confirmed by the instant enema, which shows diffuse granularity and ulceration throughout the entire colon.

with chronic large-volume watery diarrhea. The mucosa may appear normal macroscopically, although loss of vascular pattern and of friability has been reported in 20% of patients undergoing colonoscopy, and there is one report of nodularity detected by DCE.[26] The diagnosis is based on biopsy. In microscopic colitis, there are diffuse inflammatory changes extending into the lamina propria, whereas in collagenous colitis, there is a thick subepithelial deposit of collagen. The rectum is usually involved, so that rectal biopsy should be diagnostic.

Minimal change colitis describes colitis, usually ulcerative, in which the mucosal change is minimal, so that results of the DCE may appear entirely normal.[27] In a large review of patients with colitis, only 8 cases were found in which results of the DCE and sigmoidoscopy were normal but colonoscopy detected widespread minimal colitis. In all cases, rectal biopsy results were abnormal.

These conditions emphasize the value of rectal biopsy coupled with DCE in the diagnosis or exclusion of colitis.

COMPLICATIONS

Acute Colitis

The evaluation of an acute attack of colitis remains an important function of radiologic investigation. Acute deterioration in the patient's condition may be due to an overall increase in the area of inflamed bowel or in the severity of the inflammation. This change, therefore, may be due to progression of the disease—for example, when distal colitis becomes extensive but remains granular—or it may be due to a granular mucosa becoming ulcerated with or without extension of involvement. Recognition of ulceration is important because it is associated with significant complications, notably perforation or toxic megacolon, that urgently require surgical intervention. Extension of colitis without ulceration may be managed medically. Surgical treatment can then be undertaken electively only when the response to medical treatment has been inadequate.

The initial investigation should be a plain film of the abdomen. *If* the colon is devoid of gas or residue—an "empty abdomen"—then extensive active colitis is probably present (Fig. 17–21). The extent of fecal residue is good evidence of a normally functioning colon. Intraluminal gas, which increases with the severity of the colitis, shows the mucosal edge and width of the bowel.[5] An irregular edge suggests ulceration, and when there is dilatation greater than 5 cm, the ulceration probably extends down into the muscle layer.[28] This condition may progress to perforation or toxic megacolon and places the patient in a high-risk category.

FIGURE 17–22

TOXIC MEGACOLON. *A*, The plain film shows a dilated transverse colon with "mucosal islands."

B, The resected specimen shows dilatation localized to a short segment. Most of the mucosa has been sloughed, and a few polypoid mucosal remnants form the mucosal islands.

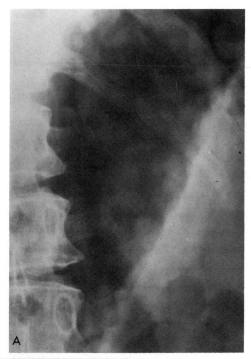

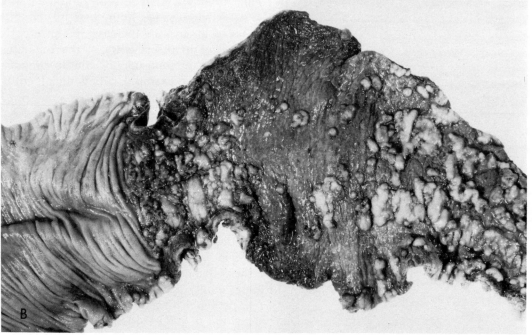

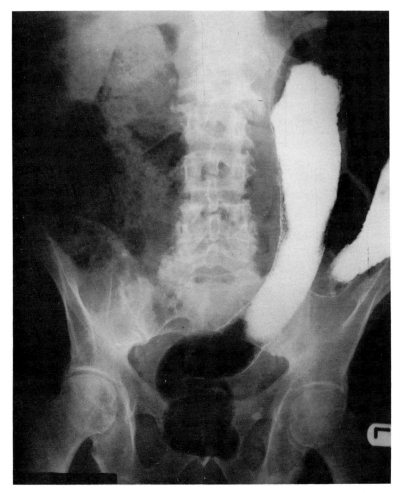

FIGURE 17–23

FECAL STASIS. Active disease in the left colon with a normal right colon containing a large fecal residue. (From Bartram, C.I.: Radiology in the current assessment of ulcerative colitis. Gastrointest. Radiol. 1:383, 1977, with permission.)

In overt toxic megacolon, the colon may measure 8 cm in width,[29] with edematous mucosal remnants forming "mucosal islands" (Fig. 17–22). The bowel wall may appear thickened from subserosal edema, and the small bowel may be dilated as a condition secondary to a profound ileus.

An instant enema is safe to perform, provided the abdominal film does not show any acute complication or early dilatation. The plain film may provide enough evidence of the state of the colitis for an immediate management decision to be made, but if any disparity exists between the patient's condition and the plain film findings, an instant enema should be performed.

Fecal Stasis

Fecal stasis may occur when the patient has severe active distal disease with a normal proximal colon. Residue may accumulate and become impacted proximally, causing pain and the paradoxical situation of diarrhea from retention with overflow (Fig. 17–23).[30]

Stricture

Stricture formation is related to extensive involvement of more than 5 years' duration.[16] Strictures occur most commonly in the sigmoid and may be single or multiple (Fig. 17–24). They are not fibrotic in origin and are due to localized thickening of the muscularis mucosae. Most strictures in ulcerative colitis are benign,[31] with a symmetric configuration, regularly tapering ends, and a mucosal texture that is constant throughout the narrowed segment and similar to that in the adjacent colon. Any irregularity or eccentricity of the lumen suggests malignancy (Fig. 17–25).[32] Endoscopic biopsy is indicated when any doubt arises radiologically (Fig. 17–26), and it is usually indicated to detect dysplasia because most patients with strictures fall into the risk category for cancer (see the following section).

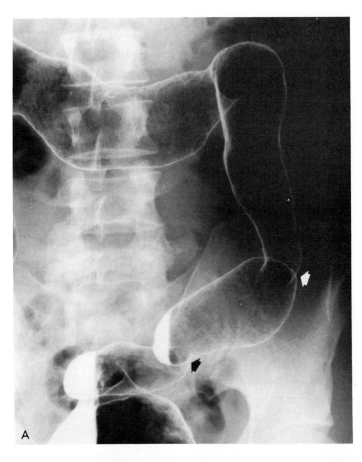

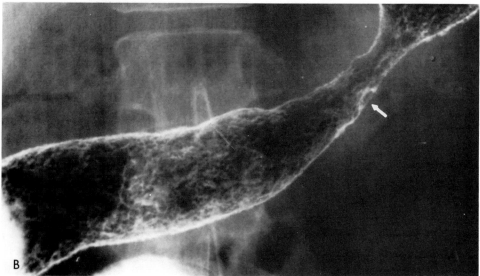

FIGURE 17–24

STRICTURES IN ULCERATIVE COLITIS. A, Total, long-standing colitis with two short, benign strictures (arrows) in the descending colon. (From Bartram, C.I.: Radiology in the current assessment of ulcerative colitis. Gastrointest. Radiol. 1:383, 1977, with permission.)

B, Stricture of the distal transverse colon. Note that the mucosa within the strictured segment is granular and is identical to the mucosa distally and proximally. There are also inflammatory polyps (arrow).

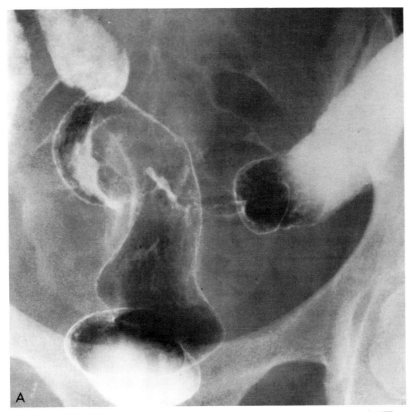

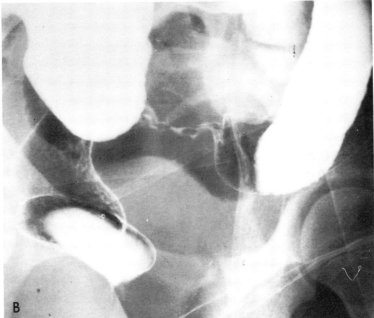

FIGURE 17–25

MALIGNANT STRICTURES. *A*, Annular adenocarcinoma in a patient with ulcerative colitis. There is an irregular lumen with shouldered margins.

B, Malignant stricture due to adenocarcinoma in another patient.

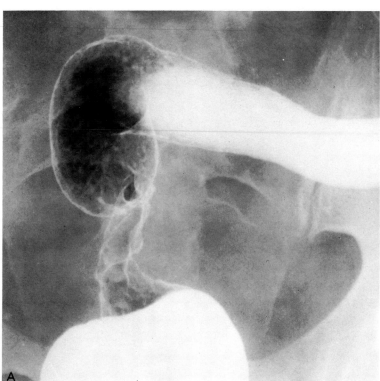
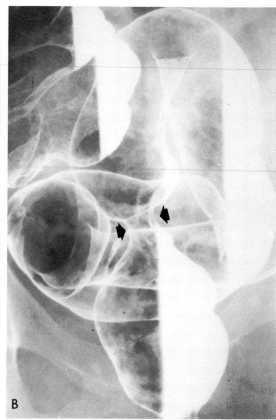

FIGURE 17–26

DIFFICULTY IN DISTINGUISHING BENIGN FROM MALIGNANT STRICTURES. *A,* Asymmetric and irregular stricture suggests carcinoma. However, this proved to be a benign stricture.

B, Smooth, tapered stricture *(arrows)* in the rectum with no radiologic suggestion of malignancy. Nevertheless, this stricture proved to be a carcinoma.

Malignancy

Cancer is an uncommon complication of ulcerative colitis. However, tumors are more likely to develop in patients with ulcerative colitis, and at an earlier age, than in the general population.[33] The tumors associated with ulcerative colitis show a different distribution from cancers in the general population. Rectosigmoid tumors are less common, and the lesions are more evenly distributed around the colon.[34] Synchronous growths are more common and have been reported in 34% of cases.[35] Most of the tumors are annular in shape (Fig. 17–27). Polypoid growths are rare (Fig. 17–28A). Scirrhous carcinomas are a feature of colitic carcinoma (Fig. 17–28B), although they are uncommon.[36]

The risk of cancer in ulcerative colitis is not uniform, and a high-risk group of patients can be identified.[37] The following factors define this group:

1. Extent of the disease. Many studies have shown that cancer is associated with total colitis.[38–40]

2. Duration of disease. The increased risk of carcinoma starts approximately 10 years after the onset of the disease. Thereafter, the risk of carcinoma is approximately equal to 10% for every 10 years of disease.[16, 37, 41] Carcinoma frequently develops in patients with quiescent or minimally active colitis.

3. Age of onset. If colitis begins in childhood, the risk of cancer may be greater than if it starts in adulthood.[33, 41]

4. Epithelial dysplasia. Severe dysplasia is usually present in the colon of patients whose colitis is complicated by cancer.[42] Persistent severe dysplasia is considered an indication for colectomy.[37]

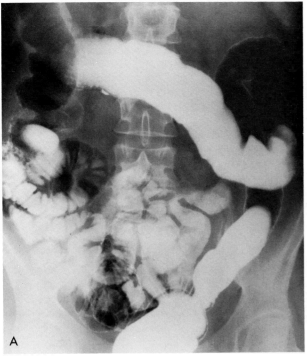

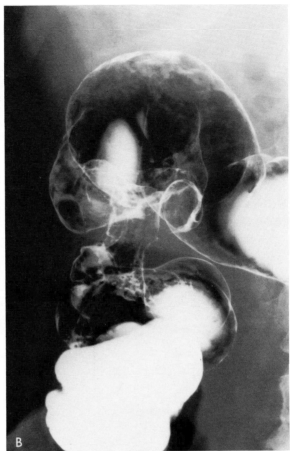

FIGURE 17–27

THE DEVELOPMENT OF COLITIC CARCINOMA. *A,* Total active colitis of 11 years' duration.

B, Three years later, there is an annular carcinoma in the ascending colon.

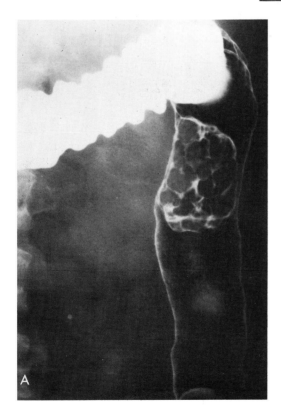

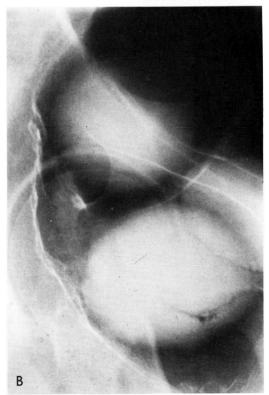

FIGURE 17–28

COLITIC CARCINOMAS. *A,* Unusual polypoid carcinoma in ulcerative colitis.

B, Flat infiltrating carcinoma along the lateral wall of the rectum in a patient with a long history of ulcerative colitis.

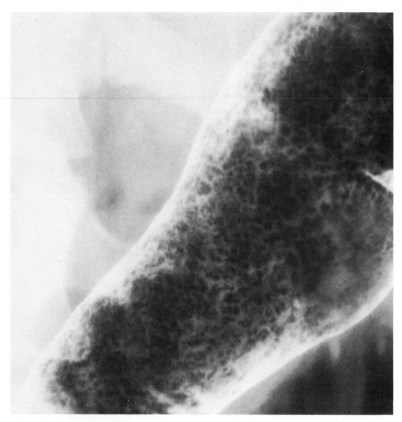

FIGURE 17–29

DYSPLASIA IN ULCERATIVE COLITIS. The mucosal surface of the distal transverse colon is covered by a raised polygonal pattern characteristic of mucosal dysplasia.

Dysplasia in a flat mucosa cannot be recognized radiologically.[43] When the dysplasia becomes elevated and villous in form, it may become visible as a nodular, polygonal pattern (Fig. 17–29).[44–46]

A localized, nodular, elevated lesion, often resembling a villous adenoma, is termed a "macrodysplastic lesion" or a "dysplasia-associated lesion or mass" (Fig. 17–30).[47] These lesions are important markers of dysplasia and represent a high risk for cancer (Fig. 17–31). Butt and associates reported that in 34 patients undergoing colectomy, 51 cancers and 65 macrodysplastic lesions were found.[47, 47a] Only one cancer occurred with a flat mucosa. Of 28 patients with dysplasia but no cancer, eight had a flat mucosa, but in 20 patients, 40 macrodysplastic lesions were found. This series therefore suggests that most patients with dysplasia should have a radiologically detectable lesion.

The management of high-risk patients requires regular radiologic and endoscopic surveillance to detect the presence of dysplasia,[37] particularly when young patients are involved.[48] The role of the radiologist is to determine the extent of the colitis and the configuration of the colon to aid the endoscopist and to draw attention to any area suspicious for dysplasia or carcinoma. It should be noted that lymphoma has also been reported as a rare complication of chronic ulcerative colitis.[49]

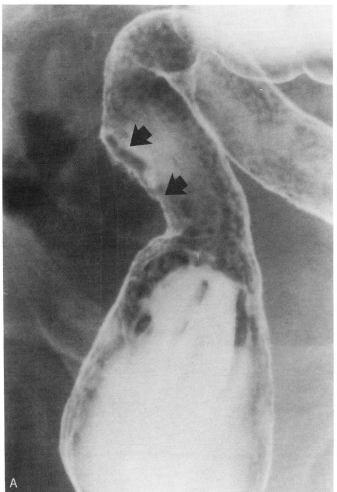

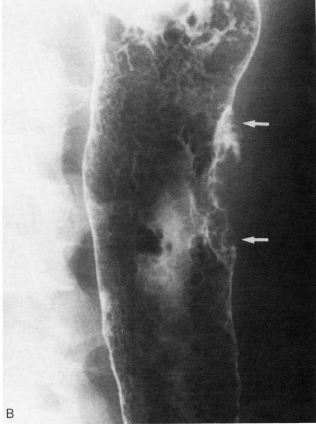

FIGURE 17–30

DYSPLASIA-ASSOCIATED MASS. *A,* A plaque-like lesion *(arrows)* along the right lateral wall of the rectum. On resection, this was a dysplastic mass.

B, In another patient, there is a large macrodysplastic lesion *(arrows)* in the descending colon surrounding dysplastic mucosa. In the same patient, there was a carcinoma in the sigmoid colon.

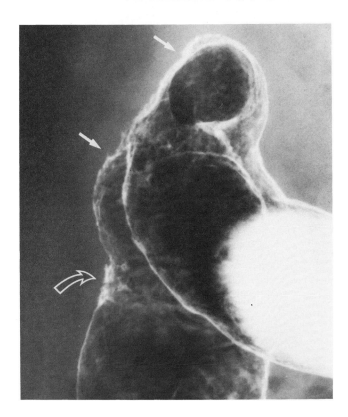

FIGURE 17–31

CARCINOMA AND DYSPLASIA. In this patient with a 12-year history of ulcerative colitis, there is an infiltrative plaque-like carcinoma at the hepatic flexure *(solid arrows)*. Proximal to the carcinoma is a small macrodysplastic lesion *(open arrow)*.

CROHN'S DISEASE

Crohn's disease is a patchy chronic inflammatory process that may affect any part of the gastrointestinal tract. It is characterized histologically by the presence of noncaseating granulomas, fissuring ulceration, and transmural inflammation, with focal collections of lymphocytes scattered across all layers of the bowel wall and extending into the serosa and peri-intestinal fat. Hyperplasia of the lymphoid tissue occurs (Fig. 17–32), with an obstructive lymphedema that leads to widening of the submucosa. Crypt abscesses in the mucous membrane are not as common as in ulcerative colitis.[9]

Clinical Course

In contrast to ulcerative colitis, Crohn's disease is more of a chronic disorder. Acute episodes with toxic megacolon may occur, but chronic ill health, diarrhea, and abdominal pain are typical. The transmural inflammation has two important consequences: fistulization and formation of strictures. It has been suggested that patients may be divided into two main groups on the basis of these changes. Fistulae result from the fissuring ulceration. Because the serosa is also inflamed, adjacent structures become adherent, and any penetrating ulcer forms a fistula rather than free perforation. Strictures result from fibrosis within

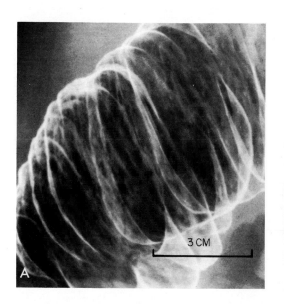

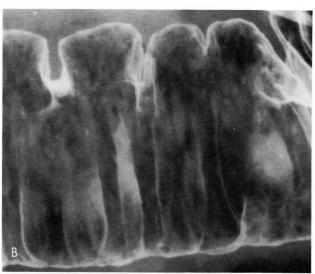

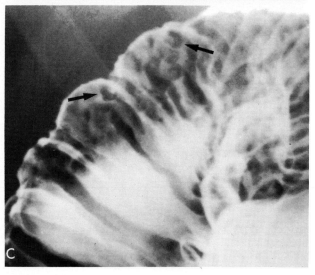

FIGURE 17–32

A to C, Lymphoid hyperplasia in the early stages of Crohn's disease. The very fine nodularity of the colon is due to enlargement of the lymph follicles. Some of the follicles have small central collections of barium, which probably represent superficial ulceration. (A, From Laufer, I., and deSa, D.: Lymphoid follicular pattern: A normal feature of the pediatric colon. AJR *130*:51–55, 1978, with permission, © by American Roentgen Ray Society. B, From Laufer, I.: Air-contrast studies of the colon in inflammatory bowel disease. CRC Crit. Rev. Diagnost. Imaging 9:421, 1977, with permission.)

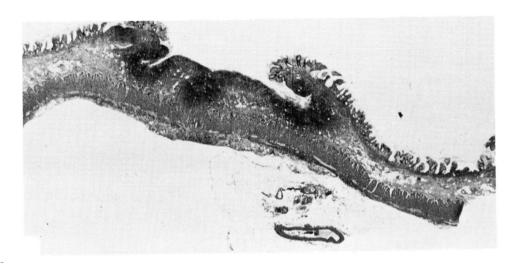

FIGURE 17–33

APHTHOID ULCERS IN CROHN'S DISEASE. This histologic section shows a superficial ulcer with transmural inflammation. The ulcer has elevated margins and is surrounded by normal mucosa. (From Laufer, I., and Costopoulos, L.: Early lesions of Crohn's disease. AJR 130:307–311, 1978, with permission, © by American Roentgen Ray Society.)

the bowel wall that is associated with chronic deep ulceration.

The aims of surgery have changed over the decades. Surgical intervention is now more conservative. Limited resection or strictureplasty is used to treat local complications or cases that fail to respond to medical treatment. These surgical procedures are based on the need to resect the minimal amount of bowel to relieve the main clinical problem while minimizing the probability of recurrent disease.

Crohn's disease is predominantly ileocolic (55%), with involvement limited to the colon in 15% of patients, and to the small bowel alone in 30% of patients.[50] The disease may remain relatively constant in extent but may fluctuate in activity. After resection and ileocolic anastomosis, there is a predilection for recurrence in the distal small bowel, beginning at the anastomosis. Overall, about 50% of cases recur at 10 years, although endoscopy frequently shows superficial ulceration localized only to the anastomosis without clinical symptoms of recurrence. Local resections of colon are frequently required, so that proctocolectomy and ileostomy may be preferred to ileorectal anastomosis.

No age group is exempt from Crohn's disease. Although it is most common in young adults, the disease is seen in children, in whom growth failure is an important complication, and in the elderly, in whom the distal colon is often affected, complicating pre-existing diverticular disease.

Radiologically, Crohn's disease of the colon presents problems in diagnosis and assessment that are similar to those of ulcerative colitis. Its chronic transmural inflammatory nature, however, makes fistula formation common, so that there is a greater emphasis on the diagnosis of chronic complications. There may be a slightly increased risk of malignancy, but this risk is much lower than in ulcerative colitis, and cancer surveillance is not usually undertaken. Patients with Crohn's disease often exhibit a great variety of mucosal lesions. For analysis, however, it is convenient to divide the radiologic features into early, advanced, and complicated stages.

Early Changes

Superficial lesions may be seen tangentially on filled single contrast studies. Marshak described small irregular nodules along the contour of the bowel with a diameter of about 5 mm and possibly with central ulceration and some distortion of haustral anatomy.[51] These lesions are probably the "aphthoid ulcers," which were first described by Lockhart-Mummery and Morson,[52] and which are very superficial ulcers over foci of lymphocytic infiltration (Fig. 17–33). Macroscopically, the ulcer crater is formed of yellowish slough surrounded by a reddened inflamed rim. Typically, the aphthoid ulcer is discrete, is set in normal mucosa, and is separated and distinct from other lesions. The double contrast image mirrors the macroscopic appearance.[53] Barium adheres to the sloughed ulcer base, which appears as a dense and irregular barium collection. The reddened rim is hyperemic and not well coated with barium, so that there is usually a radiolucent halo around the ulcer. The adjacent mucosa is normal.[53, 54] Reference to the mucosal line confirms that the ulcers are superficial and barely project beyond the contour (Fig. 17–34).

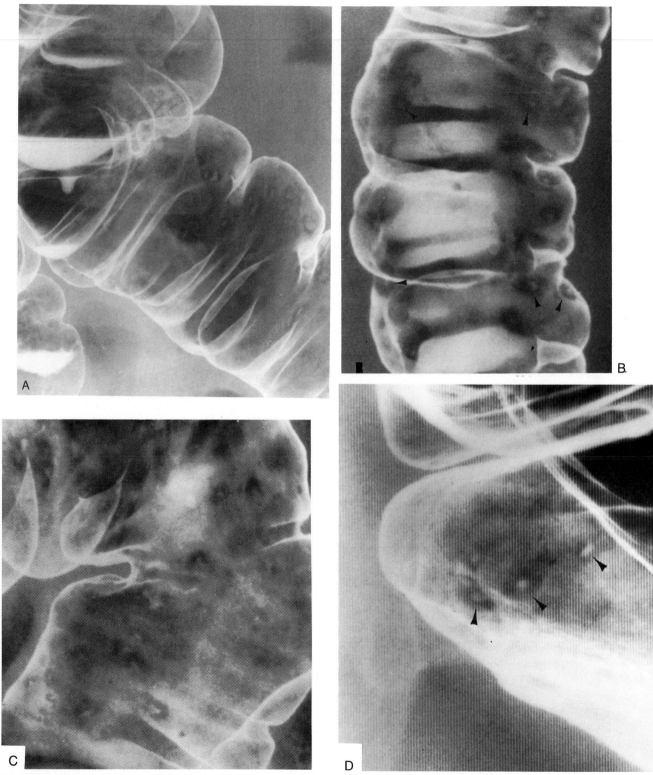

FIGURE 17–34

EXAMPLES OF APHTHOID ULCERS THROUGHOUT THE COLON. *A*, Proximal transverse colon.

B, Descending colon. (From Laufer, I., and Costopoulos, L.: Early lesions of Crohn's disease. AJR *130*:307–311, 1978, with permission, © by American Roentgen Ray Society.)

C, Sigmoid.

D, Rectum.

Aphthoid ulceration may be the only evidence of involvement, with lesions diffusely scattered throughout the bowel, or they may be associated with more advanced disease, in which case they are usually found in the boundary zone between normal and obviously involved bowel (Fig. 17–35). Aphthoid ulceration has been reported in 44% of colonic Crohn's disease.[54]

Although aphthoid ulceration is typical of Crohn's disease, it is not pathognomonic, because colitis may be associated with similar lesions due to *Yersinia,* *Shigella,* amebiasis, ischemia, Behçet's, herpes, and cytomegalovirus infections.[55] In *Yersinia* and *Shigella* infections, there are typically small pinpoint ulcers on the apex of lymphoid follicles, so that the ulcer in relation to the halo is much smaller than in Crohn's disease.

Pathologically, lymphatic obstruction and submucosal edema are early changes, but they are not as apparent in the colon as in the small bowel. The

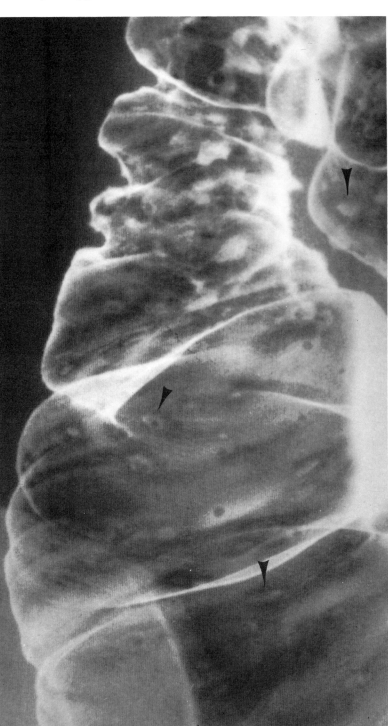

FIGURE 17–35

APHTHOID ULCERS IN ASSOCIATION WITH MORE SEVERE DISEASE. There is obvious involvement by Crohn's disease of the distal ascending colon and hepatic flexure. Multiple aphthoid ulcers are seen in the proximal ascending colon and in the proximal transverse colon *(arrowheads).* Note the normal appearance of the mucosa between the aphthoid ulcers. (From Laufer, I., and Costopoulos, L.: Early lesions of Crohn's disease. AJR *130*:307–311, 1978, with permission, © by American Roentgen Ray Society.)

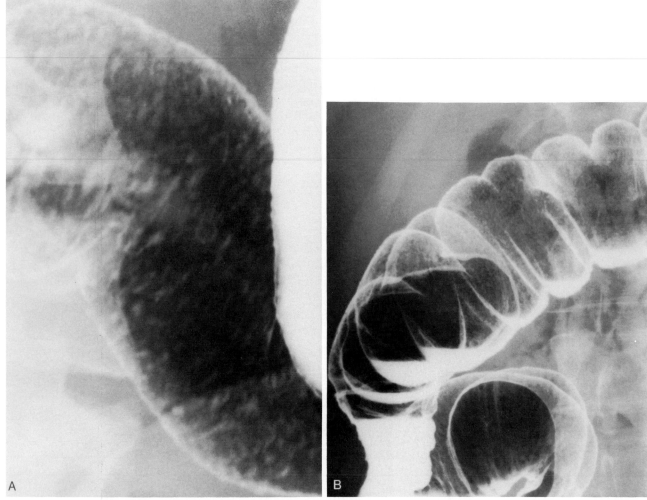

FIGURE 17–36

DIFFUSE MUCOSAL ABNORMALITIES IN CROHN'S DISEASE. *A*, Confluent aphthoid ulceration in the transverse colon with almost complete obliteration of the haustral folds. Note the transverse orientation of the ulcers with swollen intervening mucosa.

B, An unusual example of granular mucosa due to recurrence of Crohn's disease in the colon following ileocolic anastomosis.

haustral pattern, folds, and bowel wall may appear entirely normal, with scattered aphthoid ulceration and intervening normal mucosa. Once these ulcers become confluent, some alteration in contour may be expected (Fig. 17–36A). A granular mucosal texture similar to ulcerative colitis is seen occasionally in early Crohn's colitis (Fig. 17–36B).[56] Should the aphthoid ulceration become confluent, it can be difficult to distinguish from a coarse granular texture.

ADVANCED DISEASE

Discontinuous Ulceration

As previously mentioned, the tendency for discontinuity of ulceration is a hallmark of Crohn's disease.

Even in the earliest stages, the aphthoid ulcers are separated by a normal mucosa. As the ulcers enlarge, large patches of normal mucosa can still be identified in between them (Fig. 17–37). With further progression, larger segments of colon become involved (Fig. 17–38), but discontinuous involvement has been demonstrated in 90% of our patients with Crohn's disease.[57] The tendency toward discontinuity may be manifested only by a few aphthoid ulcers in the colon of a patient with extensive small bowel disease (Fig. 17–39).

The large ulcers may be indistinguishable from the ulcers in ulcerative colitis, but in Crohn's disease, the intervening mucosa tends to be normal and is not granular.

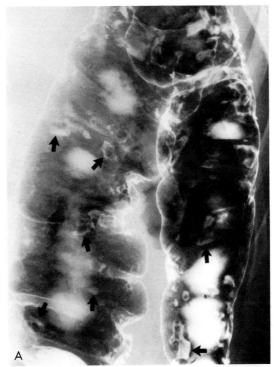

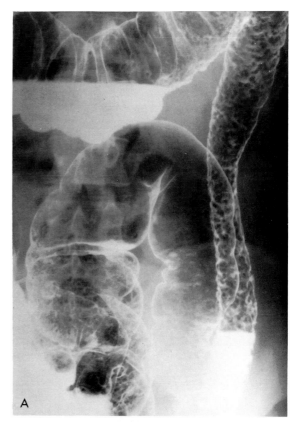

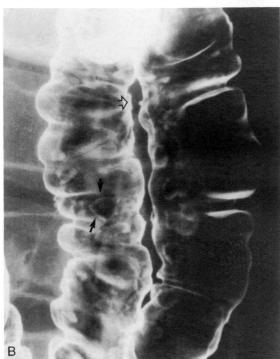

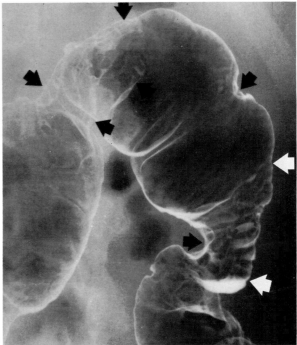

FIGURE 17–37

DISCONTINUOUS ULCERATION IN CROHN'S DISEASE. *A,* In the region of the splenic flexure, there are large ulcers with normal intervening mucosa. Note the discontinuous nature of the ulceration along the inferior aspect of the transverse colon.

B, Another example of discontinuous ulceration with serpiginous ulceration at the splenic flexure. A ring shadow representing an ulcer is seen en face *(solid arrows).* Shallow ulcers can be seen in profile protruding from the mucosal line *(open arrow).*

FIGURE 17–38

A, Variability of the lesions in Crohn's disease. There are postinflammatory polyps in the splenic flexure, confluent ulceration in the descending colon, and separated discrete ulcers in the sigmoid.

B, Typical skip lesions *(arrows)* separated by intervening normal mucosa. (From Laufer, I., and Hamilton, J. The radiologic differentiation between ulcerative and granulomatous colitis by double contrast radiology. Am. J. Gastroenterol. *66:*259–269, 1976, with permission, © by American College of Gastroenterology.)

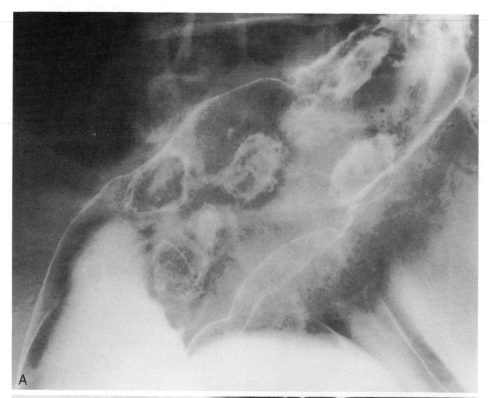

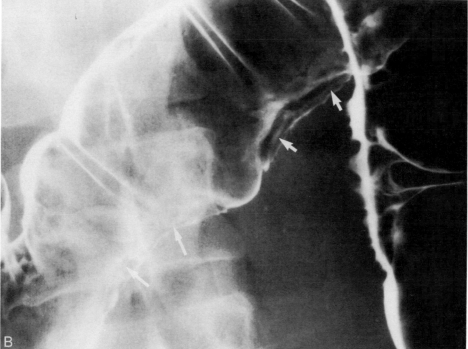

FIGURE 17–39

LARGE ULCERS IN CROHN'S DISEASE. *A,* In the sigmoid colon, there are multiple large but shallow ulcers.

    B, In another patient, there is linear ulceration *(arrows)* on the antimesenteric aspect of the transverse colon with a normal background mucosa.

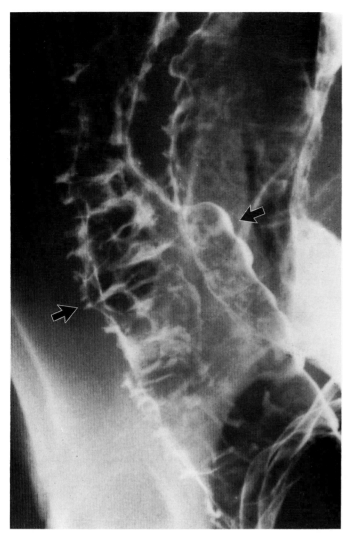

FIGURE 17-40

DEEP ULCERATION IN CROHN'S COLITIS WITH ASYMMETRIC LESIONS. *Arrows* indicate a segment that is ulcerated on the lateral aspect but is unaffected on the medial side.

Asymmetry

In addition to discontinuity, asymmetric involvement is a major hallmark of Crohn's disease. In the early stages, it may be manifested by involvement of one wall of the bowel, while the opposite wall remains completely normal (Fig. 17–40). In more advanced disease with fibrous scarring, it may be manifested as sacculation of the bowel wall as the involved segment contracts and causes the remaining uninvolved portion to balloon out (Fig. 17–41).[58] This sacculation may resemble the sacculation seen in the small and large bowel in patients with scleroderma (see Chapter 16, Fig. 16–23). In scleroderma, however, the intervening mucosa has a normal appearance, whereas in sacculation due to Crohn's disease, there are mucosal thickening and nodularity.

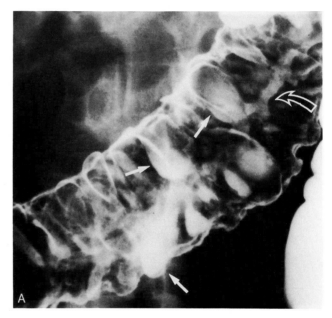

FIGURE 17-41

SACCULATION IN CROHN'S DISEASE. *A,* In the presence of active disease with linear ulceration *(open arrow),* multiple small sacculations *(solid arrows)* are seen.

B, In chronic disease, there is extensive sacculation of the transverse colon due to asymmetric fibrosis. The intervening mucosa has a nodular appearance.

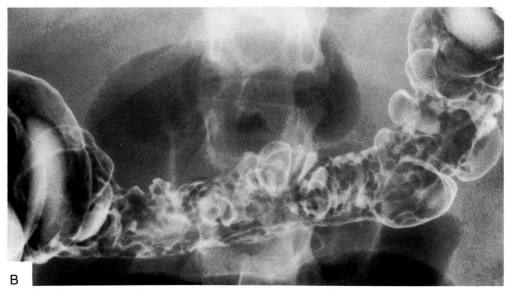

Other Manifestations

There are numerous other manifestations of Crohn's disease, particularly in its more advanced stages. Serpiginous longitudinal and transverse ulcers are a frequent finding and produce the typical cobblestone mucosa (Fig. 17–42). A stricture is a frequent development in Crohn's disease (Fig. 17–43). However, the possibility of carcinoma need rarely be considered in the presence of colonic strictures in Crohn's disease.[59]

Fistulae and abscesses are well-recognized features of Crohn's disease. Fistulae may be better demonstrated by the thin barium used in a single contrast enema. Therefore, when a study is performed primarily to demonstrate a fistula, we usually prefer the single contrast study.

Welin and Welin described a transverse stripe as being characteristic of colonic Crohn's disease (Fig. 17–44).[60] In some cases, the stripe was a manifestation of transverse ulceration; in others, it was caused by a stripe of contrast material being caught between two transverse folds. Intramural or paracolonic sinus tracts are also a feature of Crohn's disease, particularly in patients with diverticulosis (Fig. 17–45).[61] Meyers and co-workers have shown that these sinus tracts develop because of granulomatous inflammation involving the base of the diverticula.[62] However, these sinus tracts are not specific for Crohn's disease, because they are also found in patients with acute diverticulitis (see Chapter 16, Fig. 16–6D) and are rarely found in patients with carcinoma.[63]

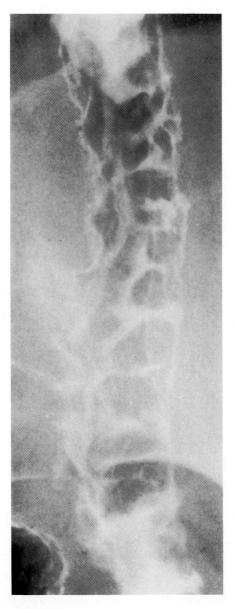

FIGURE 17–42

Cobblestoned mucosa in Crohn's colitis.

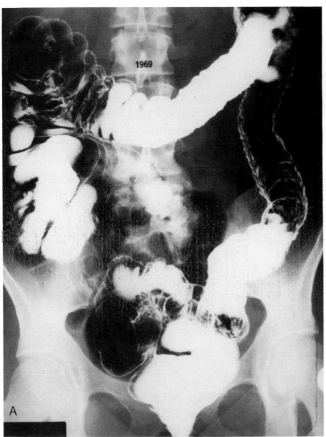

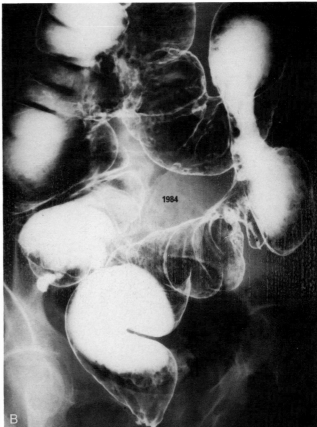

FIGURE 17–43

DEVELOPMENT OF STRICTURES. A, An examination in 1969 shows extensive involvement of the left colon by Crohn's disease.

B, Fifteen years later, the disease is in remission, and several strictures have developed, with postinflammatory polyps in the transverse and descending colon. Note the sacculation of the descending and sigmoid colon.

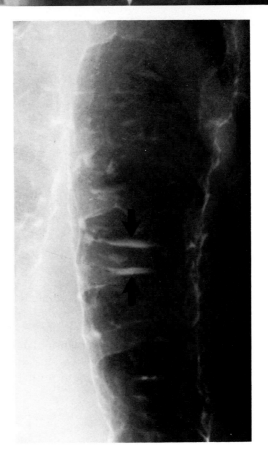

FIGURE 17–44

The transverse stripe, which according to Welin and Welin[60] is pathognomonic of Crohn's disease.

Rectal Disease

Endoscopically and histologically, rectal disease is found in approximately 50% of patients with colonic Crohn's disease.[64] However, it may be difficult to demonstrate this condition radiologically because signs of the disease tend to be patchy and asymmetric. We have been able to demonstrate rectal disease radiographically in 37% of patients with granulomatous colitis. These patients represented 75% of those with endoscopic or histologic evidence of rectal involvement.[57]

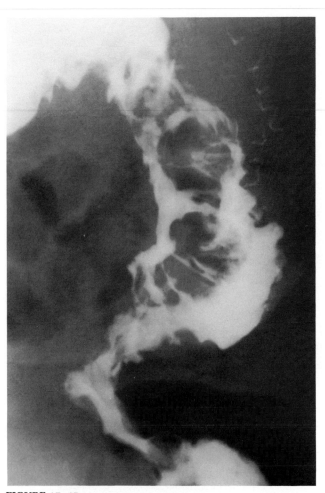

FIGURE 17–45

INTRAMURAL TRACKING DUE TO CROHN'S DISEASE. There is an intramural track along the medial aspect of the descending colon. This area was resected, and examination of pathologic features showed Crohn's colitis with an intramural track connecting the bases of diverticula.

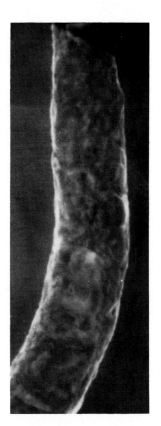

FIGURE 17–46

Diffuse mucosal thickening with loss of haustration in a patient with chronic granulomatous colitis.

Some patients with chronic disease due to granulomatous colitis may have total involvement of the colon manifested by only slight narrowing of the colon and mucosal thickening (Fig. 17–46). These cases may be particularly difficult to distinguish from those of ulcerative colitis, although careful double contrast study may show some patches of uninvolved colon.

Rectal involvement in Crohn's disease differs from rectal involvement in ulcerative colitis. Deep or "collar stud" ulcers are seen in Crohn's disease, but they are rarely seen in the rectum in ulcerative colitis, although they may be seen in the more proximal portions of the colon.[65] In addition, rectal sinus tracts are a characteristic feature of Crohn's disease (see Chapter 18).

Polypoid Lesions

Polypoid lesions in Crohn's disease are similar to those in ulcerative colitis and include pseudopolyps due to extensive ulceration, inflammatory polypoid masses (Fig. 17–47), and postinflammatory polyps, which may be sessile, pedunculated, or filiform (see Chapter 15, Fig. 15–21). Neoplastic polyps are rare in Crohn's disease.

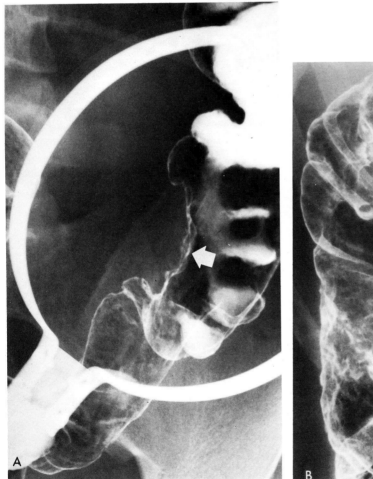
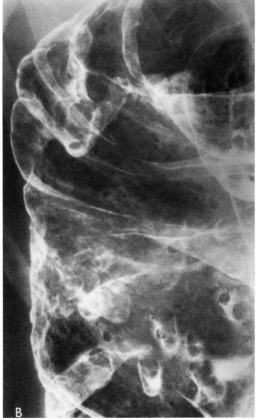

FIGURE 17–47

POLYPOID LESIONS. *A,* Inflammatory, sessile, polypoid mass *(arrow)* in a patient with granulomatous colitis.
 B, Multiple sessile and pedunculated postinflammatory polyps in a patient with a previous history of severe granulomatous colitis.

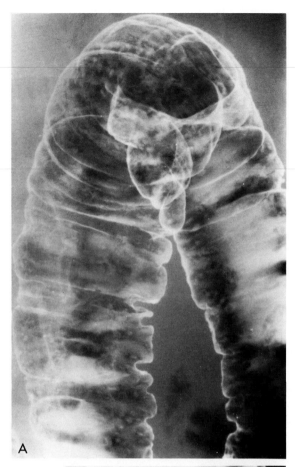

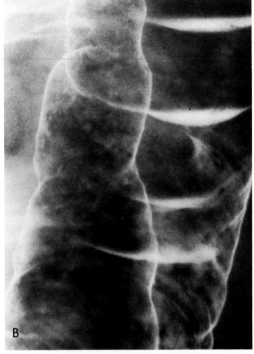

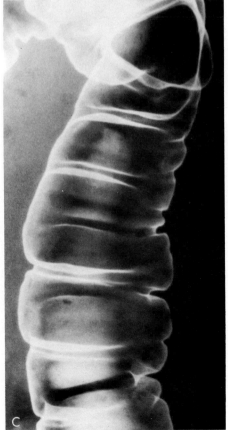

FIGURE 17–48

REVERSIBILITY IN THE EARLY STAGES OF CROHN'S DISEASE. *A,* Diffuse aphthoid ulceration at the splenic flexure.

B, Several months later, there is marked improvement, although a few superficial ulcers remain.

C, Following an additional several months, the appearance of the colon has returned entirely to normal.

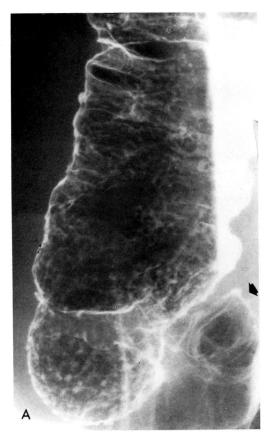

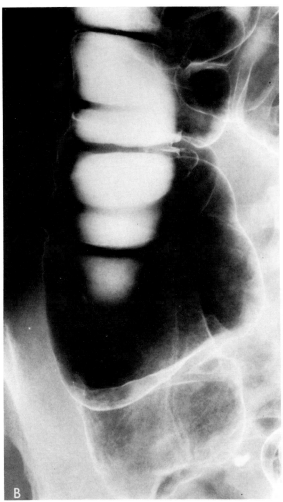

FIGURE 17–49

REVERSIBILITY IN CROHN'S DISEASE. *A,* Extensive involvement of the right colon and terminal ileum *(arrow)* by Crohn's disease.

B, Six months later, the appearance of the colon has returned to normal.

REVERSIBILITY

Reversibility of lesions is a much more frequent occurrence in the colon than in the small bowel. As mentioned previously, the aphthoid ulcers of Crohn's disease are unstable lesions that usually progress to more extensive disease, but not infrequently regress (Fig. 17—48). Even the more advanced lesions of Crohn's disease may regress either spontaneously or after medical treatment (Fig. 17–49). Hywel-Jones and co-workers reported the cases of 11 patients in whom radiographic regression of the colonic lesions occurred.[66] Brahme found temporary regression in only 7% of 86 patients with Crohn's disease.[67] Definitive permanent healing after medical treatment was not observed in that series.

Rarely, when the lesions of Crohn's disease regress, the colon may heal completely with no radiologic evidence of scarring (see Fig. 17–49). This outcome is uncommon, however, and more frequently, there is some evidence of scarring (Fig. 17–50). The sacculation described previously is also a manifestation of focal colonic scarring. This scarring is understandable in view of the transmural inflammation that is characteristic of Crohn's disease. This process appears in marked contrast to the mucosal involvement in ulcerative colitis, which frequently heals completely without residual scarring, even when there has been extensive and deep ulceration.

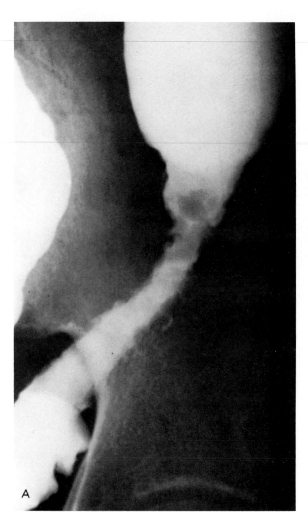 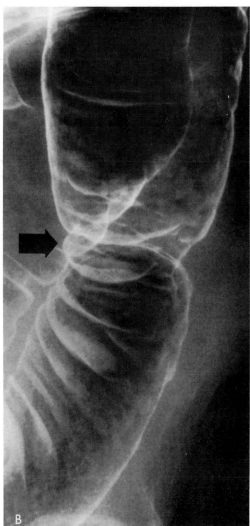

FIGURE 17–50

SCARRING IN CROHN'S COLITIS. *A*, Segmental disease in the distal descending colon, with narrowing and deep ulceration.

B, Two years later, the patient was asymptomatic, and there was marked regression with minimal narrowing and shortening along the medial aspect *(arrow)*, resulting in retraction and convergence of the folds.

TERMINAL ILEUM

Double contrast views of the terminal ileum can frequently be obtained during the course of the routine double contrast enema. When the terminal ileum is not visualized during the routine examination, it is often filled on a postevacuation film. Alternatively, the terminal ileum can be examined by the small bowel enema technique with rectal insufflation of air as the terminal ileum is filled. Double contrast views show the normal circular folds, which are thin, deli-

cate, and straight (see Chapter 12, Figs. 12–2, 12–4, and 12–10). The early lesions of Crohn's disease involving the small bowel can be demonstrated using these techniques. In some patients, mucosal and submucosal inflammation may be manifested as thickening and slight nodularity of the circular folds (Fig. 17–51). In others, the typical aphthoid ulcers of Crohn's disease can be seen (Fig. 17–51B). In more advanced cases, the typical features of ulceration, cobblestoned mucosa, and stricture are demonstrated (Fig. 17–52).

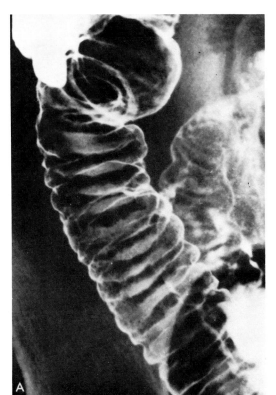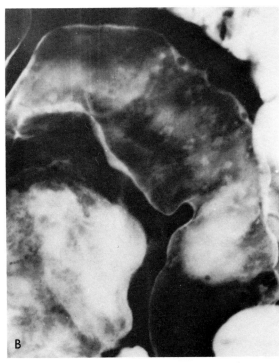

FIGURE 17–51

EARLY LESIONS IN THE TERMINAL ILEUM. *A,* Enlargement and nodularity of the valvulae conniventes due to granulomatous inflammation.

B, Aphthoid ulcers in the terminal ileum. (Courtesy of L. Costopoulos, M.D., Edmonton, Alberta. From Laufer, I., and Costopoulos, L.: Early lesions of Crohn's disease. AJR *130:*307–311, 1978, with permission, © by American Roentgen Ray Society.)

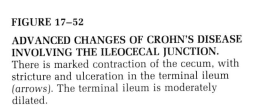

FIGURE 17–52

ADVANCED CHANGES OF CROHN'S DISEASE INVOLVING THE ILEOCECAL JUNCTION. There is marked contraction of the cecum, with stricture and ulceration in the terminal ileum *(arrows).* The terminal ileum is moderately dilated.

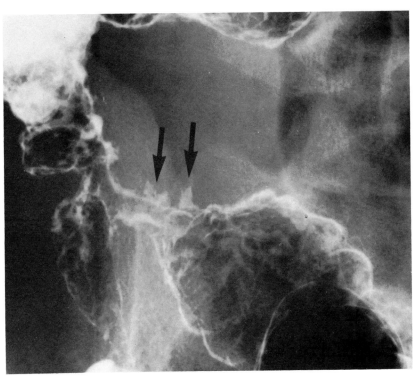

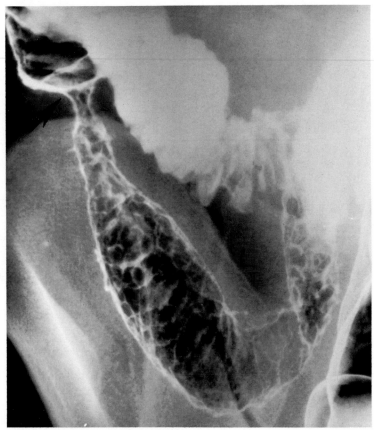

FIGURE 17–53

RECURRENT CROHN'S DISEASE FOLLOWING ILEOCOLIC ANASTOMOSIS. Typical cobblestoning is seen and involves the neoterminal ileum to the anastomosis with the ascending colon (*arrow*).

Patients with previous ileocolic anastomoses are particularly easy to examine with the double contrast technique (Fig. 17–53). The absence of the ileocecal valve facilitates the visualization of the neoterminal ileum.

The early lesions must be differentiated from lymphoid hyperplasia in the terminal ileum (Fig. 17–54). Lymphoid hyperplasia is probably a normal variant that results in tiny nodular filling defects best visualized in the terminal ileum. There is no associated ulceration. Inflammation of the terminal ileum is also a feature of *Yersinia* enterocolitis.[68, 69] This condition is manifested by swelling of the mucosa of the terminal ileum, which returns to normal within a 2-

month period (Fig. 17–55). Inflammatory changes in the terminal ileum can also be caused by a periappendiceal abscess, which is characterized by a soft tissue mass in the ileocecal area, with swelling of ileal mucosa. However, the mucosal abnormalities in the small bowel are relatively minor compared with the soft tissue mass. Patients with Crohn's disease frequently have a mass in the right lower quadrant, but it is invariably accompanied by extensive mucosal ulceration, frequently with formation of fistulae.

Disease of the terminal ileum may also have a number of indirect manifestations on the colon. Berridge has described a medial cecal defect that appears to be characteristic of Crohn's disease (Fig. 17–56).[58]

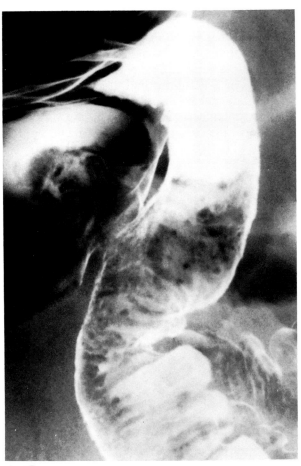

FIGURE 17–54

LYMPHOID HYPERPLASIA IN THE TERMINAL ILEUM. There are tiny nodular filling defects due to lymph follicles. There is no associated enlargement of the folds, ulceration, or spasm.

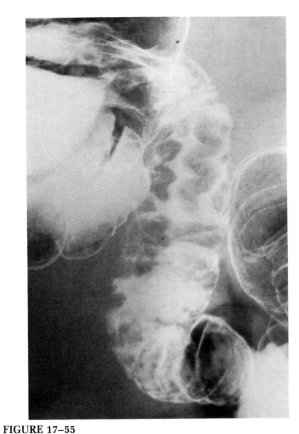

FIGURE 17–55

***YERSINIA* ENTERITIS.** There are marked swelling and tortuosity of the folds in the terminal ileum in this patient with proven *Yersinia* enteritis. The appearance returned to normal within 2 months.

FIGURE 17–56

MEDIAL CECAL DEFECT IN CROHN'S DISEASE. There is compression on the medial aspect of the cecum by the diseased terminal ileum and its affected mesentery.

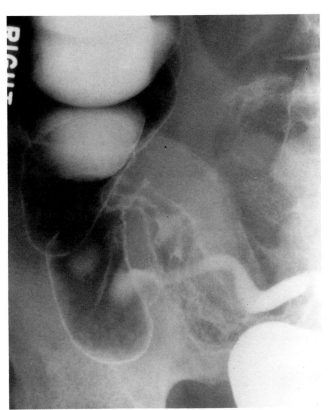

This defect is due not to intrinsic cecal involvement, but rather to small bowel disease, with compression of the medial aspect of the cecum resulting from thickening of the bowel wall and mesentery. Similar effects may be produced in other parts of the colon, and they appear to be particularly common in the sigmoid, which is frequently affected by disease in the small bowel (Fig. 17–57). Presumably, these effects represent the pathogenesis of ileosigmoid fistulae, which are so common in this condition.[70]

GASTRODUODENAL CROHN'S DISEASE

Involvement of the stomach and duodenum in Crohn's disease has been illustrated in Chapter 10. In previous studies, gastroduodenal involvement was reported in 2% to 3% of patients with Crohn's disease.[71, 72] However, these cases invariably represent advanced disease, characterized clinically by gastric outlet obstruction and radiologically by deformity and narrowing of the antrum and proximal duodenum

(Fig. 17–58).[73] Endoscopic series report gastroduodenal involvement in a much higher proportion of patients, approaching 75% of patients with Crohn's disease involving the stomach.[74]

The early lesions of Crohn's disease are the same in the upper gastrointestinal tract as elsewhere.[75] These lesions consist of mild thickening of the folds due to granulomatous inflammation (Fig. 17–59) and to aphthoid ulceration (Fig. 17–60).[76] The aphthoid ulcers are indistinguishable from gastric or duodenal erosions of other causes.[77]

The stomach and duodenum are usually involved in continuity.[78] Because of the transmural nature of the disease, definitive diagnosis by endoscopic biopsy is often difficult.[79] We have found these subtle changes of gastroduodenal Crohn's disease in 20% to 40% of patients with Crohn's disease of the small or large bowel. Esophageal involvement is less common and has been noted in isolated case reports.[80] With increasing use of double contrast technique, subtle involvement of the esophagus in Crohn's disease is being seen more frequently (see Chapter 5).[75]

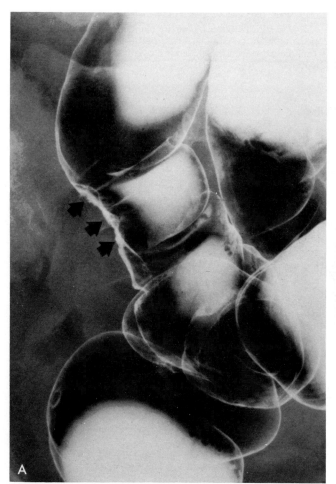

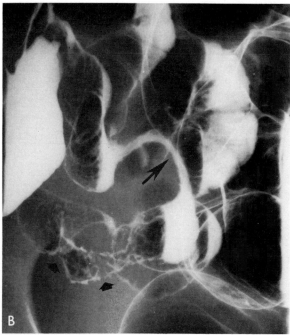

FIGURE 17–57

A and B, Involvement of the lateral aspect of the sigmoid colon (A) by extensive disease in the terminal ileum (B), characterized by stricture (arrow) and cobblestoned mucosa (arrows).

FIGURE 17–58

ADVANCED GASTRODUODENAL CROHN'S DISEASE. This appearance is typical, with deformity and narrowing of the distal antrum extending to involve the duodenal cap and proximal portion of the descending duodenum. Note the normal distensibility of the distal duodenum.

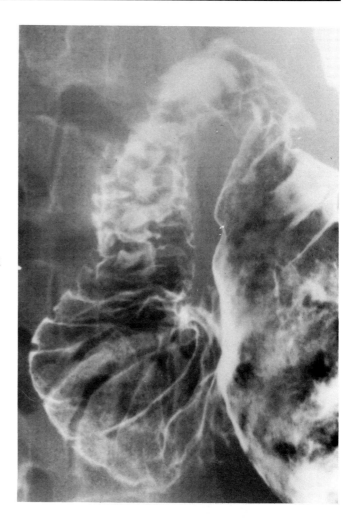

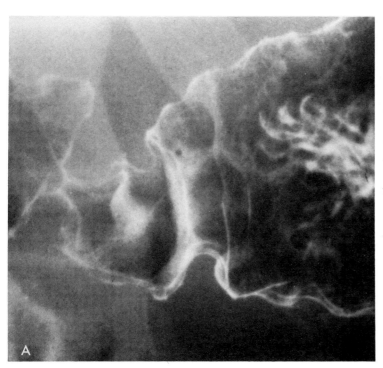

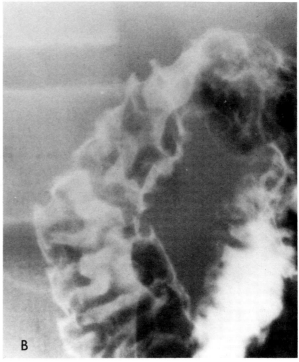

FIGURE 17–59

A and B, Thickening of the folds as a result of Crohn's disease involving the stomach (A) and duodenum (B).

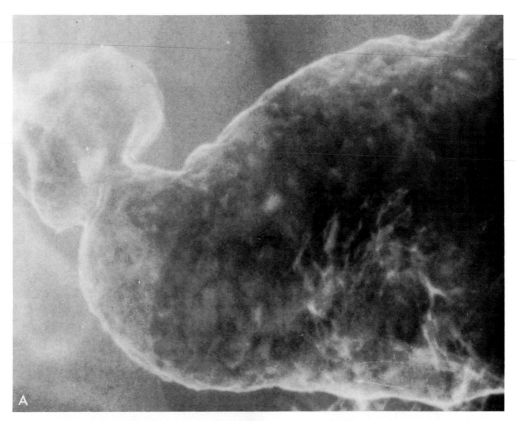

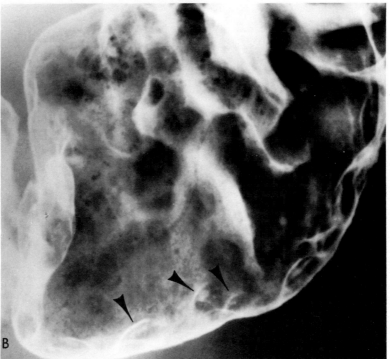

FIGURE 17–60

A and *B*, Two examples of erosive gastritis (*arrowheads* in *B*) due to Crohn's disease. (From Laufer, I., et al.: Multiple superficial gastric erosions due to Crohn's disease of the stomach: Radiologic and endoscopic diagnosis. Br. J. Radiol. 49:726, 1976, with permission.)

DIFFERENTIAL DIAGNOSIS OF COLITIS

Colitis may have no known cause or may be due to a variety of specific agents. The colon is limited in its ability to respond; therefore, it is not surprising that there may be some overlap in the radiologic findings in various types of colitis.

In North America and Europe, the vast majority of cases of colitis are idiopathic, although with the spread of AIDS, infectious colitis is becoming a more frequent problem. On the basis of a number of clinical, radiologic, and pathologic features, idiopathic colitis may be subdivided into ulcerative and granulomatous colitis. However, before relegating a patient with colitis into the idiopathic group, the various specific types of colitis must be excluded by the appropriate bacteriologic and histologic studies.

ULCERATIVE VERSUS GRANULOMATOUS COLITIS

In the majority of cases, the differential diagnosis is reduced to the distinction between ulcerative and granulomatous colitis. This distinction is clinically significant, because it affects the treatment of the disease, the approach to surgery, and the prognosis regarding recurrent disease and the development of carcinoma.

The specific features of the two diseases have been described in detail. In general, ulcerative colitis can be described as a disease with mucosal inflammation starting in the rectum and extending proximally to a variable extent. The involvement is confluent and symmetric, and the terminal ileum is normal. The major complications are toxic megacolon and carcinoma, the latter of which has a markedly increased incidence in patients who have had the disease for 10 years or more. By comparison, granulomatous colitis can be described as a transmural inflammatory process that involves the entire gastrointestinal tract in a discontinuous distribution. The discontinuity is manifested by discrete ulceration with intervening normal mucosa, or by skip lesions consisting of larger diseased segments separated by normal segments. There is a particular tendency to involve the terminal ileum and right colon. The complications are fistula and abscess.

Table 17-1 lists the incidence of various radiologic findings in a group of patients having either ulcerative or granulomatous colitis. This table demonstrates a number of radiologic findings that are relatively specific for each condition. In ulcerative colitis, these findings are a granular mucosa, diffuse rectal disease, continuous inflammation, ulcers on a granular mucosa, and a normal terminal ileum. In granulomatous colitis, the findings are patchy rectal disease with punched-out ulcers, discontinuous disease, ulcers on a normal mucosa, and involvement of the terminal ileum. These criteria have allowed these two diseases to be distinguished in at least 95% of patients.[81] We have found the differentiation easier to make in the early stages of disease, because the early manifestations are particularly distinctive. In the later stages, when the disease is chronic or when there have been numerous exacerbations and remissions, the distinction may be more difficult. For instance, ulcerative colitis in remission may become discontinuous, whereas chronic granulomatous colitis may involve the entire colon. Nevertheless, in most cases, the distinction can still be made by careful examination of the mucosal surface.

TABLE 17-1. Radiologic Features of Ulcerative and Granulomatous Colitis			
Radiologic Finding		Ulcerative Colitis (23 Patients)	Granulomatous Colitis (27 Patients)
Mucosal surface	Granular	19 (83%)	0
	Normal	4* (17%)	19 (70%)
Rectum	Diffuse disease	19 (18%)	0
	Patchy disease	0	3 (11%)
	Punched-out ulcers	0	5 (19%)
Continuity	Continuous	22 (96%)	5 (19%)
	Discontinuous	1 (4%)	22 (81%)
Ulcers	On granular mucosa	4 (17%)	0
	On normal mucosa	0	19 (70%)
Terminal ileum	Normal	17 (74%)	12 (44%)
	Abnormal	0	15 (55%)
	Indeterminate	6	0

*In two patients, rectal disease has never been documented radiologically or endoscopically. The two other patients had had rectal disease in the past but were examined during remission, when the rectum appeared normal radiologically and endoscopically.

From Laufer, I., and Hamilton, J.D.: The radiologic differentiation between ulcerative and granulomatous colitis by double contrast radiology. Am. J. Gastroenterol. 66:259-269, 1976, with permission, © by American College of Gastroenterology.

INFECTIONS AND INFESTATIONS

The incidence and etiologic factors of the infective colitides vary geographically, although with travel, migration, and opportunistic infection in AIDS, a wide range of infective disorders may be seen in any country. Infections may be categorized as noninvasive because of the release of an enterotoxin, or invasive because of penetration of the mucosa by the organism, causing cellular damage with ulceration and inflammation. In the early stages, the radiologic features are often nonspecific, and appropriate laboratory investigation is essential to exclude an infective agent.

Amebiasis

Entamoeba histolytica is a simple protozoan, existing either as a commensal in cystic form, or as an invasive trophozoite, which invades the mucosa and causes cell destruction. Four clinical forms are recognized.[82]

Diffuse Colitis. Aphthoid ulcers, similar to those occurring in Crohn's disease, may be seen (Fig. 17–61A), or the colitis may resemble ulcerative colitis with a granular mucosa. Ulceration is most common in the rectosigmoid or proximal colon, and the patchy distribution may suggest Crohn's disease.

Typhloappendicitis. Appendicitis that is secondary to amebiasis and involves the cecum causes plain film changes of a soft tissue mass in the right iliac fossa with dilated cecum and air–fluid level.

Ameboma. In 1.5% to 8.4% of cases, segmental strictures develop as a result of extensive local necrosis with an inflammatory granuloma reaction.[82] Amebomas occur most often at the cecum and flexures, and they are often multiple (Fig. 17–61B).[83] Compared with neoplastic strictures, amebomas tend to be longer with tapering ends, although short-shouldered lesions indistinguishable from cancers may be found. The response to antiamebic therapy is rapid and diagnostic.

Fulminating Colitis. Toxic megacolon may complicate severe infections. Deep ulceration may result in perforations.

Amebiasis must always be excluded by examination of fresh stool specimens or rectal biopsies for trophozoites in any patient presenting with colitis, even in patients from nonendemic areas. Persistent strictures may occur in patients with severe ulceration despite adequate medical treatment, so that a post-treatment DCE is recommended.[84]

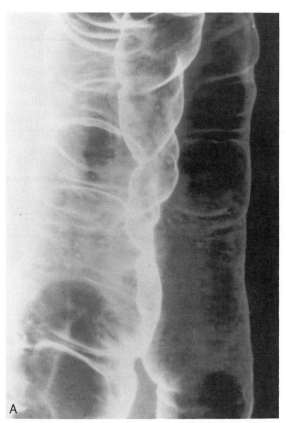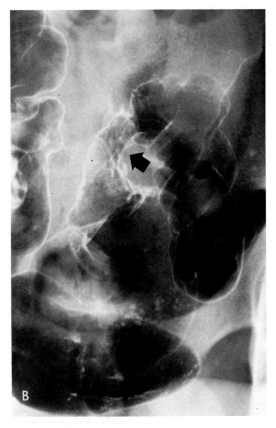

FIGURE 17–61

AMEBIASIS. *A*, Extensive aphthous ulceration due to amebiasis in a male homosexual. (Courtesy of Dr. Harvey Goldstein, San Antonio, Texas.)

B, Ameboma in the sigmoid *(arrow)*, with narrowing and an irregular surface suggestive of carcinoma.

Tuberculosis

Infection may be primary from *Mycobacterium bovis* acquired by drinking nonpasteurized milk, or secondary to pulmonary infection, although the incidence of associated pulmonary disease is now much lower than in the earlier part of the century. The chest radiograph is often normal.[85] Ileocecal involvement is most common, and patients present with abdominal pain, a mass of the right iliac fossa, and fever.[86]

The mycobacteria in the submucosa cause an inflammatory reaction characterized by caseating necrosis. Ulceration may be extensive and variable in form with a tendency toward transverse orientation. A hypertrophic response leads to a gross inflammatory reaction with fibrosis and thickening of the bowel wall (Fig. 17–62).[87] A mixed appearance of ulceration and narrowing with a thickened bowel wall is typical in the acute stage (Fig. 17–63A). Complications include perforation and tuberculous peritonitis. Contraction of the cecal pole, a patulous ileocecal valve (Fig. 17–63B), ulceration, strictures, mucosal nodularity from inflammatory masses, and bowel wall thickening with sharp demarcation of affected from normal bowel are typical radiologic features (Fig. 17–64).[87, 88] Occasionally, localized colonic strictures, sinus tracts, or fistulae may be seen. Segmental lesions in the distal colon may mimic carcinoma.[89] Residual deformity of the ileocecal region is common, even when the disease has been adequately treated (Fig. 17–63B).

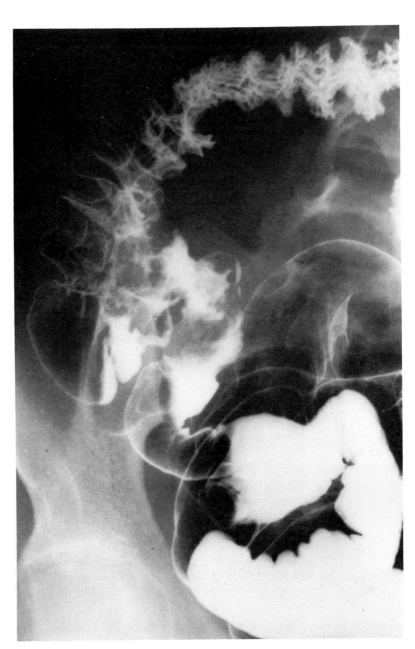

FIGURE 17–62

Ileocecal tuberculosis with florid irregular ulceration and thickening of the bowel wall.

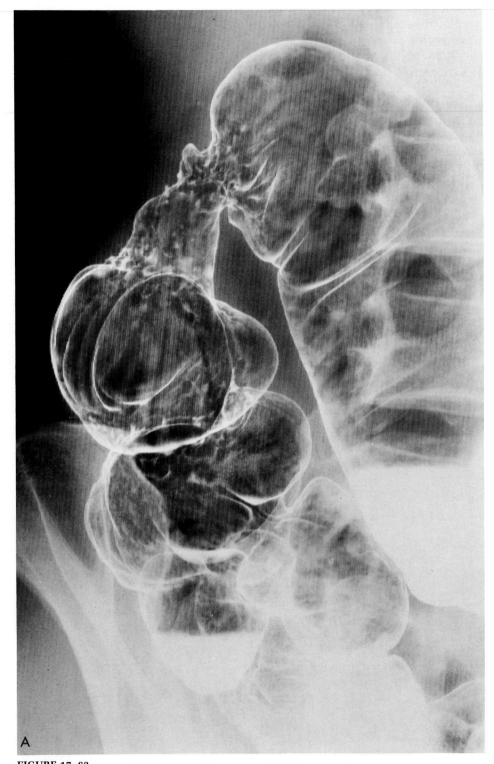

A

FIGURE 17–63

TUBERCULOUS COLITIS. *A*, Multiple short strictures and superficial ulcers in the ascending colon. At the hepatic flexure, there is a longer stricture with deeper ulceration.

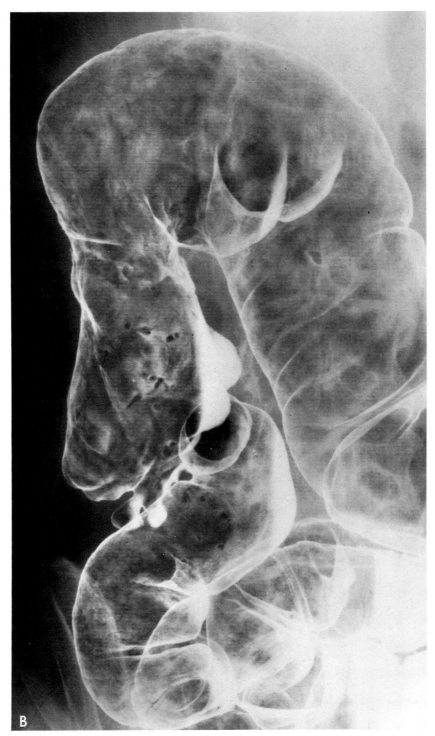

FIGURE 17–63 *Continued*

B, Residual deformity of the ileocecal area and postinflammatory polyposis without active ulceration. (Courtesy of M. Maruyama, M.D., Tokyo. From Maruyama, M.: Diagnosis of ileocecal tuberculosis—A clinico-pathological study on 12 operated cases (in Japanese). Stomach and Intestine 9:865, 1974, with permission.)

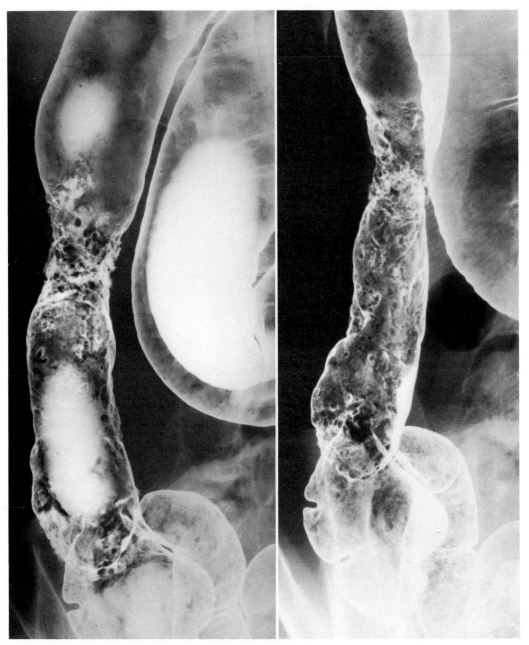

FIGURE 17–64

Tuberculous colitis with ulceration and narrowing affecting the right side of the colon. (Courtesy of M. Maruyama, M.D., Tokyo. From Maruyama, M.: Diagnosis of ileocecal tuberculosis—clinico-pathological study on 12 operated cases [in Japanese]. Stomach and Intestine 9:865, 1974, with permission.)

Yersinia Enterocolitis

Yersinia infection involves mainly the distal small bowel, although diffuse edema with aphthoid ulcers in the colon has been reported.[90] As with *Shigella* infection, these aphthoid ulcers tend to differ from those found in Crohn's disease: They are smaller, well defined, and situated on top of elevated lymphoid follicles.

Pseudomembranous Enterocolitis

Pseudomembranous enterocolitis is related to the use of broad-spectrum antibiotics allowing overgrowth with *Clostridium difficile*, which releases an enterotoxin. This enterotoxin results in mucosal damage and necrosis. Sigmoidoscopy is usually abnormal. The pseudomembrane forms slightly raised yellowish plaques, which may be scattered or confluent. Where the membrane has become separated, the underlying mucosa is ulcerated. These changes are reflected by results of the DCE. The plaques are seen as small elevated lesions (Fig. 17–65).[91] Where the membrane is confluent, the surface is shaggy, and the plaques cannot be defined. In some areas, the appearance of the colon may simulate ulcerative colitis (Fig. 17–66). The whole colon is involved, and plain film changes of dilated, air-filled small bowel loops with thickened walls indicate small bowel involvement.[92] Occasionally, the rectum may be spared even in the presence of proximal disease.[93]

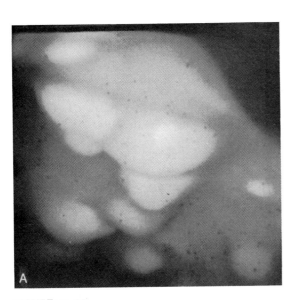

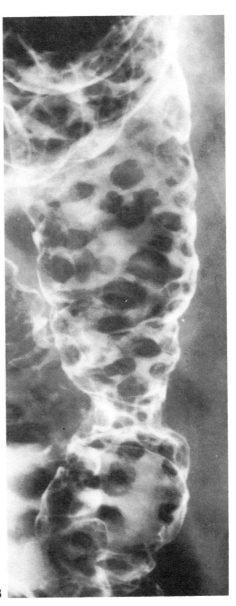

FIGURE 17–65

PSEUDOMEMBRANOUS COLITIS. *A*, An endoscopic photograph shows multiple plaque-like protrusions within the colon. (Courtesy of the Upjohn Company.)

B, The double contrast study in another patient shows the corresponding radiographic appearance with multiple polypoid filling defects representing pseudomembrane in the descending colon.

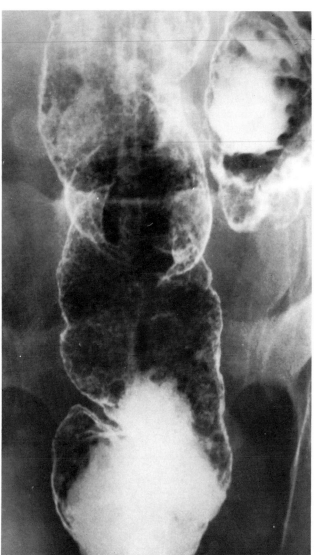

FIGURE 17–66

PSEUDOMEMBRANOUS COLITIS WITH PLAQUES IN THE PROXIMAL SIGMOID COLON. The distal rectosigmoid has a somewhat granular appearance, suggestive of ulcerative colitis. (Courtesy of Dr. L. Berger, Royal Free Hospital, London, England.)

Cytomegalovirus

Cytomegalovirus is a variety of the herpes virus and is a common cause of illness in immunocompromised patients. Vasculitis from viral invasion of the mucosa leads to ulceration, which may be deep and complicated by hemorrhage or perforation. The colitis may be segmental, often involving the cecum, or it may be diffuse. The mucosal changes vary from granularity to ulceration, which may be either superficial or deep in configuration. Computed tomography (CT) shows that the bowel wall is thickened with inflammation of the mesentery.[94]

Schistosomiasis

In the early stages, the mucosa may be granular or superficially ulcerated. The inflammatory response is characterized by granuloma formation progressing to the presence of ova in the submucosa, predominantly in the distribution of the inferior mesenteric vein. This process results in a very prominent inflammatory polyposis in the distal colon.[95] Calcification may be seen in the bowel wall on plain films or on CT images and is usually associated with calcification of the bladder wall.

Other Infections

Venereal Proctitis. Venereal proctitis may be caused by a variety of organisms,[96] including those of chlamydial, lymphogranuloma venereum (LGV), gonococcal, and herpes simplex infections. These conditions are discussed in Chapter 18.

***Campylobacter (Helicobacter)* Infection.** *Campylobacter jejuni* is a common cause of food poisoning. Plain films may show an ileus (Fig. 17–67A). The DCE may reveal diffuse colitis with a granular or finely ulcerated mucosa (Fig. 17–67B). In other cases, the appearance resembles Crohn's disease, with aphthoid ulceration and segmental distribution.[97]

***Salmonella* Enteritis.** There are only a few reports of DCE findings of *Salmonella* enteritis. Granular or diffuse ulcerative colitis may be present with enlarged Peyer's patches in the terminal ileum.[98]

***Shigella* Infection.** *Shigella sonnei* and *S. dysenteriae* are common cancers of severe infective colitis. The infection may begin with small, discrete aphthoid ulcers in the distal colon and proceed to more extensive deep ulceration.[98]

***Escherichia coli* Infection.** Pathogenic *Escherichia coli* is a common cause of food poisoning, but radiologic studies are seldom performed. Diffuse granular colitis may be present, or the radiographic appearance may suggest ischemic colitis with wall thickening, "thumbprinting," and spasm.[99]

***Strongyloides stercoralis* Infection.** *Strongyloides stercoralis* predominantly affects the small bowel and rarely causes colitis. Diffuse involvement with a granular or ulcerated mucosa has been reported.[100]

ISCHEMIC COLITIS

Patients with ischemic colitis typically present with severe abdominal pain, tenderness over the affected colon, and melena. The region of the splenic flexure is commonly affected as a result of insufficiency of the marginal artery between the superior and inferior mesenteric artery distribution.[101] However, in about 20% of cases, other parts of the colon,[102] and even the

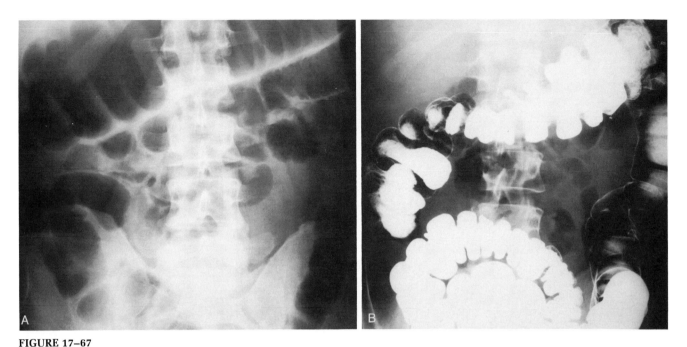

FIGURE 17–67

CAMPYLOBACTER **COLITIS.** *A,* A plain film of the abdomen shows a marked colonic ileus.

B, An instant enema performed 2 days later, after the patient's condition had improved, shows a fine granular mucosal pattern with residual blunting of the haustra in the transverse colon.

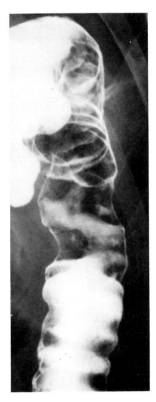

FIGURE 17–68

Ischemic colitis with "thumbprinting" in the proximal descending colon.

rectum,[103] may be involved. The spectrum of radiologic changes is related to the duration and severity of the ischemia. Early changes involve exudation and hemorrhage into the submucosa, resulting in polypoid "thumbprinting" (Fig. 17–68),[104] which may be seen on plain films and contrast studies. Anoxic changes in the smooth muscle of the affected segment cause considerable spasm, which is not relieved by intravenous smooth muscle relaxants. Gas insufflation during double contrast studies can distend the affected segment and temporarily obliterate the thumbprinting (Fig. 17–69).[105] There is a short transition zone in which the abnormal bowel funnels into the normal colon. Double contrast studies help to distinguish ischemic colitis because the en face detail shows that the mucosal surface is relatively intact. Ulceration develops with progressive mucosal damage (Fig. 17–70).

If the overall damage has been slight, complete repair occurs, and the colon becomes entirely normal, indicating transient ischemic colitis. A stricture results from healing of transmural disease with fibrosis. The strictures are eccentric, with tapering ends, and they exhibit marked sacculation (Fig. 17–71). Massive ischemic damage leads to a gangrenous bowel wall, with toxic megacolon, which is complicated by perforation or portal gas. Serial examinations in ischemic colitis have shown that thumbprinting is seen in 75%, and linear ulceration in 60%, of patients. If these signs disappear by 10 days, then the colitis is tran-

FIGURE 17–69

ISCHEMIC COLITIS. *A*, The plain film shows a narrowed descending colon with small "thumbprints."

B, An instant enema performed immediately after the plain film shows a narrowed, spastic descending colon, but the thumbprinting has been obliterated. (From Bartram, C.I.: Obliteration of thumbprinting with double-contrast enemas in acute ischemic colitis. Gastrointest. Radiol. 4:85, 1979, with permission.)

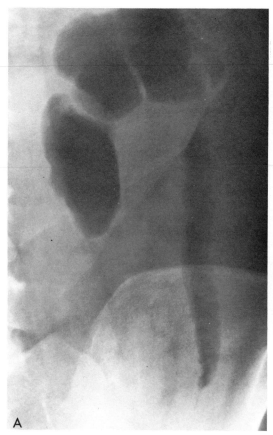

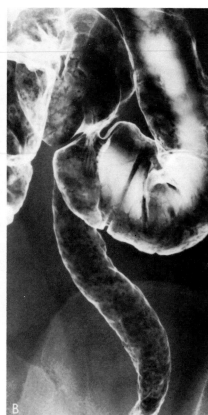

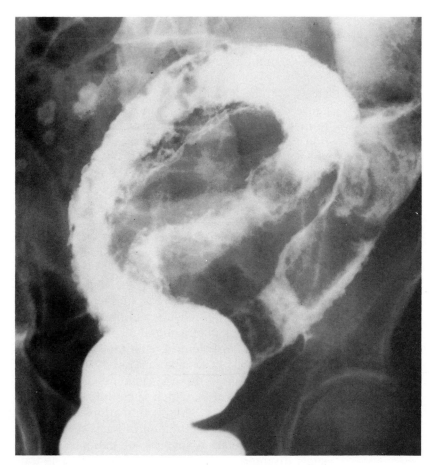

FIGURE 17–70

Severe ischemic colitis in the sigmoid with extensive mucosal ulceration. Toxic megacolon developed within 48 hours.

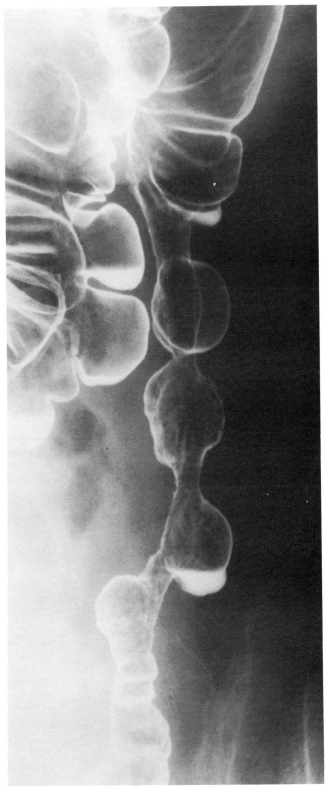

FIGURE 17–71

ISCHEMIC STRICTURE. In the descending colon, there is a long smooth stricture with acentric sacculation, which represents the sequela of ischemic colitis.

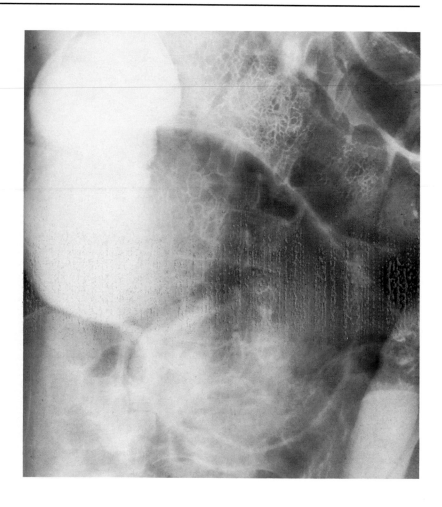

FIGURE 17–72

URTICARIAL PATTERN DUE TO MUCOSAL ISCHEMIA. There is marked colonic distention due to an ileus. The urticarial pattern seen in the transverse and right portions of the colon represents mucosal edema due to ischemia.

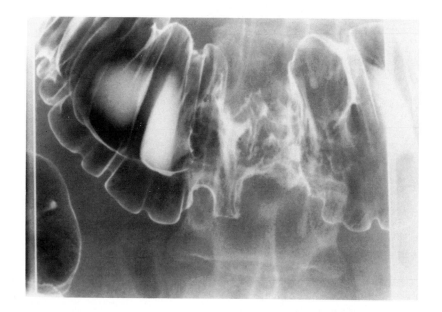

FIGURE 17–73

FOCAL ISCHEMIC COLITIS SIMULATING CARCINOMA. There is a focal area of ischemic colitis in the transverse colon due to vasculitis from intravenous drug abuse. The focal nature of the lesion may resemble a carcinoma.

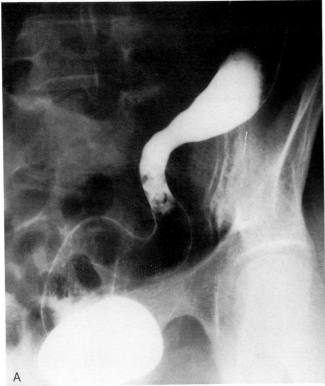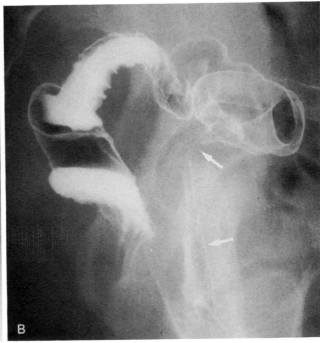

FIGURE 17–74

RADIATION COLITIS. *A,* A smooth stricture is present in the rectosigmoid 10 years after radiation treatment for carcinoma of the cervix.

B, The rectum and sigmoid are involved by radiation change. There is a fistula from the sigmoid to the vagina *(arrows).*

sient, but persistence of either for more than 20 days is associated with stricture formation.[106]

Any type of colonic obstruction, typically carcinoma, distends the colon and so reduces mucosal blood flow, causing about 10% of the cases of ischemic colitis. An "urticarial" pattern has been described as an early manifestation of ischemia proximal to an obstruction.[107] A similar pattern due to mucosal ischemia may be seen in patients with marked colonic distention of any cause, including an ileus (Fig. 17–72). In other cases, an ischemic lesion may mimic a carcinoma (Fig. 17–73).[108]

The instant enema is the preferred examination for suspected ischemic colitis. Plain films are needed to evaluate fulminating cases. A follow-up DCE is recommended in all cases to exclude stricture formation. If a stricture is present, a further examination is recommended after 6 to 9 months to show its final state because strictures may regress substantially during this period. The radiographic evaluation of changes in ischemic colitis have been extensively documented by Reeders and colleagues.[109]

RADIATION COLITIS

Most radiation-induced large bowel complications affect the sigmoid and rectum following treatment of cervical or uterine carcinoma. Doses in excess of 4500 rads increase the incidence of damage, and damage is more likely with combined intracavitary and external-beam treatments. Overall, the incidence of complications is about 5%.[110]

The initial effect of radiation is transient proctocolitis, 6 to 24 months after treatment. Later effects result from endarteritis, with fibrosis and telangiectasia causing stricturing, ulceration, and formation of fistula. These effects may develop several years later. The strictures are usually smooth and symmetric with a narrow lumen (Fig. 17–74A). Short strictures may simulate carcinoma. Ulceration occurs most often in the anterior wall of the rectum, where penetration of the ulcer creates the typical rectovaginal fistula (Fig. 17–74B). The mucosal telangiectasia results in rectal bleeding.

MISCELLANEOUS FORMS OF COLITIS

Behçet's Disease

The syndrome of recurrent oral and genital ulceration with ocular manifestations was described by Behçet in 1973. This syndrome is now recognized to be a multisystem disease in which intestinal ulceration may develop. The ulceration commonly occurs in the ileocecal region. The ulcers tend to be deep and "punched out." This transmural ulceration may be complicated by severe bleeding or perforation.[111] Radiologically, the ulcers are discrete, and if superficial, they may be aphthoid ulcers.

Colonic Urticaria

Colonic urticaria is a rare condition in which edema lifts up parts of the mucosal surface, resulting in a mosaic or crazy-paving effect (Fig. 17–75). This condition may be due to allergic reactions,[112] early ischemia,[107] or herpes zoster.[113]

Diversion Colitis

Once the colon is no longer functional, bacterial overgrowth results, and the bowel lumen becomes narrow. Both conditions resolve spontaneously once the bowel is reanastomosed. The mucosa in a nonfunctional loop appears slightly granular endoscopi-

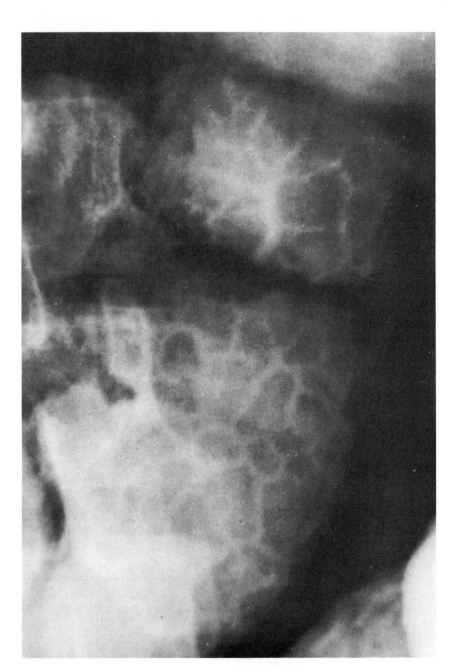

FIGURE 17–75

The mosaic mucosal pattern in urticaria of the colon.

cally and radiologically. There are reports suggesting nodularity, inflammatory polyposis, or fine ulcerations,[114] but these reports are rare. Double contrast studies may be performed on a nonfunctional loop, but barium is retained within it for some time unless the loop is washed out. A water-soluble contrast examination is preferred to outline the loop and is sufficient to exclude gross ulceration.

Graft-Versus-Host Disease

Following bone marrow transplantation, graft-versus-host disease occurs in approximately 70% of patients. Diffuse ulceration, narrowing, and loss of haustration may be seen in the colon approximately 3 to 5 weeks after transplantation as part of a generalized reaction that also involves the small bowel.[115]

Typhlitis

Typhlitis is an inflammatory or ischemic condition of the cecum and right colon occurring in patients who are immunosuppressive because of hematologic malignancy or aplastic anemia. Its appearance essentially resembles that of an ischemic lesion affecting the right colon. Because of the risk of perforation, contrast studies with water-soluble contrast are usually performed, and double contrast studies are rarely performed.[116]

SUMMARY

Although the number of macroscopic changes in the colon occurring in response to inflammatory injury from a variety of causes is limited, the nature and distribution of these changes often provide a good indication of the specific type of colitis. Double contrast studies accurately reflect all but the earliest mucosal changes. They have the additional advantages of revealing complications, such as fistulae and strictures, and providing an overall map of the extent and severity of the colitis, so that a permanent record for assessment and comparison can be maintained. Table 17–2 lists the major radiologic features of colitis and the conditions in which they are often found as well as those conditions in which they are occasionally found.

ACKNOWLEDGMENT

We are grateful to Dr. Basil C. Morson of the Department of Pathology, St. Mark's Hospital, London, for supplying the specimen photographs for this chapter.

TABLE 17–2. Summary of the Predominant Radiologic Features in Colitis		
Radiologic Feature	Commonly Found In	May Be Found In
Granular mucosa	Ulcerative colitis	Early Crohn's colitis (rare)
Ulceration		
Discrete	Crohn's disease Yersinia enterocolitis Behçet's disease	Amebiasis Ischemia Tuberculosis
Confluent shallow	Ulcerative colitis	Crohn's disease Amebiasis
Confluent deep	Crohn's disease	Ischemia Amebiasis Tuberculosis *Strongyloides* colitis
Stricture formation		
Symmetric	Ulcerative colitis Lymphogranuloma venereum	Tuberculosis
Asymmetric	Crohn's disease Ischemia Tuberculosis	
Fistula	Crohn's disease Lymphogranuloma venereum	Tuberculosis
Inflammatory polyps	Ulcerative colitis Crohn's disease Schistosomiasis Colitis cystica profunda	Ischemia (rare)
Small bowel involvement	Yersinia enterocolitis Tuberculosis Pseudomembranous enterocolitis Crohn's disease	Ulcerative colitis (backwash) Behçet's disease Ischemia
Skip lesions	Crohn's disease Tuberculosis Amebiasis	Lymphogranuloma venereum
Toxic megacolon	Ulcerative colitis	Crohn's disease Ischemia Amebiasis

REFERENCES

1. Bartram, C.I.: Radiology in Inflammatory Bowel Disease. New York, Marcel Dekker, 1983, p. 31.
2. Fraser, G.M., and Findlay, J.M.: The double contrast enema in ulcerative colitis and Crohn's disease. Clin. Radiol. 27:103, 1976.
3. Laufer, I.: Air contrast studies of the colon in inflammatory bowel disease. CRC Crit. Rev. Diagnost. Imaging 9:421, 1977.
4. Young, A.C.: The instant barium enema in procto-colitis. Proc. R. Soc. Med. 56:491, 1963.
5. Bartram, C.I.: The plain abdominal x-ray in acute colitis. Proc. R. Soc. Med. 69:617, 1976.
6. Bartram, C.I.: Radiology in the current assessment of ulcerative colitis. Gastrointest. Radiol. 1:383, 1977.
7. Roth, J.L.A., Valdes-Dapena, A., Stein, G.N., et al.: Toxic megacolon in ulcerative colitis. Gastroenterology 37:239, 1959.
8. Thomas, B.M.: The instant enema in inflammatory disease of the colon. Clin. Radiol. 30:165, 1979.

9. Morson, B.C., and Dawson, I.M.P.: Gastrointestinal Pathology. Oxford, Blackwell Scientific Publications, 1972, p. 458.
10. Welin, S., and Brahme, F.: The double contrast method in ulcerative colitis. Acta Radiol. 55:257, 1961.
11. Powell-Tuck, J., Ritchie, J.K., and Lennard-Jones, J.E.: The prognosis of idiopathic proctitis and distal colitis. Gut 17:392, 1976.
12. Lennard-Jones, J.F., Misiewicz, J.J., Parish, J.A., et al.: Prospective study of outpatients with extensive colitis. Lancet 1:1065, 1974.
13. Bartram, C.I., and Walmesley, K.: A pathological and radiological correlation of the mucosal changes in ulcerative colitis. Clin. Radiol. 29:323, 1978.
14. Laufer, I., Mullens, J.E., and Hamilton, J.: Correlation of endoscopy and double contrast radiography in the early stages of ulcerative and granulomatous colitis. Radiology 118:1, 1976.
15. Jalan, K.N., Walker, R.J., Sircus, W., et al.: Pseudopolyposis in ulcerative colitis. Lancet 11:555, 1969.
16. de Dombal, F.T., Watts, J., Watkins, G., et al.: Local complications of ulcerative colitis, strictures, pseudopolyps, and carcinoma of colon and rectum. Br. Med. J. 1:1442, 1966.
17. Zegel, H., and Laufer, I.: Filiform polyposis. Radiology 127:615, 1978.
18. Goldberger, L.E., Neely, H.R., and Stammer, J.L.: Large mucosal bridges. An unusual roentgenographic manifestation of ulcerative colitis. Gastrointest. Radiol. 3:81, 1978.
19. Hammerman, A.M., Shatz, B.A., and Susman, N.: Radiographic characteristics of colonic "mucosal bridges": Sequelae of inflammatory bowel disease. Radiology 127:611, 1978.
20. Joffe, N.: Localized giant pseudopolyposis secondary to ulcerative or granulomatous colitis. Clin. Radiol. 28:609, 1977.
21. Russell, J.G.B., and Donoghue, V.: Rectal fold thickness as an indicator of disease. Clin. Radiol. 34:427, 1983.
22. Simpkins, K.C., and Stevenson, G.W.: The modified Malmö double contrast barium enema in colitis: An assessment of its accuracy in reflecting sigmoidoscopic findings. Br. J. Radiol. 45:486, 1972.
23. Edling, N.P.G., and Eklof, O.: The retrorectal soft tissue space in ulcerative colitis: A roentgen diagnostic study. Radiology 80:949, 1963.
24. Counsell, B.: Lesions of the ileum associated with ulcerative colitis. Br. J. Surg. 185:276, 1956.
25. Sellink, J.L.: Radiological Atlas of Common Disease of the Small Bowel. Leiden, Stenfert Kroese, 1976, p. 202.
26. Glick, S.N., Teplick, S.K., and Amenta, P.S.: Microscopic (collagenous) colitis. AJR 153:995, 1989.
27. Elliott, P.R., Williams, C.B., Lennard-Jones, J.E., et al.: Colonoscopic diagnosis of minimal change colitis in patients with a normal sigmoidoscopy and normal air-contrast barium enema. Lancet 1:650, 1982.
28. Buckell, N.A., Williams, G.T., Bartram, C.I., and Lennard-Jones, J.E.: Depth of ulceration in acute colitis. Gastroenterology 79:19, 1980.
29. Hywel-Jones, J., and Chapman, M.: Definition of megacolon in colitis. Gut 10:562, 1969.
30. Lennard-Jones, J.E., Langman, M.J.S., and Avery Jones, F.: Fecal stasis in proctocolitis. Gut 3:301, 1962.
31. Hunt, R.H., Teague, R.H., Swartbrick, E.T., et al.: Colonoscopy in the management of colonic strictures. Br. Med. J. 3:360, 1975.
32. Simpkins, K.C., and Young, A.C.: The differential diagnosis of large bowel strictures. Clin. Radiol. 22:449, 1971.
33. Edwards, F.C., and Truelove, S.C.: The course and prognosis of ulcerative colitis. IV. Carcinoma of the colon. Gut 5:15, 1964.
34. Edling, N.P.G., Lagercrantz, R., and Rosenquist, H.: Roentgenologic findings in ulcerative colitis with malignant degeneration. Acta Radiol. 52:123, 1959.
35. Fennessey, J.J., Sparberg, M.B., and Kirsner, J.B.: Radiological findings in carcinoma of the colon complicating chronic ulcerative colitis. Gut 9:388, 1968.
35a. Williams, C.B., and Teague, R.: Colonoscopy. Gut 14:990, 1973.
36. Hodgson, J.R., and Sauer, W.G.: The roentgenologic features of carcinoma in chronic ulcerative colitis. AJR 86:91, 1961.
37. Lennard-Jones, J.E., Morson, B.C., Ritchie, J.K., et al.: Cancer in colitis: Assessment of the individual risk by clinical and histological criteria. Gastroenterology 73:1280, 1977.
38. Ekbom, A., Helmick, C., Zack, M., et al.: Ulcerative colitis and colorectal cancer: A population-based study. N. Engl. J. Med. 323:1228, 1990.
39. MacDougall, I.P.M.: Clinical identification of those cases of ulcerative colitis most likely to develop cancer of the bowel. Dis. Colon Rectum 7:447, 1964.
40. Hinton, J.M.: Risk of malignant change in ulcerative colitis. Gut 7:427, 1966.
41. Devroede, G., and Taylor, W.F.: On calculating cancer risk and survival of ulcerative colitis patients with the life table method. Gastroenterology 71:505, 1976.
42. Morson, B.C., and Pang, L.S.C.: Rectal biopsy as an aid to cancer control in ulcerative colitis. Gut 8:423, 1967.
43. Hooyman, J.R., MacCarty, R.L., Carpenter, H.A., et al.: Radiographic appearance of mucosal dysplasia associated with ulcerative colitis. AJR 149:47, 1987.
44. Frank, P.H., Riddell, R.H., Feczko, P.J., et al.: Radiological detection of colonic dysplasia (precarcinoma) in chronic ulcerative colitis. Gastrointest. Radiol. 3:209, 1978.
45. Kelvin, F.M., Woodward, B.H., McLeod, M., et al.: Prospective diagnosis of dysplasia (pre-cancer) in chronic ulcerative colitis. AJR 138:347, 1982.
46. Stevenson, G.W., Goodacre, R., and Jackson, M.: Dysplasia to carcinoma transformation in ulcerative colitis. AJR 143:108, 1984.
47. Blackstone, M.O., Riddell, R.H., Rogers, B.H., and Levin, B.: Dysplasia-associated lesion or mass (DALM) detected by colonoscopy in long-standing ulcerative colitis: An indication for colectomy. Gastroenterology 80:366, 1981.
47a. Butt, J.H., Konishi, F., Morson, B.C., et al.: Macroscopic lesions in dysplasia and carcinoma complicating ulcerative colitis. Dig. Dis. Sci. 28:18, 1983.
48. Lennard-Jones, J.E.: Compliance, cost, and common sense limit cancer control in colitis. Gut 27:1403, 1986.
49. Bartolo, D., Goepel, J.R., and Parsons, M.A.: Rectal malignant lymphoma in chronic ulcerative colitis. Gut 23:164, 1982.
50. Mekhjian, H.A., Switz, D.M., Melnyk, C.S., et al.: Clinical features and natural history of Crohn's disease. Gastroenterology 77:898, 1979.
51. Marshak, R.H.: Granulomatous disease of the intestinal tract (Crohn's disease). Radiology 114:3, 1975.
52. Lockhart-Mummery, H.E., and Morson, B.C.: Crohn's disease of the large intestine. Gut 5:493, 1964.
53. Laufer, I., and Costopoulos, L.: Early lesions of Crohn's disease. AJR 130:307, 1978.
54. Simpkins, K.C.: Aphthoid ulcers in Crohn's colitis. Clin. Radiol. 28:601, 1978.
55. Max, R.J., and Kelvin, F.M.: Nonspecificity of discrete colonic ulceration on double-contrast barium enema study. AJR 134:1265, 1980.
56. Joffe, N.: Diffuse mucosal granularity in double-contrast studies of Crohn's disease of the colon. Clin. Radiol. 32:85, 1981.
57. Laufer, I., and Hamilton, J.: The radiological differentiation between ulcerative and granulomatous colitis by double contrast radiology. Am. J. Gastroenterol. 66:259, 1976.
58. Berridge, F.R.: Two unusual radiological signs of Crohn's disease of the colon. Clin. Radiol. 22:444, 1971.
59. Greenstein, A.J., and Janowitz, H.D.: Cancer in Crohn's disease. Am. J. Gastroenterol. 64:122, 1976.
60. Welin, S., and Welin, G.: A pathognomonic roentgenologic sign of regional ileitis (Crohn's disease). Dis. Colon Rectum 16:473, 1973.
61. Marshak, R.H., Janowitz, H.D., and Present, D.H.: Granulomatous colitis in association with diverticula. N. Engl. J. Med. 283:1080, 1970.
62. Meyers, M.A., Alonso, D.R., Morson, B.C., et al.: Pathogenesis of diverticulitis complicating granulomatous colitis. Gastroenterology 74:24, 1978.
63. Ferrucci, J.T., Jr., Ragsdale, B.D., Barrett, P.J., et al.: Double tracking in the sigmoid colon. Radiology 120:307, 1976.

64. Korelitz, B.I., and Sommers, S.C.: Differential diagnosis of ulcerative and granulomatous colitis by sigmoidoscopy, rectal biopsy and cell counts of rectal mucosa. Am. J. Gastroenterol. *61*:460, 1974.

65. Deveroede, G.J.: The differential diagnosis of colitis. Can. J. Surg. *17*:369, 1974.

66. Hywel-Jones, J., Lennard-Jones, J.E., and Young, A.C.: Reversibility of radiological appearances during clinical improvement in colonic Crohn's disease. Gut *10*:738, 1969.

67. Brahme, F.: Granulomatous colitis: Roentgenologic appearance and course of the lesion. AJR *97*:35, 1967.

68. Vantrappen, G., Ayg, H.O., Ponette, E., et al.: Yersinial enteritis and enterocolitis: Gastroenterological aspects. Gastroenterology *72*:220, 1977.

69. Ekberg, O., Sjostrom, B., and Brahme, F.J.: Radiological findings in *Yersinia* ileitis. Radiology *123*:15, 1977.

70. Herlinger, H., O'Riordan, D., Saul, S., and Levine, M.S.: Nonspecific involvement of bowel adjoining Crohn disease. Radiology *159*:47, 1986.

71. Kusakeioglu, O., and Norton, R.A.: Granulomatous duodenitis, clubbed digits and psoriasis: Report of a case. Lahey Clin. Found. Bull. *16*:191, 1967.

72. Wilder, W.M., and Davis, W.D.: Duodenal enteritis. South. Med. J. *59*:884, 1966.

73. Legge, D.A., Carlson, H.C., and Judd, E.S.: Roentgenologic features of regional enteritis of the upper gastrointestinal tract. AJR *110*:355, 1970.

74. Tanaka, M., Kimura, K., Sakai, H., et al.: Long-term follow-up for minute gastroduodenal lesions in Crohn's disease. Gastrointest. Endosc. *32*:206, 1986.

75. Levine, M.S.: Crohn's disease of the upper gastrointestinal tract. Radiol. Clin. North Am. *25*:79, 1987.

76. Laufer, I., Trueman, T., and deSa, D.: Multiple superficial gastric erosions due to Crohn's disease of the stomach: Radiologic and endoscopic diagnosis. Br. J. Radiol. *49*:726, 1976.

77. Laufer, I., Hamilton, J., and Mullens, J.E.: Demonstration of superficial gastric erosions by double contrast radiology. Gastroenterology *68*:387, 1975.

78. Nugent, F.W., and Roy, M.A.: Duodenal Crohn's disease: An analysis of 89 cases. Am. J. Gastroenterol. *84*:249, 1989.

79. Gad, A.: The diagnosis of gastroduodenal Crohn's disease by endoscopic biopsy. Scand. J. Gastroenterol. Suppl. *167*:23, 1989.

80. Cynn, W.S., Chon, H.K., Gureghian, P.A., et al.: Crohn's disease of the esophagus. AJR *125*:359, 1975.

81. Williams, H.J., Stephens, D.H., and Carlson, H.C.: Double contrast radiography: Colonic inflammatory disease. AJR *137*:315, 1981.

82. Cardosa, J.M., Kimura, K., Stoopen, M., et al.: Radiology of invasive amebiasis of the colon. AJR *128*:935, 1977.

83. Middlemiss, H.: Tropical Radiology. London, William Heineman, 1961, p. 128.

84. Martinez, C.R., Gilman, R.H., Rabbani, G.H., and Koster, F.: Amebic colitis: Correlation of proctoscopy before treatment and barium enema after treatment. AJR *138*:1089, 1982.

85. Werbeloff, L., Novis, B.H., Banks, S., et al.: The radiology of tuberculosis of the gastrointestinal tract. Br. J. Radiol. *46*:329, 1973.

86. Palmer, K.R., Patil, D.H., Riordan, J.F., and Silk, D.B.A.: Abdominal tuberculosis in urban Britain—a common disease. Gut *26*:1296, 1985.

87. Balthazar, E.J., Gordon, R., and Hulnick, D.: Ileocecal tuberculosis: CT and radiologic evaluation. AJR *154*:499, 1990.

88. Carrera, F., Young, S., and Lewick, A.M.: Intestinal tuberculosis. Gastrointest. Radiol. *1*:147, 1976.

89. Balthazar, E.J., and Bryk, D.: Segmental tuberculosis of the distal colon: Radiographic features in 7 cases. Gastrointest. Radiol. *5*:75, 1980.

90. Lachman, R., Soong, J., Wishon, G., et al.: *Yersinia* colitis. Gastrointest. Radiol. *2*:133, 1977.

91. Stanley, R.J., Melson, G.L., and Tedesco, F.J.: The spectrum of radiographic findings in antibiotic-related pseudomembranous colitis. Radiology *111*:519, 1974.

92. Strada, M., Meregaglia, D., and Donzelli, R.: Double-contrast enema in antibiotic-related pseudomembranous colitis. Gastrointest. Radiol. *8*:67, 1983.

93. Rubesin, S.E., Levine, M.S., Glick, S.N., et al.: Pseudomembranous colitis with rectosigmoid sparing on barium studies. Radiology *170*:811, 1989.

94. Balthazar, E.J., Megibow, A.J., Fazzini, E., et al.: Cytomegalovirus colitis in AIDS: Radiographic findings in 11 patients. Radiology *155*:585, 1985.

95. Medina, J.T., Seaman, W.B., Gazman-Acosta, C., et al.: The roentgen appearance of *Schistosomiasis mansoni*. Radiology *85*:628, 1978.

96. Sider, L., Mintzer, R.A., Mendelson, E.B., et al.: Radiographic findings of infectious proctitis in homosexual men. AJR *138*:667, 1982.

96a. Fataar, S., Bassiony, H., Hamed, M.S., et al.: Radiographic spectrum of rectocolonic calcification from schistosomiasis. AJR *142*:933, 1984.

97. Tielbeek, A.V., Rosenbusch, G., Muytjens, H.L., et al.: Roentgenologic changes of the colon in *Campylobacter* infection. Gastrointest. Radiol. *10*:358, 1985.

98. Farman, J., Rabinowitz, J.G., and Meyers, M.A.: Roentgenology of infectious colitis. AJR *119*:375, 1973.

99. Shortsleeve, M.J., Wilson, M.E., Finkelstein, M., et al.: Radiologic findings in hemorrhagic colitis due to *Escherichia coli* 0157:H7. Gastrointest. Radiol. *14*:341, 1989.

100. Drasin, G.F., Moss, J.P., and Cheng, S.H.: *Strongyloides stercoralis* colitis: Findings in four cases. Radiology *126*:619, 1978.

101. Griffiths, J.D.: Surgical anatomy of the distal colon. Ann. R. Coll. Surg. Engl. *19*:241, 1956.

102. Tomchik, F.S., Wittenberg, J., and Ottinger, L.W.: The roentgenographic spectrum of bowel infarction. Radiology *96*:249, 1970.

103. Kilpatrick, Z.M., Farman, J., Yesner, R., et al.: Ischemic proctitis. JAMA *205*:74, 1968.

104. Boley, S.J., Schwartz, S., Lash, J., et al.: Reversible vascular occlusion of the colon. Surg. Gynecol. Obstet. *116*:53, 1963.

105. Bartram, C.I.: Obliteration of thumbprinting with double-contrast enemas in acute ischemic colitis. Gastrointest. Radiol. *4*:85, 1979.

106. Iida, M., Matsui, T., Fuchigami, T., et al.: Ischemic colitis: Serial changes in double-contrast barium enema examination. Radiology *159*:337, 1986.

107. Greenberg, H.M., Goldberg, H.I., and Axel, L.: Colonic "urticaria" pattern due to early ischemia. Gastrointest. Radiol. *6*:145, 1981.

108. Brandt, L.J., Katz, H.J., Wolf, E.L., et al.: Simulation of colonic carcinoma by ischemia. Gastroenterology *88*:1137, 1985.

109. Reeders, J.W., Tytgat, G.N., Rosenbusch, G., et al.: Ischemic Colitis. The Hague, Martinus Nijhoff, 1984.

110. Allen-Mersch, T.G., Wilson, E.J., Hope-Stone, H.F., and Mann, C.V.: Has the incidence of radiation-induced bowel damage following treatment of uterine carcinoma changed in the last 20 years? J. R. Soc. Med. *79*:387, 1986.

111. O'Connell, D.J., Courtney, J.V., and Riddell, R.: Colitis of Behçet's syndrome: Radiologic and pathologic features. Gastrointest. Radiol. *5*:173, 1980.

112. Berk, R.N., and Millman, S.J.: Urticaria of the colon. Radiology *99*:539, 1971.

113. Menuck, L.S., Brahme, F., Amberg, J., and Sherr, H.P.: Colonic changes of herpes zoster. AJR *127*:273, 1976.

114. Scott, R.L., and Pinstein, M.L.: Diversion colitis demonstrated by double-contrast barium enema. AJR *143*:767, 1984.

115. Fisk, J.D., Shulman, H.M., Greening, R.R., et al.: Gastrointestinal radiographic features of human graft-vs.-host disease. AJR *136*:329, 1981.

116. Taylor, A.J., Dodds, W.J., Gonyo, J.E., et al.: Typhlitis in adults. Gastrointest. Radiol. *30*:363, 1985.

RECTUM

Marc S. Levine, M.D.
Igor Laufer, M.D.

18

Because the rectum is inaccessible to fluoroscopic palpation or compression, the conventional single contrast barium enema has been ineffective in diagnosing inflammatory or neoplastic lesions in this area.[1] As a result, the rectum has traditionally been considered the domain of the endoscopist rather than the radiologist. However, it is now recognized that endoscopy also has limitations in evaluating the rectum and that significant abnormalities may remain undetected.[2-5] This is partly because proctosigmoidoscopy is often done by examiners who are not expert in performing the procedure or in interpreting the findings.[6] Even experienced examiners can miss lesions in endoscopic "blind spots" behind a valve of Houston or on the posterior wall of the distal rectum near the anal verge (see Figs. 18–7 and 18–24).[3, 4] Other lesions can be missed because of patient discomfort, anatomic variation, or distortion of the rectosigmoid by underlying disease that prevents complete insertion of the sigmoidoscope. For all of these reasons, the rectum should be carefully evaluated during the routine barium enema examination, even in patients who have recently undergone or are about to undergo endoscopy. The major advantage of double contrast technique is that it permits visualization of the rectum in double contrast without an overlying column of barium, so that lesions can be demonstrated both en face and in profile.

TECHNIQUE

A complete study of the rectum is included in the routine double contrast enema (see Chapter 12). A high-quality examination of the rectum requires drainage of excess barium through the enema tip prior to final air insufflation.[7] This is best accomplished by placing the patient in a prone or left lateral position with the head of the table elevated 20 to 40 degrees and gently depressing the enema tip between the patient's legs to facilitate drainage of barium from the rectum.[8] It should be recognized that the enema tip itself may obscure lesions in the distal rectum (see Fig. 18–19). In patients with adequate sphincter tone, the tip therefore should be removed prior to obtaining spot films of the rectum. Early removal of the enema tip results not only in greater diagnostic accuracy in evaluating the rectum but in better patient acceptance of the procedure.[9]

After the enema tip has been removed, spot films of the rectum should be obtained in prone, supine, and lateral projections. Frontal views often provide better mucosal detail because of decreased scatter. However, lateral views permit better delineation of perirectal disease involving the anterior wall of the rectosigmoid owing to inflammatory conditions, en-

dometriosis, or metastatic tumor (see later section, "Extrinsic Abnormalities"). Additional spot films may be obtained in appropriate projections when rectal lesions are suspected at fluoroscopy.

Two of the routine overhead radiographs included in the double contrast enema—the prone, angled view of the rectosigmoid and the prone, cross-table lateral view of the rectum—are particularly helpful for evaluating this region.[10, 11] Some small lesions near the rectosigmoid junction may be visible only on the prone, angled view, whereas larger lesions that are suspected on other views may be demonstrated conclusively only on the angled view (see Fig. 18–21). The prone, cross-table lateral view is ideal for demonstrating abnormalities involving the anterior or posterior wall of the rectum.

A double contrast enema may be performed on patients with poor or absent sphincter tone by inflating a balloon in the rectum at the beginning of the examination and applying gentle traction on the enema tip to prevent leakage of barium and air. It is safe to use a balloon as long as there is no history of rectal disease or pelvic irradiation. The balloon should be inflated only under fluoroscopic guidance, and no more than 100 cc of gas should be injected into the balloon. When a balloon is used, it is still possible to evaluate the rectum by deflating the balloon at the end of the study and obtaining frontal and lateral spot films of the rectum at that time. Otherwise, proctoscopy is required to rule out rectal disease.

Recently, there has been considerable interest in the use of defecography or excretory proctography to evaluate patients with rectal prolapse, incontinence, or other defecation disorders.[12, 13] However, this subject is beyond the scope of this text.

NORMAL APPEARANCES

The normal anatomy of the rectum is well demonstrated on double contrast studies. There are usually three prominent transverse folds, known as the valves of Houston, which are best seen on lateral views of the rectum (Fig. 18–1A).[14] The largest of these folds has been called the fold of Kohlrausch (Fig. 18–1B). When the distal rectum is partially collapsed, the columns of Morgagni may also be recognized as relatively straight, 2- to 4-mm-wide folds extending 2 to 3 cm from the anorectal junction (Fig. 18–2). Aside from these normal structures, the rectal mucosa usually has a smooth, featureless appearance. On lateral views, the posterior wall of the rectum generally lies 1 cm or less from the curve of the sacrum, but there is considerable variation, particularly in older patients, in whom a presacral space of 1 to 2 cm may

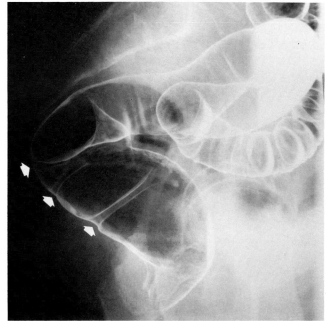

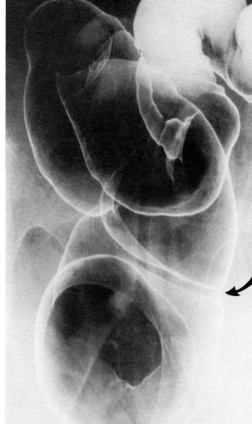

FIGURE 18–1

NORMAL ANATOMY OF RECTUM. *A,* Lateral view showing valves of Houston *(arrows).*

B, Prone, angled view showing prominent valve of Kohlrausch *(arrow).*

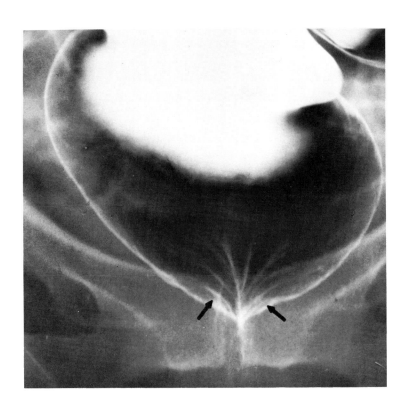

FIGURE 18–2

Rectal columns of Morgagni, appearing as thin, straight folds *(arrows)* near anorectal junction.

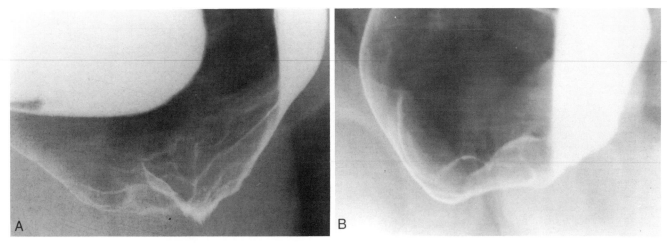

FIGURE 18–3

A and *B*, Two examples of internal hemorrhoids manifested by lobulated folds near anorectal junction.

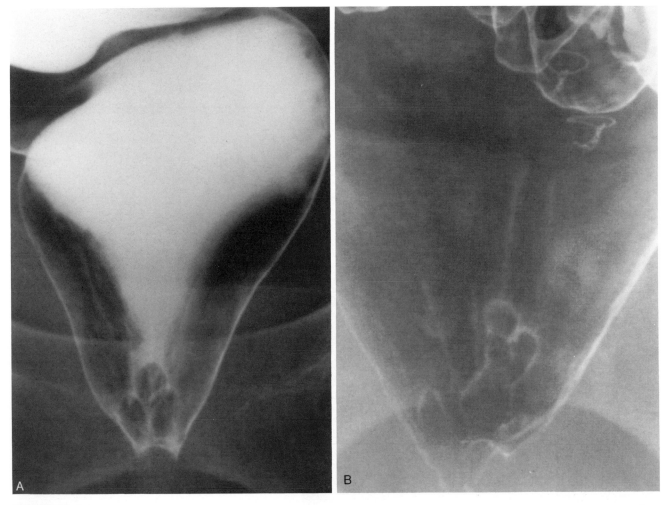

FIGURE 18–4

A and *B*, Two examples of internal hemorrhoids manifested by small submucosal nodules in distal rectum.

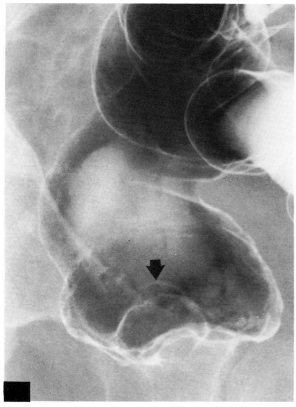

FIGURE 18–5

Large internal hemorrhoids manifested by a polypoid mass
(*arrow*) in distal rectum. Proctoscopy is required in this patient,
because a polypoid carcinoma could produce similar findings.

be observed as a normal finding.[15] A sharp angulation
almost always occurs at the rectosigmoid junction, as
the distal rectum heads anteriorly and inferiorly.

INTRINSIC ABNORMALITIES

Hemorrhoids

Hemorrhoids are a common source of rectal bleeding
in older patients. They may be classified as internal
or external, depending on their location above or
below the anorectal junction. Although external hemorrhoids are readily detectable by visual inspection,
internal hemorrhoids may be diagnosed by digital
examination of the rectum, by proctoscopy, or by
double contrast barium enema. In many cases, the
patient is already known to have hemorrhoids, and a
barium enema is performed to search for other more
proximal sources of rectal bleeding. Nevertheless, it
is important to be aware of the radiographic appearance of internal hemorrhoids, so that they can be
differentiated from other more serious pathologic lesions.

Internal hemorrhoids are typically manifested on
double contrast enemas by lobulated folds extending
3 cm or less from the anorectal junction (Fig. 18–3)
or by multiple, small submucosal nodules (usually
two to four) in the distal rectum, often resembling a
small cluster of grapes (Fig. 18–4).[16, 17] Much less
frequently, internal hemorrhoids may appear as lobulated folds extending more than 3 cm from the
anorectal junction or as solitary nodules or polypoid
lesions in the distal rectum (Fig. 18–5).[17] However,
proctitis, rectal tumors, or hypertrophied anal papillae may produce similar findings (Fig. 18–6).[17, 18]
Thus, any lesions that have an atypical appearance
for internal hemorrhoids on double contrast enema
should be evaluated by proctoscopy to rule out other
pathologic conditions.

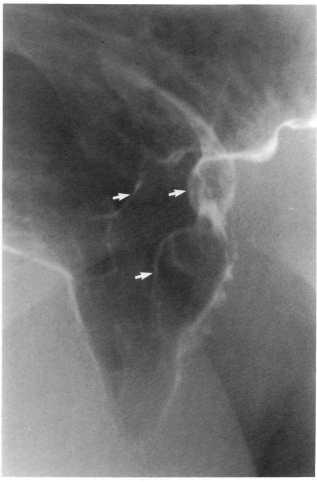

FIGURE 18–6

Rectal carcinoma with irregular, lobulated folds (*arrows*) in distal
rectum, raising the possibility of prominent hemorrhoids.
However, the folds extend farther proximally from the anorectal
junction than expected for most internal hemorrhoids. (From
Levine, M.S., et al.: Internal hemorrhoids: Diagnosis with double-
contrast barium enema examinations. Radiology *177*:141–144,
1990, with permission.)

Neoplastic Lesions

Polyps

Because they are predominantly located in the distal colon, polyps are particularly common in the rectosigmoid region. Rectal polyps are more likely to be missed at endoscopy if they lie just beyond the anal verge or behind a valve of Houston (Fig. 18–7).[3] These polyps are usually hyperplastic or adenomatous. Hyperplastic polyps tend to be smooth, rounded elevations less than 5 mm in size, whereas adenomatous polyps tend to be larger and more lobulated.[19] Occasionally, small villous tumors may be indistinguishable from tubular adenomas (Fig. 18–8). It is important to visualize all surfaces of the rectum in double contrast, because polyps can easily be obscured by the barium pool (Fig. 18–9). The radiologic aspects of polyps are discussed in more detail in Chapter 13.

Rectal polyps occasionally may be simulated by a variety of see-through artifacts projected over the rectum, such as calcified uterine fibroids, phleboliths, injection granulomas, and lymphangiographic contrast in pelvic lymph nodes (Fig. 18–10). However, the true nature of these findings is easily recognized by visualizing the rectum in other projections.

Double contrast enemas performed 2 weeks or less from the time of biopsy or resection of rectal polyps occasionally may reveal areas of shallow ulceration or deformity at the biopsy or polypectomy sites (Figs. 18–11 to 18–13).[20–22] The radiographic findings erroneously may suggest Crohn's disease or other inflammatory conditions involving the rectum. However, some postbiopsy or postpolypectomy ulcers may have a ring-like appearance that should distinguish these lesions from the aphthous ulcers of Crohn's disease (Figs. 18–11 and 18–12).[21] A hot (electrocoagulation)

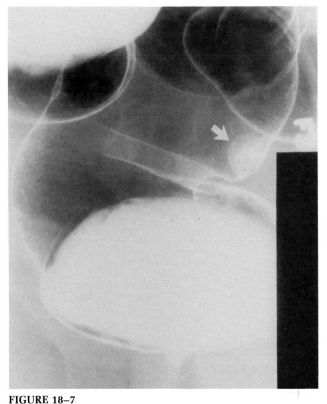

FIGURE 18–7

Rectal polyp *(arrow)* missed at proctoscopy because of its location behind valve of Houston.

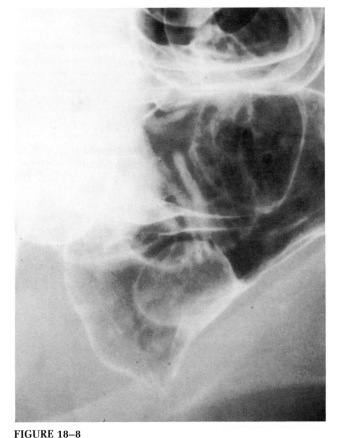

FIGURE 18–8

Villous adenoma in rectum. Note smooth surface of polyp, which has none of the radiologic features of a villous tumor.

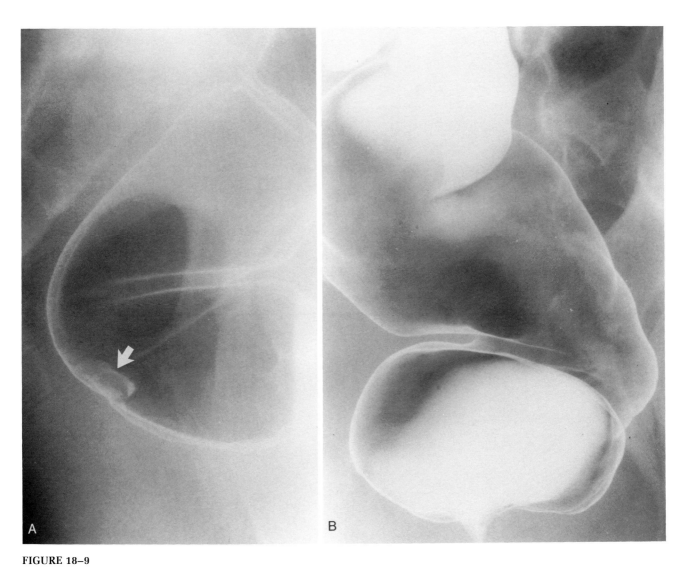

FIGURE 18–9

IMPORTANCE OF PROJECTION FOR DEMONSTRATING RECTAL POLYPS. *A,* Lateral view shows sessile polyp *(arrow)* on posterior wall of rectum.

B, Prone view shows no evidence of polyp, which is obscured by barium pool on dependent surface (the anterior wall).

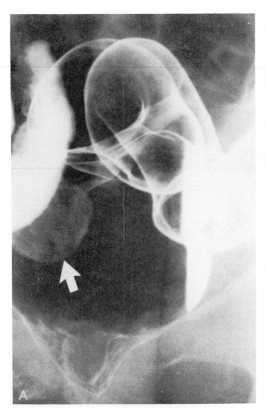

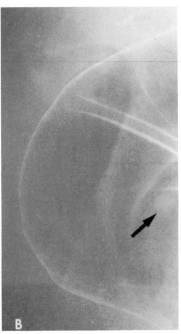

FIGURE 18–10

PELVIC CALCIFICATIONS *(ARROWS)*, MIMICKING RECTAL POLYPS. *A,* Calcified uterine fibroid.

B, Phlebolith.

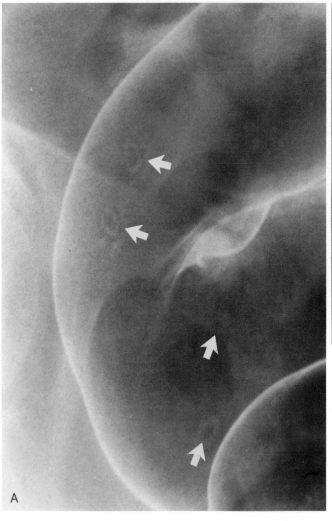

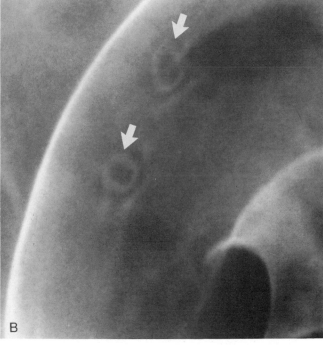

FIGURE 18–11

MULTIPLE RECTAL ULCERS AT SITES OF BIOPSIES TAKEN 4 DAYS EARLIER. *A,* Note characteristic ring-like appearance of ulcers *(arrows)* with surrounding radiolucent halos.

B, Close-up view better delineates these ring-like ulcers *(arrows)*, which should be differentiated from the aphthous ulcers of Crohn's disease. *(B,* From Lev-Toaff, A.S., et al.: Ringlike rectal ulcers after biopsy or polypectomy. AJR 148:285–286, 1987, with permission, © by American Roentgen Ray Society.)

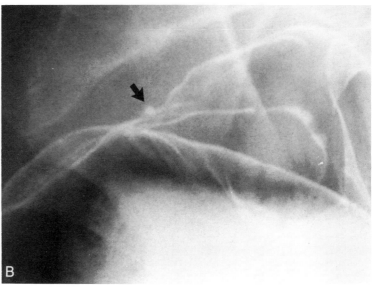

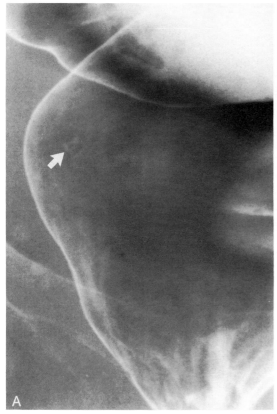

FIGURE 18–12

RECTAL ULCER AT SITE OF POLYPECTOMY DONE THREE DAYS EARLIER. *A,* Frontal view shows tiny, ring-like ulcer *(arrow)* with faint halo surrounding ulcer. (From Lev-Toaff, A.S., et al.: Ringlike rectal ulcers after biopsy or polypectomy. AJR *148:*285–286, 1987, with permission, © by American Roentgen Ray Society.)

B, Lateral view shows ulcer in profile *(arrow)*. Note deformity and puckering of adjacent rectal wall.

biopsy of a polyp may also result in a "fried egg" appearance, with an irregular, peripheral area representing the partially coagulated base of the polyp and a smooth, domed center representing the point of separation from the resected fragment (Fig. 18–13).[22] When these lesions are encountered, it is important to ascertain whether or not there has been a recent biopsy or polypectomy, so that unnecessary follow-up studies can be avoided.

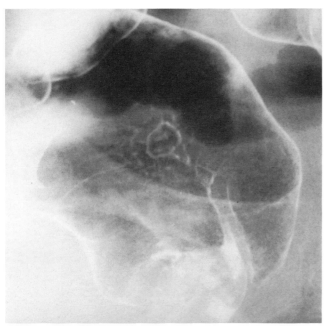

FIGURE 18–13

"Fried egg" appearance following electrocoagulation biopsy of rectal polyp. Note irregular periphery representing coagulated base of polyp and smooth, domed center at point of separation from resected fragment. (Courtesy of Henry Degryse, M.D., Antwerp, Belgium.)

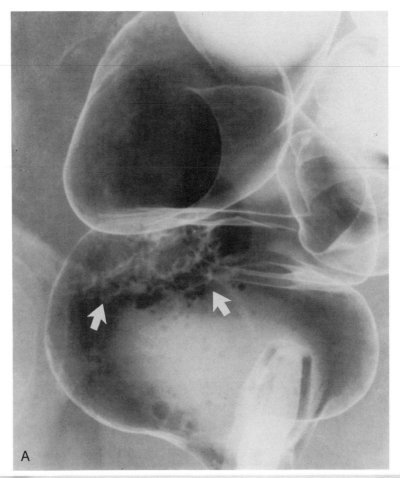

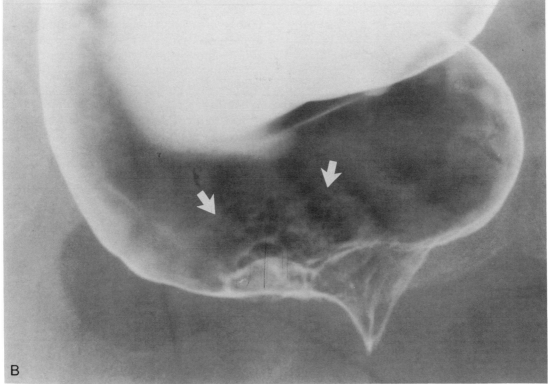

FIGURE 18–14

A and B, Two examples of carpet lesions (arrows) in rectum, manifested by finely nodular or reticular surface pattern of mucosa. Both patients had tubular adenomas with varying degrees of villous change. (A, From Rubesin, S.E., et al.: Carpet lesions of the colon. Radiographics 5:537–552, 1985, with permission.)

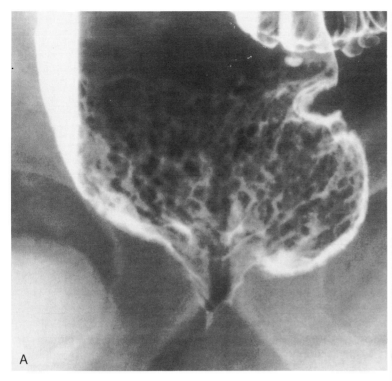

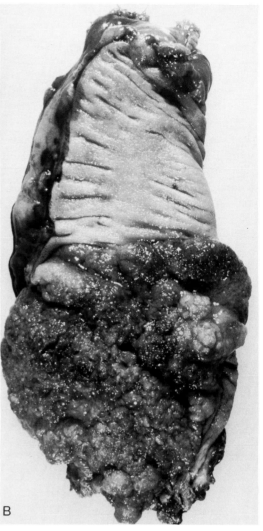

FIGURE 18–15

A, Extensive carpet lesion of distal rectum, causing diffuse coarsening and irregularity of mucosa.

B, Surgical specimen from similar case showing flat, carpet-like growth involving entire circumference of distal rectum. (From Rubesin, S.E., et al.: Carpet lesions of the colon. Radiographics 5:537–552, 1985, with permission.)

Carpet Lesions

Carpet lesions of the colon are defined as flat, lobulated lesions that may involve a considerable surface area of the bowel with little or no protrusion into the lumen.[23] For reasons that are unclear, they are found predominantly in the rectum and cecum.[23] Most carpet lesions are benign adenomas with varying degrees of villous change (tubulovillous adenomas).[23] Resection is warranted because of the risk of malignant degeneration.

Carpet lesions of the rectum may be recognized en face by a nodular or reticular surface pattern of the mucosa (Fig. 18–14).[23, 24] They may be relatively extensive lesions, involving the entire circumference of the rectum (Fig. 18–15). Despite their large size, these lesions may cause only minimal alteration in the appearance of the mucosa, so that they can be missed at endoscopy.[5] One or more repeat endoscopic examinations therefore may be required when the double contrast enema arouses suspicion of a carpet lesion of the rectum.

Malignant Tumors

Nearly 50% of all colonic carcinomas missed on single contrast barium enemas are located in the rectum.[25] Double contrast technique is therefore particularly important for detecting lesions in this location. Like malignant tumors elsewhere in the colon, rectal carcinomas may be polypoid (Figs. 18–16 and 18–17), ulcerated (Fig. 18–18), plaque-like (Fig. 18–19), or annular lesions (Fig. 18–20).[4] In general, polypoid lesions on the dependent wall of the rectum appear as filling defects in the barium pool, whereas those on the nondependent wall are etched in white (Fig. 18–17; see Chapter 2). Lesions near the rectosigmoid junction may be seen exclusively or to best advantage on prone, angled views (Fig. 18–21), whereas lesions on the posterior wall may be seen best on prone, cross-table lateral views. In any case, lesions that are visible on one projection may be partially or completely obscured by the barium pool in other projections, so that all the spot films and overhead radiographs must be scrutinized carefully to avoid missing polypoid or plaque-like lesions in the rectum.

Because colorectal cancer often results from malignant degeneration of preexisting adenomatous polyps, early rectal cancers are virtually always polypoid lesions, and they may be indistinguishable radiographically from benign-appearing polyps (Fig. 18–22). Not surprisingly, some early lesions may be detected as incidental findings in asymptomatic patients. The patient illustrated in Figure 18–23 had a double contrast enema because of right lower quadrant pain. The polypoid lesion in the rectum, which proved to be an early cancer, was detected as a fortuitous finding.

Some rectal cancers may be located at endoscopic "blind spots" discussed previously (Fig. 18–24; see previous section, "Polyps").[4] Others can be missed if the sigmoidoscope is not advanced to its full extent, particularly if angulation or fixation of the bowel by tumor prevents complete insertion of the scope. The patient illustrated in Figure 18–20 had undergone sigmoidoscopy twice in the previous 1½ years without detection of the lesion. In one study, 91% of rectal carcinomas were diagnosed on double contrast enema, whereas 86% were diagnosed on proctoscopy.[4] Thus, the double contrast enema detects most rectal cancers, including some that are missed at proctoscopy.

Primary scirrhous carcinoma of the rectum is a rare type of malignancy characterized by a linitis plastica appearance due to an extensive desmoplastic response incited by the tumor. Some lesions may be

Text continued on page 664

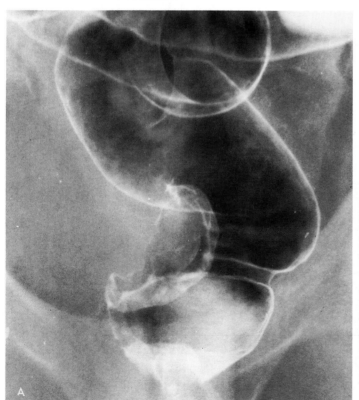
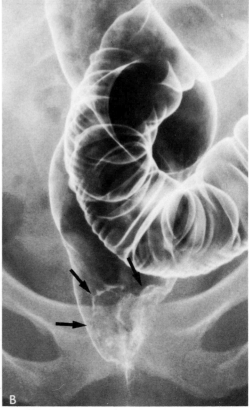

FIGURE 18–16

A and *B,* Two examples of polypoid carcinomas *(arrows in B)* in rectum.

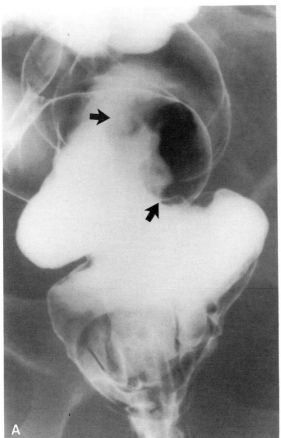

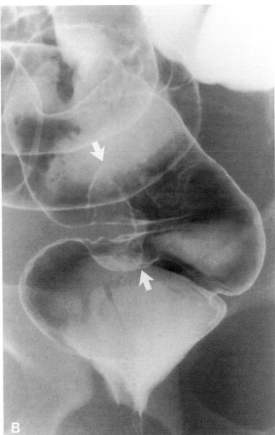

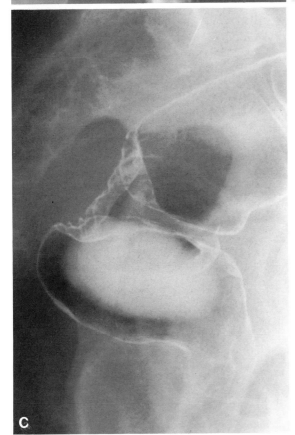

FIGURE 18–17

POLYPOID RECTAL CARCINOMA. *A,* Supine view shows
lesion as irregular filling defect *(arrows)* in barium pool, so it
must be located on posterior wall.

B, Prone view shows lesion etched in white *(arrows)* on
nondependent surface.

C, Lateral view confirms location of mass on posterior wall.

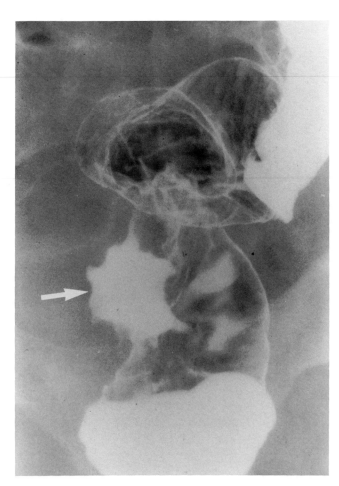

FIGURE 18–18

Rectal carcinoma containing large area of ulceration *(arrow)*.

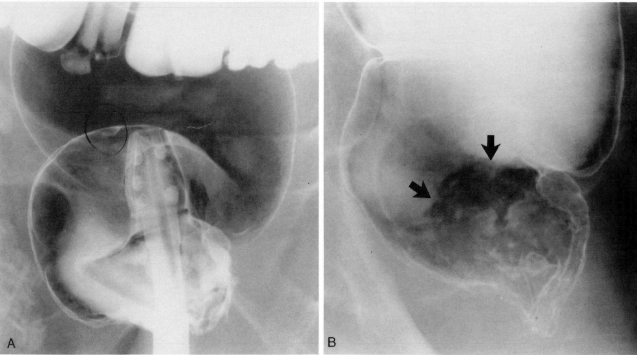

FIGURE 18–19

RECTAL CARCINOMA OBSCURED BY ENEMA TIP. *A*, Initial view shows small polyp *(circle)* in proximal rectum. However, the enema tip prevents adequate visualization of distal rectum.

B, Another view after removal of enema tip shows plaque-like cancer *(arrows)* that had been obscured by tip. (From Evers, K., et al.: Double-contrast enema examination for detection of rectal carcinoma. Radiology *140*:635–639, 1981, with permission.)

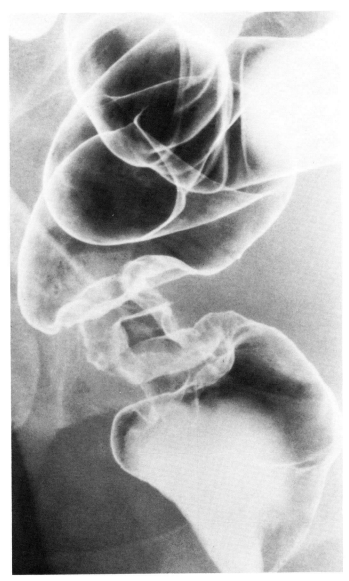

FIGURE 18–20

Annular carcinoma in proximal rectum, which was missed at sigmoidoscopy. Angulation caused by the tumor apparently prevented the sigmoidoscope from reaching the cancer.

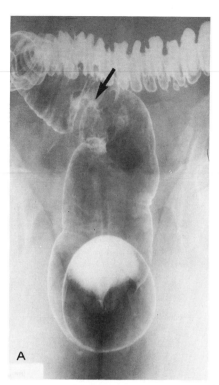

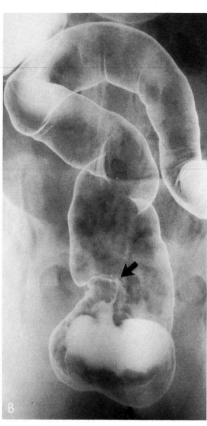

FIGURE 18–21

TWO EXAMPLES OF POLYPOID CARCINOMAS *(ARROWS)* BEST SEEN ON PRONE, ANGLED VIEW. *A*, Carcinoma of rectosigmoid junction.

   B, Carcinoma of rectum.

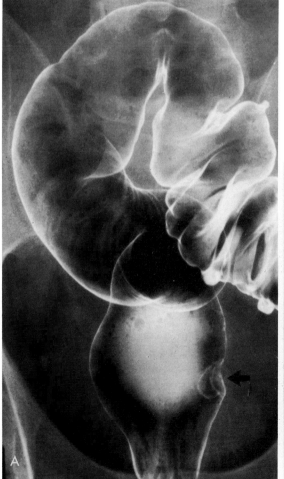

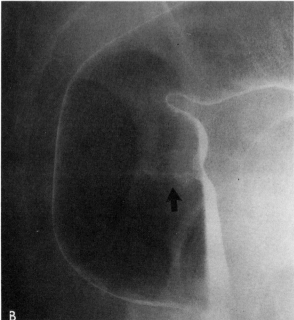

FIGURE 18–22

EARLY RECTAL CARCINOMA. *A*, Frontal view shows small, sessile polyp *(arrow)* in rectum. Note slight retraction of base of polyp.

   B, Polyp *(arrow)* is barely visible on prone, cross-table lateral view.

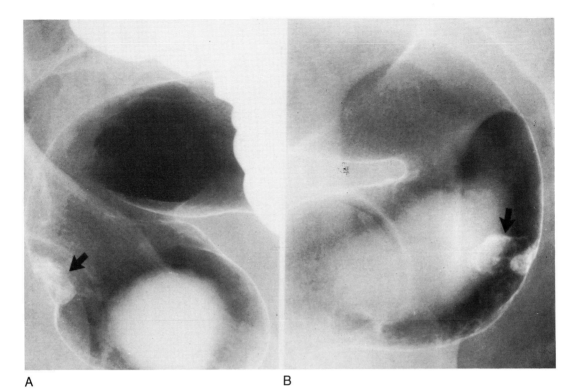

A   B

FIGURE 18–23

A and *B*, Early, asymptomatic rectal carcinoma appearing as a sessile, polypoid lesion *(arrows)*. This patient presented with right lower quadrant pain. The rectal tumor was an incidental finding.

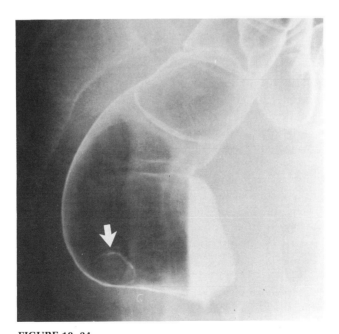

FIGURE 18–24

Small, polypoid rectal carcinoma *(arrow)* missed at sigmoidoscopy. This lesion probably was not detected by the endoscopist because of its location at a potential blind spot on posterior wall of rectum just inside anal verge.

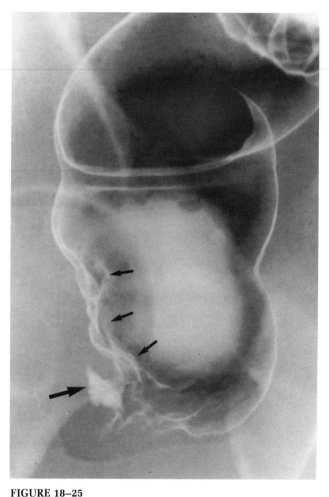

FIGURE 18–25

Cloacogenic carcinoma appearing as plaque-like lesion (*small arrows*) on posterolateral wall of distal rectum with area of ulceration (*large arrow*). (Courtesy of Seth N. Glick, M.D., Philadelphia, Pennsylvania.)

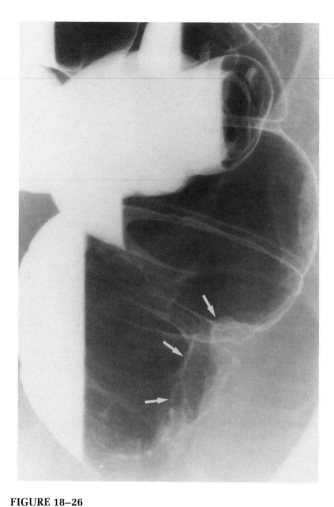

FIGURE 18–26

Plaque-like carcinoma (*arrows*) in distal rectum. Note resemblance to the cloacogenic carcinoma illustrated in Figure 18–25.

associated with narrowing and rigidity of the rectosigmoid with a smooth contour and effaced mucosal folds, whereas others may be associated with an irregular rectal contour and distorted, spiculated folds.[26, 27] The latter findings erroneously may suggest that the rectosigmoid colon has been encased by metastatic tumor (see later section, "Extrinsic Abnormalities"). Cloacogenic carcinoma is another unusual malignancy arising from the transitional cloacogenic zone of the anorectal junction. These tumors typically appear as plaque-like or polypoid lesions involving the distal rectum near the anal verge (Fig. 18–25).[28, 29] However, adenocarcinoma of the distal rectum or even squamous cell carcinoma of the anus invading the rectum may produce similar findings (Figs. 18–26 and 18–27).[30] Other malignant tumors that rarely may involve the rectum are carcinoid, lymphoma, and leiomyosarcoma (Fig. 18–28).[31–33] However, pathologic specimens are required for a definitive diagnosis.

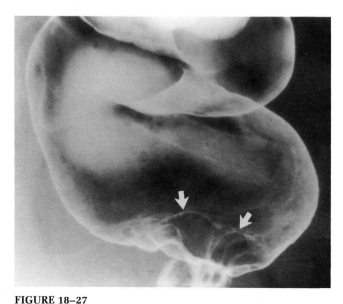

FIGURE 18–27

Squamous cell carcinoma of the anus invading the distal rectum (*arrows*).

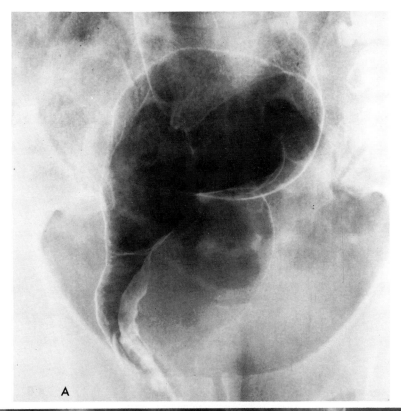

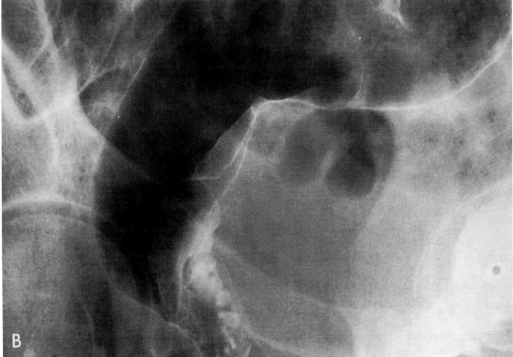

FIGURE 18–28

A and *B*, Leiomyosarcoma of the rectum, appearing as giant submucosal mass.

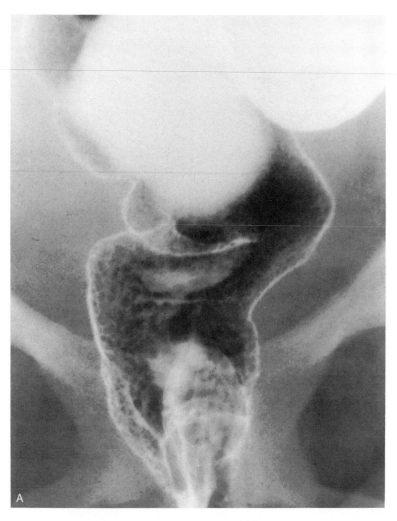

FIGURE 18–29

ULCERATIVE PROCTITIS. *A*, Frontal view shows coarse granularity of rectum due to chronic inflammation.

B, Lateral view in another patient shows stippling of mucosa in distal rectum due to superficial ulceration.

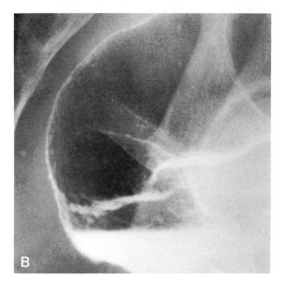

Inflammatory Conditions

Ulcerative Proctitis

Ulcerative proctitis is a mild variant of ulcerative colitis, in which involvement is limited to the rectum. Conventional single contrast barium enemas usually reveal no abnormalities in these patients.[34] With double contrast techniques, however, inflammatory changes can readily be demonstrated in the rectum, even in its most distal portion (Fig. 18–29).[35] As in patients with ulcerative colitis, ulcerative proctitis is initially manifested by a granular-appearing rectum due to mucosal edema and hyperemia (Fig. 18–29A). As the disease progresses, areas of shallow ulceration may be superimposed on a diffusely granular background mucosa (Fig. 18–29B).

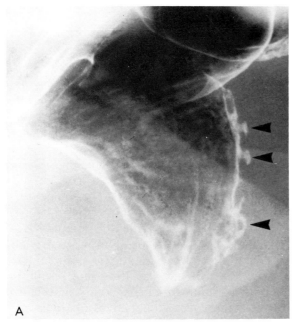

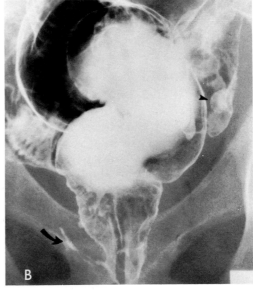

FIGURE 18–30

RECTAL INVOLVEMENT BY CROHN'S DISEASE.
A, Deep, collar-button ulcers (arrowheads) in the
rectum. When found in the rectum, these ulcers are
characteristic of Crohn's disease rather than
ulcerative colitis.

B, Ulcers and a sinus tract (arrow) in the rectum.
Inflammatory polyps (arrowhead) are also present.

C, More severe disease with narrowing, ulceration,
and multiple perirectal fistulae (arrows).

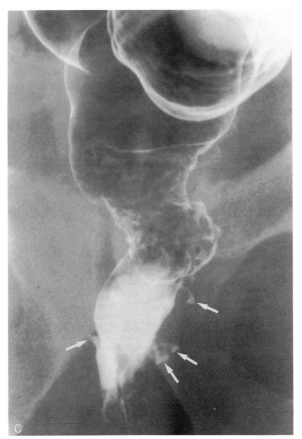

Crohn's Disease

The rectum is involved endoscopically in about 50%
of patients with granulomatous colitis.[36, 37] However,
the involvement tends to be patchy and asymmetric
rather than the diffuse involvement seen in ulcerative
colitis. As in the remainder of the colon, early Crohn's
disease in the rectum may be manifested radiographically by discrete "aphthous" ulcers separated by
normal mucosa (see Fig. 17–34).[38] In more advanced
disease, there may be relatively deep, collar-button
ulcers in the rectum as well as perirectal or perianal
fistulae (Fig. 18–30).[39] These findings are rarely seen
in the rectum in ulcerative colitis.[40] Thus, it is usually
possible to differentiate Crohn's disease and ulcerative colitis involving the rectum on double contrast
enemas.

Venereal Proctitis

Venereal proctitis has become a relatively common disease in homosexual men. Gonorrhea and herpes simplex are the most common organisms responsible for this condition.[41] Both gonococcal and herpetic proctitis may be manifested by edema, spasm, and ulceration.[42, 43] Some patients with anorectal herpes may have discrete aphthous ulcers indistinguishable from those of Crohn's disease involving the rectum (Fig. 18–31A).[44] Lymphogranuloma venereum is another less common cause of venereal proctitis characterized by diffuse rectosigmoid narrowing, deep ulcers, and perirectal fistulae (Fig. 17–31B).[45] Although the possibility of venereal proctitis may be suspected from the clinical history, stool cultures are required for a definitive diagnosis.

Other Forms of Proctitis

Injury to the rectosigmoid colon frequently occurs as the result of pelvic irradiation for cervical carcinoma or other malignant tumors.[46] In the acute phase, the mucosa may have a granular or ulcerated appearance indistinguishable from that of ulcerative proctitis (Fig. 18–32).[47] In the chronic phase, there may be diffuse narrowing and loss of haustration, producing a rigid, tubular structure that has a smooth, featureless appearance (Fig. 18–33).[46] The rectum is usually spared in patients with ischemic colitis. When it is involved, however, the appearance may be similar to that of ulcerative proctitis (Fig. 18–34).[48]

Some patients may have nonspecific proctitis on double contrast enemas with nodular mucosa or thickened, edematous valves of Houston, producing

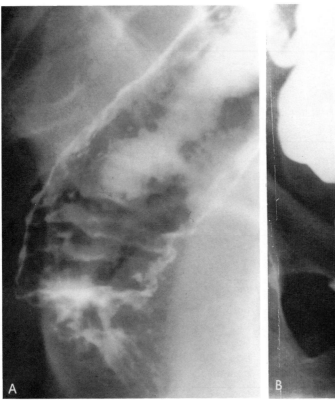
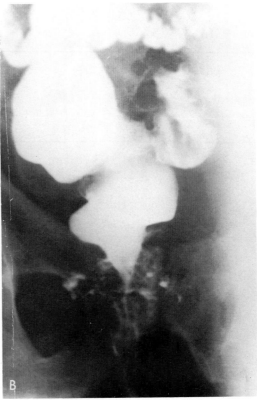

FIGURE 18–31

VENEREAL PROCTITIS. *A*, Herpetic proctitis with multiple aphthous ulcers in rectum. Rectal involvement by Crohn's disease could produce identical findings. (Courtesy of Francis J. Scholz, M.D., Burlington, Massachusetts. From Shah, S.J., and Scholz, F.J.: Anorectal herpes: Radiographic findings. Radiology 147:81–82, 1983, with permission.)
   B, Lymphogranuloma venereum with narrowing of distal rectum and multiple anorectal fistulae.

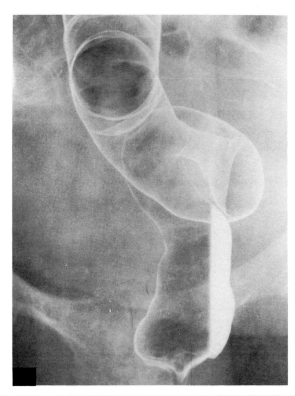

FIGURE 18–32

Acute radiation proctitis with minimal granularity of mucosa.

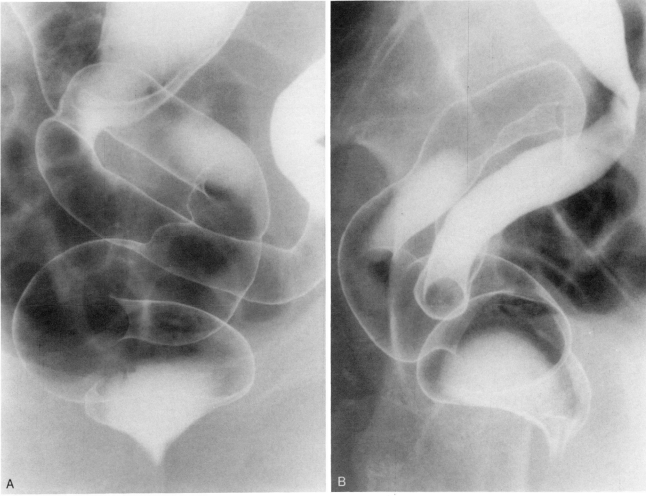

FIGURE 18–33

CHRONIC RADIATION CHANGES IN RECTOSIGMOID COLON WITH DIFFUSE NARROWING AND LOSS OF HAUSTRATION.
A, Frontal view.
  B, Steep oblique view.

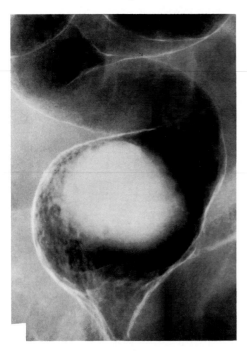

FIGURE 18–34

Ischemic proctitis with coarse granularity of rectal mucosa.

FIGURE 18–35

Nonspecific proctitis with nodular mucosa and thickened folds in rectum, producing "boggy" appearance. (From Rubesin, S.E., et al.: Carpet lesions of the colon. Radiographics 5:537–552, 1985, with permission.)

a "boggy" rectum (Fig. 18–35). Other patients with proctitis may have enlarged lymphoid follicles in the rectum, a condition known as "follicular proctitis" (Fig. 18–36).[49] In our experience, mild forms of proctitis may even be caused by the laxatives that the patient takes for the barium enema examination.

Solitary Rectal Ulcer Syndrome and Colitis Cystica Profunda

Solitary rectal ulcer syndrome is a benign clinical entity in which a persistent, nonhealing ulcer is classically found on the anterior wall of the rectum in young patients with rectal bleeding.[50] However, the name of the condition is misleading, because some patients may have multiple ulcers and others

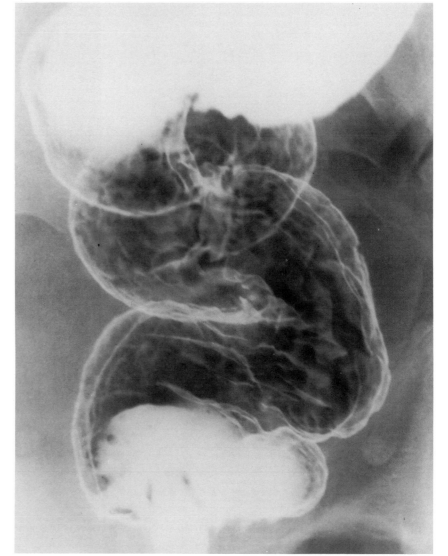

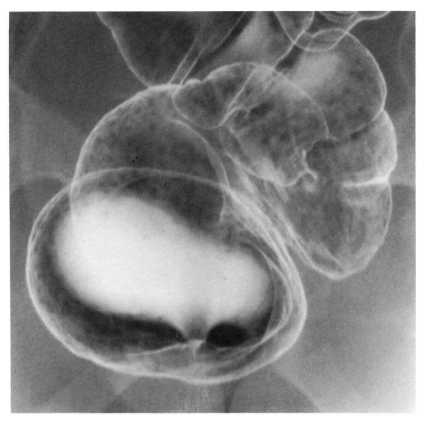

FIGURE 18–36

Follicular proctitis with enlarged lymphoid follicles appearing as multiple small nodules in rectum.

may have localized proctitis without ulceration.[50] Although the pathogenesis is uncertain, there frequently is a history of rectal straining or prolapse, so that ulceration of the anterior rectal wall may be traumatic or ischemic in origin. The diagnosis may be confirmed by rectal biopsy, which reveals classic histopathologic findings (fibromuscular obliteration of the lamina propria and thickening and fraying of the muscularis mucosae).[50]

The diagnosis of solitary rectal ulcer syndrome may be suggested radiographically by the presence of a discrete, benign-appearing ulcer on the anterior rectal wall near the first valve of Houston (Fig. 18–37). In the majority of patients, however, double contrast enemas demonstrate thickened, edematous valves of Houston or nodular mucosa without ulcers (Fig. 18–38).[51, 52] The latter findings therefore should raise the possibility of solitary rectal ulcer syndrome, particularly in young patients with rectal bleeding.

Proctoscopy and biopsy can then be performed for a definitive diagnosis.

Colitis cystica profunda is an unusual condition characterized by the presence of mucus-filled, epithelial-lined cysts in the submucosa. Some investigators have reported an association between a localized form of colitis cystica profunda involving the rectum and solitary rectal ulcer syndrome, possibly due to extension of regenerating surface epithelium into the submucosa.[50, 53] The lesions of colitis cystica profunda may appear radiographically as one or more lobulated submucosal masses in the rectum (Fig. 18–39).[53, 54] Although it is a benign condition, pathologists occasionally have mistaken these mucus-filled cysts for invasive mucinous adenocarcinoma. Thus, it is important to be aware of the association between solitary rectal ulcer syndrome and colitis cystica profunda, so that unnecessary radical surgery can be avoided in these patients.

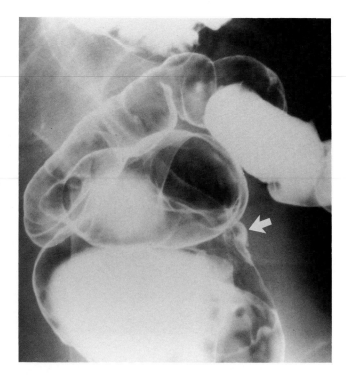

FIGURE 18–37

Solitary rectal ulcer syndrome with single, discrete ulcer *(arrow)* on anterior wall of rectum. (Courtesy of Harvey N. Goldstein, M.D., San Antonio, Texas.)

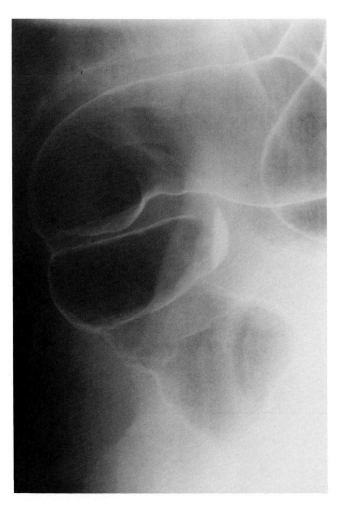

FIGURE 18–38

Solitary rectal ulcer syndrome with thickened, edematous valves of Houston but no ulcers. (From Levine, M.S., et al.: Solitary rectal ulcer syndrome: A radiologic diagnosis? Gastrointest. Radiol. *11:*187, 1986, with permission.)

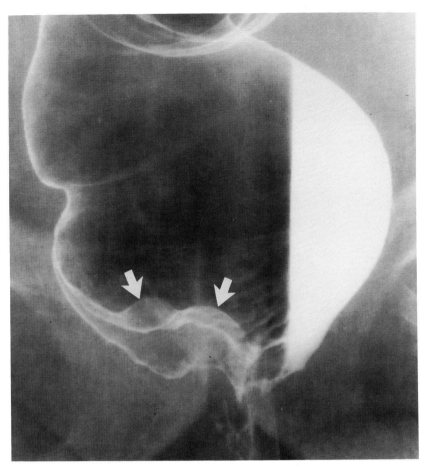

FIGURE 18–39

Solitary rectal ulcer syndrome with localized colitis cystica profunda. Note slightly lobulated submucosal-appearing mass *(arrows)* in distal rectum near anal verge due to mucus-filled, epithelium-lined cysts in submucosa. (From Levine, M.S., et al.: Solitary rectal ulcer syndrome: A radiologic diagnosis? Gastrointest. Radiol. 11:187, 1986, with permission.)

EXTRINSIC ABNORMALITIES

Various types of perirectal disease are well demonstrated on double contrast studies. Extrinsic compression of the rectosigmoid colon may be caused by soft tissue masses (uterine or ovarian tumors; Figs. 18–40 and 18–41), fluid collections (ascites, hematomas, lymphoceles, and others), or even accumulation of fat in the pelvis (pelvic lipomatosis; Fig. 18–42).[55, 56] A pelvic mass may be manifested by a smooth, gently sloping indentation on the anterior border of the rectosigmoid that usually is most obvious on lateral projections (Fig. 18–40). In some patients, the findings may be quite subtle (Fig. 18–41A) and may be easiest to recognize on prone, cross-table lateral views (Fig. 18–41B). Less frequently, extrinsic compression of the lateral borders of the rectosigmoid colon may

be seen best on frontal projections (Fig. 18–42). Regardless of the location of the mass, the absence of irregularity, spiculation, tethering, or ulceration generally indicates that it is compressing the bowel and not invading it.[57]

Because the rectosigmoid colon directly abuts the most dependent portion of the peritoneal cavity, it is the most common site of involvement by intraperitoneal seeding of metastatic tumor from ovarian, gastric, colonic, or pancreatic carcinoma.[58, 59] These metastatic deposits in the rectovesical space (the pouch of Douglas in a woman) may incite a marked desmoplastic response in the wall of the bowel, causing mass effect, irregularity, spiculation, or tethering of the anterior border of the rectosigmoid (Fig. 18–43). Although these changes may be recognized en face (Fig. 18–43B), they are best seen in profile on lateral

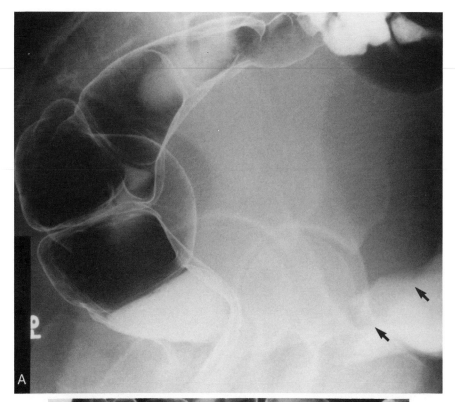

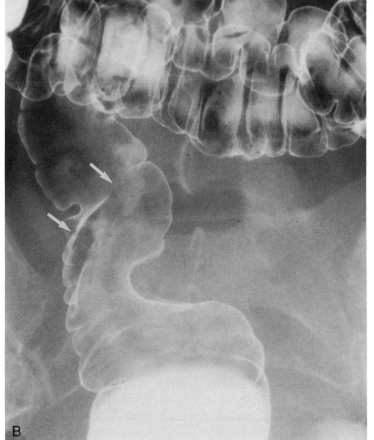

FIGURE 18–40

EXTRINSIC COMPRESSION OF RECTOSIGMOID BY UTERINE FIBROIDS. *A*, Lateral view shows smooth, gently sloping indentation on anterior border of rectosigmoid. Also note impression on bladder *(arrows)*.

B, Frontal view shows area of mass effect en face *(arrows)*, but findings are more subtle in this projection.

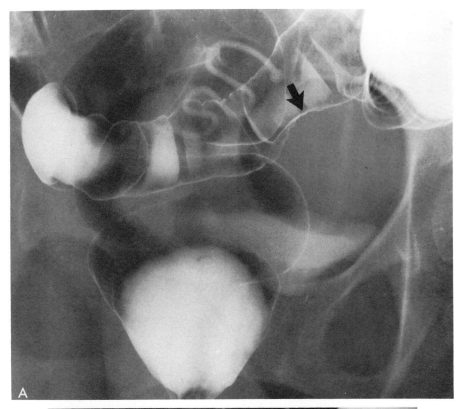

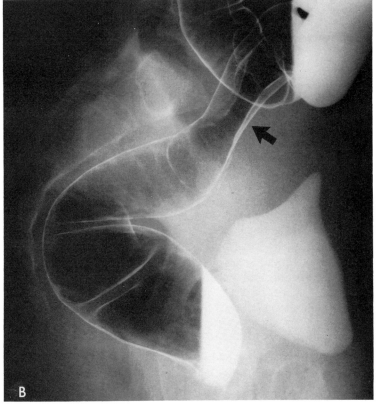

FIGURE 18–41

SUBTLE AREAS OF MASS EFFECT ON RECTOSIGMOID. *A,* Slight displacement of sigmoid colon *(arrow)* by small pelvic mass. *B,* Cross-table lateral view showing minimal compression of rectosigmoid *(arrow)* by pelvic mass.

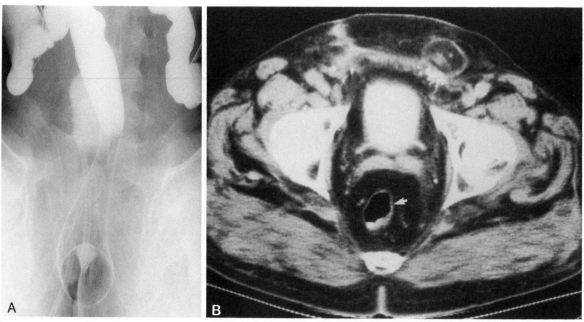

FIGURE 18–42

EXTRINSIC COMPRESSION OF RECTOSIGMOID BY FAT IN PELVIS. *A,* Prone, angled view shows smooth, symmetric compression of lateral walls of rectosigmoid colon.

B, Computed tomography scan shows marked amount of adipose tissue surrounding rectum *(arrow)* in this patient with pelvic lipomatosis.

views of the rectum (Fig. 18–43A). Involvement of the rectovesical space by inflammatory conditions such as appendicitis, diverticulitis, Crohn's disease, and tubo-ovarian abscess may produce similar radiographic findings (Fig. 18–44).[55] In the latter patients, spread of inflammation to the serosa of the bowel may result in thickened, spiculated folds (Fig. 18–45). The rectosigmoid is also a common site of colonic involvement by endometriosis.[60] These hormonally stimulated endometriosis implants may cause mass effect, crenulation, and tethering of the anterior border of the rectosigmoid due to bleeding and subsequent fibrosis in the wall of the bowel (Figs. 18–46 and 18–47A).[61] Additional implants may be found in the sigmoid and cecum (Fig. 18–47). Thus, intraperitoneal metastases, inflammatory diseases, and endometriosis may produce similar changes in the rectosigmoid colon, so that the clinical history is essential for differentiating these conditions.

Pelvic malignancies such as cervical, uterine, and bladder cancer may directly invade the rectum, causing mass effect and tethered, spiculated folds on its anterior or lateral walls or, in advanced cases, circum-

ferential narrowing of the bowel (Fig. 18–48). However, these tumors tend to involve the distal portion of the rectum below the level of the peritoneal reflection, whereas intraperitoneal metastases to the rectosigmoid rarely extend below this level. Although prostatic carcinoma may also invade the distal rectum (Fig. 18–49), this malignancy tends to spread superiorly to the seminal vesicles before invading the rectum.[62] As a result, the majority of patients have localized rectosigmoid involvement with sparing of the distal rectum (Fig. 18–50). Invasion of the bowel wall may be manifested by mass effect and spiculated, tethered folds on the anterior border of the rectosigmoid, mimicking the appearance of intraperitoneal metastases.[62] However, prostatic carcinoma often spreads posteriorly around the bowel, causing circumferential narrowing and widening of the presacral space (Fig. 18–50), whereas intraperitoneal seeding of the rectosigmoid almost always produces abnormalities that are confined to the anterior border of the bowel. Thus, it is often possible to suggest the nature and origin of malignant spread to the rectosigmoid colon on radiologic criteria.

Text continued on page 684

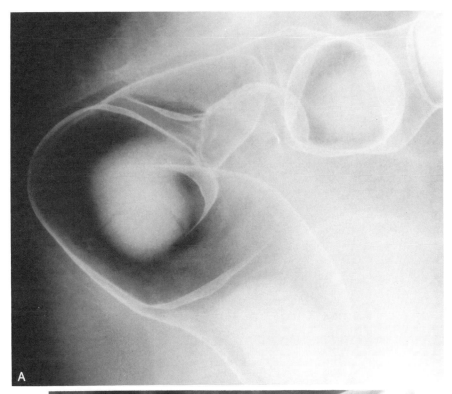

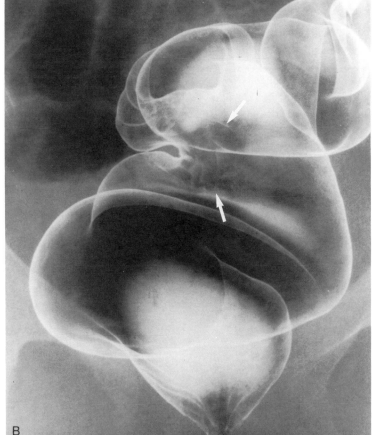

FIGURE 18–43

INTRAPERITONEAL-SEEDED METASTASIS TO RECTOSIGMOID COLON. *A,* Lateral view shows area of mass effect, spiculation, and irregularity on anterior border of rectosigmoid due to metastatic seeding.

B, This metastatic deposit can also be recognized en face by pleated, tethered appearance of mucosa *(arrows)* on frontal view.

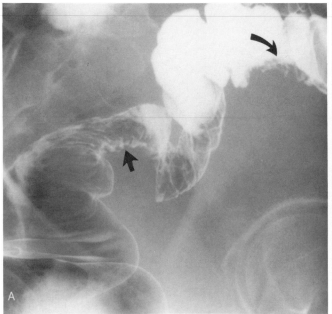

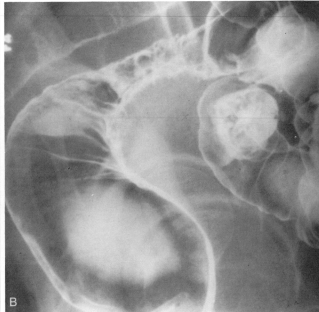

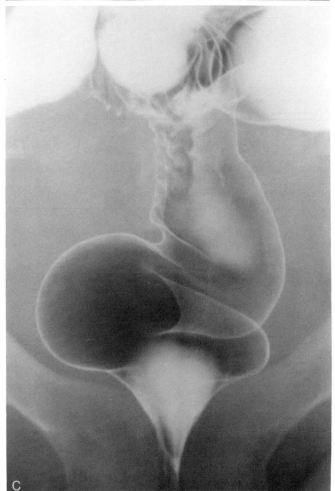

FIGURE 18–44

**RECTOSIGMOID INVOLVEMENT BY INFLAMMATORY
CONDITIONS IN RECTOVESICAL SPACE.** *A,* Sigmoid
diverticulitis *(curved arrow)* with extension of inflammatory
process to rectosigmoid *(straight arrow).*

   B, Crohn's disease with findings indistinguishable from those
of metastatic disease or endometriosis involving rectosigmoid
colon.

   C, Tubo-ovarian abscess with mucosal pleating seen en face on
frontal view of rectum.

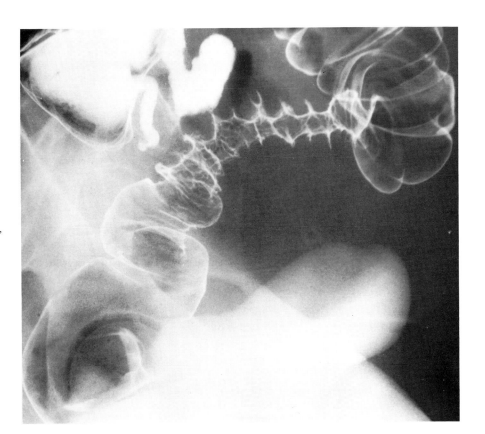

FIGURE 18–45

Tuberculous tubo-ovarian abscess involving sigmoid colon. Note thickened, spiculated folds.

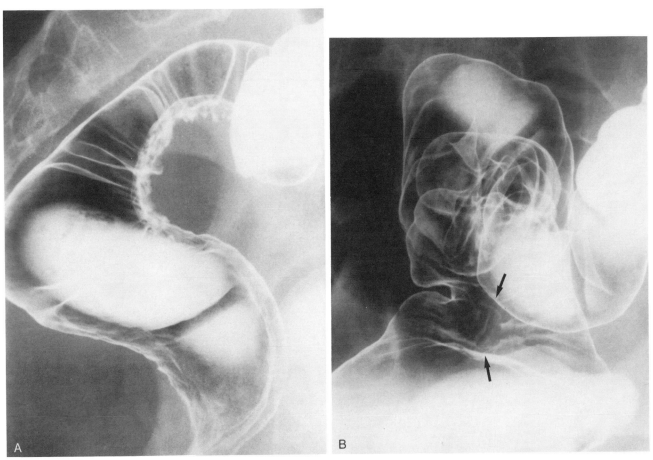

FIGURE 18–46

RECTOSIGMOID INVOLVEMENT BY ENDOMETRIOSIS. *A,* Lateral view shows mass effect on anterior border of rectosigmoid colon with spiculated, tethered mucosal folds.

B, Frontal view shows mucosal pleating en face *(arrows).* Intraperitoneal metastases or inflammatory processes in rectovesical space may produce identical findings, so that the clinical history is essential for differentiating these conditions.

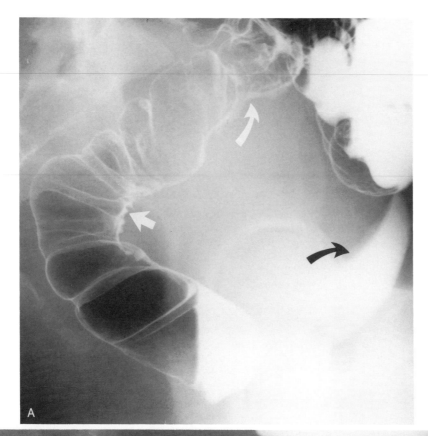

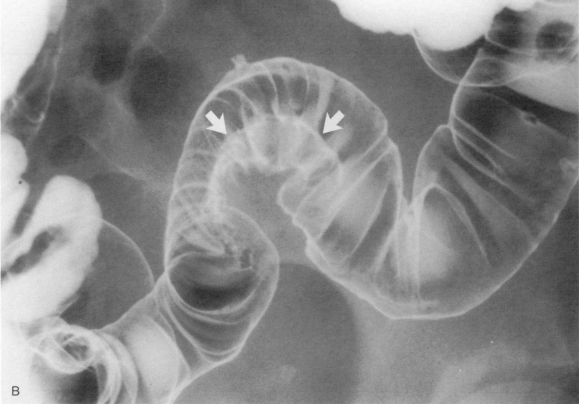

FIGURE 18–47

COLONIC INVOLVEMENT BY ENDOMETRIOSIS. *A*, Lateral view shows spiculation and tethering of anterior border of rectosigmoid *(straight white arrow)*. Also note pelvic mass compressing sigmoid colon *(curved white arrow)* and bladder *(curved black arrow)*.

B, Endometriosis implant in sigmoid colon *(arrows)* in another patient. Note mucosal pleating in this region.

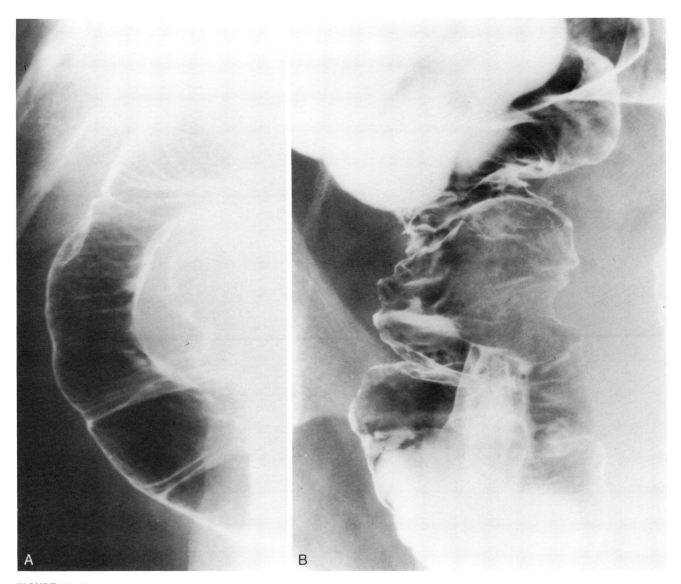

FIGURE 18–48

RECTAL INVASION BY CERVICAL CARCINOMA. *A*, Lateral view shows mass effect and irregular mucosa on anterior border of rectum.

  B, Frontal view also shows area of mass effect and pleated mucosal folds in rectum. Unlike in patients with intraperitoneal metastases to rectosigmoid, note how rectum is involved below level of peritoneal reflection.

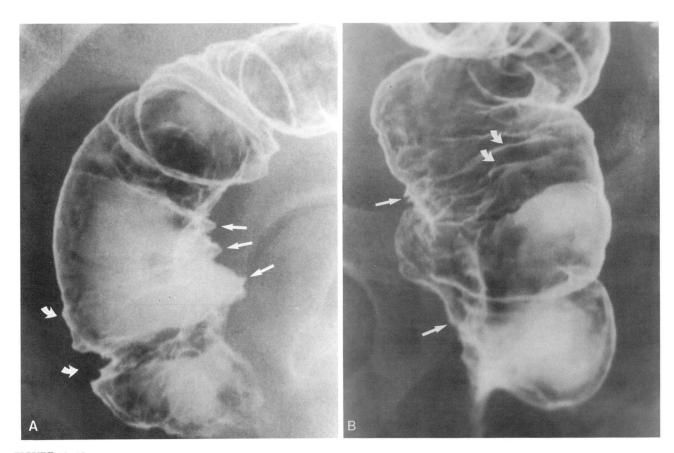

FIGURE 18–49

RECTAL INVASION BY PROSTATIC CARCINOMA. *A*, Lateral view shows flattening and spiculation of anterior border of rectum *(straight arrows)*. Mild circumferential extension is seen distally *(curved arrows)*.

B, Frontal view shows mass effect and spiculation along right lateral wall of rectum *(straight arrows)* and mucosal pleating en face *(curved arrows)*. (From Rubesin S.E., et al.: Rectal involvement by prostatic carcinoma: Barium enema findings. AJR *152*:53–57, 1989, with permission, © by American Roentgen Ray Society.)

FIGURE 18–50

RECTOSIGMOID INVASION BY PROSTATIC CARCINOMA. *A,* Lateral view shows mass effect and spiculated contour along anterior border of rectosigmoid *(black arrows)* with widening of presacral space *(double white arrow).* Note sparing of distal rectum.

B, Oblique view shows narrowing of rectosigmoid and mucosal pleating en face. Although intraperitoneal metastases could produce similar findings, circumferential narrowing of rectosigmoid colon and widening of presacral space should suggest the correct diagnosis. (U: Opacified ureter from intravenous urography.) (*A* and *B,* From Rubesin, S.E., et al.: Rectal involvement by prostatic carcinoma: Barium enema findings. AJR 152:53–57, 1989, with permission, © by American Roentgen Ray Society.)

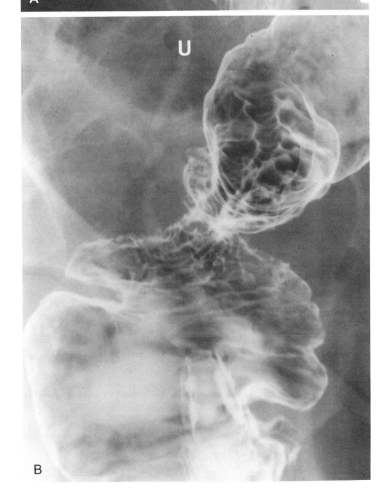

REFERENCES

1. Cooley, R.N.: The diagnostic accuracy of radiologic studies of the biliary tract, small intestine and colon. Am. J. Med. Sci. 246:610, 1963.
2. Simpkins, K.C., and Young, A.C.: The radiology of colonic and rectal polyps. Br. J. Surg. 55:731, 1968.
3. Laufer, I., Smith, N.C.W., and Mullens, J.E.: The radiologic demonstration of colorectal polyps undetected by endoscopy. Gastroenterology 70:167, 1976.
4. Evers, K., Laufer, I., Gordon, R.L., et al.: Double-contrast enema examination for detection of rectal carcinoma. Radiology 140:635, 1981.
5. Glick, S.N., Teplick, S.K., Balfe, D.M., et al.: Large colonic neoplasms missed by endoscopy. AJR 152:513, 1989.
6. Kirsner, J.B.: Problems in the differentiation of ulcerative colitis and Crohn's disease of the colon: The need for repeated diagnostic evaluation. Gastroenterology 68:187, 1975.
7. Miller, R.E.: Barium enema examination with large bore tubing and drainage. Radiology 82:905, 1964.
8. Miller, R.E., and Peterson, G.H.: Drainage of the rectum: A simple maneuver to improve the accuracy of colon examinations. Radiology 128:506, 1978.
9. Maglinte, D.D.T., Miller, R.E., and Chernish, S.M.: Early rectal tube removal for improved patient tolerance during double-contrast barium enema examination. Radiology 155:525, 1985.
10. Dysart, D.N., and Stewart H.R.: Special angled roentgenography for lesions of the rectosigmoid. AJR 96:285, 1966.
11. Niizuma, S., and Kobayashi, S.: Rectosigmoid double contrast examination in the prone position with a horizontal beam. AJR 128:519, 1977.
12. Goei, R.: Anorectal function in patients with defecation disorders and asymptomatic subjects: Evaluation with defecography. Radiology 174:121, 1990.
13. Goei, R., and Baeten, C.: Rectal intussusception and rectal prolapse: Detection and postoperative evaluation with defecography. Radiology 174:124, 1990.
14. Cohen, W.N.: Roentgenographic evaluation of the rectal valves of Houston in the normal and ulcerative colitis. AJR 104:580, 1968.
15. Kattan, K.R., and King, A.Y.: Presacral space revisited. AJR 132:437, 1979.
16. Thoeni, R.F., and Venbrux, A.C.: The anal canal: Distinction of internal hemorrhoids from small cancers by double-contrast barium enema examination. Radiology 145:17, 1982.
17. Levine, M.S., Kam, L.W., Rubesin, S.E., et al.: Internal hemorrhoids: Diagnosis with double-contrast barium enema examinations. Radiology 177:141, 1990.
18. Heiken, J.P., Zuckerman, G.R., and Balfe, D.M.: The hypertrophied anal papilla: Recognition on air-contrast barium enema examinations. Radiology 151:315, 1984.
19. Ott, D.J., and Gelfand, D.W.: Colorectal tumors: Pathology and detection. AJR 131:691, 1978.
20. Millward, S.F., Chapman, A., Somers, S., et al.: Rectal biopsy as a cause of rectal ulceration. Radiology 156:42, 1985.
21. Lev-Toaff, A.S., Levine, M.S., Laufer, I., et al.: Ringlike rectal ulcers after biopsy or polypectomy. AJR 148:285, 1987.
22. Bartram, C.I., and Hall-Craggs, M.A.: Interventional colorectal endoscopic procedures: Residual lesions on follow-up double-contrast barium enema study. Radiology 162:835, 1987.
23. Rubesin, S.E., Saul, S.H., Laufer, I., et al.: Carpet lesions of the colon. RadioGraphics 5:537, 1985.
24. Herman, T.E., Koehler, R.E., and Lee, J.K.T.: Focal irregularity of the rectal mucosa. AJR 133:677, 1979.
25. Cooley, R.N., Agnew, C.H., and Rios, G.: Diagnostic accuracy of the barium enema study in carcinoma of the colon and rectum. AJR 84:316, 1960.
26. Balthazar, E.J., Rosenberg, H.D., and Davidian, M.M.: Primary and metastatic scirrhous carcinoma of the rectum. AJR 132:711, 1979.
27. Oliver, T.W., Somogyi, J., and Gaffney, E.F.: Primary linitis plastica of the rectum. AJR 140:79, 1983.
28. Kyaw, M.M., Gallagher, T., and Haines, J.O.: Cloacogenic carcinoma of the anorectal junction: Roentgenologic diagnosis. AJR 115:384, 1972.
29. Hertz, I., Train, J., and Keller, R.: Cloacogenic carcinoma. J. Clin. Gastroenterol. 3:367, 1981.
30. McConnell, E.M.: Squamous carcinoma of the anus: A review of 96 cases. Br. J. Surg. 57:89, 1970.
31. Sato, T., Sakai, Y., Sonoyama, A., et al.: Radiologic spectrum of rectal carcinoid tumors. Gastrointest. Radiol. 9:23, 1984.
32. Ioachim, H.L., Weinstein, M.A., Robbins, R.D., et al.: Primary anorectal lymphoma. Cancer 60:1449, 1987.
33. Marshak, R.H., and Lindner, A.E.: Leiomyosarcoma of the colon. Am. J. Gastroenterol. 54:155, 1970.
34. Fennessy, J.J., Sparberg, M., and Kirsner, J.B.: Early roentgen manifestations of mild ulcerative colitis and proctitis. Radiology 87:848, 1966.
35. Laufer, I.: The radiologic demonstration of early changes in ulcerative colitis by double contrast technique. J. Can. Assoc. Radiol. 26:116, 1975.
36. Laufer, I., and Hamilton, J.D.: The radiologic differentiation between ulcerative and granulomatous colitis by double contrast radiology. Am. J. Gastroenterol. 66:259, 1976.
37. Korelitz, B.I., and Sommers, S.C.: Differential diagnosis of ulcerative and granulomatous colitis by sigmoidoscopy, rectal biopsy and cell counts of rectal mucosa. Am. J. Gastroenterol. 61:460, 1974.
38. Laufer, I., and Costopoulos, L.: Early lesions of Crohn's disease. AJR 130:307, 1978.
39. DuBrow, R.A., and Frank, P.H.: Barium evaluation of anal canal in patients with inflammatory bowel disease. AJR 140:1151, 1983.
40. Devroede, G.J.: Differential diagnosis of colitis. Can. J. Surg. 17:369, 1974.
41. Quinn, T.C., Corey, L., Chaffee, R.G., et al.: The etiology of anorectal infections in homosexual men. Am. J. Med. 71:395, 1981.
42. Goodman, K.J.: Radiologic findings in anorectal gonorrhea. Gastrointest. Radiol. 3:223, 1978.
43. Sider, L., Mintzer, R.A., Mendelson, E.B., et al.: Radiographic findings of infectious proctitis in homosexual men. AJR 139:667, 1982.
44. Shah, S.J., and Scholz, F.J.: Anorectal herpes: Radiographic findings. Radiology 147:81, 1983.
45. Annamunthodo, H., and Marryatt, J.: Barium studies in intestinal lymphogranuloma venereum. Br. J. Radiol. 34:53, 1961.
46. Meyer, J.E.: Radiography of the distal colon and rectum after irradiation of carcinoma of the cervix. AJR 136:691, 1981.
47. Gelfand, M.D., Tepper, M., Katz, L.A., et al.: Acute irradiation proctitis in man. Gastroenterology 54:401, 1968.
48. Kilpatrick, Z.M., Farman, J., Yesner, R., et al.: Ischemic proctitis. JAMA 205:74, 1968.
49. Flejou, J.F., Potet, F., Bogomeletz, W.V., et al.: Lymphoid follicular proctitis: A condition different from ulcerative proctitis? Dig. Dis. Sci. 33:314, 1988.
50. Rutter, K.R., and Riddell, R.H.: The solitary ulcer syndrome of the rectum. Clin. Gastroenterol. 4:505, 1975.
51. Feczko, P.J., O'Connell, D.J., Riddell, R.H., et al.: Solitary rectal ulcer syndrome: Radiologic manifestations. AJR 135:499, 1980.
52. Levine, M.S., Piccolello, M.L., Sollenberger, L.C., et al.: Solitary rectal ulcer syndrome: A radiologic diagnosis? Gastrointest. Radiol. 11:187, 1986.
53. Rosengren, J.E., Hildell, J., Lindstrom, C.G., et al.: Localized colitis cystica profunda. Gastrointest. Radiol. 7:79, 1982.
54. Miller, D.L.G., O'Malley, B.P., and Richmond, H.: Colitis cystica profunda. J. Can. Assoc. Radiol. 34:70, 1983.
55. Schulman, A., and Fataar, S.: Extrinsic stretching, narrowing, and anterior indentation of the rectosigmoid junction. Clin. Radiol. 30:463, 1979.

56. Farman, J., Faegenburg, D., Dallemand, S., et al.: Pelvic lipomatosis. Am. J. Gastroenterol. *60*:640, 1973.
57. Gedgaudas, R.K., Kelvin, F.M., Thompson, W.M., et al.: The value of the preoperative barium-enema examination in the assessment of pelvic masses. Radiology *146*:609, 1983.
58. Meyers, M.A.: Distribution of intra-abdominal malignant seeding: Dependency on dynamics of flow of ascitic fluid. AJR *119*:198, 1973.
59. Meyers, M.A.: Intraperitoneal spread of malignancies and its effect on the bowel. Clin. Radiol. *32*:129, 1981.
60. Fagan, C.F.: Endometriosis: Clinical and roentgenographic manifestations. Radiol. Clin. North Am. *12*:109, 1974.
61. Gordon, R.L., Evers, K., Kressel, H.Y., et al.: Double-contrast enema in pelvic endometriosis. AJR *138*:549, 1982.
62. Rubesin, S.E., Levine, M.S., Bezzi, M., et al.: Rectal involvement by prostatic carcinoma: Barium enema findings. AJR *152*:53, 1989.

INDEX

Note: Numbers in *italics* refer to illustrations; numbers followed by (t) indicate tables.

DATE DUE

DEMCO 38-296